LIPPINCOTT'S
REVIEW SERIES

Medical-
Surgical
Nursing

LIPPINCOTT'S REVIEW SERIES

Medical-Surgical Nursing

J.B. LIPPINCOTT COMPANY
Philadelphia

New York · London · Hagerstown

Sponsoring Editor: **Donna L. Hilton, RN, BSN**
Coordinating Editorial Assistant: **Susan Perry**
Project Editor: **Melissa McGrath**
Indexer: **Alexandra Nickerson**
Designer: **Doug Smock**
Production Manager: **Helen Ewan**
Production Coordinator: **Maura Murphy**
Compositor: **Pine Tree Composition, Inc.**
Printer/Binder: **R. R. Donnelley & Sons Company**
Cover Printer: **The Lehigh Press, Inc.**

6 5 4 3 2 1

Library of Congress Cataloging-in-Publication Data

Lippincott's review series : medical-surgical nursing.
   p.   cm.
  Includes bibliographical references and index.
  ISBN 0-397-54775-7
  1. Nursing—Outlines, syllabi, etc. 2. Surgical nursing—
—Outlines, syllabi, etc. 3. Nursing—Examinations, questions, etc.
4. Surgical nursing—Examinations, questions, etc. I. J. B.
Lippincott Company. II. Title: Medical-surgical nursing.
  [DNLM: 1. Nursing Care—examination questions. 2. Nursing Care—
—outlines. 3. Surgical Nursing—examination questions. 4. Surgical
Nursing—outlines. WY 18 L764]
RT52.L57 1992
610.73'076—dc29
DNLM/DLC
for Library of Congress   91–30000
                                        CIP

Any procedure or practice described in this book should be applied by the health-care practitioner under appropriate supervision in accordance with professional standards of care used with regard to the unique circumstances that apply in each practice situation. Care has been taken to confirm the accuracy of information presented and to describe generally accepted practices. However, the authors, editors, and publisher cannot accept any responsibility for errors or omissions or for any consequences from application of the information in this book and make no warranty, express or implied, with respect to the contents of the book.

Every effort has been made to ensure drug selections and dosages are in accordance with current recommendations and practice. Because of ongoing research, changes in government regulations, and the constant flow of information on drug therapy, reactions, and interactions, the reader is cautioned to check the package insert for each drug for indications, dosages, warnings, and precautions, particularly if the drug is new or infrequently used.

CONTRIBUTING AUTHORS

Nu-Vision, Inc.
Paula S. Cokingtin, RN, EdD, President
Kathy D. Robinson, RN, MSN, Vice President
Carolyn H. Brose, RN, EdD, Vice President
Linda N. Kohlman, RN, MN, Associate

Martha Bogart, RN, MS
  Teaching Associate
  School of Nursing
  University of Kansas Medical Center
  Kansas City, Kansas

Jan E. Carter, RN, MN, OCN
  Oncology Clinical Nurse Specialist
  Bethany Medical Center
  Kansas City, Missouri

Barbara Clancy, RN, EdD
  Professor
  School of Nursing
  University of Kansas Medical Center
  Kansas City, Kansas

Shirley Cudney, RN, C, GNP, MA
  Associate Professor
  College of Nursing
  Montana State University
  Bozeman, Montana

Mary Ersek, RN, MN
  Doctoral Candidate
  School of Nursing
  University of Washington
  Seattle, Washington

Joan Farrell, RN, PhD
  Dean
  College of Health
  University of North Florida
  Jacksonville, Florida

Pamela Gotch, RN, MSN, CDE
  Clinical Specialist—Endocrine/Diabetes
  Findling, Norton, Shaker, SC
  Milwaukee, Wisconsin

Jacquelyn Grinde, RN, MS
  Staff Nurse
  United Hospital
  St. Paul, Minnesota

Peggi Guenter, RN, MSN, CNSN

Doctoral Student
School of Nursing
University of Pennsylvania
Philadelphia, Pennsylvania

Deborah Kenny, RN, MSN, EdM

Critical Care Instructor
Staff Development, Nursing Service
University of Kansas Medical Center
Kansas City, Kansas

Melva Kravitz, RN, PhD

Director of Nursing
Shriners Burns Institute
Galveston, Texas

Larry Lancaster, RN, MSN, EdD

Associate Professor and Chairman
Department of Adult Health
Vanderbilt University School of Nursing
Nashville, Tennessee

Joan LeSage, RN, PhD

Chairperson
Gerontological Nursing
Rush-Presbyterian—St. Luke's Medical Center
Chicago, Illinois

Barbara Martin, RN, MS

Professor of Nursing
The University of Tulsa
College of Nursing and Applied Health Sciences
Tulsa, Oklahoma

Jewel McKay, RN, MSN

Director
Discharge Planning
Baptist Medical Center, Montclair
Birmingham, Alabama

Linda Pachucki-Hyde, RN, MS, CDE

Clinical Specialist—Endocrine/Diabetes
Findling, Norton, Shaker, SC
Milwaukee, Wisconsin

Pam Patterson, RN, MS

Ambulatory Care Manager and
Clinical Nurse Specialist
Jack and Renee Breslin Cancer Center
Lansing, Michigan

Jill Pendarvis, RNC, MA

Assistant Professor
Intercollegiate Center for Nursing Education
Spokane, Washington

Sharon B. Roth, RN, MS

Practitioner–Teacher
Department of Geriatric/Gerontological Nursing
Rush-Presbyterian—St. Luke's Medical Center
Chicago, Illinois

Mariah Snyder, RN, PhD, FAAN

Professor
School of Nursing
University of Minnesota
Minneapolis, Minnesota

Judith Sweeney, RN, MSN

Assistant Professor
School of Nursing—Vanderbilt University
Nashville, Tennessee

Lydia L. Tordecilla, RN, MS

Practitioner–Teacher
Department of Geriatric/Gerontological Nursing
Rush-Presbyterian—St. Luke's Medical Center
Chicago, Illinois

Kuei-Shen Tu, RN, MSN

Assistant Professor
School of Nursing
University of Alabama at Birmingham
Birmingham, Alabama

Nancy Williamson, RN, MSN

Assistant Professor
Medical College of Georgia
Augusta, Georgia

Jean Winter, RN, EdD
Assistant Professor
School of Nursing
Adelphi University
Garden City, New York

Mary Young, RN, MAN
Professor Emeritus of Nursing
Central Missouri State University
Warrensburg, Missouri

Neoma Youtsey, RN, MN
Instructor
School of Nursing
St. Luke's Hospital
Kansas City, Missouri

REVIEWERS

Martha Banyon, RN, EdD

Associate Professor of Nursing
University of Alabama at Birmingham
Birmingham, Alabama

Diane M. Billings, RN, EdD

Professor of Nursing
Indiana University
School of Nursing
Indianapolis, Indiana

Rebecca E. Boehne, RN, MSN

Critical Care Preceptor Trainer
U.S. Veterans Affairs Medical Center
Portland, Oregon

Karen M. Brubakken, RN, MS, CS

Clinical Nurse Specialist—Surgical
Community Memorial Hospital
Menomonee Falls, Wisconsin

Betty Chang, RN, DNSc

Professor
School of Nursing
University of California, Los Angeles
Los Angeles, California

Barbara Erickson, RN, PhD, CCRN

Associate Professor and Coordinator
Adult Critical Care Nursing Project
Seton Hall University
South Orange, New Jersey

Mary Fitzgerald, RN, MSN

Associate Professor of Nursing
University of Nevada
Las Vegas, Nevada

Ruth H. Franklin, RN, PhD, MPH

Assistant Professor—College of Nursing
Program Director
Geriatric Education and Health Management
  Program
University of New Mexico
Albuquerque, New Mexico

Deanne E. Grimes, RN, DrPH

Assistant Professor
School of Nursing
University of Texas Health Science Center
  at Houston
Houston, Texas

Donna D. Ignatavicius, RN, MS

Director of Nursing
William Hill Manor
Easton, Maryland

Marquerite R. Kinney, RN, DNSc, FAAN

Professor of Nursing
University of Alabama at Birmingham
Birmingham, Alabama

Jane Lancour, RN, MSN

President
JML & Associates
Irvine, California

Pamela D. Larsen, RN, MS, CRRN
Fort Collins, Colorado

Patricia P. Lillis, RN, DSN
Associate Professor
Medical College of Georgia
School of Nursing
Augusta, Georgia

Marilyn Lowe, MSN, RNC
Perinatal Clinical Specialist
Methodist Hospital
Omaha, Nebraska

Kenneth P. Miller, RN, PhD
Assistant Professor
Department of Physiological Nursing
University of California
San Francisco, California

Patricia Gonce Morton, RN, PhD
Assistant Professor
School of Nursing
University of Maryland
Baltimore, Maryland

Ayda G. Nambayan, RN, MEd, OCN
Assistant Professor
School of Nursing
University of Alabama at Birmingham
Birmingham, Alabama

Mary Oberg, RN, MN
Assistant Professor of Nursing
Avila College
Kansas City, Missouri

Joyce Olson, RN, MS, CDE
Pediatric Clinical Nurse Specialist
University of Kansas Medical Center
Kansas City, Kansas

Linda Pachucki-Hyde, RN, MS, CDE
Clinical Specialist—Endocrine/Diabetes
Findling, Norton, Shaker, SC
Milwaukee, Wisconsin

Phyllis M. C. Patterson, RN, MS, CS, OCN
Clinical Nurse Specialist—Hematology
University Hospital
University of Michigan
Ann Arbor, Michigan

Jeanne Salyer, RN, MSN
Doctoral Student
School of Nursing
Medical College of Virginia
Virginia Common Wealth University
Richmond, Virginia

Linda Sarna, RN, MN
Lecturer
School of Nursing
University of California, Los Angeles
Los Angeles, California

Suzanne Shaffer, RN, MN, OCN
Hematology Clinical Nurse Specialist
Kansas University Medical Center
Kansas City, Kansas

Dobrah Wright Shpritz, RN, MS, CCRN
Instructor—Undergraduate Studies
School of Nursing
University of Maryland
Baltimore, Maryland

Gail W. Snyder, RN, MSN
Instructor
Austin Community College
Austin, Texas

Clare Marie Tack, RN, MSN, CCRN
Staff Nurse
Frankford Hospital
Philadelphia, Pennsylvania

Rose Utley, RN, MS, CEN
Instructor
School of Nursing
University of Michigan
Ann Arbor, Michigan

Connie A. Walleck, RN, MS, CNRN
Associate Director of Clinical Nursing
Maryland Institute for Emergency Medical
  Services Systems
Baltimore, Maryland

INTRODUCTION

Lippincott's Review Series is designed to help you in your study of the key subject areas in nursing. The series consists of four books, one in each core nursing subject area:

Medical-Surgical Nursing
Pediatric Nursing
Maternal-Newborn Nursing
Mental Health and Psychiatric Nursing

Each book contains a comprehensive outline content review, chapter study questions and answer keys with rationales for correct and incorrect responses, and a comprehensive examination and answer key with rationales for correct and incorrect responses.

Lippincott's Review Series was planned and developed in response to your requests for outline review books that address each major subject area and also contain a self-test mechanism. These books meet the need for comprehensive subject review books that will also assist you in identifying your strong and weak areas of knowledge. Each book is a complete source for review and self-assessment of a single core subject—all four together provide an excellent comprehensive review of entry-level nursing.

Each book is all-inclusive of the content addressed in major textbooks. The content outline review uses a consistent nursing process format throughout and addresses nursing care for well and ill clients. Also included are such necessary additional topics as developmental and life-cycle issues, health assessment, patient teaching, and other concepts including growth and development, nutrition, pharmacology, and anatomy, physiology, and pathophysiology.

You can use the books in this series in several different ways. Overall, you can use them as subject reviews to augment general study throughout your basic nursing program and as a review to prepare for the National Council Licensure Examination (NCLEX-RN). How you use each book depends on your individual needs and preferences and on whether you review each chapter systematically or concentrate only on those chapters whose subject areas are particularly problematic or challenging. You may instead choose to use the comprehensive examination as a self-assessment opportunity to evaluate your knowledge base before you review the content outline. Likewise, you can use the study questions for pre- or post-testing after study, followed by the comprehensive examination as a means of evaluating your knowledge and competencies of an entire subject area.

Regardless of how you use the books, one of the strengths of the series is the self-assessment opportunity it offers in addition to guidance in studying and reviewing content. The chapter study questions and comprehensive examination questions have been carefully developed to cover all topics in the outline review. Most importantly, each question is categorized according to the components of the National Council of State Boards of Nursing Licensing Examination (NCLEX).

▶ Cognitive Level: Knowledge, Comprehension, Application, or Analysis
▶ Client Need: Safe, Effective Care Environment (Safe Care); Physiological Integrity (Physiologic); Psychosocial Integrity (Psychosocial); and Health Promotion and Maintenance (Health Promotion)
▶ Phase of the Nursing Process: Assessment, Analysis (Dx), Planning, Implementation, Evaluation

For those questions not related to a client need or to a phase of the nursing process, NA (not applicable) will be used, as in questions that test knowledge of a basic science.

Unlike the NCLEX examination that tests the cumulative knowledge needed for safe practice by an entry-level nurse, these practice tests systematically evaluate the knowledge base that serves as the building block for the entire nursing educational process. In this way, you can prepare for the NCLEX examination throughout your course of study. Good study habits throughout your educational program are not only the best way to ensure on-going success, but also will prove the most beneficial way to prepare for the licensing examination.

Keep in mind that these books are not intended to replace formal learning. They cannot substitute for textbook reading, discussion with instructors, or class attendance. Every effort has been made to provide accurate and current information, but class attendance and interaction with an instructor will provide invaluable information not found in books. Used correctly, these books will help you increase understanding, improve comprehension, evaluate strengths and weaknesses in areas of knowledge, increase productive study time, and as a result help you improve your grades.

MONEY BACK GUARANTEE—Lippincott's Review Series will help you study more effectively during coursework throughout your educational program and help you prepare for quizzes and tests, including the NCLEX exam. If you buy and use any of the four volumes in Lippincott's Review Series and fail the NCLEX exam, simply send us verification of your exam results and your copy of the review book to the address below. We will promptly send you a check for our suggested list price.

Lippincott's Review Series
J. B. Lippincott Company
227 East Washington Square
Philadelphia, PA 19106-3780

CONTENTS

Nursing Process and Health Assessment

I. Overview of the nursing process

A. Definitions

1. *Nursing* involves diagnosis and treatment of human responses to actual or potential health problems (ANA, 1980).
2. The science of nursing is built on a systematic step-by-step

method of problem solving known as the *nursing process* (Luck-mann and Sorensen, 1986).

B. **Steps of the nursing process**

1. *Assessment* involves collecting and organizing data about a patient's health status.
2. *Nursing diagnosis* encompasses identifying, delineating, and validating the patient's responses to health situations (problems or strengths) that lie within the scope of nursing practice.
3. *Planning* involves establishing expected outcomes (goals and objectives) and planning ways to address the patient's problems or support his or her strengths.
4. *Implementation* refers to carrying out the plan of care.
5. *Evaluation* involves comparing the patient's responses to nursing care with the expected outcomes.

II. Overview of nursing health assessment

A. **Definition**

1. Assessment, the first step of the nursing process, refers to systematic appraisal of all factors relevant to a patient's health.
2. Health assessment components include:
   a. Collection of information through health history, physical examination, and records and reports
   b. Analysis of information: comparing patient data with baseline data
   c. Synthesis of information from all sources to form a complete clinical picture and discover relationships among data

B. **Purposes: nursing health assessment elicits data that can be used to:**

1. Survey the patient's health status: wellness checks
2. Identify latent or occult (nondetected) disease
3. Screen for specific type of disease (e.g., diabetes or hypertension [case finding])
4. Determine functional impact of disease (human response to actual or potential health problem)
5. Evaluate the effectiveness of the health care plan

III. Health history

A. **Purposes**

1. Through the health history, the nurse elicits detailed, accurate, and chronologic health record as seen from the patient's perspective.
2. The health history also helps the nurse establish contact with a patient and develop good rapport.
3. It also helps focus and guide subsequent physical examination.
4. Health history information helps the nurse gain insight into the patient's functional status.

B. **Data collection techniques**
  1. Provide privacy and comfort for the patient.
  2. Greet the patient and introduce yourself.
  3. Establish a verbal contract with the patient that delineates the purpose of the history-taking session, the patient's role, and a time limit for the interview.
  4. Ask open-ended questions to explore problem areas (e.g., "Tell me about any problems you may have with your breathing.")
  5. Ask progressively more specific questions after identifying a particular problem (symptom analysis).
  6. Guide the interview to obtain essential information without discouraging the patient's discussion.

IV. **Health history components**
  A. **Biographic information** (*Note:* If this information already is in the patient's record, do not repeat it.)
    1. Date and time of interview
    2. Patient's name, address, telephone number, and Social Security number
    3. Name, address, and telephone number of person to contact in case of emergency or other situation
    4. Gender, race, ethnic origin, and religious preference
    5. Age, birthdate, birthplace, and marital status
    6. Occupation and level of education
    7. Health insurance, usual source of health care, and source of referral

  B. **Reliability of data**
    1. This component involves a description of patient behaviors that lead the interviewer to believe that the patient is a reliable, partially reliable, or unreliable source of information (e.g., "Responded promptly to all questions; maintained eye contact; dates consistent. Patient reliable.").
    2. This is the only section of the health history in which the nurse draws a conclusion from data.

  C. **Health and illness patterns**
    1. The patient's reason for seeking health care, including:
       a. Brief statement, usually in the patient's own words, of the overriding problem for which he or she is seeking help
       b. Duration of the problem
    2. Current health status or concern: details of the patient's reason for seeking health care, including:
       a. A detailed chronologic picture of the problem, beginning with when the patient last felt well and ending with a description of the current condition
       b. For multiple problems, each described in a separate paragraph

    c.   For each problem, a symptom analysis that includes bodily location (e.g., pain in lower right abdomen), quality (e.g., sharp), quantity (e.g., "The pain is about a 6 on a 10-point scale."), chronology (onset, duration, constant or intermittent, etc.), setting (precipitating circumstances, place, activity, persons present, etc.), aggravating and alleviating factors (e.g., "When I stand up straight, the pain is worse; when I curl up, it goes away."), and associated manifestations (e.g., vomiting, headache)

    d.   In case of acute infections, information on possible exposure or incubation period

    e.   In both acute and chronic illnesses, observations of whether and when the patient stopped working or went to bed

    f.   The patient's perception of whether the problem is getting better or worse

    g.   Information on previous treatments, including medications (prescribed and over the counter), the prescribing practitioner, treatment setting (e.g., hospital, clinic)

3. Past health status: health information not specifically associated with the current problem; usually considered to be any problem occurring more than 6 months to 1 year previously and includes:

    a.   General health and strength compared to 1 year ago: stability of weight, appetite

    b.   Past illnesses: childhood illnesses, acute infectious diseases, illnesses not requiring hospitalization, illness requiring hospitalization or surgery

    c.   Accidents and injuries

    d.   Sexual history: sexual performance, menstrual history, pregnancies (*Note:* This information also may appear in the review of systems.)

    e.   Immunizations

    f.   Allergies, including eczema, hives, and itching (with description of reaction); treatments

    g.   Geographic exposure: areas of residence, foreign travel

    h.   Psychiatric history: history of "nervous breakdown," depression, dementia

4. Status of physiologic systems: subjective information on the patient's perceptions of major body system functions, including current status and any related past symptoms (positives), or lack of symptoms (negatives), with a symptom analysis of any positive findings:

    a.   General: weakness, fatigue, malaise, fever, chills, recent weight loss or gain

    b.   Integument: pruritus, pigmentary and other color changes, bleeding and bruising tendencies, lesions, excessive dryness, change in texture or character of hair or nails, use of hair dyes or any possibly toxic agents

c. Head: headache, head injury, syncope, dizziness

d. Eyes: pain, recent change in appearance or vision, eyeglasses or contact lenses and recent change in prescription, diplopia, photophobia, blind spots, itching, burning, discharge, conjunctivitis, infection, glaucoma, cataracts, diabetes, hypertension

e. Ears: hearing acuity, earaches, tinnitus, vertigo, discharge, infection, mastoiditis

f. Nose and sinuses: sense of smell, sinus pain, epistaxis, nasal obstruction, discharge, postnasal drip, frequency of head colds, sneezing, use of nose drops or sprays

g. Oral cavity: toothache, recent extractions, state of dental repair; dry mouth, soreness or bleeding of lips, gums, mouth, tongue, or throat; disturbed taste sensation; hoarseness; tonsillectomy

h. Neck: pain, limitation of motion, thyroid enlargement

i. Lymph nodes: tenderness or enlargement of neck, axillary, epitrochlear, or inguinal nodes; duration and progress of abnormality

j. Breasts: pain, lumps, nipple discharge, surgery, mammography and breast self-examination, and timing with regard to menstrual cycle, estrogen replacement therapy

k. Respiratory: chest pain (and its relationship to respirations), pleurisy, frequent sneezing, cough, sputum production (character and amount), hemoptysis, wheezing (and its location in the chest), stridor, asthma, bronchitis, pneumonia, tuberculosis or contact therewith, night sweats, date of recent chest radiograph, smoking history

l. Cardiovascular: precordial or retrosternal pain or discomfort, palpitations, dyspnea (and how it relates to exertion), orthopnea (assessing the number of pillows the patient needs under his or her head to sleep comfortably), paroxysmal nocturnal dyspnea, edema, cyanosis; history of heart murmur, rheumatic fever (and its manifestations), hypertension (and usual blood pressure, if known), or coronary artery disease; most recent ECG and results

m. Gastrointestinal: appetite, food intolerances, dysphagia (with solids, liquids, or both), heartburn, postprandial pain or distress, biliary colic, jaundice, other abdominal pain or distress, belching, nausea, vomiting, hematemesis or flatulence; change in character or color of stools (bleeding, melena, clay colored, diarrhea, constipation) or change in bowel habits; use of laxatives (type, frequency); rectal conditions (pruritus, hemorrhoids, fissures, fistula);

ulcers; gallbladder disease; hepatitis; appendicitis; colitis; parasites; hernia; radiographs (where and when obtained, results)

n. Renal and urinary: renal colic, frequency of urination, nocturia, polyuria, oliguria, urine retention, hesitancy, urgency, dysuria, narrowing of urine stream, dribbling, incontinence, hematuria, albuminuria, pyuria, kidney disease, facial edema, renal calculi, cystoscopy, and results

o. Male reproductive: testicular pain, change in scrotum; puberty (onset, voice change, erections, emissions); libido and satisfaction with sexual relations

p. Female reproductive: menstrual history (menarche, last period, cycle and duration, amount of flow, premenstrual pain, dysmenorrhea, and intermenstrual bleeding), vaginal discharge, dyspareunia, obstetric history (gravida/para, miscarriages, abortions, complications), menopause and associated symptoms, contraceptive methods used, libido and satisfaction with sexual relations

q. Venereal: gonorrhea, syphilis, herpes, AIDS (date of onset, treatments and their effectiveness, any complications)

r. Peripheral vascular: intermittent claudication, varicose veins, thrombophlebitis

s. Musculoskeletal: joint pain, stiffness, swelling (location, migratory nature, relation to known cardiac involvement); rheumatoid arthritis, gout, bursitis; limitations in function or range of motion; flat feet, osteomyelitis, fractures; muscle pain, cramps; back pain (location and radiation, especially to extremities), stiffness, limitation of motion, sciatica or disk disease

t. Neurologic: loss of consciousness, convulsions, meningitis, encephalitis, stroke, seizures, or other neurologic problems; use of medication for seizure control; cognitive disturbances (recent or remote memory loss, hallucinations, disorientation, speech and language dysfunction, or inability to concentrate); change in sleep pattern; motor problems (gait, balance, coordination), tics, twitching, tremors; muscle weakness, spasms; paralysis, muscle wasting, activity intolerance; sensory disturbances (pain, insensitivity to temperature or touch, paresthesias); neuralgic pain (head, neck, trunk, extremities)

u. Hematopoietic and immune systems: bleeding tendencies of skin or mucous membranes; anemia; blood type, transfusions and reaction; blood dyscrasias, low platelet count, exposure to toxic agents or radiation; unexplained systemic infections and lymph node swelling

v. Endocrine and metabolic: nutritional and growth history;

thyroid dysfunction (e.g., goiter), adrenal problems, or diabetes; changes in tolerance to heat and cold; relationship between appetite and weight; excessive voiding or excessive thirst; changes in skin (e.g., pigmentation, texture); changes in body contour, hair distribution, shoe or glove size; unexplained weakness

5. Family health status, covering grandparents, parents, brothers, sisters, spouse, and children, and including:
   a. Age and health status or age at death and cause of death
   b. History of heart disease, hypertension, stroke, diabetes, gout, kidney disease or calculi, thyroid disease, asthma or other allergic disorders, blood problems, cancer, epilepsy, mental illness, arthritis, alcoholism, obesity
   c. Hereditary diseases such as hemophilia or sickle cell disease
   d. Family history presented as a genogram or diagram of the "family tree" with added notations regarding family negatives (diseases not present in the family)

6. Developmental considerations: overview of the patient's growth history, including pertinent physical and cognitive developmental milestones and factors

7. Functional history
   a. Status of patient's mobility in relationship to activities and demands of daily living (e.g., [Shanas' Index of Incapacity]: "Can you go out of doors? Can you walk up and down stairs? Can you get out of the house? Can you wash and bathe yourself? Can you dress yourself? Can you put on your shoes? Can you cut your toenails?") (Carnevali and Patrick, 1979)
   b. Patient's preferred lifestyle (e.g., "Is there anything you cannot do now compared with last year? Do you travel now? Did you in the past? Where did you travel?")
   c. The patient's home and neighborhood environment (e.g., "Who buys and carries the groceries? Who cooks? Who does the housekeeping? Do you feel safe in and around your home?")

D. Health promotion and protection patterns
   1. Health beliefs, encompassing:
      a. Expectations of health care
      b. Promotive, preventive, and restorative practices (e.g., breast self-examination, seat belt use)
      c. What client considers an illness
   2. Personal habits, including:
      a. Use of tobacco, alcohol, street drugs
      b. Use of prescribed and over-the-counter medications
      c. Use of caffeine
      d. Hygiene

          e.   Elimination patterns

    3. Sleep and wake patterns

    4. Exercise and activity

    5. Recreation

    6. Nutrition, including:
        a.   Height and weight
        b.   24-hour dietary recall, including number of portions and portion sizes

    7. Stress and coping patterns

    8. Socioeconomic status, encompassing:
        a.   Educational level
        b.   Financial status

    9. Environmental health patterns, including:
        a.   Home conditions: living arrangements, housing
        b.   General environmental conditions: neighborhood, region

    10. Occupational health patterns, covering:
        a.   Exact nature of work, or of previous work if retired
        b.   Exposure to toxic agents, fatigue, abnormal surroundings

E. **Role and relationship patterns**

    1. Self-concept, including:
        a.   Self-expectations (short- and long-range goals)
        b.   Perceived strengths and weaknesses

    2. Cultural influences

    3. Spiritual and religious influences

    4. Family role and relationship patterns

    5. Sexuality and reproductive patterns, including:
        a.   Menstrual history and puberty history
        b.   Sexual activity (past and present)
        c.   Pregnancies (miscarriages, live births)

    6. Social support patterns (family, friends, agencies)

    7. Emotional health status

F. **Conclusion: Complete the health history by asking "Is there anything else you'd like to tell me?" This allows the patient to end the interview by discussing feelings and concerns.**

V. Physical examination

  A. **General principles**

    1. Physical examination is the second component of a complete nursing health assessment.

    2. Perform a complete or partial physical examination after obtaining a careful comprehensive or problem-related history; history findings help focus the physical examination.

    3. Examine the patient in a quiet, warm, well-lit room; consider privacy and comfort needs.

    4. Explain what you plan to do, what the patient likely will feel, and what you expect from the patient.

5. Use appropriate draping for examination, exposing only the portions of the body being examined.
6. Always compare body sides for symmetry and, where appropriate, compare distal to proximal areas; the patient's body can serve as its own control.
7. Visualize underlying structures and organs when performing the examination.
8. Use anatomical landmarks to locate specific structures and to report significant findings (e.g., thorax, heart, abdomen).
9. When possible, examine the patient while standing at his or her right side.

B. Assessment techniques
1. The nurse uses four basic techniques in physical assessment: inspection, auscultation, palpation, and percussion.
2. Inspection: Inspection, the most important of all techniques (but the most commonly slighted), starts at the initial client encounter. The nurse begins each portion of an examination with inspection, using the eyes and other senses as appropriate.
3. Auscultation: This technique involves listening (usually through a stethoscope) to sounds produced in the body, particularly in the heart, lungs, vessels, stomach, and intestines.
4. Palpation: In this technique, the nurse uses different parts of the hand to detect characteristics of pulsations, vibrations, texture, shape, temperature, and movement. Palpation can confirm and amplify findings observed during inspection.
5. Percussion: Sharply tapping the body surface with the fingers or hands produces sounds that vary in quality depending on the density of underlying structures (e.g., organ borders, fluid, or gas). This technique also is done to elicit tenderness and assess reflexes.

C. Vital signs
1. Normal temperature readings range from 35.8 to 37.3°C (96.4 to 99.1°F). Subnormal readings are common in elderly patients. These patients and others (e.g., those receiving certain medications or experiencing shock) may not exhibit significant temperature elevation in response to an infectious process.
2. Normal pulse findings are 60 to 80 beats per minute, regular, full, and strong.
3. Normal respiratory rate ranges from 16 to 20 breaths per minute.
4. The significance of blood pressure readings is as follows:
   a. Diastolic: normal, less than 85 mmHg; high normal pressure, 85 to 89 mmHg; mild hypertension, 90 to 104 mmHg; moderate hypertension, 105 to 114 mmHg; severe hypertension, 115 mmHg and above
   b. Systolic (when diastolic is less than 90 mmHg): normal,

less than 140 mmHg; borderline isolated systolic hypertension, 140 to 159 mmHg; isolated systolic hypertension,
160 mmHg or above

    c.   A difference of 5 to 10 mmHg between arms is common;
systolic pressure usually is 10 mmHg higher in legs than in
arms.

    d.   Changing positions from recumbent to standing can cause
a 10 to 15 mmHg drop in systolic pressure and a slight rise
(5 mmHg or so) in diastolic pressure.

    e.   In elderly patients, check blood pressure in the lying, sit-
ting, and standing positions to detect excessive postural
hypotension related to antihypertensive drugs or age-
related physiologic changes.

5.   When assessing a patient's vital signs, keep in mind that they
normally may vary somewhat with the time of day; for example:

    a.   Diurnal body temperature variation of 0.5 to 2°F; lowest
during sleep and highest from noon to early evening

    b.   Blood pressure decreased during sleep and fluctuating
throughout the day with no predictable pattern

    c.   Pulse rate decreased during sleep and increased during the
day in response to activity and stress

D. **Height and weight**

1.   Weight is related to body frame size: small, medium, or large.
2.   Adipose tissue measurements (e.g., triceps skinfold thickness)
help determine body fat percentage.
3.   Elderly patients, particularly females, commonly lose height with
aging due to osteoporotic kyphosis.

E. **General appearance**

1.   Race
2.   Sex
3.   General physical development
4.   Nutritional status
5.   Mental alertness
6.   Evidence of pain, restlessness
7.   Body position
8.   Apparent age
9.   Clothing, hygiene, grooming

F. **Integument**

1.   Inspection

    a.   Color of skin and mucous membranes (complexion, jaun-
dice, cyanosis, erythema)

    b.   Pigmentation

    c.   Lesions and scars (distribution, type, configuration, size),
superficial vascularity

    d.   Moisture

        e.   Edema
        f.   Hair distribution
        g.   Nails

  2. Palpation
        a.   Temperature
        b.   Texture and consistency, elasticity, turgor, mobility
        c.   Tenderness

  3. Normal findings
        a.   No lesions
        b.   Skin warm, slightly moist, smooth, finely textured, with good turgor
        c.   Hair distribution characteristic for gender and age
        d.   Nails present and smooth
        e.   Mucous membranes moist and pink

  4. Gerontologic considerations: common age-related differences in elderly patients include:
        a.   Skin wrinkled, drier (loss of subcutaneous fat and diminished sweat gland activity), and increasingly fragile
        b.   Turgor decreased (cannot be used to assess level of hydration)
        c.   Hair grayer, sparser on head, axilla, extremities, and pubic area; increased facial hair in women; bristly hair in nose and ears of men
        d.   Mucous membranes possibly drier and paler
        e.   Nails possibly horny and tough in response to decreased peripheral circulation
        f.   Common benign lesions: senile lentigines ("age" or "liver spots"); seborrheic keratoses (yellowish or brownish wart-like lesions with oily scale); cherry angiomas (small bright or dark red papules)

G. Head

  1. Inspection
        a.   Skull size and shape
        b.   Symmetry of face
        c.   Scalp: flaking, lesions, masses, deformities, swelling, tenderness
        d.   Hair color, distribution, nits on hair shafts

  2. Palpation
        a.   Hair texture
        b.   Scalp
        c.   Skull shape: bony overgrowths, symmetry

  3. Normal findings
        a.   Skull normocephalic
        b.   Face symmetric
        c.   Scalp clear
        d.   No alopecia or foreign bodies in hair

4. Gerontologic considerations: Nose and ears commonly appear larger in proportion to head size.

H. **Eyes and vision**
1. Vision testing
   a. Test visual acuity with a Snellen chart; test a patient wearing corrective lenses with and without the lenses.
   b. Test visual peripheral fields.
2. Inspection
   a. Globes: Observe for protrusion.
   b. Palpebral fissures: Assess symmetry and width.
   c. Lid margins: Observe for scaling, secretions, erythema, position of lashes.
   d. Conjunctivae: Inspect for congestion; note color.
   e. Sclerae and irises: Observe color.
   f. Pupils: Note size, shape, symmetry, reaction to light and accommodation.
   g. Eye movement: Assess extraocular movements; note nystagmus or convergence.
3. Palpation
   a. Evaluate strength of the upper lids by attempting to open the patient's closed lids against his or her resistance.
   b. Assess tenderness and tension of eyeballs.
4. Fundoscopic examination (with an ophthalmoscope)
   a. Locate the red reflex.
   b. Check the transparency of the anterior and posterior chambers, cornea, and lens.
   c. Examine the retina (color, pigmentation, hemorrhages, and exudates); optic disk (color, distinction of margins, pigmentation, degree of elevation, cupping); macula (color); and blood vessels (diameter, atriovenous [AV] ratio, origin and course, venous–arterial crossings).
5. Normal findings
   a. Central vision 20/20 OU (both eyes), visual fields unrestricted
   b. No ptosis or lid lag
   c. Eyes move in conjugate fashion
   d. Anterior and posterior chambers, lens and cornea transparent; sclera and conjunctiva clear
   e. Lacrimal system unobstructed
   f. Pupils equal, round, and reactive to light and accommodation (PERRLA)
   g. Red reflex present bilaterally
   h. Bilateral well-marginated discs revealed on fundoscopic examination
   i. C–D ratio 1:4, vessels to all four quadrants
   j. AV ratio 2:3

        k.   No arterial narrowing, venous engorgement, AV nicking, hemorrhages, or exudate

    6. Gerontologic considerations

        a.   Assess for entropion, ectropion, lens opacity, and eye dryness.

        b.   Entropion in elderly patients can cause discomfort and damage to the eye.

        c.   Fundoscopic examination may be difficult in an elderly patient because the pupil commonly is small (3 cm), with limited ability to dilate without a medicinal dilator.

I.   **Ears and hearing**

    1. Hearing assessment

        a.   Test gross hearing acuity with whispered words or a watch.

        b.   With a tuning fork (512 to 1024 Hz), perform the Weber (bone conduction) and Rinne (air conduction to bone conduction ratio) tests.

    2. Inspection

        a.   Pinna: Assess size, shape, placement on head, and color; note any lesions or masses.

        b.   External canal: With an otoscope, check for discharge, impacted cerumen, inflammation, masses, and foreign bodies.

        c.   Tympanic membrane: With an otoscope inserted inferiorly into the distal portion of the tympanic canal, assess color, luster, shape, position, transparency, and integrity; note any scarring; locate landmarks (cone of light, umbo, handle and short process of malleus, pars flaccida, and pars tensa).

    3. Palpation: Examine pinna for tenderness, consistency of cartilage, swelling, and pain.

    4. Normal findings

        a.   Weber test not referred (or lateralized)

        b.   Rinne test positive (air conduction greater than bone conduction)

        c.   External ear appearance normal

        d.   Canals clear without discharge

        e.   Tympanic membranes pearly gray and intact, with landmarks visible

    5. Gerontologic considerations: Moderate hearing loss (especially of high-frequency sounds) and difficulty with sound discrimination are common in elderly patients.

J.   **Nose and sinuses**

    1. Inspection

        a.   Observe position of the nose on the face.

        b.   Note any discharge.

        c.   Assess airway patency; note any nasal obstruction.

        d.   Perform a speculum examination of interior structures: nasal septum (assessing position, noting any bleeding or perforation), mucous membranes (noting hydration and color), and turbinates (assess color, note any swelling).

2. Palpation: Apply fingertip pressure to the frontal and maxillary sinuses to assess for tenderness.

3. Normal findings
- a. Nose symmetrically placed on face
- b. Nasal passages patent with septum in midline
- c. Mucous membrane moist and dark pink without perforation or bleeding
- d. Sinuses nontender

4. Gerontologic considerations: Elderly patients commonly exhibit pale nasal mucosa.

K. **Mouth and pharynx**

    1. Inspection (*Note:* Use a penlight and tongue depressor when examining inside the patient's mouth.)
- a. Lips: Observe color, moisture; note abnormal pigmentation, masses, ulcerations, or fissures.
- b. Teeth: Note number, arrangement, and general condition.
- c. Gingivae: Assess color and texture; note discharge, swelling, retraction, or bleeding.
- d. Buccal mucosa: Assess for discoloration, vesicles, ulcerations, or masses.
- e. Pharynx: Note any inflammation, exudate, or masses.
- f. Tongue (both at rest and protruded): Assess size, color, moisture, and symmetry; note any lesions, deviations from midline, fasciculations, or tremors.
- g. Salivary glands: Assess patency.
- h. Uvula: Assess position on phonation; should be midline.
- i. Soft palate: Observe symmetry on phonation, intactness.
- j. Tonsils: Note presence or absence, size, ulcerations, exudate, or inflammation.
- k. Note breath odor.
- l. Assess voice volume; note any hoarseness.
- m. Check the patient's ability to swallow.

    2. Palpation (*Note:* Wear a glove when putting your fingers inside the patient's mouth.)
- a. Oral cavity: Palpate for masses and ulcerations.
- b. Tongue: Grasp the tongue with a gauze sponge to retract and palpate it and to inspect its undersurface and the floor of the oral cavity.
- c. Gag reflex: Attempt to elicit bilaterally.

    3. Normal findings
- a. No lesions of lips, gums, tongue, or buccal mucosa

   b. Tongue pink, moist, well papillated, and in midline, both at rest and on protrusion

   c. Salivary glands unobstructed

   d. Pharynx not injected

   e. Tonsils nonobstructing

   f. Uvula in midline

   g. Palate elevating symmetrically on phonation

   h. Gag reflex present bilaterally

   i. Teeth present with no caries

   j. Gums clear

  4. Gerontologic considerations

   a. Assess hydration status by observing for a small saliva pool under the tongue.

   b. If the patient wears dentures, be sure he or she removes them before you examine the mouth.

L. **Neck**

 1. Inspection

   a. All areas of neck anteriorly and posteriorly: Assess muscle symmetry and range of motion; note any masses, unusual swelling, or pulsations.

   b. Thyroid: Observe for enlargement.

   c. External jugular veins: Note distention.

 2. Palpation

   a. Cervical nodes and salivary glands: Palpate for enlargement, tenderness.

   b. Trachea: Note deviation from midline.

   c. Thyroid: Palpate for nodules, masses, or irregularities.

   d. Carotid arteries: Note amplitude and symmetry of pulsations.

 3. Auscultation: Listen for bruits over the carotid arteries and the thyroid.

 4. Normal findings

   a. Neck symmetric with no tenderness or limitation of movement

   b. Trachea in midline

   c. Thyroid nonpalpable

   d. No bruits auscultated

 5. Gerontologic considerations: Elderly patients are at risk for heart irregularities (reflex drop in pulse rate or blood pressure if carotid arteries are palpated at level of carotid sinuses); to prevent this, palpate well below the upper border of the thyroid cartilage.

M. **Lymph nodes**

 1. Inspection: Note observable nodes.

 2. Palpation

   a. Feel for palpable nodes: Assess size, shape, mobility, and consistency; note tenderness or inflammation.

       b.   Locations to palpate: cervical, supra, and infraclavicular; axillary central, lateral, subscapular, and pectoral groups; inguinal (horizontal and vertical); and epitrochlear.

  3. Normal findings: no palpable or tender nodes

  4. Gerontologic considerations: Elderly patients may exhibit shotty nodes in inguinal areas.

N. **Female breasts**

  1. Inspection

       a.   With the patient sitting and her arms at her side, inspect the nipples and areolae for position, pigmentation, inversion, discharge, crusting, and masses; note any supernumerary nipples.

       b.   Observe the size, shape, color, symmetry, surface contour, skin characteristics, and level of breasts; note any retraction or dimpling of skin or nipples, new pigmentation, engorged veins, swelling, or any tendency of a breast to cling to the thorax.

       c.   Repeat these observations with the patient's hands above or behind her head, with her hands pressed firmly on her hips, with the patient leaning forward from the hips, and with the patient supine.

  2. Palpation

       a.   Palpate the breasts with the patient in both sitting and supine positions; when the patient is supine, and for a patient with large breasts, place a pad under the ipsilateral scapula of the breast being palpated, and raise the arm on that side over the patient's head.

       b.   Palpate one breast at time, using the palmar aspects of your fingers in a rotating motion and moving in concentric circles from the periphery of the breast to the nipple. Assess skin texture, moisture, and temperature; note any masses. Be sure to include the tail of Spence (breast tissue extending into the axillary region in the upper outer quadrant of the breast).

       c.   Gently squeeze, milk, and then invert the nipple to check for any expressible discharge and to detect any mass beneath the nipple.

       d.   Repeat these steps for the other breast, and compare findings on both sides.

       e.   Conclude by applying lotion for lubrication, then—using the palmar surface of the fingers—sweeping both breasts superiorly to inferiorly, compressing them against the thorax; note any masses.

  3. Normal findings

       a.   Nipples symmetric with no erosion, discharge, or recent inversion

   b.   Breasts symmetric although possibly varying in size
   c.   Tissue soft, lobular, and homogenous
    4.   Gerontologic considerations
   a.   In postmenopausal women, the breasts may feel nodular or stringy on palpation.
   b.   Half of all deaths from breast cancer occur in women age 65 or older.
O.   **Male breasts** (*Note:* Although this examination is brief, it should not be omitted.)
    1.   Inspection: Observe the nipples and areolae for ulceration, nodules, swelling, or discharge.
    2.   Palpation: Palpate the areolae, noting nodules and tenderness.
    3.   Normal findings
   a.   Nipples symmetric with no erosion or discharge
   b.   No masses, discharge, or tenderness
P.   **Thorax and lungs**
    1.   Inspection
   a.   Posterior chest: With the patient seated, observe spine for mobility and structural deformity; symmetry, posture, mobility of thorax, and intercostal spaces (bulges or retraction) on respiration; anteroposterior diameter in relation to lateral diameter of chest.
   b.   Anterior chest: With the patient supine, inspect for structural deformities; assess the width of the costal angle; note rate and rhythm of breathing; observe for respiratory abnormalities (e.g., bulging or retraction of intercostal spaces, use of accessory muscles), and asymmetry.
    2.   Palpation
   a.   Posterior chest: With the patient seated, palpate the ribs and costal margins for symmetry, mobility, and tenderness, and the spine for tenderness and vertebral position. Assess respiratory excursion (note the distance that your thumbs part) and symmetry of motion and fremitus with the patient's arms crossed and scapulae separated.
   b.   Anterior chest: With the patient supine, assess as for the posterior chest, comparing symmetric areas and gently displacing female breasts if necessary.
    3.   Percussion
   a.   Posterior chest: With the patient seated with his or her arms across the chest and the scapulae separated, percuss symmetric areas, comparing sides. Begin across the top of each shoulder and proceed downward between the scapulae and then under the scapulae, both medially and laterally in axillary lines; note and localize abnormal percussion sounds (Table 1–1). Percuss for diaphragmatic

TABLE 1-1.
Review of Percussion Notes

Flat sounds: soft, high pitched, and of short duration (e.g., thigh)

Dull sounds: medium in intensity, pitch, and duration (e.g., liver)

Resonant sounds: loud, low pitched, and of long duration (e.g., normal lung)

Hyperresonant sounds: very loud, lower in pitch, and longer in duration (e.g., emphysematous lung)

Tympanic sounds: loud and musical (e.g., gastric air bubble, intestine)

excursion on complete exhalation and inhalation, marking points where resonance changes to dullness; note symmetry and levels.

b. Anterior chest: With the patient supine with his or her arms at sides, percuss from just below the clavicles along the midclavicular line (displacing female breasts as necessary), then move laterally. Note intercostal spaces where you detected hepatic dullness on the right side and cardiac dullness and gastric air bubble tympany on the left side.

4. Auscultation

a. Posterior chest: With the patient seated as for percussion, ask him or her to breathe somewhat more deeply than normal with mouth open. With a stethoscope, listen over the same areas and in the same pattern as for percussion, comparing from side to side and moving from apices to lung bases.

b. Anterior chest: Auscultate over the same areas and in the same pattern as for percussion, comparing sides and proceeding from lungs apices to bases. Note the distribution of vesicular and bronchovesicular sounds, both posteriorly and anteriorly (Table 1–2).

5. Normal findings

a. Respiratory rate 12 to 18 breaths per minute

b. Thorax symmetric; costal angle less than 90 degrees; transverse diameter 1:2 to 5:7; expansion 3 to 5 cm, symmetric, free and easy; no bulges or retractions in intercostal spaces

c. Diaphragm position and excursion 3 to 6 cm

d. Fremitus felt throughout lung fields, diminishing near periphery

e. Percussion resonant over symmetric areas of lung to expected lung borders (fifth intercostal space [ICS] anteriorly, seventh ICS laterally, T_{10} posteriorly); dullness between the third and fifth left intercostal spaces (LICS; heart)

TABLE 1–2.
Review of Vocal Sounds

Breath sounds

Vesicular sounds: longer on inspiration than expiration, of low pitch and soft intensity on expiration, and heard over most of the peripheral lung

Bronchovesicular sounds: equal in duration on inspiration and expiration, of medium pitch and intensity on expiration, and heard near the mainstem bronchi (anteriorly, below the clavicles at sternal borders to near the level of the second ICS; posteriorly, between the clavicles and between T1 and T4)

Bronchial (tracheal, tubular) sounds: shorter on inspiration than expiration, of high pitch and loud intensity on expiration, and heard over the trachea. (*Note:* Bronchial sounds heard over a lung are always abnormal.)

Adventitious sounds

Crackles: discrete, noncontinuous sounds most commonly heard on inspiration in dependent right and left lung bases and may clear on coughing (formerly called rales and crepitations); may be of two types: fine crackles (soft, short, high pitched) or coarse crackles (louder, slightly longer, lower pitched)

Gurgles: loud gurgling and bubbling sounds heard during both inspiration and expiration, possible produced by secretions in the trachea and large bronchi

Wheezes: continuous musical sounds of greater duration that may be heard during inspiration or expiration

Pleural rubs: loud, low pitched, and confined to a relatively small area of the chest wall; produced by inflamed pleura

Altered voiced sounds (spoken sounds that change when transmitted through airless lung tissue)

Bronchophony: voiced sound "99" heard louder and clearer than usual

Egophony: gives nasal bleating quality to voiced sounds; the patient's "ee" sounds like "ay"

Whispered pectoriloquy: whispered sounds (e.g., "1, 2, 3" or "99," heard louder and clearer than usual)

---

    f.   No adventitious sounds (crackles, gurgles, wheezes, or friction rubs), enhanced voiced sounds (egophony, bronchophony, or whispered pectoriloquy), or bronchial breath sounds

  6. Gerontologic considerations

    a.   Elderly patients may have "barrel chest" (AP-transverse diameter ratio of 1:1) in the absence of emphysema due to skeletal changes.

    b.   In elderly patients, crackles may be auscultated at the lung bases in the absence of congestive heart failure. Such crackles should clear with deep breathing or coughing; however, elderly adults tend not to breathe as deeply or cough as productively as younger adults due to decreased rib mobility and reduced vital capacity.

Q. Heart

  1. Inspection

    a.   Precordium: Look for lifts, heaves, thrusts, or pulsations.

    b.   Apical impulse: Observe for visible palpations (occurs in about 50% of patients).

2. Palpation
   a. Using the palms, palpate all auscultatory areas, noting vibrations or thrills.
   b. Locate the apical impulse, and assess the rate and strength of pulsations.
3. Percussion: Percuss the heart's borders in the 3rd to 5th LICS, noting areas of cardiac dullness.
4. Auscultation
   a. Listen with the stethoscope's diaphragm (best for high-pitched sounds) and bell (best for low-pitched sounds) in each auscultatory area.
   b. Identify S1 and S2 (lub-dub).
   c. Determine which sound is louder. (Normally, S2 is loudest in the aortic and pulmonic areas, S1 is louder than or equal to S2 in the tricuspid area, and S1 is loudest in the mitral area.)
   d. Listen for physiologic split in S2.
   e. Determine systolic phase (between S1 and S2) and diastolic phase (between S2 and S1): diastolic should be longer than systolic at a heart rate of 120 beats per minute or less.
   f. Note extra sounds or murmurs.
   g. Determine heart rate and rhythm.
5. Normal findings
   a. AP rate 60 to 80 beats per minute, regular
   b. No thrills, heaves, or abnormal pulsations
   c. Apical impulse 5 LICS at or medial to the midclavicular line (palpated within one ICS and no more than 1 to 2 cm wide; 7 to 9 cm from the sternal border)
   d. Left cardiac border dullness 9 to 12 cm from the sternal border
   e. S1 and S2 heard in expected locations with expected intensities (S2 split common in supine position on inspiration); no extra sounds or murmurs
6. Gerontologic considerations
   a. Dysrhythmias become more common with aging; they may or may not be significant.
   b. Stiffened valves may cause murmurs or S4 ("Ten-nes-see").
   c. S3 ("Ken-tuck-y") in elderly patients usually is pathologic.

R. Peripheral circulation
1. Inspection
   a. Jugular veins: With the patient supine, observe the neck for internal jugular venous pulsations; if present, note their characteristics and relationship to inspiration. With the patient sitting, observe for distended jugular veins.

   b. Carotid arteries: Observe for pulsations (timed with apical impulse).
   c. Extremities (arterial): Observe color, noting pallor or rubor; hair distribution, noting abnormal absence; and skin characteristics, noting shiny or thin skin and any circumscribed lesions on feet and toes.
   d. Extremities (venous): Observe color, noting abnormal brown pigmentation; look for skin lesions on the lower legs, varicosities, and edema.

2. Palpation
   a. Extremities (arterial): Assess the temperature of the skin. Palpate pulses (radial, femoral, posterior tibial, dorsalis pedis), comparing sides. Check capillary refill times in fingernails and toenails. Perform Allen's test on radial and ulnar arteries.
   b. Extremities (venous): Palpate the skin over the tibia and at the medial malleoli for pitting edema. Compress the calf between your two hands placed anteriorly and posteriorly; note any pain that this maneuver elicits.

3. Auscultation: Listen over the carotid, abdominal, and femoral arteries for bruits.

4. Normal findings
   a. Jugular veins soft and undulating, decreasing on inspiration when supine; not observable when sitting
   b. Carotid artery pulsations synchronous with apical impulse
   c. In extremities, skin warm with no discoloration, lesions, varicosities, or edema
   d. Pulses 2+ bilaterally on a scale of 0 to 3+
   e. Capillary refill immediate; hands pink immediately in response to Allen's test
   f. No calf tenderness elicited
   g. No bruits auscultated over the carotid, abdominal, or femoral artery

5. Gerontologic considerations
   a. Elderly persons commonly experience thickening, hardening, and loss of elasticity in vessel walls.
   b. Gradual pink or purple discoloration on the toes and feet is common in elderly persons.

S. Abdomen

1. Inspection
   a. Skin: scars, striae, and rashes
   b. General contour and symmetry
   c. Visible peristalsis, aortic pulsations and hernias (umbilical, inguinal, and incisional)

2. Auscultation (*Note:* Auscultate the abdomen before percussing and palpating to avoid stimulating intestinal activity and altering bowel sounds.)
   a. Bowel sounds: Listen in all quadrants; note frequency, pitch, and duration.
   b. Auscultate for bruits over abdominal aorta and the renal, iliac, and femoral arteries.
3. Percussion
   a. Percuss in all quadrants; note areas of tympany or dullness.
   b. Percuss along the right midclavicular line, starting below the umbilicus and moving upward, to locate the liver borders.
   c. Percuss in the left upper quadrant for gastric air bubble.
   d. With the patient sitting, strike the back at the costovertebral angles (CVA); note tenderness or pain.
4. Palpation
   a. Abdomen: Palpate lightly in all quadrants; follow with deep palpation. Assess organ location and abdominal muscle tone; note unusual masses, pulsations, tenderness, or pain.
   b. Kidney: Palpate kidneys bimanually slightly below the umbilicus; note size, shape, and any tenderness.
   c. Abdominal aorta: Palpate for contour and pulsations.
   d. Lymph nodes: Palpate inguinal and femoral areas bilaterally; note enlargement.
5. Normal findings
   a. No scars; abdominal wall flat and symmetric; no incisional, umbilical, or inguinal hernias
   b. Bowel sounds intermittent (every 5 to 35 seconds) and gurgling with no hyperactive or tinkling sounds; rushing sounds over the ileocecal valve (in the right lower quadrant) 4 to 7 hours after eating; no bruits
   c. Liver dullness 6 to 12 cm at RMCL; tympany of gastric air bubble over left anterior lower border of thorax; tympany in all quadrants
   d. No CVA tenderness
   e. Muscle tone normal; abdomen soft with no masses or tenderness
   f. Aorta width 2.5 to 4 cm; soft, pulsatile
   g. Pole of right kidney may be palpable
6. Gerontologic considerations
   a. Elderly patients commonly exhibit diminished peristalsis.
   b. In elderly patients, the liver may be 1 to 2 cm below the right costal margin due to an enlarged lung field.

T. Male genitalia and hernias (*Note:* Wear gloves during examination.)
   1. Inspection
      a. Pubic hair: Assess distribution; note any nits or lice.

    b.   Penis: Retract the foreskin, if present. Note any ulcerations, masses, or scarring on the glans penis. Inspect the urethral meatus for location, lesions, and discharge.

    c.   Scrotum: Inspect anterior and posterior aspects, assessing size, contour, and symmetry; note ulcerations, masses, redness, or swelling.

    d.   Inguinal areas: Look for bulges, with and without the patient bearing down, or when raising his head off the bed.

2. Palpation

    a.   Penis: Palpate the shaft for lesions, nodules, or masses; if present, note tenderness, contour, size, and degree of induration.

    b.   Scrotum: Palpate each testis and epididymis, assessing size, shape, and consistency. Note any masses of unusual tenderness. Also note any nodules or tenderness of the spermatic cord and vas deferens.

    c.   Inguinal and femoral areas: Assess for hernias.

3. Normal findings

    a.   Normal male pubic hair distribution with no infestations

    b.   No penile lesions, masses, or discharge

    c.   Testes symmetric without masses or undue tenderness; the left testis may be slightly larger and hang lower than the right testis

    d.   No inguinal or femoral hernias

4. Gerontologic considerations

    a.   In elderly men, pubic hair commonly thins and scrotal skin loses tone, causing the scrotum to appear more pendulous.

    b.   Some degree of testicular atrophy and softening commonly occurs with aging.

U. **Female genitalia** (*Note:* Wear gloves during examination.)

    1. Inspection and palpation (performed almost simultaneously)

        a.   Place the patient in lithotomy position; drape properly.

        b.   Assess pubic hair distribution; note any nits or lice.

        c.   Inspect the labia majora, mons pubis, and perineum; note skin color and integrity.

        d.   Separate the labia majora, and inspect the clitoris, urethral meatus, and vaginal opening; note abnormal color, ulcerations, swelling, nodules, or discharge.

    2. Normal findings

        a.   Normal female pubic hair distribution with no infestations

        b.   Outlet, vagina, and perineum free of masses, edema, tenderness, nodules, lesions, and discharge

    3. Gerontologic considerations

        a.   In elderly women, pubic hair becomes gray, more sparse, and brittle.

        b.   External genitalia typically atrophy somewhat.

        c.   Weakened muscle tone with aging increases the likelihood of cystocele.

V.   **Rectum** (*Note:* Wear gloves during examination.)

   1.   Inspection

        a.   With the patient lying in left Sims' position and properly draped, spread the buttocks and examine the anus and the perianal and sacral regions. Note any inflammation, nodules, scars, lesions, ulcerations, rashes, bleeding, fissures, or hemorrhoids.

        b.   Check for bulges when the patient bears down.

        c.   If necessary, use an alternative position for examination: for a male patient, standing and bent over the table; for a female patient, the lithotomy position.

   2.   Palpation

        a.   Ask the patient to bear down; slowly insert your lubricated index finger of gloved hand through the anal sphincter; assess sphincter tone. Then, gently rotate your index finger to palpate the rectum and rectal walls anteriorly and posteriorly; note any nodules, masses, or tenderness.

        b.   Palpate for fecal impaction.

        c.   In a male patient, anteriorly palpate the two lateral lobes of the prostate gland for irregularities, nodules, swelling, or tenderness.

        d.   Withdraw your finger gently; test any fecal material on the glove for occult blood.

   3.   Normal findings

        a.   Sphincter closes around finger

        b.   Wall of rectum smooth and moist; soft stool may be present

        c.   No hemorrhoids, fissures, or fistulas

        d.   Stool guaiac test negative

        e.   Male prostate 2.5 to 4 cm in size with a small groove separating the lobes; feels firm, smooth, nonmovable, nontender, and rubbery

   4.   Gerontologic considerations: Most older men exhibit some degree of prostatic enlargement.

W. **Musculoskeletal system**

   1.   Inspection

        a.   Observe the patient's ability to perform functional tasks of daily living (e.g., grasping objects, performing personal hygiene, bathing, dressing, bending, sitting, rising from sitting to standing, and walking up and down stairs as well as on a level surface).

        b.   Note any pain the patient experiences while performing functions or being examined.

        c.   Examine the arms and legs; note size, symmetry, muscle mass, and any deformities.

    d. Assess the spine for range of motion (flexion, extension, lateral flexion, and rotation) and lateral or anterior–posterior curvature.

    e. Assess all major joints, noting any limitations to active range of motion, swelling, or redness.

    f. Neck: Assess flexion, extension, lateral rotation.

    g. Shoulders: Assess flexion, extension, and rotation.

    h. Elbows: Assess flexion, extension, supination, and pronation.

    i. Wrists: Assess flexion, extension, and ulnar and radial deviation.

    j. Fingers: Assess flexion, extension, abduction, and adduction.

    k. Hips: Assess flexion, extension, and rotation.

    l. Knees: Assess flexion and extension.

    m. Ankles: Assess dorsiflexion, plantar flexion, inversion, and eversion.

    n. Toes: Assess flexion, extension, abduction, and adduction.

2. Palpation

    a. Palpate the joints of the neck and upper and lower extremities, noting tenderness, swelling, temperature, limitations to passive range of motion, and crepitation.

    b. Palpate muscles to assess size, tone, and any tenderness.

    c. Palpate the spine, noting bony deformities and crepitation.

3. Percussion: Directly percuss the spine with the ulnar surface of the fist from the cervical to lumbar region; note any pain or tenderness.

4. Normal findings

    a. No limitation to function

    b. No gross deformities or abnormal postures

    c. Range of joint motion unrestricted in extremities and spine

    d. Muscle mass symmetric with no hypertrophy or atrophy; tone normal

    e. No joint pain, crepitus, bony overgrowths, or tenderness in extremities or spine

5. Gerontologic considerations

    a. Elderly patients commonly exhibit diminished joint flexibility and decreased muscle mass and strength.

    b. Other common age-related musculoskeletal problems include degenerative joint changes, mild scoliosis or kyphosis, stooped body posture, and some degree of functional limitation.

X. Neurologic system

1. Components of neurologic examination include:

    a. Mental status

    b. Cranial nerve function

    c. Cerebellar function

      d.   Motor function

      e.   Sensory function

      f.   Reflexes

2. Mental status: Observed during history taking, includes:

      a.   State of consciousness: alert, somnolent, stuporous, comatose

      b.   Orientation to person, place, and time

      c.   Memory: immediate, recent, remote

      d.   Cognition: calculations, current events, response to proverbs

      e.   Judgment and problem-solving ability

      f.   Emotion: mood, affect, congruence of responses

3. Cranial nerve function

      a.   Olfactory (CN I): With the patient's eyes closed, present various odors, occluding one nostril at a time. Note the patient's ability to identify the odors.

      b.   Optic (CN II): Test visual acuity and visual fields, and examine the optic disc with an ophthalmoscope.

      c.   Oculomotor (CN III), trochlear (CN IV), and abducens (CN VI): Assess extraocular motion by evaluating the six cardinal positions of gaze (parallelism, nystagmus), performing the cover–uncover test (movement of eye when uncovered or opposite eye when contralateral eye covered), and corneal light reflex (symmetry of reflection of light on pupil); check size and shape of pupils and pupillary reaction to light and accommodation (PERRLA).

      d.   Trigeminal (CN V): Motor—Assess the patient's ability to chew, assess strength of bite. Sensory—Assess the patient's ability to distinguish light touch and pain when you lightly stroke his or her face with a cotton wisp and gently prick the skin with a sterile pin on forehead (to assess the ophthalmic branch), cheek (to assess the maxillary branch), and chin (to assess the mandibular branch).

      e.   Facial (CN VII): Motor—Assess symmetry of facial movements as the patient smiles, frowns, grimaces, clenches his or her teeth, and so forth. Sensory—Ask the patient to identify various distinct flavors placed on the anterior two thirds of the tongue.

      f.   Acoustic (CN VIII): Cochlear branch—Assess hearing acuity. Vestibular branch—Perform the Romberg test to evaluate equilibrium.

      g.   Glossopharyngeal (CN IX): Test for the gag reflex by gently touching the posterior pharyngeal wall with a tongue blade.

      h.   Vagus (CN X): As the patient speaks, check movement of the uvula (noting any deviation from midline) and palate (noting asymmetric elevation).

    i.   Spinal accessory (CN XI): Assess strength of the sternoclei-domastoid (SCM) and upper trapezius muscles by asking the patient to move the head against resistance of your hand. Also observe and palpate contraction of SCM muscle on the opposite side; ask the patient to shrug the shoulders against resistance of your hands.

    j.   Hypoglossal (CN XII): Test strength and articulation of the tongue by having the patient push the tongue to the side of the mouth against resistance applied to the cheek. Ask the patient to stick out the tongue and then return it to the mouth while you observe for deviation, asymmetry, tremors, and fasciculations.

4. Cerebellar function (coordination and balance)

    a.   Assess posture, gait, and balance; have the patient walk forward and backward in a straight line.

    b.   Perform the Romberg test; stand close to the patient to provide support if necessary.

    c.   Assess coordination in the upper extremities by having the patient perform the finger-to-nose test.

    d.   Assess coordination in the lower extremities by having the patient tap the toes and slide the heel down the contralateral shin.

5. Motor function

    a.   Muscle mass: Assess symmetry and distribution distally and proximally, and circumference of extremities bilaterally.

    b.   Tone: Evaluate resistance of muscles in response to passive motion during flexion and extension of extremities.

    c.   Strength: Assess hand squeeze and evaluate muscle strength in each extremity against resistance during flexion and extension (also abduction and adduction where appropriate), comparing bilaterally.

    d.   Observe for involuntary movements (tics, fasciculations, tremors, or twitching) and abnormal postures (e.g., fetal, decerebrate).

6. Sensory function: With the patient's eyes closed, assess:

    a.   Light touch: Have the patient indicate response to cotton wisp lightly stroked on skin at representative dermatomes (i.e., backs of hands, forearms and upper arms, torso, thigh, tibia, and dorsal portion of foot); compare bilaterally and distal to proximal.

    b.   Pain: Repeat the pattern of light touch assessment, using a sterile safety pin to elicit sharp sensation; alternate with the pin's rounded end for contrast.

    c.   Vibration: Place a vibrating low-pitched tuning fork (128 Hz) over the sternum, then quickly on the distal interphalangeal joint of a finger; ask the patient to identify whether vibration sensation in the finger is 100%, 75%, 50%, or 25% of that felt in the sternum, and to indicate when vibration is no longer felt. Repeat this procedure in a great toe. If vibration sense is impaired in the finger or toe, proceed to assessment in more proximal bony prominences (wrist and elbow or medial malleolus, patella, anterior iliac spine, and spinous processes).

    d.   Position sense: With your fingers placed on the lateral surface of the patient's digit (finger, great toe), move it up or down; ask the patient which direction the digit is pointing.

    e.   Stereognosis: Ask the patient to identify small objects placed in his or her hand, one hand at a time.

    f.   Graphesthesia: Ask the patient to identify a number that you trace in his or her palm with your fingertip.

7.   Deep tendon reflexes: Striking with a reflex hammer, compare reflex amplitude bilaterally, grading on scale of 0 to 4+ (4+ = hyperactive; 2+ or 3+ = average; 1+ = diminished; 0 = no response).

    a.   Brachioradialis (C5, C6): Strike the radius tendon about 1 to 2 inches above the wrist; observe for flexion and supination of the forearm.

    b.   Biceps (C5, C6): Place your thumb or forefinger at the base of the biceps tendon and strike it; observe for flexion of the arm at the elbow.

    c.   Triceps (C7, C8): Strike the triceps tendon, just above the elbow; observe for slight elbow extension.

    d.   Patellar or quadriceps (L2, L3, L4): Sharply strike the patellar tendon; observe for extension of knee.

    e.   Achilles or ankle jerk (S1, S2): Support the patient's foot in the dorsiflexed position; tap the Achilles tendon, and observe for plantar flexion.

8.   Superficial cutaneous reflexes

    a.   Abdominal: Stroke the abdomen above (T8, T9, T10) and below (T10, T11, T12) the umbilicus bilaterally; observe for contraction of abdominal muscles and deviation of the umbilicus toward the stimulus.

    b.   Cremasteric (L1, L2): In a male patient, stroke the inner surface of the thigh; observe for prompt elevation of the testis on the ipsilateral side.

    c.   Plantar (L4, L5, S1, S2): Extend the patient's legs with the feet relaxed; stroke the lateral aspect of the sole from the heel to the ball of the foot, curving medially across the ball; observe for flexion of toes.

9.   Normal findings

    a.   Mental status: alert, quiet, able to follow three-step instructions; oriented to person, place, and time; judgment and intellectual performance within normal limits

  b. Cranial nerve function: CN I through XII grossly normal

  c. Cerebellar function: Romberg test negative, no clumsiness of movement, coordination normal

  d. Motor: no atrophy, tremors, or weakness

  e. Muscle tone: no flaccidity, rigidity, or spasticity

  f. Muscle strength: +5 (on a scale of 0 to +5)

  g. Sensory function: light touch, pain, vibration and position sense normal; stereognosis and graphesthesia normal bilaterally

  h. Reflexes: deep tendon reflexes +2 (on a scale of 0 to +4) (brachioradialis, biceps, triceps, patella, ankle); superficial reflexes present (abdominal, cremasteric); plantar reflexes normal (toes flex)

 10. Gerontologic considerations

  a. Many elderly patients exhibit moderate recent memory loss.

  b. The sense of smell tends to become less keen with aging.

  c. Common age-related vision changes include diminished peripheral vision, color discrimination (especially greens and blues), pupil size, accommodation, and upward gaze.

  d. Many elderly patients experience moderate hearing loss (particularly of high-frequency sounds) and diminished ability for sound discrimination. These changes may interfere with the ability to follow instructions associated with testing; the elderly patient may need more time to respond or react to verbal stimuli.

  e. Age-related changes in cerebellar function may include drifting during the Romberg test; wide-based, slowed gait; and diminished sense of equilibrium, especially when moving rapidly.

  f. Elderly patients commonly exhibit some degree of muscle atrophy and decreased muscle strength.

  g. Age-related sensory changes may include diminished pain perception and diminished sense of touch, temperature, vibration, and position.

  h. Reflexes commonly become diminished or absent.

VI. Laboratory studies: The third part of a complete health assessment, laboratory study results fall into three basic categories: urinalysis, hematology, and blood chemistry.

 A. Urinalysis

  1. Protein

   a. Normal values in young adults range from 0 to 5 mg/100 mL.

   b. Normal values rise slightly with aging.

  2. Glucose

   a. Normal values in young adults range from 0 to 15 mg/100 mL.

   b. Normal values decline slightly with aging.
  3. Specific gravity
   a. Normal value in young adults is 0.032.
   b. Normal value declines to 1.024 by age 80.

B. **Hematology**
  1. Hemoglobin (Hgb)
   a. Normal values: men, 13 to 18 g/100 mL; women, 12 to 16 g/100 mL.
   b. Normal value drops to 1 to 2 g/100 mL in elderly men; no change documented in elderly women.
  2. Hematocrit (Hct)
   a. Normal values: men, 45% to 52%; women, 37% to 48%.
   b. Specific changes in elderly are not documented to date; a slight decline has been hypothesized.
  3. Leukocytes
   a. Normal values in young adults range from 4,300 to 10,800/cu mm.
   b. Total count drops to 3,100 to 9,000/cu mm with aging.
  4. Lymphocytes
   a. Normal values in young adults: T-lymphocytes, 500 to 2,400/mL; B-lymphocytes, 50 to 200/mL.
   b. Both T- and B-lymphocyte counts drop somewhat in elderly patients.
  5. Platelets
   a. Normal values range from 150,000 to 350,000/cu mm.
   b. No changes in platelet number have been detected in elderly patients, but changes in platelet characteristics have been documented.
  6. Prothrombin time (PT)
   a. Normal time ranges from 11 to 15 seconds.
   b. No change has been identified in healthy elderly patients.

C. **Blood chemistry**
  1. Albumin
   a. Normal values range from 3.5 to 5.0 g/100 mL; before age 65, level tends to be higher in men than in women.
   b. After age 65, values equalize and decline at the same rate; however, this rate of decline has not been documented.
  2. Beta globulin
   a. Normal value ranges from 2.3 to 3.5 g/100 mL.
   b. Normal value increases slightly with aging.
  3. Total serum protein
   a. Normal values range from 6.0 to 8.4 g/100 mL.
   b. No change has been identified in elderly patients; increased B-globulin balances decreased albumin.
  4. Sodium
   a. Normal values range from 135 to 145 mEq/L.
   b. No change has been identified in elderly patients.

5. Potassium
   a. Normal values range from 3.5 to 5.5 mEq/L.
   b. Normal value increases slightly in elderly patients.
6. Carbon dioxide
   a. Normal values range from 24 to 30 mEq/L.
   b. No change has been identified in elderly patients.
7. Chloride
   a. Normal values range from 100 to 106 mEq/L.
   b. No change has been identified in elderly patients.
8. Blood urea nitrogen (BUN)
   a. Normal values: men, 10 to 25 mg/100 mL; women, 8 to 20 mg/100 mL.
   b. Values increase in elderly patients; sometimes as high as 69 mg/100 mL.
9. Creatinine
   a. Normal values range from 0.6 to 1.5 mg/100 mL.
   b. Increases in elderly men sometimes as high as 1.9 mg/100 mL.
10. Creatinine clearance
    a. Normal values range from 104 to 125 mL/min.
    b. Formula for calculating age-referenced interval in men: 140 minus age times body weight (in kg), divided by 72 times serum creatinine; in women, age-referenced interval is 85% of this figure.
11. Glucose tolerance
    a. Normal findings: 1 hour, 160 to 170 mg/100 mL; 2 hours, 115 to 125 mg/100 mL; 3 hours, 70 to 110 mg/100 mL.
    b. In elderly patients, fasting plasma glucose rises more quickly in the first 2 hours, then drops to baseline more slowly.
12. Triglycerides
    a. Normal values in younger adults range from 40 to 150 mg/100 mL.
    b. Normal values in elderly patients range from 20 to 200 mg/100 mL.
13. Cholesterol
    a. Normal values range from 120 to 220 mg/100 mL.
    b. In men, values tend to increase up to age 50, then decrease. In women, values tend to be lower than those in men until age 50, then higher up to to age 70; values decrease after age 70.
14. High-density lipoproteins (HDL)
    a. Normal values range from 80 to 310 mg/100 mL; values are consistently higher in women than in men.
    b. This difference diminishes with aging.
15. Thyroxine (T$_4$)

        a.   Normal values range from 4.5 to 13.5 mcg/100 mL.

        b.   Values decrease by about 25% in elderly patients.

16. Triiodothyronine (T_3)
    a. Normal values range from 90 to 230 mg/100 mL.
    b. Values decrease by about 25% in elderly patients.
17. Thyroid-stimulating hormone (TSH)
    a. Normal values range from 0.5 to 5.0 mcg U/mL.
    b. Values increase slightly in elderly patients.
18. Alkaline phosphatase
    a. Normal values range from 13 to 39 IU/L.
    b. Values increases by 8 to 10 IU/L in elderly patients.
19. Acid phosphatase
    a. Normal values: young men, 0.13 to 0.63 U/mL; young women, 0.01 to 0.56 U/mL.
    b. No age-related changes have been identified.
20. Serum glutamicoxaloacetic transaminase (SGOT)
    a. Normal values range from 0 to 40 U/L.
    b. No age-related changes have been identified.
21. Creatinine kinase (CK)
    a. Normal values range from 17 to 148 U/L.
    b. Values increases slightly in elderly patients.
22. Lactate dehydrogenase (LDH)
    a. Normal values range from 45 to 90 U/L.
    b. Values increase slightly in elderly patients.

Bibliography

American Nurses Association (1980). *Nursing: A social policy statement*. Kansas City: Author.

Bates, B. (1987). *A guide to physical examination and history taking* (4th ed.). Philadelphia: J. B. Lippincott.

Brunner, L. S., & Suddarth, D. S. (1988). *Textbook of medical-surgical nursing* (6th ed.). Philadelphia: J. B. Lippincott.

Brunner, L. S., & Suddarth, D. S. (1986). *The Lippincott manual of nursing practice* (4th ed.). Philadelphia: J. B. Lippincott.

Carnevali, D. L., & Patrick, M. (1979). *Nursing management for the elderly*. Philadelphia: J. B. Lippincott.

Garner, B. (1989). Guide to changing lab values in elders. *Geriatric Nursing, 10*(3), 144–145.

Luckmann, J., & Sorensen, K. C. (1986). *Basic nursing: A psychophysiologic approach* (3rd ed.). Philadelphia: W. B. Saunders.

Malasanos, L., Barkauskas, V., & Stoltenberg-Allen, K. (1990). *Health assessment* (4th ed.). St. Louis: C. V. Mosby.

Morton, P. G. (1989). *Health assessment in nursing*. Springhouse, PA: Springhouse Corporation.

U.S. Department of Health and Human Services, Public Health Service, National Institutes of Health (1984). *Report of the Joint National Committee on Detection, Evaluation, and Treatment of High Blood Pressure*.

STUDY QUESTIONS

1. To give accountable care that meets the needs of the individual patient, the nurse uses a problem-solving method that includes which of the following steps?
   a. assessment, planning, nursing action, evaluation
   b. planning, intervention, evaluation, reassessment
   c. assessment, analysis and diagnosis, planning, implementation, evaluation
   d. analysis, diagnosis, planning, implementation, evaluation

2. Ms. Montgomery has come to the nursing clinic for a comprehensive health assessment. Which of the following statements would be the best way to begin a history interview once Ms. Montgomery's biographic data have been obtained?
   a. "What brought you to the clinic today?"
   b. "Would you describe your health as good?"
   c. "Are you healthy?"
   d. "Describe your health, now and in the past."

3. Mr. Cugat has come to the nursing clinic for a blood pressure check. Based on readings of 150/86 mmHg, how would you classify Mr. Cugat's blood pressure?
   a. systolic borderline; diastolic normal
   b. systolic normal; diastolic high normal
   c. systolic hypertensive; diastolic high normal
   d. systolic borderline; diastolic high normal

4. After examining Mr. Robertson's mouth and pharynx, the nurse records the following assessment data: "No lesions of lips, gums, tongue, or buccal mucosa. Pharynx not injected; tonsils nonobstructing; uvula in midline; palate elevates symmetrically on phonation."

Which of the following statements represents the best critique of this summary?
   a. It is a complete, concise recording.
   b. It lacks important data.
   c. It is biased.
   d. It uses inappropriate terminology.

5. Documentation of skin assessment for Mr. Lorah, age 80, reads as follows: "Brownish, oily, wartlike lesions 1 cm or smaller interspersed with dark red papules scattered over anterior and posterior torso. Skin dry with poor turgor. Hair distribution over extremities sparse with bristly hairs in ears and nose. Nails horny. Mucous membranes pale." Which of the following statements provides the best analysis of this data?
   a. Mr. Lorah's skin characteristics are common in men aged 80.
   b. Mr. Lorah is dehydrated and anemic.
   c. The description of the lesions is highly indicative of malignancy.
   d. Descriptions of hair and nails do not belong in a skin assessment.

6. When performing a routine blood pressure check in an elderly man, the nurse measures blood pressure with the patient in which position(s)?
   a. lying down
   b. sitting
   c. lying down and sitting
   d. lying down, sitting, and standing

7. What is the primary reason that early detection of the eye condition entropion is so important?
   a. The conjunctiva and lower cornea may become irritated.
   b. If it is not treated, the lid muscles may lose their tone.
   c. It can lead to glaucoma if not corrected.
   d. It can lead to conjunctival dryness.

8. When teaching self-breast examination to a woman, the nurse should stress which of the following points?

a. Half of all breast cancer deaths occur in women between ages 35 and 45.
b. The "tail of Spence" area must be included in self-examination.
c. The position of choice for the self-breast examination is supine.
d. The woman should place a pad under the contralateral scapula of the breast being palpated.

9. Ms. Jellenik, aged 40, has come to the nursing clinic for a routine health assessment. To prevent discomfort and injury during otoscopic examination, which of the following should be avoided?
   a. tipping her head away from the examiner and pulling her ear up and back
   b. inserting the otoscope inferiorly into the distal portion of the external canal
   c. inserting the otoscope superiorly into the proximal two thirds of the external canal
   d. bracing the examiner's hand against the patient's head

10. To avoid a reflex drop in pulse rate or blood pressure in Ms. Jellenik, where should the nurse assess the carotid pulse?
    a. at the suprasternal notch
    b. at the angle of the jaw
    c. lateral to the esophagus
    d. well below the upper border of the thyroid cartilage

11. Which of the following examinations does *not* require the nurse to wear gloves?
    a. oral
    b. rectal
    c. breast
    d. genital

12. To ensure a patient's safety during the Romberg test, which of the following measures should the nurse take?
    a. Stand close to provide support if the patient loses her balance.
    b. Allow the patient to keep her eyes open.
    c. Allow the patient to brace herself by spreading her feet apart.

d. Instruct the patient to hang on to a piece of furniture.

13. During abdominal examination, the nurse performs the four physical examination techniques in what sequence?
    a. Do auscultation immediately after inspection and before palpation and percussion.
    b. Start with percussion, then follow with inspection, auscultation, and palpation.
    c. Palpate first, then inspect, percuss, and auscultate.
    d. The standard sequence—inspection, palpation, percussion, and auscultation—is used.

14. Mr. Sumlin, aged 75, was hospitalized 2 days ago when he began to complain of dyspnea and shortness of breath on exertion. His radiographs show lung consolidation, indicating pneumonia. When assessing Mr. Sumlin's lungs, the nurse would expect to find all the following *except*
    a. bronchial breath sounds
    b. bronchophony
    c. increased tactile fremitus
    d. decreased voice sounds

15. Which of the following assessments performed on Mr. Sumlin would not be congruent with the others?
    a. memory
    b. sensory
    c. orientation
    d. judgment

16. Which of the following hematology results for Mr. Sumlin might indicate restoration of homeostasis and good prospects for recovery?
    a. Hgb 17 g/100 mL; Hct 50%; leukocytes 15,000/mL
    b. Hgb 10 g/100 mL; Hct 40%; leukocytes 5,000/mL
    c. Hgb 13 g/100 mL; Hct 46%; leukocytes 4,300/mL
    d. Hgb 21 g/100 mL; Hct 55%; leukocytes 2,000/mL

ANSWER KEY

1. **Correct response: c**
   The five steps of the nursing process represent the most recent evolution in the definition of the nursing process and are the framework used for organizing the NCLEX-RN test. Some authors still define the nursing process in four steps: assessment, planning, implementation, and evaluation.
   a, b, and d. These responses do not include all steps of the nursing process.
   Knowledge/Safe care/Assessment

2. **Correct response: d**
   Asking the patient to describe her health status gives her the opportunity to share her personal perspective of her health and allows expression of strengths as well as health problems.
   a. This is an ambiguous question to which the patient might answer, "my car" or any similarly disingenuous reply.
   b. This is a leading question that puts words in the patient's mouth.
   c. This is a yes/no question that can elicit little information from the patient.
   Application/Psychosocial/Assessment

3. **Correct response: d**
   The Joint National Committee on High Blood Pressure uses the following guidelines to classify blood pressure:
   - Diastolic: normal pressure, below 85 mmHg; high normal pressure, 85 to 89 mmHg; mild hypertension, 90 to 104 mmHg; moderate hypertension, 105 to 114 mmHg; severe hypertension, 115 mmHg or above
   - Systolic (when diastolic is below 90 mmHg: normal, below 140 mmHg; borderline isolated systolic hypertension, 140 to 159 mmHg; isolated systolic hypertension, 160 mmHg or above.
   Comprehension/Health promotion/ Implementation

4. **Correct response: b**
   This summary lacks data about the tongue surface, whether the tongue has tremors at rest or with protrusion, salivary gland condition, condition of teeth, and presence or absence of the gag reflex.
   a. The summary is not complete.
   c. It is not biased because the data listed are presented objectively.
   d. The terminology used is appropriate.
   Analysis/Physiologic/Assessment

5. **Correct response: a**
   All these findings are normal in elderly men.
   b. Because poor turgor and pale mucous membranes are normal age-related changes, they do not necessarily indicate dehydration and anemia.
   c. The lesions described (seborrheic keratoses and cherry angiomas) are benign and commonly seen on aging skin.
   d. Skin assessment includes hair, nails, and mucous membranes.
   Analysis/Physiologic/Assessment

6. **Correct response: d**
   Elderly patients should have blood pressure checked when lying, sitting, and standing to detect excessive postural hypotension, a common age-related manifestation.
   Comprehension/Health promotion/ Implementation

7. **Correct response: a**
   Entropion, inward turning of the lid margin, can cause irritation of the conjunctiva from the eyelashes.
   b, c, and d. These complications are not related to entropion.
   Comprehension/Physiologic/Assessment

8. **Correct response: b**
   The tail of Spence, an extension of the upper outer quadrant of breast tissue, can develop breast tumors.

a. Half of breast cancer deaths occur in women over age 65.

c. The correct position for self-breast examination is not limited to just the supine position; the sitting position with hands at sides, above head, and on hips is also recommended.

d. A pad is placed under the ipsilateral (same side) scapula of the breast being palpated.

Knowledge/Health promotion/ Implementation

9. *Correct response: c*
   In the superior position, the speculum of the otoscope is nearest the tympanic membrane, and the most sensitive portion of the external canal is the proximal two thirds. Therefore, it is important to avoid these structures in the examination.

   a, b, and d. All other techniques listed are safe and appropriate.

Application/Safe care/Assessment

10. *Correct response: d*
    By palpating well below the upper border of the thyroid cartilage, the carotid sinus will be avoided.

    a, b, and c. The suprasternal notch, jaw, and esophagus are not landmarks associated with locating the carotid artery.

Application/Physiologic/Assessment

11. *Correct response: c*
    Breast examination normally does not involve contact with a patient's body fluids and thus does not require the nurse to wear gloves for protection.

    a, b, and d. Although this question may seem elementary, in the era of such diseases as AIDS and hepatitis, it has become increasingly important to protect patients and health care providers against contamination from body

fluids and excrement by wearing gloves.

Application/Safe care/Assessment

12. *Correct response: a*
    During the Romberg test, the patient is asked to stand with feet together and eyes shut and still maintain her balance with a minimum of sway. Should she lose her balance, having your arm close around her shoulder will prevent a fall.

    b, c, and d. These actions all would interfere with the proper execution of the test.

Application/Self care/Assessment

13. *Correct response: a*
    In abdominal assessment, auscultating before palpating and percussing avoids altering bowel sounds through manipulation.

    b. Although the bladder should be empty for an abdominal examination, percussion does not precede inspection and auscultation; therefore, this answer is incorrect.

    c. This answer is incorrect because tender areas are always palpated last.

    d. This answer is incorrect because the usual sequence of examination is altered in an abdominal assessment.

Application/Physiologic/Assessment

14. *Correct response: d*
    Because sound waves are transmitted more readily through solid tissue, lung consolidation would produce increased voice sounds.

    a, b, and c. All these findings would be expected.

Analysis/Physiologic/Assessment

15. *Correct response: b*
    All these items are included in neurologic assessment. However, all except sensory function are also components of the mental status examination. Sensory function is a separate component of a neurologic assessment.

    a, c, and d. Memory, orientation, and judgment are all parts of a neurologic assessment and a mental status examination.

Analysis/Psychosocial/Assessment

16. *Correct response: c*

All these hematology values are well within normal ranges for an elderly man.

a. Leukocyte count is abnormally high.

b. Hgb and Hct are too low.

d. Hgb and Hct are too high, and the leukocyte count is too low.

Analysis/Health promotion/Assessment

Patient Education

I. Essential concepts

A. Philosophy

1. Patient education can be defined as an ongoing process of assisting a person to incorporate learned behaviors related to health into his or her lifestyle.
2. Patient education is an integral component of comprehensive health care.
3. Teaching is a form of communication directed toward providing instruction and imparting knowledge.
4. Learning involves gaining knowledge or skills that can result in modification of behavior.
5. All interactions between health care providers and patients and their families or significant others contribute to the process and objectives of teaching and learning.
6. Effective teaching incorporates:

    a.   Recognizing patients' and families' or significant others' perceptions of learning needs

    b.   Setting priorities for learning

    c.   Addressing quality of life issues

7. The American Nurses' Association's Standards of Nursing Practice defines health education as an essential component of nursing care directed toward promotion, maintenance, and restoration of health and adaptation to residual effects of illness.

8. Nurse practice acts have clarified professional responsibility to provide patient education in standards of practice.

9. Basic standards of nursing practice encompass:

    a.   Commitment to patient care and well-being

    b.   Broad knowledge and experiential base in both wellness and illness

    c.   Integration of education into a total approach to patient care

    d.   Promotion of health in individuals, families, and communities

10. The Patient's Bill of Rights, developed by the American Hospital Association in 1972, established standards for health care, including recognition of patients' right to information and promotion of their participation in health care.

11. Mounting evidence indicates that patients' health knowledge may be instrumental in decreasing length of hospital stays and frequency of readmission for the same condition.

B. Trends in patient education

1. Milestones in the health promotion movement include the following:

    a.   Halbert Dunn's 1959 Theory of High Level Wellness stated that there is more than one optimal level of wellness; each person has the potential to achieve his or her own personal level of wellness.

    b.   The World Health Organization, in 1974, defined health as a state of complete physical, mental, and social well-being, not merely as the absence of disease or infirmity.

    c.   Over the past two decades in the United States, the focus of public health policy has shifted from disease treatment to disease prevention and health promotion.

    d.   Published in 1979, *Healthy People: The Surgeon General's Report on Health Promotion and Disease Prevention* introduced a set of national goals for improving the health of Americans by 1990.

    e.   Published in 1980 by the Office of the Surgeon General, *Promoting Health/Preventing Disease: Objectives For The Nation* focused on health promotion, health protection, and preventive health services.

2. Wellness programs now are promoted throughout the country in both community and corporate settings.
3. Self-responsibility for health is increasingly promoted in the media as more links are established between lifestyle and disease.
4. Today's better-informed health care consumer expects more technologically sophisticated care and health education.
5. Increased longevity demands more health care dollars and expands the population needing health education.
6. The advent of the current prospective payment system (diagnosis-related groups [DRGs]) has resulted in higher acuity of hospitalized patients and earlier discharge, leading to changes in home care expectations and education needs.
7. Advances in self-testing and self-monitoring equipment and treatment modalities available for home use require more extensive education of patients and family members.
8. More complex testing (e.g., MRI, CT) necessitates increasingly detailed patient education and preparation.

C. **Health education needs**
1. Health education needs vary according to patient population.
2. Needs of the well population include information on:
   a. Health maintenance
   b. Promoting a higher level of wellness
   c. Illness prevention
   d. Recognizing early warning signs of illness
   e. Treatment for medical emergencies
   f. Recognizing and treating tobacco, alcohol, or drug abuse
   g. Proper nutritional habits
   h. Weight control
   i. A regular exercise program
   j. Stress management
   k. Breast self-examination or testicular self-examination
3. Needs of the episodically ill or acutely ill population include information on:
   a. Pathophysiology and cause of the condition and ways to prevent or minimize recurrence
   b. Self-care measures, including medication use
   c. Necessary procedures and treatments, including purpose and expectations
   d. Expectations for convalescence (e.g., length of hospitalization, schedule for resuming normal activities)
   e. Possible long-term effects of illness, likelihood of recurrence
   f. Follow-up care
   g. Appropriate items listed under well population education needs (see Section I.C.2)

4. Needs of the chronically ill population include information on:
    a. Management of illness
    b. Promotion of optimal level of functioning; necessary life-style changes
    c. Pathophysiology and cause of disease, its treatment, and preventive measures
    d. Disease complications
    e. Appropriate items listed under well population education needs (see Section I.C.2)

D. Characteristics of adult learners
1. As defined by Knowles & Associates (1984), *andragogy* refers to the art and science of helping adults learn.
2. Assumptions about adult learners include that they:
    a. Are self-directing
    b. Enter educational activity with more and different experiences than younger learners
    c. Are ready to learn when they need to know information in order to perform more effectively in some aspect of life or to cope more effectively with a situation
    d. Enter educational activities with a life-centered (task-centered, problem-centered) orientation to learning
    e. Are motivated by internal needs (e.g., self-esteem, increased job satisfaction, better quality of life, greater self-confidence, self-actualization)
3. Elements of the andragogy model important to the educational process include:
    a. Climate conducive to learning: comfortable physical environment, mutual respect and trust, collaborativeness, supportiveness and humanness, openness and authenticity
    b. Learner involvement in identifying learning needs
    c. Learner involvement in formulating learning objectives
    d. Learner involvement in designing learning plans
    e. Teacher assistance in helping the learner carry out learning plans
    f. Learner involvement in evaluating learning

II. Learning process
  A. Readiness for learning
1. A patient's readiness for learning depends on physical and emotional adaptation to illness, recognition of needs, and level of cognition.
2. Basic physical needs (e.g., food, sleep, comfort) must be met before learning can occur.
3. Learning is reduced when the environment is not conducive to focusing on tasks (e.g., sensory underload or overload).

4. Emotional needs must be recognized and addressed, such as:
   a. Anxiety
   b. Fear
   c. Distrust
   d. Anger
   e. Depression
5. Learning readiness also depends on mastery of emotional, physical, and psychologic tasks essential for development.
6. Emotional maturity is measured by Erikson's developmental stages, which outline tasks specific to each maturation period:
   a. Infant: trust vs. mistrust
   b. Toddler: autonomy vs. shame and doubt
   c. Preschooler: initiative vs. guilt
   d. School-aged child: industry vs. inferiority
   e. Adolescent: identity vs. role confusion
   f. Young adult: intimacy vs. isolation
   g. Middle-aged adult: generativity vs. stagnation
   h. Older adult: integrity vs. despair
7. Tasks may not be completed at each stage, affecting adjustment to later crises in life and affecting ability to learn.
8. The stress of hospitalization may result in regression to an earlier developmental stage.
9. Jean Piaget's last two stages describe levels of cognition necessary for adults to accommodate and assimilate new information:
   a. A child in the *concrete stage* (approximately first grade to early adolescence) can think abstractly and make rational judgments; concrete objects or observable phenomena must be within sight for this process to occur.
   b. A person in the *formal operations stage* (adolescence) is capable of hypothetical and deductive reasoning.

B. **Motivation for learning**
   1. Theories of motivation for learning include:
      a. *Needs theory*: Maslow's hierarchy of needs implicates the drive to satisfy personal needs ranging from basic survival to self-actualization.
      b. *Cognitive dissonance theory*: Inconsistency experienced in ideas or beliefs creates a tendency to seek resolution of disagreement.
      c. *Attribution theory*: Success or failure is attributed to internal or external, stable or unstable, controllable or uncontrollable factors; locus of control concept is central to the theory.
      d. *Competence theory*: Persons have a general tendency to strive toward certain types of goals by developing skills or acquiring knowledge.

2. The *health belief model* asserts that motivation for learning depends on the person's perception of his or her susceptibility to disease and of disease severity. Under this theory, a person becomes motivated to learn if he or she:
   a. Believes that he or she is susceptible to the disease in question
   b. Believes that this disease would have serious effects on his or her life
   c. Is aware of certain actions to take and believes that these actions may reduce the likelihood of contracting the disease or may reduce disease severity
   d. Believes that the threat of taking action is not as great as the threat of the disease

C. **Learning styles**
   1. Learning styles refer to a person's preferred method for learning, as influenced by:
      a. Educational training
      b. Intelligence
      c. Personal preferences
   2. Learning styles can be broadly classified as visual, auditory, and tactile.
   3. Visual learners learn by:
      a. Seeing tasks performed
      b. Reading informational material
      c. Looking at pictures
   4. Auditory learners learn by listening to spoken information.
   5. Tactile learners learn by:
      a. Performing tasks
      b. Touching and taking apart or putting together equipment or models
   6. The nurse can identify a patient's learning style by:
      a. Observing the patient's behavior
      b. Asking the patient about his or her preferred methods for learning
      c. Experimenting with different learning tools

D. **Learning domains**
   1. Learning behaviors fall into three broad *learning domains*: cognitive, psychomotor, and affective.
   2. Categorizing what a patient needs to learn into these domains helps the nurse develop teaching plans and evaluate learning.
   3. Tasks to be learned require certain abilities and actions that fall into one, two, or all three of the learning domains. Each domain has specific characteristics necessary for learning.
   4. The cognitive domain reflects:
      a. Intellectual ability

   b. Abstract thinking
   c. Knowledge acquisition
   d. Concept development
  5. The psychomotor domain includes:
   a. Physical activity
   b. Use of motor skills
   c. Proficiency performance
  6. The affective domain incorporates:
   a. Expression of feelings
   b. Expression of attitudes
   c. Expression of beliefs

E. **Enhancing learning: To help ensure optimal learning, the nurse should:**

  1. Arrange for personal pacing; move at the patient's pace and be flexible.
  2. Compensate for altered ability to learn in older adults, such as:
   a. Decline in recent recall memory capacity: Use the patient's experiences and knowledge from the past as a reference point for addition of new knowledge.
   b. Increased difficulty organizing complex material: Allow the patient more time to absorb material; use a stepped approach to learning.
   c. Reduced ability to discriminate between stimuli: Eliminate extraneous stimuli.
  3. Clarify structure through such strategies as:
   a. Presenting information in a way that applies to present lifestyle
   b. Creating memorable encounters to reinforce learning
   c. Progressing from basic or easy concepts to more difficult ones.
  4. Vary the teaching resources used; for example:
   a. Use the patient's preferred resources.
   b. Incorporate group discussions to draw on peers' knowledge and experiences.
  5. Provide prompt feedback that includes:
   a. Emphasizing abilities
   b. Reinforcing positive learning
   c. Focusing on behaviors, not on progress or personalities
   d. Offering specific suggestions for behavior changes
  6. Consider the patient's preferred learning style.

F. **Barriers to learning**

  1. Low literacy level interferes with a patient's ability to read and comprehend written materials.
  2. Certain physical disabilities can hinder learning, including:
   a. Visual impairment

b.　Hearing impairment
c.　Motor deficits
d.　Pain
e.　Chronic illness

3.　Socioeconomic or cultural factors that may cause barriers to learning include:
   a.　Beliefs about health and wellness
   b.　Ethnic background
   c.　Religious beliefs
   d.　Support systems and home environment
   e.　Financial concerns

4.　Communication barriers may include:
   a.　Inappropriate use of medical or nursing jargon by health care professionals
   b.　The health care professional's inability to speak the patient's primary language

5.　Schedule problems that can interfere with learning include:
   a.　Patient fatigue resulting from frequently interrupted rest
   b.　Overfrequency of scheduled activities

III.　Teaching process

A.　General principles: The nurse should:

1.　Establish a good teacher–learner rapport by:
   a.　Developing a trusting relationship
   b.　Using effective communication techniques (e.g., asking open-ended questions)
   c.　Understanding the patient's unique cultural or ethnic needs

2.　Plan the optimum timing of teaching by:
   a.　Recognizing the patient's "most teachable" moments
   b.　Scheduling teaching sessions to allow the patient adequate periods of uninterrupted rest
   c.　Controlling the teaching environment

3.　Use the nursing process in patient teaching (see Section IV) by:
   a.　Assessing learning needs, beginning with what the patient knows
   b.　Developing nursing diagnoses to address learning needs
   c.　Involving the patient and family or significant other in goal setting
   d.　Planning and implementing the teaching plan
   e.　Evaluating learning and teaching

B.　Teaching methods

1.　For maximum effectiveness, the nurse should match teaching methods to the patient's primary learning style (see Section II.C).

2.　Effective teaching methods for a visual learner may include:
   a.　Demonstration

  b. Role playing

 3. Effective teaching methods for an auditory learner may include:

  a. Discussion (individual or group)

  b. Lectures

  c. Case studies

 4. Effective teaching methods for a tactile learner may include:

  a. Return demonstration

  b. Practice of learned skills

C. **Teaching tools**

 1. The nurse also should use teaching tools appropriate to the patient's primary learning style.

 2. Visual tools may include:

  a. Printed materials

  b. Transparencies

  c. Slides and filmstrips

  d. Videotapes

  e. Closed-circuit TV

  f. Physical models

  g. Computer-assisted instruction

 3. Auditory tools include audiocassette tapes.

 4. Psychomotor tools include:

  a. Physical models

  b. Disease-specific self-treatment or self-monitoring equipment

  c. Computer-assisted instruction

D. **Barriers to teaching**

 1. Teaching may be impeded by inadequate teaching time available because of such factors as:

  a. Lack of support from supervisor

  b. Overly heavy workload

  c. Inadequate staffing

 2. Another barrier to teaching may be the nurse's lack of knowledge about the subject and effective teaching strategies, which can result from:

  a. Inadequate knowledge base

  b. Inadequate preparation for teaching

  c. Improper development of teaching objectives

  d. Overambitious presentation of material

  e. Lack of involvement of the patient's family or significant others

  f. No evaluation of learning outcomes

 3. Poor communication between members of health care team can cause:

  a. Improper coordination of patient teaching

  b. Duplication or gaps in material presented

c. Inadequate reporting of the patient's learning needs and progress in learning
4. Communication barriers affecting teaching are similar to those affecting learning (see Section II.F).

IV. Applying the nursing process to patient education

A. Assessment

1. The nurse assesses the patient's readiness for learning by evaluating:
   a. Personal learning goals
   b. Stages in adaptation to illness
   c. Emotional maturity
   d. Past life experiences with health and illness
2. The nurse assesses the patient's motivation for learning by evaluating:
   a. Health beliefs
   b. Religious and sociocultural practices
   c. Perception of learning needs; the gap between what the patient knows and what he or she wants to know
3. The nurse assesses the patient's ability to learn by evaluating:
   a. Physical condition
   b. Intellectual abilities
   c. Barriers to learning
   d. Learning styles
4. Assessment data are collected by interviewing the patient or, if appropriate, the patient's family members or significant others.
5. Principles of conducting a successful interview include:
   a. Setting the stage: Providing privacy, if possible, in a quiet, relaxed environment; minimizing interruptions
   b. Listening attentively
   c. Observing the patient's nonverbal cues
   d. Asking open-ended questions
   e. Evaluating the patient's use of terms to help guide the level of teaching
   f. Having a self-awareness of attitudes and beliefs

B. Nursing diagnoses (related to learning)

1. Anxiety
2. Impaired Communication: Verbal
3. Ineffective Individual Coping
4. Ineffective Family Coping: Compromised
5. Ineffective Family Coping: Disabling
6. Decisional Conflict
7. Fatigue
8. Fear
9. Anticipatory Grieving
10. Altered Health Maintenance

11. Health-Seeking Behaviors
12. Hopelessness
13. Knowledge Deficit
14. Noncompliance
15. Pain
16. Powerlessness
17. Altered Role Performance
18. Self-Esteem Disturbance
19. Sleep Pattern Disturbance
20. Social Isolation
21. Altered Thought Processes

C. **Planning and implementation: Nursing interventions related to patient education include:**
   1. Formulate learning goals:
       a. Involve the patient and family members or significant others in development.
       b. Facilitate realistic goal setting.
       c. Use behavioral objectives—measurable statements of expectations.
       d. Include the three learning domains (see Section II.D).
   2. Develop a teaching plan:
       a. Include content to be taught based on learning goals.
       b. Determine teaching strategies and tools based on the patient's primary learning styles.
       c. Incorporate the patient's learning strengths into the plan.
       d. Involve family members or significant others and members of the health care team in planning.
       e. Determine teaching priorities; teach survival information, including correct method for medication administration, before discharge from hospital.
       f. Develop a contract with the patient to meet learning goals.
   3. Determine teaching content:
       a. Include what the patient needs to know for survival, maintenance of health, and prevention of disease.
       b. Include information about the disorder, including causes, complications, and treatments.
       c. Include information about any tests to be performed.
       d. Include discharge information necessary for self-care and for reporting signs and symptoms of complications.
   4. Implement the teaching plan:
       a. Reinforce positive learning.
       b. Redirect teaching to meet the patient's changing needs as teaching progresses.
       c. Promote compliance.
       d. Involve the patient and family members or significant others in teaching.

5. Refer the patient and family members or significant others to appropriate agencies or resources for more information and support, as necessary.

D. Evaluation

1. Evaluation involves ongoing assessment of the patient's and family members' or significant others' learning.
2. Purposes of evaluation include:
    a. To reinforce desirable behavior
    b. To redirect undesirable behavior
    c. To measure the patient's progress in achieving learning goals
    d. To provide direction in restructuring teaching strategies
    e. To provide necessary documentation and accountability for quality education
    f. To identify effective and ineffective teaching strategies
3. Evaluation should determine expected outcomes to be measured in terms of patient behavior.
4. The patient's evaluation should cover:
    a. Knowledge
    b. Application of learning
    c. Attitude
    d. Compliance
5. The teacher's evaluation should cover:
    a. Use of teaching strategies
    b. Use of teaching tools
    c. Effectiveness of teaching
6. Methods of evaluation include:
    a. Interviews
    b. Direct observation and anecdotal notes
    c. Tests (written or oral)
    d. Checklists
    e. Situation simulation

E. Documentation

1. Proper documentation of patient education enhances communication by:
    a. Promoting continuity of teaching: material taught, patients' perceptions, need for follow-up
    b. Promoting assessment of standards of care
2. Documentation should meet the mandate of the 1976 Joint Commission for the Accreditation of Hospitals, covering:
    a. The teaching provided to the patient
    b. The patient's understanding of the information taught
    c. The patient's response to teaching
    d. Assessment of progress toward learning goals

Bibliography

Brunner, L., & Suddarth, D. (1988). *Textbook of medical-surgical nursing* (6th ed.). Philadelphia: J. B. Lippincott.

Brunner, L., & Suddarth, D. (1986). *The Lippincott manual of nursing practice* (4th ed.). Philadelphia: J. B. Lippincott.

Cahill, M. (Ed.) (1987). *Patient teaching*. Springhouse, PA: Springhouse Corp.

Gessner, B. (1989). Adult education: The cornerstone of patient teaching. *Nursing Clinics of North America, 24* (3), 589–595.

Knowles, M., & Associates (1984). *Andragogy in action: Applying modern principles of adult learning*. San Francisco: Jossey-Bass.

Knox, A. (1986). *Helping adults learn*. San Francisco: Jossey- Bass.

Luckman, J., & Sorenson, K. (1987). *Medical-surgical nursing: A psychophysiologic approach* (3rd ed.). Philadelphia: W. B. Saunders.

Pender, N. (1987). *Health promotion in nursing practice*. Norwalk, CT: Appleton & Lange.

Redman, B. (1988). *The process of patient education*. St. Louis: C. V. Mosby.

Ruzicki, D. (1989). Realistically meeting the educational needs of hospitalized acute and short-stay patients. *Nursing Clinics of North America, 24* (3), 629–637.

U.S. Department of Health and Human Services, Public Health Service, National Institutes of Health. (1984). *The 1984 report of the Joint National Committee on Detection, Evaluation, and Treatment of High Blood Pressure*.

STUDY QUESTIONS

1. When teaching varied patient populations, the education plans are developed around specific health education needs. In the education plan, the inclusion of which of the following distinguishes the episodically or acutely ill or the chronically ill from the well population?
   a. maintenance of health
   b. promotion of higher level of wellness
   c. discussion of pathophysiology or cause of disease
   d. recognition of early warning signs of illness

2. Which of the following elements is *not* important in the educational process as outlined in the andragogy model?
   a. learner involvement in the identification of learning needs
   b. teacher determination and evaluation of learning
   c. learner involvement in the formulation of learning objectives
   d. teacher assistance in helping the learner carry out learning plan

3. Mr. Thomas, aged 75, was admitted to an acute care facility with an exacerbation of his chronic obstructive pulmonary disease (COPD). He has been referred to a nurse for planning of self-care instruction. The nurse determined that Mr. Thomas had been taking his theophylline only when he had difficulty breathing rather than as prescribed. The nurse would be expected to select which of the following settings to teach this patient correct medication administration?
   a. hospital
   b. ambulatory clinic
   c. home
   d. community health clinic

4. In assessing Mr. Thomas's learning needs regarding the use of in-home oxygen therapy, the nurse should evaluate all the following parameters *except*
   a. comfort level
   b. past experience with health and illness

c. dietary habits
d. perception of learning needs

5. Recognizing that physiologic changes occur in older adults that can affect learning, the nurse should modify patient teaching to specifically enhance learning for Mr. Thomas in which of the following ways?
   a. Create memorable encounters to reinforce learning.
   b. Progress from basic to more difficult concepts.
   c. Use resources that are preferred by the patient.
   d. Reduce input that requires discrimination between stimuli.

6. In evaluating Mr. Thomas's ability to safely use in-home oxygen, the nurse would employ all the following strategies *except*
   a. redirecting undesirable behaviors
   b. comparing his skill level with that of others in the class
   c. measuring his progress in meeting learning goals
   d. determining the need to restructure teaching

7. Because he lives alone, Mr. Thomas must understand at a cognitive level and be able to perform at a psychomotor level. Which of the following nursing diagnoses would prohibit safe performance?
   a. Impaired Gas Exchange
   b. Sensory and Perceptual Alterations: Visual
   c. Anticipatory Grieving
   d. Anxiety

8. In the United States, several trends have had a direct effect on the increase in development of patient education programs. Which of the following would *not* have an influence on this increase in program development?
   a. escalation of health care costs
   b. low literacy levels of the patient population

c. health promotion movement

d. technologic advances in health care

9. Ms. Davis, aged 45, was diagnosed with a malignant tumor of the breast after a biopsy was performed. The treatment selected was a modified radical mastectomy. During her recovery from a modified radical mastectomy, the nurse is assessing Ms. Davis's progress and learning readiness. Of the following parameters, which would *not* be a predictor of learning readiness?

a. physical needs

b. emotional maturity

c. cognitive level

d. concept development

10. As the nurse further evaluates Ms. Davis's adaptation to her diagnosis and to the proposed adjuvant chemotherapy, based on the health belief model, which of the following nursing diagnoses would be most likely to motivate her to initiate chemotherapy?

a. Anxiety

b. Knowledge Deficit

c. Health-Seeking Behaviors

d. Hopelessness

11. After determining that Ms. Davis has a knowledge deficit regarding the role of adjuvant chemotherapy in the treatment of breast cancer and that she does not display health-seeking behaviors, which of the following health beliefs is *not* valid in planning interactions with her?

a. her belief that cancer can have serious effects on her life

b. her belief that the threat of chemotherapy is not as great as the threat of cancer

c. her belief that she is susceptible to the consequences of cancer

d. her belief that it is the health care professional's responsibility to determine her treatment

12. In evaluating Ms. Davis's response to a discussion about health beliefs, the nurse recognizes her use of abstract thinking. Which of the following categories does this behavior demonstrate?

a. attribution motivation theory

b. cognitive learning domain

c. generativity task

d. psychomotor learning domain

13. Which of the following statements does *not* provide justification for the role of nursing in addressing patients' health education needs?

a. The American Nurses Association's Standards of Nursing Practice defines health education as an essential component of nursing care.

b. Nurses have a broad knowledge and experiential base in both wellness and illness.

c. Nurse practice acts have clarified professional responsibility in providing patient education.

d. Nurses have expressed interest in being patient educators from the inception of nursing.

14. In formulating learning goals, which of the following does *not* illustrate an important factor to be considered at this stage of the teaching process?

a. involvement of patients and their families or significant others in the development of goals

b. inclusion of teaching methods appropriate to patients' learning styles

c. consideration of the primary learning domains in which to focus teaching

d. use of behavioral objectives in formulating goals

15. In the implementation of a predischarge teaching plan for a patient newly diagnosed with diabetes, the nurse must relate the concepts of andragogy. Which of the following does *not* reflect awareness of these concepts?

a. Include content to be taught based on the patient's learning goals.

b. Include family members or significant others in the teaching.

c. Include all information needed to live at an optimal level of wellness with diabetes.

d. Include information that is perceived by the patient as necessary to reduce the severity of illness.

16. In evaluating documentation of patient teaching, the nurse should check that documentation includes which of the following?
   a. assessment of progress toward learning goals
   b. resolution of underlying disease progress
   c. progression of physical therapy activities
   d. ability to perform activities of daily living

ANSWER KEY

1. **Correct response: c**
   This answer is appropriate to a specific illness. To include it in general education of well population is not appropriate because perception of need to know would not be present.
   a, b, and d. These areas are appropriate for both well and ill populations.
   Comprehension/Physiologic/Planning

2. **Correct response: b**
   Involvement of the learner in his or her own evaluation is a primary element of adult learning.
   a, c, and d. These answers all reflect elements of adult learning.
   Knowledge/Safe care/Implementation

3. **Correct response: a**
   This patient's exacerbation may result from improper medication administration. Teaching in the hospital setting should incorporate survival teaching, including administration techniques.
   b, c, and d. Chronically ill patients are often taught skills during the nonacute phase of illness outside the hospital setting, but in the hospital, survival skills are taught to all patients regardless of acuity.
   Comprehension/Health promotion/ Implementation

4. **Correct response: c**
   Even though this is important in overall assessment, it is not important in home oxygen therapy learning.
   a. This reflects the patient's ability to learn.
   b. This reflects readiness to learn.
   d. This reflects willingness to learn.
   Analysis/Safe care/Assessment

5. **Correct response: d**
   Older adults often have decreased ability to discriminate between stimuli.

   a, b, and c. These factors are important to the enhancement of learning but are not specific to the older adult.
   Application/Physiologic/Implementation

6. **Correct response: b**
   The only appropriate measure of skill level is the one that demonstrates understanding of safe equipment use.
   a, c, and d. These answers reflect primary purposes for performing evaluation.
   Application/Safe care/Evaluation

7. **Correct response: b**
   If the patient is unable to see the oxygen equipment clearly, he or she cannot safely administer an accurate flow of oxygen.
   a, c, and d. These factors all have the potential to influence understanding or performance; they do not prohibit or preclude safe performance.
   Analysis/Safe care/Analysis (Dx)

8. **Correct response: b**
   Although a low literacy level affects patient teaching methods, it does not increase the number of education programs developed.
   a, c, and d. These all have had an impact on the number of patient education programs developed at the national and local levels.
   Knowledge/Health promotion/Assessment

9. **Correct response: d**
   This answer is not a measure of learning readiness but a component of a learning domain.
   a, b, and c. These all are used in evaluating learning readiness.
   Comprehension/Psychosocial/Assessment

10. **Correct response: c**
    In order to be motivated to take action,

a patient must have a perception of his or her need to know.

a, b, and d. These factors have the potential to immobilize the patient or hamper decision making.

Analysis/Psychosocial/Analysis (Dx)

11. **Correct response: d**

The patient always should be involved in decision making regarding treatment based on adequate knowledge.

a, b, and c. These answers all reflect the health belief model, which proposes that motivation to learn requires certain patient beliefs regarding health and illness.

Analysis/Physiologic/Planning

12. **Correct response: b**

Abstract thinking is present in the cognitive learning domain.

a. This is an inappropriate answer.

c. This reflects a developmental stage that is a measure of emotional maturity.

d. This is a learning domain that does not include abstract thinking.

Application/Physiologic/Evaluation

13. **Correct response: d**

Interest is not justification for practice.

a, b, and c. Knowledge, standards of practice, and nurse practice acts are necessary prerequisites for incorporation into nursing practice.

Application/Health promotion/Analysis (Dx)

14. **Correct response: b**

Teaching methods are appropriate in developing a teaching plan, not in formulating learning goals.

a and c. These factors are important in the development of learning goals that reflect patients' perception of need.

d. This allows measurement of learning through the use of behavioral objectives.

Application/Health promotion/Planning

15. **Correct response: c**

It is important during the acute phase of illness to teach only what is necessary for survival or safe care.

a, b, and d. These interventions reflect awareness of the concepts of andragogy.

Analysis/Physiologic/Implementation

16. **Correct response: a**

This is an appropriate area in which to document supporting teaching and learning that has occurred.

b, c, and d. These are all important points to be documented but do not address evaluation of patient teaching.

Application/Health promotion/Evaluation

Homeostasis

I.   Essential concepts: anatomy and physiology

A.   Cellular composition

1. Cells are composed of protoplasm, which consists mainly of:
   a. Water
   b. Electrolytes
   c. Proteins
   d. Lipids
   e. Carbohydrates
2. A cell has three major parts:
   a. Cell membrane
   b. Cytoplasm
   c. Nucleus
3. The cell membrane completely envelops the cell and acts as a diffusion barrier for water and water-soluble substances (i.e., ions, glucose), while allowing lipid-soluble molecules (i.e., oxygen, carbon dioxide) to readily permeate the lipid bilayer.
4. Cell membrane proteins act as receptors for hormones and other chemical messengers that regulate cellular activity.
5. The cell membrane consists of a bilayer of lipid molecules; phospholipids (75%), glycolipids (5%), and cholesterol (25%).
6. Two types of cell membrane proteins (glycoproteins) float in this lipid bilayer:

a. Integral (structural) proteins protrude through the cell and provide a structural pathway through which water and water-soluble molecules can diffuse between extracellular and intracellular pathways.

b. Peripheral proteins are entirely or almost entirely on the inside of the membrane, normally attached to one of the integral proteins; they function almost entirely as enzymes.

7. The cytoplasm is a fine granular substance that contains the nucleus and highly organized structures known as organelles; principle organelles include:

a. Mitochondria: The cell's "powerhouse" extracts energy from nutrients and oxygen and in turn provides it in usable form (ATP) to energize essentially all cellular functions. Numbers vary from hundreds to thousands per cell, depending on cellular energy requirements; erythrocytes do not contain mitochondria, however.

b. Endoplasmic reticulum: In this continuous network of tubular and flat vascular structures, the rough (granular) type has small granular particles—ribosomes—attached to the entire surface, which play a role in protein synthesis; the smooth (agranular) type, which has no attached ribosomes, is involved in synthesis of nonprotein substances such as steroids and lipids.

c. Golgi apparatus: Closely related to the endoplasmic reticulum, this organelle processes transported substances from the endoplasmic reticulum to form secretory vesicles, lysosomes, and other cytoplasmic components.

d. Lysosomes: This intracellular digestive system digests most constituents of cells and tissues down to basic building blocks (amino acids or dipeptides, sugars, and fatty acids); these products diffuse across the lysosome membrane and are neutralized in biosynthesis.

e. Microtubules and microfilaments: These filamentous structures function in cell support and cell mobility.

f. Centriole: This organelle plays a role in cell division and reproduction.

8. The nucleus, the cell's control center and its largest structure, contains large quantities of deoxyribonucleic acid (DNA).

9. The nucleus governs chemical reactions within the cell and cell reproduction and transmits genetic information.

10. Nucleoli, smaller spherical bodies within the nucleus, contain large quantities of ribonucleic acid (RNA).

11. The size of the nucleoli reflects the overall rate of protein synthesis for either growth or secretion.

B. **Principles of homeostasis**

1. Homeostasis refers to the state of equilibrium in the body's internal environment; the cells, tissues, organs, and fluids.
2. Maintenance of homeostasis depends primarily on normal cellular function.
3. Cellular activities related to homeostasis include:
   a. Energy production
   b. Reproduction
   c. Intracellular digestion
4. The control of substances moving in and out of cells is central to maintaining homeostasis.
5. Normal organ function depends on collective action of cells that comprise it.

C. **Cellular repair**

1. Mechanisms of cellular repair include adaptation, regenerative healing, and replacement healing.
2. Adaptation is the desired outcome in managing actual or perceived stress to reestablish equilibrium.
3. Health represents successful adaptation to stress; illness, maladaptive or unsuccessful outcome to stress.
4. Regenerative healing occurs when damaged cells and tissues are replaced by new cells and tissues identical or nearly identical to the damaged cells and tissues.
5. The ability of cells to regenerate depends on cell type:
   a. *Labile cells* (e.g., gastrointestinal [GI] mucosal cells, respiratory tract cells, epithelial cells of skin) multiply constantly to replace worn-out cells.
   b. *Stable cells* (e.g., in the liver, renal tubules, pancreas, salivary and endocrine glands) may regenerate but only after injury occurs.
   c. *Permanent cells* (e.g., myocardial cells and neurons in the central nervous system) do not regenerate.
6. Replacement healing occurs with replacement cells such as connective tissue, resulting in scar formation.
7. This healing can take two forms:
   a. In *primary intention*, the wound heals well with well-approximated edges and minimal granulation tissue.
   b. In *secondary intention*, the wound is large and gaping with more necrotic material; fills from bottom upward with granulation tissue.
8. During replacement healing, abnormal scar formation can cause contractures and strictures, which may interfere with normal physiologic function.
9. Factors affecting cellular repair include:
   a. Age: Elderly patients may have decreased blood flow to

skin, organ atrophy and diminished function, and altered immunity; these effects slow cellular repair and increase the risk of infection.

b. Nutritional status: Adequate protein and caloric intake is essential to optimal cellular; a person with cellular injury has greater protein and calorie needs.

c. Infection: The presence of infection slows cellular repair.

d. Chronic illness: Various chronic conditions can predispose a patient to cellular injury (e.g., uncontrolled diabetes mellitus).

e. Nature of wound: Incisional wounds made under aseptic conditions are less prone to infection than traumatic wounds, which typically involve microorganism invasion.

f. Extent of wound and associated blood loss: The greater the extent, the slower the healing process in most cases.

g. Tissue involved: Tissues with good blood supply heal faster (e.g., wounds of the hands and head tend to heal more quickly than those of adipose tissue or lower extremities).

h. Psychosocial factors (e.g., stress, fatigue): These factors can impair healing.

II. Disruption of cellular function

A. Pathophysiology

1. Stress is defined as a state resulting from a change in the environment that is perceived as threatening to homeostasis.

2. A stimulus that evokes this state is known as a stressor.

3. Psychosocial sources of stress include:

   a. Daily stressors (e.g., traffic jams, arguments, school difficulties)

   b. Major complex occurrences involving large groups or nations; includes events such as war, terrorism, and economic depression

   c. Major life events (e.g., death, marriage, birth, divorce, retirement)

4. Physiologic sources of stress include:

   a. Hypoxia (inadequate cellular oxygenation): This leading cause of cell death may result from diminished blood supply to tissue, reduced oxygen-carrying capacity of blood (i.e., hemoglobin), or ventilation–perfusion problems.

   b. Temperature extremes (heat or cold): Extreme heat increases metabolic activity of cells, subsequently destroying enzymes and coagulating cytoplasmic protein; cold causes vasoconstriction, which decreases blood supply to tissues, and blood stasis, which may lead to thrombus formation.

   c. Trauma: Wounds can disrupt cells and tissues; the outcome of wound healing is related to the type and extent of injury, tissue involved, and mechanism of injury (e.g., blunt vs. penetrating wound).

d. Radiation: Exposure to ionizing radiation can cause cell mutation, damage enzymes, and interrupt cell division.

e. Chemical agents: Various chemicals can injure or destroy cells; damage depends on the nature of the exposure and on cellular susceptibility to the chemical.

f. Infectious agents: Viruses, bacteria, rickettsiae, mycoplasma, fungi, and protozoa may cause disease.

g. Nutritional imbalances: Deficiency or excess of one or more essential nutrients increases stress on cells and tissues.

h. Immune system dysfunction: Immunodeficiency occurs with hypoactivity; hypersensitivity, with hyperactivity.

5. Insults at either the cellular or organ level may result in pathologic (disease) processes.

6. Responses of the internal environment to diseases are termed pathophysiologic processes.

7. The inflammatory response occurs when limits of adaptive capability are exceeded or when no adaptive response is possible; may be reversible or irreversible if cell death occurs.

8. Transient vasoconstriction occurs immediately after injury, followed by vasodilation.

9. Blood flow is increased to the injury site, resulting in local heat and redness.

10. As vascular permeability increases, plasma leaks into inflamed tissues, producing swelling.

11. Swelling causes pressure on nerve endings or possibly direct irritation of nerve endings by chemical mediations such as histamines or kinins.

12. Loss of function usually is attributed to pain and swelling.

13. Plasma elements left in tissue include white blood cells, platelets, and red blood cells.

14. White blood cells (leukocytes) migrate to the injury site; their primary purpose is phagocytosis (engulfing organisms and removing of cellular debris).

15. Fibrinogen from leaked plasma coagulates, forming a fibrin wall that helps prevent the spread of infection.

16. Systemic responses to cellular injury include:

a. Temperature elevation, caused by endogenous pyrogens released from neutrophils and macrophages

b. Leukocytosis

c. Malaise, loss of appetite, aching, and weakness

17. Response to cellular injury is either acute or chronic:

a. Acute responses usually last less than 2 weeks and are characterized by vascular congestion with inflammatory exudate.

     b. Chronic responses, which usually last weeks to months, are characterized by proliferative exudate; a continued cycle of cellular infiltration, necrosis, and fibrosis may cause scarring.

18. Pathologic cellular adaptation results from excessive physiologic stress or pathologic stimuli in effort to preserve the cell; types of maladaptation include:

     a. Atrophy: Cell size shrinks through loss of cell substances; predisposing factors include aging, inadequate nutrition, and diminished workload, such as will occur in paralysis and loss of neural innervation.

     b. Hypertrophy: Cell size increases, resulting in increased organ size; predisposing factors include increased functional demand, as with hypertension, in which the heart muscle enlarges in effort to pump blood more efficiently through vasoconstricted or atherosclerotic arterioles.

     c. Hyperplasia: Number of cells increases in organ or tissue; predisposing factors are related to hormonal influences and tissue removal or destruction (e.g., breast changes in a pregnant female, regeneration of liver cells).

     d. Metaplasia: A reversible change occurs in which one adult cell type (epithelial or mesenchymal) is replaced by another cell type; predisposing factors include stress to highly specialized cells, as occurs with changes in epithelial cells of trachea and bronchi in a habitual cigarette smoker.

B. Assessment

1. The nursing health history should focus on factors predisposing the patient to cellular injury, such as:

     a. Age

     b. Stress

     c. Chronic disease

     d. Current medications and treatments

     e. Nutritional status

     f. Psychosocial status (e.g., ask "Is your household income adequate to secure basic needs such as housing, health care, food, and transportation? Do you have an adequate support network?")

     g. Completion and currency of immunizations

     h. Recent exposures to illness; type of illness and causative agent

     i. Recent travel (In certain areas of the world, particular disorders are endemic.)

     j. Contact with animals or any animal or insect bites

     k. List of drug allergies

2. Physical examination should focus on assessing for signs of local inflammation, such as:
   a. Heat
   b. Redness
   c. Swelling
   d. Pain at injury site
   e. Loss of function or any involuntary cessation of movement
3. The nurse also should assess for systemic signs of inflammation, including:
   a. Fever: Patient may be agitated, restless, and diaphoretic; adult patient also may experience chills.
   b. Elevated heart rate and respiratory rate
   c. Anorexia and weight loss
   d. Malaise and generalized weakness
   e. Enlarged lymph nodes
4. Assessment also should include the nature of the wound.
5. Systems review should evaluate:
   a. Any abnormal discharges from body orifices or skin lesions
   b. Any change in normal body function
   c. Presence, color, and odor of purulent drainage
6. Document all deviations from normal.
7. If acquired immunodeficiency syndrome (AIDS) is suspected, the nurse also should assess for:
   a. Kaposi's sarcoma: vascular tumors, most commonly occurring on the legs or toes, appearing as purple or dark brown plaques or nodules
   b. *Pneumocystis carinii*, marked by coughing and shortness of breath at rest
   c. Opportunistic infections (e.g., white coating on the oral mucosa points to *Candida* infection)
8. Significant laboratory data include:
   a. Complete blood count (CBC)
   b. Culture and sensitivity, to determine growth of any microorganisms and evaluate appropriate antibiotic therapy
   c. Human immunovirus (HIV) assay
   d. Electrolytes, blood urea nitrogen (BUN), creatinine levels

C. **Nursing diagnoses**
   1. Activity Intolerance
   2. High Risk for Altered Body Temperature
   3. Diarrhea
   4. Impaired Gas Exchange
   5. High Risk for Infection
   6. Knowledge Deficit
   7. Altered Nutrition: Less Than Body Requirements
   8. Pain

    9.   Impaired Skin Integrity

    10. Social Isolation

D. **Planning and implementation**

    1. Help guard against development of infection by:

        a.   Using and promoting correct handwashing technique (the most important procedure in preventing the spread of microorganisms); washing hands properly after any contact with urine, feces, blood, or other potential infection sources

        b.   Based on the risk of infections disease, wearing masks, gowns, gloves, and goggles to prevent the spread of microorganisms

        c.   Maintaining aseptic technique for all indwelling lines and surgical wounds

        d.   Monitoring for signs and symptoms of inflammation and infection

        e.   Administering antibiotics as prescribed

    2. Provide pain reduction by:

        a.   Administering analgesics or narcotics as prescribed; assess for relief of pain 30 minutes after administration

        b.   Administering anti-inflammatory agents as prescribed

        c.   Positioning the patient to promote comfort

        d.   Teaching the patient to splint the wound as appropriate

        e.   Elevating or supporting the injured area to promote venous return

        f.   After an injury, first applying cool packs to the site, then warm packs, to reduce swelling

    3. Promote adequate nutritional intake by:

        a.   Ensuring a diet high in protein and calories with vitamin supplements as need to optimize tissue repair

        b.   Monitoring dietary intake to detect deficiencies

        c.   Monitoring serum albumin and total protein to identify any nutritional deficits

        d.   Providing nutritional supplementation as necessary

    4. Maintain normothermia by:

        a.   Monitoring vital signs every 4 hours and as needed

        b.   Implementing measures to decrease temperature, such as administering antipyretics, reducing the room temperature, and providing tepid baths and cool compresses. (Extreme temperature elevations may necessitate using a cooling blanket.)

        c.   Encouraging increased oral fluid intake to compensate for insensible losses (e.g., diaphoresis) as appropriate

        d.   Obtaining cultures as ordered

5. Maintain skin integrity by:
   a. Promoting good blood supply to the injury area; avoiding tourniquets and tight dressings
   b. Elevating the injured area to increase venous return to the heart, aid wound drainage, and decrease the risk of thrombus formation
   c. Preventing pressure points on bony prominences through frequent patient repositioning
   d. Keeping the patient's skin clean and dry
   e. Assessing the skin every shift for signs of breakdown

6. Promote adequate rest by:
   a. Clustering necessary activities to allow uninterrupted periods of rest
   b. Teaching the patient energy conservation techniques, such as maintaining good posture and avoiding overreaching and overactivity
   c. Providing bedrest and limiting physical activity
   d. Limiting visitors and long conversations

7. Promote gas exchange by:
   a. Having the patient cough, turn, and deep breathe every 2 hours
   b. Having the patient ambulate as tolerated
   c. Auscultating lung sounds every shift and as needed
   d. Assessing respiratory rate and pattern
   e. Assessing cough
   f. Evaluating the color, odor, amount, and consistency of any sputum
   g. Monitoring arterial blood gas (ABG) values
   h. Suctioning as necessary to clear secretions
   i. Monitoring capillary refill time
   j. Assessing level of consciousness

8. Maintain normal bowel function by:
   a. Assessing the usual frequency, character, amount, and consistency of stool
   b. Assessing for fluid volume deficit
   c. Keeping the perineal area clean and dry to prevent skin breakdown
   d. Reinforcing the principles of handwashing (after each bowel movement)
   e. Sending stool specimens to the laboratory maintaining enteric precautions
   f. Assessing for recent antibiotic therapy
   g. Assessing dietary intake

9. Increase knowledge of the HTLV III virus by:
   a. Reviewing universal precautions with staff

    b.   Teaching the patient to use condoms with sexual intercourse and avoid direct mouth contact with the penis, vagina, or rectum

    c.   Teaching the patient to avoid sexual practices that cause cuts or tears in the rectum, penis, or vagina

    d.   Teaching the patient to avoid sex with prostitutes and other high-risk persons

    e.   Teaching a patient who abuses intravenous drugs to avoid using contaminated needles or syringes (if he or she is unable to stop using drugs)

10. Combat the patient's sense of social isolation by:

    a.   Providing accurate information about disease transmission to allay fears or clear up misconceptions

    b.   Assessing the patient's normal patterns of communication

    c.   Observing for diminished interpersonal interactions, hostility, or depression

    d.   Encouraging verbalization of feelings and concerns

    e.   Collaborating with the patient to identify available support systems and effective coping mechanisms

    f.   Providing care in an accepting, nonjudgmental manner

    g.   Providing for diversional activities to relieve boredom

11. Assess discharge needs, covering:

    a.   Home environment: adequacy of heating and cooling systems, availability of stove and refrigerator, stairs in house and their relationship to rooms used

    b.   Finances: resources available to buy food, medications, and health insurance

    c.   Support system: availability, reliability (family, friends, neighbors)

    d.   Self-care: capability to care for self—prepare meals, bathe properly, administer medications, and ambulate with assistance

12. Contact social services, rehabilitation services, or home health care services as needed.

13. Provide patient and family teaching, covering:

    a.   Signs and symptoms of infection to watch for and report

    b.   Specifics of any drug therapy; use a medication calendar to clearly describe the drug, its dosage, and the time and length of therapy (for antibiotics)

    c.   Follow-up wound care; instruct on dressing changes and whether it is appropriate to shower

    d.   Activity limitations

    e.   Stress-reduction measures

    f.   Follow-up appointments with the physician

    g.   Maintenance of proper nutrition

    h.   The need to keep all immunizations up to date

E. Evaluation

1. The patient displays no signs or symptoms of infection or inflammation.
2. The patient reports relief of pain; reduction of swelling observed.
3. The patient maintains adequate nutritional intake.
4. The patient is normothermic.
5. The patient displays no signs of skin breakdown; maintenance of circulation as evidenced by warm, pink extremities with palpable distal pulses.
6. The patient verbalizes feelings of being rested.
7. The patient's lungs are clear on auscultation.
8. The patient's ABG values remain within normal ranges.
9. The patient passes stools of normal pattern, color, and consistency.
10. The patient maintains adequate hydration, as evidenced by normal BUN and hematocrit and normal skin turgor, moist mucous membranes.
11. The patient verbalizes knowledge of prevention and transmission of AIDS.
12. The patient verbalizes diminished sense of social isolation.

Bibliography

Brunner, L. S., & Suddarth, D. S. (1988). *Textbook of medical-surgical nursing* (6th ed.). Philadelphia: J. B. Lippincott.

Cotran, R. S., Kumar, V., & Robbins, S. L. (1989). *Robbins' pathologic basis of disease* (4th ed.). Philadelphia: W. B. Saunders.

Guyton, A. C. (1986). *Human physiology and mechanisms of disease* (3rd ed.) Philadelphia: W. B. Saunders.

Luckmann, J., & Sorensen, K. C. (1987). *Medical-surgical nursing: A psychophysiologic approach* (3rd ed.). Philadelphia: W. B. Saunders.

Sodeman, W. A., & Sodeman, T. M. (1985). *Sodeman's pathologic physiology mechanisms of disease* (7th ed.). Philadelphia: W. B. Saunders.

STUDY QUESTIONS

1. Which of the following structures is responsible for providing energy for nearly all cellular functions?
    a. Golgi apparatus
    b. mitochondria
    c. nucleus
    d. rough endoplasmic reticulum

2. Which of the following statements about the cell membrane is correct?
    a. It acts as a receptor for hormones.
    b. It extracts energy from nutrients and oxygen.
    c. It governs cell reproduction.
    d. It is involved in the synthesis of nonprotein substances.

3. Which of the following nursing diagnoses would most likely lead the nurse to believe that the patient is experiencing a systemic response to cellular injury?
    a. Altered Body Temperature
    b. Impaired Skin Integrity: Actual
    c. Altered Oral Mucous Membrane
    d. Acute Pain

4. The most important factor in preventing the spread of a microorganism is
    a. using correct handwashing technique
    b. maintaining aseptic technique on Foley catheter insertion
    c. wearing masks, gowns, and gloves when caring for AIDS patients
    d. cleansing spills of blood with sodium hypochloride

5. Ms. Lee is admitted with a hemoglobin level of 6.8, blood pressure 82/50 mmHg, pulse 136, and respirations 32 and shallow. The nurse would base Ms. Lee's care on which of the following assumptions regarding the probable consequences of her clinical status?
    a. vasodilation
    b. GI bleeding
    c. tissue hypoxia
    d. metabolic acidosis

6. Numerous factors can influence cellular repair. In planning care for a patient with cellular injury, the nurse should consider that
    a. Tissue with good blood supply (e.g., adipose tissue) may heal faster.
    b. The presence of infection may slow the healing process.
    c. Nutritional needs remain unchanged for the well-nourished adult.
    d. Age is an insignificant factor in cellular repair.

7. Appropriate nursing interventions for reducing pain due to cellular injury include
    a. administering anti-inflammatory agents as prescribed
    b. elevating the injured area to decrease venous return to the heart
    c. keeping the skin clean and dry
    d. applying warm packs initially, followed by cool packs to reduce swelling

8. Mr. Mobry has been admitted with fever of unknown origin. He feels weak and achy and has been anorexic. These symptoms are indicative of
    a. local signs of inflammation
    b. metaplasia
    c. psychosocial stress
    d. systemic signs of inflammation

9. Julie Brown, aged 16, recently moved to a new city because of her parents' divorce. She is admitted with weight loss, insomnia, and lack of interest in school. Based on Julie's symptoms, all the following diagnoses would be appropriate *except*
    a. Dysfunctional Grieving
    b. Ineffective Individual Coping
    c. Altered Nutrition: Less Than Body Requirements
    d. Sensory and Perceptual Alterations: Visual

10. Mr. Atwater, a 22-year-old medical student, is admitted with bacterial pneumonia. He is febrile, diaphoretic, and short of breath. His past medical history

is significant for asthma. Based on these findings, the most important nursing intervention consideration would be to
a. Maintain adequate oxygenation.
b. Prevent fluid volume excess.
c. Reduce pain.
d. Teach risk factors related to AIDS.

11. Which of the following statements regarding stress and adaptation in planning health promotion strategies is true?
a. Health represents a pathologic adaptation to stress.
b. Illness represents an unsuccessful outcome to stress.
c. Sources of stress are always physiologic.
d. The inflammatory response occurs concurrently with the adaptive process.

12. During hospitalization, maintaining optimum respiratory function is essential to reduce the risk of infections. Which of the following evaluation statements demonstrates adequate respiratory function?
a. The patient exhibits bilateral rales on auscultation.
b. The patient displays these ABG values: pH, 7.35 to 7.45; PO_2, 80 to 100 mmHg; PCO_2, 35 to 45 mmHg.
c. The patient maintains respiratory rate of 32 to 36 breaths per minute.
d. The patient exhibits pursed-lip breathing at rest.

13. An appropriate plan of care for a hyperthermic patient would include:
a. antiemetic administration
b. axillary temperature measurement every 4 hours
c. fluid restriction of 2,000 mL/day
d. reduction of room temperature

14. When preparing to teach a patient about sources of stress that predispose to pathologic disruption of cellular function, the nurse would cover all the following nursing diagnoses *except*
a. Hyperthermia
b. Ineffective Family Coping: Compromised
c. Altered Nutrition: Less Than Body Requirements
d. Dysreflexia

15. Mrs. Aiken sustained a laceration to her left anterior thigh in a car accident. The wound has healed slowly. At dismissal, the nurse's evaluation criteria for primary intention replacement healing would include which of the following?
a. The patient displays well-approximated wound edges with minimal granulation tissue.
b. The patient displays abnormal scar formation at the wound site.
c. The patient's wound is filled from the bottom upward with granulation tissue.
d. The patient exhibits no approximation of wound edges.

16. Which of the following would be an appropriate measure of progress toward health in an older patient with herpes zoster who is struggling with decisions about moving into a retirement home and giving up her car?
a. The patient resolves conflict in decision about living arrangements.
b. The patient demonstrates a general reduction of malaise and weakness.
c. The patient exhibits regenerative healing with stable cells.
d. The patient experiences fulfilling life experiences, such as her granddaughter's wedding.

ANSWER KEY

1. **Correct response: b**
   Mitochondria act as the cell's "power house."
   a. Golgi apparatus processes and transports substances from the endoplasmic reticulum.
   c. The nucleus is the "control center" of the cell.
   d. The rough endoplasmic reticulum plays a role in protein synthesis.
   Knowledge/Physiologic/Assessment

2. **Correct response: a**
   Cell membrane proteins attached to the lipid bilayer act as receptors for messages that regulate cellular activity.
   b. The mitochondria extracts energy.
   c. The nucleus governs cell reproduction.
   d. The smooth endoplasmic reticulum is involved in synthesis of nonprotein substances.
   Knowledge/Physiologic/Assessment

3. **Correct response: a**
   Temperature elevation is caused by endogenous pyrogens released from neutrophils and macrophages.
   b, c, and d. These other diagnoses all represent local responses.
   Comprehension/Physiologic/Analysis (Dx)

4. **Correct response: a**
   Handwashing remains the most effective procedure in limiting microorganisms and the incidence of nosocomial infections.
   b. Aseptic technique is essential with all indwelling lines, especially catheters.
   c. Masks, gowns, and gloves are necessary only when the likelihood of exposure to blood or body fluids is high.
   d. Spills of blood from AIDS patients should be cleansed with sodium hypochloride.
   Application/Safe care/Implementation

5. **Correct response: c**
   Tissue hypoxia will result from the diminished oxygen-carrying capacity of the blood (hemoglobin), making the patient susceptible to impaired skin integrity.
   a. Vasoconstriction, not vasodilation, would occur.
   b. GI bleeding would be a cause, not a consequence.
   d. Respiratory acidosis, not metabolic acidosis, would most likely occur.
   Analysis/Physiologic/Implementation

6. **Correct response: b**
   Infection impairs wound healing.
   a. Tissues of the head and hand have good blood supply, not adipose tissue.
   c. Nutritional needs increase for all patients undergoing cellular repair.
   d. Elderly persons have a slower reparative process because of diminished organ functioning and altered immunity.
   Application/Health promotion/Planning

7. **Correct response: a**
   Anti-inflammatory agents will help reduce swelling and thus relieve pressure on nerve endings.
   b. Elevating the injured area would increase, not decrease, venous return to the heart.
   c. Maintaining clean, dry skin aids in preventing skin breakdown.
   d. Cool packs, not warm packs, should be used initially.
   Application/Safe care/Implementation

8. **Correct response: d**
   Fever, weakness, muscle aches, and anorexia represent systemic signs and symptoms of inflammation.
   a. Local signs and symptoms include redness, heat, swelling, and pain at the area of injury.
   b. Metaplasia is a type of pathologic adaptation in which one cell type is replaced by another.
   c. Psychosocial stress may contribute

to cellular injury, but no history of this is given.

Analysis/Physiologic/Assessment

9. **Correct response: d**
   This patient exhibits no evidence of sensory and perceptual deficit.
   a, b, and c. Major life events such as death, divorce, or birth constitute a significant source of psychosocial stress that can trigger various physiologic responses.

Analysis/Psychosocial/Analysis (Dx)

10. **Correct response: a**
    Maintaining adequate oxygenation will reduce the risk of physiologic injury from cellular hypoxia—the leading cause of cell death.
    b. This patient would be more likely to experience fluid volume deficit due to fever and diaphoresis.
    c. No information regarding pain is provided in this scenario.
    d. Teaching risk factors related to AIDS may be indicated later during hospitalization.

Application/Physiologic/Implementation

11. **Correct response: b**
    Health represents successful adaptation to stress.
    a. This is simply incorrect.
    c. Sources of stress may be both psychologic and physiologic.
    d. The inflammatory response occurs when the limits of adaptive capability are exceeded or when no adaptive response is possible.

Comprehension/Health promotion/Planning

12. **Correct response: b**
    Normal ABG values reflect adequate oxygenation.
    a. Rales heard on auscultation may indicate interstitial edema or pneumonia.
    c. Normal respiratory rate ranges from 12 to 24 breaths per minute.
    d. Pursed-lip breathing is commonly seen in patients with COPD, asthma, or chest trauma.

Analysis/Safe care/Evaluation

13. **Correct response: d**
    Reducing the room temperature may help decrease body temperature.
    a. Antipyretics—not antiemetics—are indicated to reduce fever.
    b. Oral or rectal temperature measurements are generally accepted as more accurate than axillary measurements.
    c. Fluids should be encouraged, not restricted, in order to compensate for insensible losses.

Application/Safe care/Planning

14. **Correct response: d**
    Dysreflexia is an abnormal neuromuscular disorder; it has no relationship to disruption of cellular function.
    a, b, and c. These other diagnoses would predispose a patient to pathologic disruption of cellular function.

Analysis/Health promotion/Analysis (Dx)

15. **Correct response: a**
    This answer represents primary intention replacement healing.
    b, c, and d. These answers represent problems with replacement healing and would not be set up as evaluation criteria.

Application/Health promotion/Evaluation

16. **Correct response: a**
    Stresses occur from changes in environment perceived as threats to equilibrium, increasing cellular dysfunction. Resolution in this case can increase the likelihood of a return to healthy cellular function.
    b. Malaise and weakness are not common signs of herpes zoster.
    c. Labile cells would be seen in the regenerative healing process in this case.
    d. Life events (even good ones) can be psychosocial stressors.

Comprehension/Psychosocial/Evaluation

Fluid and Electrolytes

I. Basic concepts

A. Composition

1. Fluid (water and electrolytes) accounts for about 60% of an adult's total body weight.
2. *Intracellular fluid* (ICF) comprises about two thirds of this amount; *extracellular fluid* (ECF) accounts for the other one third.

B. Electrolytes

1. Potassium (K) and phosphate (PO_4) are the major electrolytes in ICF.
2. Sodium (Na) and chloride (Cl) are the major electrolytes in ECF.
3. Sodium level is the primary determinant of ECF concentration.

C. Regulatory mechanisms

1. Various mechanisms regulate fluid distribution between intracellular and extracellular compartments.

2. *Osmosis* involves fluid shifts through membrane from an area of low solute concentration to an area of higher solute concentration.

3. *Diffusion* involves fluid movement from an area of high solute concentration to one of lower solute concentration.

4. *Filtration* refers to movement of fluid out of solution, such as occurs because of blood's hydrostatic pressure (i.e., pressure of blood pushes fluids and electrolytes out of the vasculature and into the interstitial spaces).

5. *Active transport* is an energy-requiring process that transports ions across membrane against a concentration gradient (e.g., the sodium–potassium pump).

D. **Sources of fluid loss (adults)**

1. Fluid loss constantly occurs as a normal result of body functions.

2. The *kidneys* normally produce a fluid output of 1 to 2 L/day.

3. From the *skin*, sensible losses (visible perspiration) normally range from 0 to 1000 mL/hour, depending on temperature, and insensible losses (water loss by evaporation) equal about 600 mL/day; these amounts increase with fever.

4. The *lungs* produce an insensible loss (exhaled water vapor) of 300 to 400 mL/day, increased with fever.

5. Losses from the *gastrointestinal* (GI) *tract* normally range from 100 to 200 mL/day.

E. **Homeostatic mechanisms**

1. Various organ systems and mechanisms interact to maintain homeostasis—optimal fluid and electrolyte balance.

2. The *kidneys*:
   a. Filter about 170 liters of plasma per day
   b. Reabsorb HCO, secrete hydrogen ions in proximal and distal tubules, and produce ammonia (NH_3)
   c. Compensate for imbalances more slowly than the lungs; may take up to several days

3. The *cardiovascular system* maintains adequate renal perfusion.

4. The *lungs* work to maintain acid–base balance by controlling carbon dioxide (CO_2) and H_2CO_3 excretion. PCO_2 (partial pressure of CO_2) is the most powerful respiratory stimulant, followed by pH, then PO_2 (partial pressure of oxygen).

5. *Buffers* are chemical systems that maintain body pH by inactivating or releasing hydrogen ions (H^*). The primary buffer system is bicarbonate–carbonic acid (HCO_3 to H_2CO_3). A HCO_3–H_2CO_3 ratio of 20:1 is necessary to maintain body pH; disruption of the ratio will alter pH. Less important buffer systems are the phosphate buffer system (intracellular) and the protein buffer system.

6. The *pituitary gland* stores antidiuretic hormone (ADH), which promotes water retention.

7. The *adrenal cortex* produces aldosterone, which causes sodium retention and potassium loss.
8. The *parathyroid glands* secrete parathyroid hormone, which regulates calcium and phosphate balance.
9. Normal laboratory values reflecting homeostasis include:
   a. pH: 7.35 to 7.45
   b. PO_2: 75 to 100 mmHg
   c. PCO_2: 35 to 38 mmHg
   d. HCO_3: 23 to 25 mEq/L

II. FVD

A. **Description: excessive loss of water and electrolytes in equal proportion**

B. **Etiology**
1. Inadequate intake
2. Increased output such as from severe diarrhea, vomiting, or blood loss
3. Massive third-space fluid shifting, such as in ascites due to liver dysfunction, pancreatitis, or burns

C. **Assessment findings**
1. Common clinical manifestations include:
   a. Decreased skin turgor
   b. Dry skin and mucous membranes
   c. Postural hypotension
   d. Increased heart rate
   e. Extreme thirst
   f. Apprehension
   g. Renal shutdown and coma with severe FVD
2. Laboratory findings may include:
   a. Urine specific gravity above 1.020
   b. Blood urea nitrogen (BUN) elevated disproportionately to serum creatinine
   c. Elevated hematocrit

D. **Nursing diagnoses**
1. Fluid Volume Deficit
2. Knowledge Deficit

E. **Planning and implementation**
1. Monitor intake and output carefully.
2. Monitor urine specific gravity.
3. Weigh the patient daily.
4. Take vital signs every shift and p.r.n.
5. Monitor skin turgor.
6. Maintain adequate hydration through oral or IV supplementation.
7. Teach the patient to change positions slowly to minimize postural hypotension.

F. Evaluation

   1. The patient exhibits adequate hydration, as evidenced by:
      a. Elastic skin turgor
      b. Moist mucous membranes
      c. Absence of postural hypotension and tachycardia
   2. The patient's urine specific gravity, BUN, and hematocrit levels return to normal ranges.

III. FVE

A. Description: excessive retention of water and electrolytes in equal proportion

B. Etiology

   1. Excessive intake
   2. Impaired ability to excrete fluid, such as in renal disease
   3. Abnormal fluid retention, such as may occur in congestive heart failure or corticosteroid therapy
   4. Excessive sodium intake (IV or oral)

C. Assessment findings

   1. Clinical manifestations may include:
      a. Weight gain
      b. Dependent edema (e.g., in feet, ankles, and sacrum)
      c. Dyspnea and rales (particularly in patients with a history of cardiac problems)
   2. Laboratory studies may reveal decreased BUN and hematocrit.

D. Nursing diagnoses

   1. Fluid Volume Excess
   2. Knowledge Deficit

E. Planning and implementation

   1. Monitor intake and output carefully.
   2. Weigh the patient daily.
   3. Take vital signs every shift and p.r.n.
   4. Assess for edema.
   5. Assess lung sounds; if pulmonary edema occurs, elevate the head of the bed and have the patient turn, cough, and deep breathe every 2 hours.
   6. Teach the patient the fundamentals of a sodium-restricted diet, as ordered.
   7. Administer diuretics as prescribed.
   8. Restrict sodium and water as ordered.

F. Evaluation

   1. The patient's weight decreases to preimbalance level.
   2. The patient's lungs are clear on auscultation.
   3. The patient exhibits minimal or no edema.
   4. The patient demonstrates compliance with the prescribed sodium-restricted diet.

IV. Hyponatremia (sodium deficiency)

A. Description: serum sodium level below 135 mEq/L

B. Etiology

    1. Fluid loss, such as from:
        a. Vomiting
        b. Diarrhea
        c. Fistulas
        d. Diaphoresis
        e. Diuretic therapy
    2. Adrenal insufficiency
    3. Syndrome of inappropriate antidiuretic hormone excretion (SIADH)
    4. Excessive water gain from intake of sodium-deficient parenteral fluids or compulsive water drinking

C. Assessment findings

    1. Clinical manifestations may include:
        a. Anorexia
        b. Muscle cramps
        c. Nausea
        d. Altered level of consciousness: lethargy, disorientation, confusion, convulsions (with serum sodium level below 115 mEq/L)
    2. Laboratory studies reveal:
        a. Serum sodium level below 135 mEq/L
        b. Urine sodium and specific gravity low if due to sodium loss; high if due to SIADH

D. Nursing diagnoses

    1. Fluid Volume Excess
    2. High Risk for Injury
    3. Knowledge Deficit
    4. Altered Thought Processes

E. Planning and implementation

    1. Monitor intake and output carefully.
    2. Weigh the patient daily.
    3. Assess neurologic and GI status.
    4. Administer sodium supplements as ordered.
    5. Monitor for signs of fluid volume excess.
    6. Infuse hypotonic solutions cautiously.
    7. Maintain seizure precautions.
    8. Restrict fluids, as ordered, if the patient is normovolemic or hypervolemic.

F. Evaluation

    1. The patient displays adequate orientation to person, place, and time.
    2. The patient remains free of seizure activity.

3. The patient maintains his or her normal body weight.
4. Serum sodium level returns to normal range.

V. Hypernatremia (sodium excess)

A. Description: serum sodium level above 145 mEq/L

B. Etiology
   1. Water loss, such as from:
      a. Diarrhea
      b. Fever
      c. Hyperventilation
      d. Diabetes insipidus
   2. Inadequate water replacement, most commonly due to decreased intake in elderly, cognitively impaired, or comatose patients
   3. Inability to swallow
   4. Rarely, seawater ingestion or excessive oral or parenteral sodium intake

C. Assessment findings
   1. Common clinical manifestations include:
      a. Thirst
      b. Dry skin and mucous membranes
      c. Elevated body temperature
      d. Lethargy and restlessness
   2. Laboratory study results include:
      a. Serum sodium level above 145 mEq/L
      b. Elevated serum osmolality
      c. Elevated urine specific gravity

D. Nursing diagnoses
   1. High Risk for Altered Body Temperature
   2. High Risk for Fluid Volume Deficit
   3. High Risk for Injury
   4. Altered Thought Processes

E. Planning and implementation
   1. Monitor intake and output carefully.
   2. Weigh the patient daily.
   3. Assess vital signs, skin turgor, and neurologic status.
   4. Protect the patient from injury by:
      a. Repositioning frequently
      b. Securing all invasive lines
      c. Keeping bed side rails up
      d. Keeping bed brakes locked
   5. Encourage increased fluid intake as appropriate.
   6. Infuse hypotonic solution as ordered.

F. Evaluation
   1. The patient exhibits adequate orientation to person, place, and time.

2. The patient remains free from injury.
3. The patient exhibits normal body temperature and skin turgor.
4. Serum sodium level returns to normal range.

VI. Hypokalemia (potassium deficiency)

A. Description: serum potassium level below 3.5 mEq/L

B. Etiology

1. Inadequate dietary potassium intake
2. Excessive loss due to:
   a. Treatments, such as carbenicillin, amphotericin B, diuretics, or steroid therapy; parenteral fluid therapy without potassium replacement; gastric suctioning; colostomy and ileostomy
   b. GI disorders, such as diarrhea, vomiting, or fistula
3. Alkalosis
4. Hyperaldosteronism

C. Assessment findings

1. Common clinical manifestations include:
   a. Anorexia
   b. Fatigue
   c. Muscle weakness
   d. Paresthesia
2. Laboratory and diagnostic test results typically include:
   a. Serum potassium level below 3.5 mEq/L
   b. ECG changes: flattened T wave, prominent U wave, depressed ST segment

D. Nursing diagnoses

1. High Risk for Injury
2. Knowledge Deficit
3. Altered Tissue Perfusion: Cardiopulmonary

E. Planning and implementation

1. Monitor intake and output carefully.
2. Infuse parenteral potassium supplement, as ordered; always dilute first, and monitor ECG during infusion.
3. Teach the patient to eat foods high in potassium, particularly if he or she is receiving steroid, diuretic, or digitalis therapy; such foods include:
   a. Orange juice
   b. Bananas
   c. Cantaloupe
   d. Peaches
   e. Potatoes
   f. Dates
   g. Apricots

F. Evaluation

1. The patient exhibits a normal ECG pattern.

2. The patient demonstrates normal muscle strength and energy.
3. The patient verbalizes understanding of foods high in potassium.
4. Serum potassium level returns to normal range.

VII. Hyperkalemia (potassium excess)

A. Description: serum potassium level above 5.5 mEq/L

B. Etiology
   1. "Pseudohyperkalemia" from hemolysis of blood sample
   2. Decreased renal excretion due to renal failure
   3. Hypoaldosteronism
   4. Acidosis
   5. Severe tissue trauma (e.g., burns, massive infection)
   6. Excessive intake of potassium supplement (rare)

C. Assessment findings
   1. Common clinical manifestations include:
      a. Muscle weakness
      b. Paresthesias
   2. Laboratory and diagnostic studies reveal:
      a. Serum potassium level above 5.5 mEq/L
      b. EKG changes: tall, narrow, symmetrically peaked T waves and short Q–T interval with serum potassium level between 5.5 and 7.8 mEq/L; shortened P–R interval, disappearing P wave, and widened QRS complex with continued rise in potassium level

D. Nursing diagnoses
   1. Knowledge Deficit
   2. Altered Tissue Perfusion: Cardiopulmonary

E. Planning and implementation
   1. Evaluate all blood samples exhibiting potassium excess for hemolysis.
   2. Teach patients at increased risk for hyperkalemia (such as those with renal failure) to avoid high-potassium foods.
   3. Monitor the ECG for abnormalities.
   4. Prepare for and assist with aggressive therapy, as ordered, which may include:
      a. Kayexalate
      b. Parenteral sodium bicarbonate
      c. Parenteral insulin and glucose
      d. Dialysis

F. Evaluation
   1. The patient exhibits normal ECG patterns.
   2. The patient verbalizes the importance of avoiding high-potassium foods.
   3. Serum potassium level returns to normal range.

VIII. **Hypocalcemia (calcium deficiency)**
  A. Description: serum calcium level below 8 mg/dL
  B. Etiology
    1. Primary or surgical hypoparathyroidism due to thyroidectomy
    2. Pancreatitis
    3. Inadequate vitamin D intake or synthesis
    4. Renal failure
    5. Drug therapy (e.g., aminoglycosides, corticosteroids, caffeine)
    6. Insufficient calcium intake
  C. Assessment findings
    1. Clinical manifestations may include:
      a. Tetany (tingling in fingers and circumoral area; muscle spasms associated with pain in extremities and face)
      b. Positive Trousseau's sign and Chvostek's sign
      c. Seizures due to neuromuscular irritability
    2. Laboratory and diagnostic studies may reveal:
      a. Serum calcium level above 8.5 mg/dL
      b. EKG changes: prolonged Q–T interval
  D. Nursing diagnoses
    1. High Risk for Injury
    2. Pain
  E. Planning and implementation
    1. Institute and maintain seizure precautions.
    2. Administer parenteral calcium, as ordered, taking precautions to prevent tissue infiltration, which can lead to tissue necrosis and sloughing.
    3. Do not add calcium to parenteral solutions containing bicarbonate or phosphorus; this will cause precipitate formation.
    4. Administer calcium cautiously to a patient receiving digitalis; calcium potentiates the action of digitalis, increasing the risk of cardiac arrest.
    5. Maintain a relaxed, quiet environment, and promote adequate rest.
  F. Evaluation
    1. The patient exhibits no tissue necrosis from IV calcium therapy.
    2. The patient reports reduced pain from muscle spasms.
    3. The patient exhibits no signs of seizure activity.
    4. Serum calcium level returns to normal range.

IX. **Hypercalcemia (calcium excess)**
  A. Description: serum calcium level above 10.5 mg/dL
  B. Etiology
    1. Excessive calcium administration or intake
    2. Movement of calcium from bones to serum, as occurs in prolonged immobilization and malignant neoplastic diseases

      3. Decreased renal excretion due to renal failure

      4. Drug therapy with thiazide diuretics

      5. Hyperparathyroidism

C. Assessment findings

      1. Common clinical manifestations include:

          a. Anorexia

          b. Nausea and vomiting

          c. Constipation

          d. Altered level of consciousness: slurred speech, confusion, lethargy, coma

      2. Laboratory and diagnostic tests may reveal:

          a. Serum calcium level above 10.5 mg/dL

          b. EKG changes: shortened Q–T interval

D. Nursing diagnoses

      1. Constipation

      2. High Risk for Injury

      3. Knowledge Deficit

E. Planning and implementation

      1. Provide patient teaching on the causes and treatment of hypercalcemia, covering:

          a. The importance of early ambulation to reduce calcium loss from bones during hospitalization

          b. The need for daily weight-bearing activities

      2. Encourage adequate fluid intake and dietary fiber intake.

      3. Take injury prevention measures, such as:

          a. Keeping bed side rails up

          b. Keeping bed brakes locked

          c. Repositioning often

          d. Securing all invasive lines

      4. Treat the underlying cause, as ordered; therapies may include:

          a. Calcitonin for hyperparathyroidism

          b. Mithramycin and corticosteroids for malignancies

      5. Administer parenteral saline solution, as prescribed, to dilute serum calcium and inhibit tubular reabsorption of calcium.

      6. Administer parenteral phosphate, as prescribed, to enhance deposition of calcium.

F. Evaluation

      1. The patient remains injury-free.

      2. The patient demonstrates normal bowel elimination patterns.

      3. The patient verbalizes understanding of hypercalcemia and preventive measures.

      4. Serum calcium level returns to normal range.

X. Hypomagnesemia (magnesium deficiency)

  A. Description: serum magnesium level below 1.5 mEq/L

  B. Etiology

      1. Poor nutrition

2. Alcoholism
3. GI and renal losses without replacement

C. Assessment findings
1. Common clinical manifestations include:
   a. Positive Trousseau's and Chvostek's signs
   b. Tetany
   c. Facial twitching, jerking
   d. Tachycardia
   e. Hypotension
2. Symptoms typically don't occur until serum magnesium level drops below 1 mEq/L.
3. Laboratory and diagnostic tests reveal:
   a. Serum magnesium level below 1.5 mEq/L
   b. ECG changes: flattened T wave, prominent U wave, depressed ST segment

D. Nursing diagnoses
1. High Risk for Injury
2. Knowledge Deficit
3. Pain
4. Altered Tissue Perfusion: Cardiopulmonary

E. Planning and implementation
1. Teach the patient dietary sources of magnesium, including nuts, whole grains, cornmeal, spinach, bananas, and oranges; encourage increased intake of these foods.
2. Administer parenteral magnesium replacement therapy as prescribed.
3. Monitor for signs of magnesium toxicity, including:
   a. Hot, flushed skin
   b. Diaphoresis
   c. Anxiety or lethargy
   d. Hypotension
4. Institute and maintain seizure precautions.
5. Monitor ECG and pulse for abnormalities.

F. Evaluation
1. The patient remains injury-free.
2. The patient displays normal cardiac rate and rhythm.
3. The patient verbalizes knowledge of potassium-rich foods.
4. Serum magnesium level returns to normal range.

XI. Hypermagnesemia (magnesium excess)

A. Description: serum magnesium level above 2.5 mEq/L

B. Etiology
1. Renal failure
2. Overuse of magnesium-containing antacids
3. Excessive magnesium administration
4. Repeated enemas with Epsom salts (containing magnesium)

5. Severe dehydration, such as occurs in diabetic ketoacidosis

C. **Assessment findings**
   1. Clinical manifestations may include:
      a. Hot, flushed skin
      b. Diaphoresis
      c. Hypotension
      d. Lethargy, drowsiness, absent deep tendon reflexes with increasing magnesium level
      e. Possible progression to coma and cardiac arrest
   2. Laboratory studies reveal serum magnesium level above 2.5 mEq/L.

D. **Nursing diagnoses**
   1. High Risk for Injury
   2. Knowledge Deficit
   3. Altered Tissue Perfusion: Cardiopulmonary

E. **Planning and implementation**
   1. Teach the patient about the adverse effects associated with overuse of magnesium-containing antacids and cathartics.
   2. Instruct the patient to read all over-the-counter drug labels carefully for magnesium content.
   3. Monitor cardiovascular status closely.
   4. Institute safety precautions, such as:
      a. Keeping bed side rails up
      b. Keeping bed brakes locked
      c. Repositioning often

F. **Evaluation**
   1. The patient verbalizes understanding of the adverse effects associated with magnesium overdose.
   2. The patient remains injury-free.
   3. The patient exhibits normal cardiac rate and rhythm.
   4. Serum magnesium level returns to normal range.

XII. **Metabolic acidosis**
   A. **Description: an acid–base imbalance resulting from excessive absorption or retention of acid or excessive excretion of bicarbonate (HCO_3)**
   B. **Etiology**
      1. Ketoacidosis
      2. Lactic acidosis
      3. Prolonged fasting
      4. Salicylic poisoning
      5. Oliguric renal disease
      6. Abnormal HCO_3 losses, such as can occur in severe diarrhea
   C. **Assessment findings**
      1. Common clinical manifestations include:
         a. Headache

> b.   Drowsiness, confusion
> c.   Weakness
> d.   Increased respiratory rate and depth

2.   Laboratory and diagnostic studies typically reveal:
>   a.   Abnormal arterial blood gas (ABG) values: pH below 7.35 and HCO_3 below 22 mEq/L
>   b.   Diminished cardiac output with pH below 7
>   c.   Possible hyperkalemia

D.   Nursing diagnoses
1.   High Risk for Injury
2.   Altered Tissue Perfusion: Cardiopulmonary

E.   Planning and implementation
1.   Monitor cardiovascular status closely, noting:
>   a.   Blood pressure
>   b.   Pulse rate and rhythm
>   c.   Capillary refill
>   d.   Warmth and color of extremities

2.   Institute safety precautions, such as:
>   a.   Keeping bed side rails up
>   b.   Keeping bed brakes locked
>   c.   Securing all invasive lines properly

F.   Evaluation
1.   The patient remains injury-free.
2.   The patient exhibits adequate tissue perfusion, as evidenced by warm, dry, and normal-colored skin.
3.   Vital signs remain within normal ranges.
4.   ABG values return to normal ranges.

XIII.   Metabolic alkalosis

A.   Description: an acid–base imbalance characterized by excessive loss of acid or excessive gain of HCO_3

B.   Etiology
1.   Loss of hydrogen and chloride ions due to prolonged vomiting or gastric suctioning (most common cause)
2.   Excessive intake of alkali, as in antacids or baking soda

C.   Assessment findings
1.   Clinical manifestations may include:
>   a.   Belligerence, confusion
>   b.   Tetany
>   c.   Slow, shallow respirations; possibly apnea

2.   Laboratory study results include:
>   a.   ABGs: pH above 7.45 and HCO_3 above 26 mEq/L
>   b.   Hypokalemia

D.   Nursing diagnoses
1.   Ineffective Breathing Patterns
2.   High Risk for Injury

E. **Planning and implementation**
  1. Institute safety precautions, such as:
     a. Keeping bed side rails up
     b. Keeping bed brakes locked
     c. Securing all invasive lines properly
  2. Monitor respiratory rate and pattern, lung sounds, skin color, and mental status.
  3. Provide treatment to correct the underlying cause as ordered.
  4. Promote adequate hydration.
  5. Correct electrolyte deficits, particularly of potassium and sodium, as ordered.

F. **Evaluation**
  1. The patient remains injury-free.
  2. The patient's lungs are clear on auscultation.
  3. Respiratory rate and pattern are within normal ranges.
  4. ABG values return to normal ranges.

XIV. **Respiratory acidosis**
  A. **Description: an acid–base imbalance characterized by increased arterial PCO_2 and decreased blood pH**
  B. **Etiology**
  1. Chronic obstructive respiratory disorders, such as bronchial asthma and emphysema
  2. Acute disorders such as chest wall trauma, pulmonary edema, atelectasis, pneumothorax, drug overdoses, pneumonia, and Guillian-Barre syndrome
  C. **Assessment findings**
  1. Clinical manifestations may include:
     a. Dyspnea, wheezing, tachypnea
     b. Tachycardia
     c. Disorientation
  2. Laboratory studies reveal ABG abnormalities: pH below 7.35 and PCO_2 above 42 mmHg.
  D. **Nursing diagnoses**
  1. Activity Intolerance
  2. Ineffective Breathing Pattern
  3. Altered Tissue Perfusion: Cardiopulmonary
  E. **Planning and implementation**
  1. Monitor ABG values.
  2. Administer low-flow oxygen therapy to a patient with chronic PCO_2 above 50 mmHg; assess for adequacy of delivery.
  3. Position the patient in semi-Fowler's or another comfortable position to ease the work of breathing.
  4. Improve ventilation with bronchodilators; postural drainage; antibiotic therapy to treat infection; regular coughing, turning, and deep breathing; and mechanical ventilation as appropriate.

5. Maintain a quiet, relaxing environment; cluster activities to allow for periods of uninterrupted rest.
6. Keep needed items within the patient's reach.
7. Monitor cardiovascular status, noting:
    a. Blood pressure
    b. Pulse rate and rhythm
    c. Capillary refill
    d. Warmth and color of extremities
8. Maintain fluid and electrolyte balance.
9. Intervene to correct the underlying cause.

F. Evaluation
1. The patient displays normal respiratory rate and pattern.
2. The patient exhibits adequate tissue perfusion, as evidenced by stable vital signs and warm, dry, and normal-colored skin.
3. The patient reports no dyspnea on activity.
4. ABG values return to normal ranges.

XV. Respiratory alkalosis

A. Description: an acid–base imbalance characterized by decreased arterial PCO_2 and increased blood pH

B. Etiology
1. Most commonly, hyperventilation due to anxiety, hypoxia, improper mechanical ventilation
2. Fever
3. Salicylate poisoning

C. Assessment findings
1. Common clinical manifestations include:
    a. Lightheadedness
    b. Inability to concentrate
    c. Convulsions
    d. Positive Chvostek's sign
    e. Muscle twitching
2. Laboratory studies reveal ABG abnormalities: pH above 7.45 and PCO_2 below 38 mmHg.

D. Nursing diagnoses
1. Ineffective Breathing Patterns
2. High Risk for Injury

E. Planning and implementation
1. Monitor ABG values and respiratory rate and pattern.
2. Institute and maintain seizure precautions as necessary.
3. Assess sources of anxiety and intervene to help reduce anxiety.
4. Encourage slow, deep breathing; instruct the patient to breathe into and out of a paper bag, if necessary, to reverse hyperventilation.
5. Assist the patient with activities as necessary.

F.   Evaluation
1.   The patient remains injury-free.
2.   The patient demonstrates normal respiratory rate and pattern.
3.   ABG values return to normal ranges.

Bibliography

Brunner, L. S., & Suddarth, D. S. (1988). *Textbook of medical-surgical nursing* (6th ed.). Philadelphia: J. B. Lippincott.

Cotran, R. S., Kumar, V., & Robbins, S. L. (1989). *Robbins pathologic basis of disease* (3rd ed.). Philadelphia: W. B. Saunders.

Guyton, A. C. (1986). *Human physiology and mechanisms of disease* (3rd ed.). Philadelphia: W. B. Saunders.

Luckmann, J., and Sorenson, K. C. (1987). *Medical-surgical nursing: A psychophysiological approach* (3rd ed.). Philadelphia: W. B. Saunders.

Sodeman, W. A., & Sodeman, T. M. (1985). *Sodeman's pathologic physiologic mechanisms of disease* (7th ed.). Philadelphia: W. B. Saunders.

STUDY QUESTIONS

1. Ms. Bledsoe, aged 20, is admitted with seizure activity. Her electrolyte values are as follows: Na, 115 mEq/L; K, 3.0 mEq/L; Ca, 8.0 mg/dL; and Mg, 1.0 mEq/L. Which imbalances must be controlled to reduce her seizure activity?
   a. K and Ca
   b. Na and Ca
   c. Na and K
   d. Mg and K

2. Mr. Henry is admitted with altered level of consciousness. Laboratory results show pH, 7.28; PCO_2, 20 mmHg; PO_2, 65 mmHg; and HCO_3, 18 mEq/L. The most appropriate nursing diagnoses for this patient likely would be
   a. Pain
   b. Fluid Volume Excess
   c. Ineffective Breathing Pattern
   d. Ineffective Thermoregulation

3. Laboratory data on Mr. Johnson show serum Na, 128 mEq/L and K, 3.0 mEq/L. The nurse would evaluate this patient's progress based on resolution of which of the following complications?
   a. The patient exhibits decreased diuresis.
   b. The patient's urine output increases to normal level.
   c. The patient demonstrates reduced GI fluid loss.
   d. The patient exhibits resolution of diabetic ketoacidosis.

4. Which of the following homeostatic mechanisms help regulate fluid, electrolyte, and acid–base balance?
   a. cardiovascular system
   b. pituitary gland
   c. chemical buffers
   d. renal system

5. Mr. Jones has a history of COPD; laboratory tests reveal the following ABG values: PO_2, 55 mmHg and PCO_2, 60 mmHg. When attempting to improve Mr. Jones's blood gas values through improved ventilation and oxygen therapy, the nurse should understand that this patient's primary stimulus for breathing is:
   a. high PCO_2
   b. low PO_2
   c. normal pH
   d. low PCO_2

6. Evaluation of successful resolution of a fluid volume deficit may be demonstrated by which of the following?
   a. The patient demonstrates an absence of postural hypotension and tachycardia.
   b. The patient adheres to prescribed dietary sodium restrictions.
   c. The patient maintains weight loss.
   d. The patient maintains a serum sodium level above 145 mEq/L.

7. When planning care for a patient with hypocalcemia, the nurse should consider
   a. the effects of hypoirritability, such as coma
   b. the effects of hyperirritability, such as tetany
   c. the effects of bedrest
   d. the effects of certain medications (e.g., antacids and cathartics)

8. Ms. Stone is admitted with a serum calcium deficit. Assessment reveals positive Trousseau's and Chvostek's signs and irritability. Because hypocalcemia can lead to both physiologic and psychologic problems, which of the following nursing diagnoses would be most appropriate for Ms. Stone?
   a. Fear related to increased neuromuscular irritability, laryngospasm, and impending tetany
   b. High Risk for Injury related to fractures secondary to loss of calcium from bone matrix
   c. Fluid Volume Deficit related to dehydration
   d. Activity Intolerance related to skeletal muscle weakness and flaccid paralysis

9. When administering intravenous elec-

trolyte solution, the nurse should take which of the following precautions?

a. Infuse hypertonic solutions rapidly.

b. Mix no more than 80 mEq of potassium per liter of fluid.

c. Prevent infiltration of calcium, which will cause tissue necrosis and sloughing.

d. As appropriate, reevaluate the patient's digitalis dosage; he or she may need an increased dosage since IV calcium diminishes digitalis' action.

10. Teaching about the need to avoid foods high in potassium would be most important for which patient?

a. a patient receiving diuretic therapy

b. a patient with an ileostomy

c. a patient with metabolic alkalosis

d. a patient with renal disease

11. What do the following ABG values— pH, 7.38; PO_2, 78 mmHg; PCO_2, 36 mmHg; HCO_3, 24 mEq/L—indicate?

a. metabolic alkalosis

b. homeostasis

c. respiratory acidosis

d. respiratory alkalosis

12. The major electrolytes in the intracellular fluid are

a. potassium and chloride

b. potassium and phosphate

c. sodium and chloride

d. sodium and phosphate

13. Which physiologic mechanism best describes the function of the sodium–potassium pump

a. active transport

b. diffusion

c. filtration

d. osmosis

14. Laboratory tests reveal the following electrolyte values for Mr. Pomeray: Na, 135 mEq/L; Ca, 8.5 mg/dL; Cl, 102 mEq/L; K, 2.0 mEq/L. Which of these values should the nurse report to the physician because of its potential risk to the patient?

a. Ca

b. K

c. Na

d. Cl

15. A patient receiving drug therapy with furosemide (Lasix) and digitalis requires careful observation and care. In planning care for this patient, the nurse should recognize that one of the following electrolyte imbalances would be most likely to occur, requiring nursing intervention. Which one?

a. hyperkalemia

b. hypernatremia

c. hypokalemia

d. hypomagnesemia

16. Ms. Brown, aged 82, has a history of congestive heart failure, for which she receives periodic home health care. She is very independent and wants to take care of her own home as much as possible. However, recently she has experienced increased problems with fluid retention, and she was admitted to the hospital this morning with dyspnea and marked dependent edema. The nurse finds Ms. Brown crying, saying that she can't even walk across the room to go to the bathroom by herself. Based on this situation, all the following nursing diagnoses would be appropriate for identifying Ms. Brown's needs *except*

a. Powerlessness

b. Fear

c. Impaired Home Maintenance Management

d. Dysfunctional Grieving

ANSWER KEY

1. **Correct response: b**
   Hyponatremia, hypomagnesemia, and hypocalcemia all may result in neuromuscular irritability with seizure activity.
   a, c, and d. Hypokalemia commonly produces dysrhythmias, weakness, and anorexia but is not associated with seizure activity.
   Application/Health promotion/ Implementation

2. **Correct response: c**
   This patient is in partially compensated metabolic acidosis. (A pH below 7.35 indicates acidosis.) Alteration in PCO_2 points to the regulatory mechanism of acid–base balance—the lungs. Decreased HCO_3 supports metabolic acidosis; decreased PCO_2 supports attempts to compensate. Kussmaul's respirations would be a classic response to metabolic acidosis.
   a, b, and d. These diagnoses would not be expected with metabolic acidosis.
   Application/Physiologic/Analysis (Dx)

3. **Correct response: c**
   Decreased Na and K levels can result from GI fluid loss, as occurs with diarrhea and vomiting. This can lead to cardiac dysrhythmias.
   a and b. Increased fluid output would increase serum Na level.
   d. Decreased renal excretion and acidosis would increase serum K level.
   Analysis/Physiologic/Evaluation

4. **Correct response: d**
   Homeostatic mechanisms common to fluid, electrolyte, and acid–base balance are the kidneys and lungs.
   a and b. Cardiovascular and pituitary mechanisms are involved in fluid and electrolyte balance only.

   c. Chemical buffers are specific to acid–base balance.
   Application/Physiologic/Assessment

5. **Correct response: a**
   Chronically elevated PCO_2 (above 50 mmHg) is associated with inadequate response of the respiratory center to plasma CO_2. The major stimulus to breathing then becomes hypoxia.
   b, c, and d. These blood gas parameters would not be primary stimuli for breathing in this patient.
   Analysis/Safe care/Implementation

6. **Correct response: a**
   This patient would exhibit signs of adequate hydration such as stable blood pressure and pulse.
   b and c. Sodium restrictions would apply if the patient exhibited fluid volume excess, as would weight loss.
   d. Serum sodium level above 145 mEq/L would indicate hypernatremia.
   Analysis/Health promotion/Evaluation

7. **Correct response: b**
   Hyperirritability, such as tetany, is associated with hypocalcemia.
   a. In contrast, hypercalcemia may result in mental status changes, such as lethargy and coma.
   c. Prolonged bedrest is associated with calcium loss from bones in hypercalcemia.
   d. Antacid and cathartic use may potentiate hypermagnesemia.
   Comprehension/Safe care/Planning

8. **Correct response: a**
   Fear is an appropriate diagnoses to describe a typical response on painful tonic muscle spasms and laryngospasms.
   b. The loss of calcium from bone is a consequence of hypercalcemia.
   c. Dehydration commonly results from hypermagnesemia.

    d. Muscle weakness and flaccid paralysis can result from hyperkalemia.

Application/Psychosocial/Analysis (Dx)

9. *Correct response: c*
Preventing tissue infiltration is necessary to avoid skin damage.
    a. Hypertonic solutions should be infused cautiously.
    b. Potassium should be mixed at a concentration no higher than 60 mEq/L.
    d. Calcium (particularly intravenous) potentiates the action of digitalis.

Application/Safe care/Implementation

10. *Correct response: d*
Patients with renal disease are predisposed to hyperkalemia and thus should avoid foods high in potassium.
    a, b, and c. Patients receiving diuretics, with ileostomies, or with metabolic alkalosis all may be hypokalemic and thus should be encouraged to eat foods high in potassium.

Analysis/Health promotion/Planning

11. *Correct response: b*
These ABG values are within normal limits.
    a, c, and d. These ABG values indicate non of these acid–base disturbances.

Analysis/Physiologic/Evaluation

12. *Correct response: c*
Sodium and chloride are the major electrolytes in the extracellular fluid.

Knowledge/Physiologic/Assessment

13. *Correct response: a*
Active transport is a process requiring energy to transport ions against a concentration gradient, as is needed in the sodium–potassium pump.
    b, c, and d. Diffusion, filtration, and osmosis are other regulatory mechanisms involved in fluid and electrolyte balance.

Knowledge/Physiologic/Assessment

14. *Correct response: b*
Normal serum potassium level ranges between 3.5 and 5.5 mEq/L.
    a, c, and d. These Na, Ca, and Cl levels are within normal ranges.

Comprehension/Safe care/Implementation

15. *Correct response: c*
Diuretics such as furosemide may deplete serum potassium. Additionally, the action of digitalis may be potentiated by hypokalemia.
    a. These drugs are not associated with hyperkalemia.
    b. Diuretic therapy could cause hyponatremia, not hypernatremia.
    d. Hypomagnesemia generally is associated with poor nutrition, alcoholism, and excessive GI or renal losses.

Comprehension/Health promotion/Planning

16. *Correct response: d*
No evidence indicates that Ms. Brown is dysfunctional because of grief. Rather, her physiologic response to fluid retention impairs her ability to go to the bathroom.
    a, b, and c. These nursing diagnoses all reflect normal responses to the situation and Ms. Brown's need for independence.

Application/Psychosocial/Analysis (Dx)

Pain

5

I. Anatomy and physiology of pain

A. Peripheral nervous system

1. The peripheral nervous system, including spinal and cranial nerves, carries pain impulses to and from the central nervous system (CNS).
   a. Afferent nerve fibers carry impulses to the CNS.
   b. Efferent nerve fibers carry impulses from the CNS.
2. Nerve receptors on the skin surface specific for pain are known as nociceptors.
3. Different types of afferent nerve fibers conduct impulses from nociceptors to the spinal cord:
   a. A-alpha, A-beta, and A-gamma fibers (myelinated) transmit touch, pressure, heat, cold and movement impulses at speeds of up to 120 m/sec.
   b. A-delta fibers (myelinated) transmit sharp, piercing pain impulses at 30 to 60 m/sec.
   c. Type C fibers (unmyelinated) transmit aching and burning pain at 0.5 to 2 m/sec and account for more than two thirds of all fibers in the peripheral nervous system.

B. **Autonomic nervous system**
   1. The nervous system branch regulating involuntary vital functions, the autonomic nervous system comprises sympathetic and parasympathetic divisions.
   2. This system also contains two types of neurotransmitters—chemicals that modify or enable transmission of nerve impulses between synapses.
   3. Cholinergic neurotransmitters include acetylcholine.
   4. Adrenergic neurotransmitters include:
      a. Epinephrine
      b. Norepinephrine
      c. Dopamine
      d. Serotonin
   5. Sympathetic nervous system functions include:
      a. Fight, flight, or freeze response to alarm or stress (e.g., pain)
      b. Whole person response, which helps cope with stress by mobilizing defenses
      c. Control of the adrenal medullae, sweat glands, blood vessels, and piloerector muscles in hair
   6. Parasympathetic nervous system functions include:
      a. Exhaustion or shock response with intense or prolonged stress (pain); triggered when sympathetic system no longer functions
      b. Specific organ responses
      c. Control of many body functions, such as digestion and elimination

C. **Central nervous system**
   1. The CNS comprises the spinal cord and the brain.
   2. The spinal cord transmits painful stimuli to the brain and motor responses and pain perception to the periphery.
   3. The brain processes and interprets transmitted pain impulses.
   4. Spinal cord pathways (nerve tracts) consist of:
      a. Afferent tracts to the brain
      b. Efferent tracts from the brain
   5. In the substantia gelatinosa (SG), located in lamina II of the spinal cord's dorsal horn, fibers carrying information about pain from the periphery converge with large fibers and synapse with T cells and fibers from the brain that carry pain inhibitory information.
   6. The midbrain contains many centers for control, association, and relay of impulses, including:
      a. Reticular formation
      b. Medulla
      c. Hypothalamus: center for brain opiates
      d. Thalamus: relay station and center for perception of pain

  e. Limbic system: center for emotion, responses to environment
7. In the sensory cortex, tactile sensory impulses from periphery are interpreted and understood.
8. The motor cortex initiates motor responses to information reaching the sensory cortex.
9. The frontal lobes contain areas for:
  a. Attention (an essential component of the pain experience)
  b. Memory
  c. Cognition
  d. Emotion
  e. Decision making

D. **Physiology of pain**
 1. Various models and theories of pain transmission and perception have been promulgated.
 2. Gate control model
  a. Nerve fibers carry touch and pain impulses from receptors on the skin to the spinal cord.
  b. Nerve cells in the SG of the spinal cord receive these touch and pain impulses.
  c. Impulses then proceed through transmission cells (T cells) to the brain.
  d. Increased input over large fibers (A-alpha, A-beta, and A-gamma) inhibits some pain impulses over smaller fibers (A-delta and Type C fibers); thus, fewer pain impulses reach T cells for transmission to the brain.
  e. Decreased input over large fibers allows more pain impulses to reach T cells.
  f. Fibers from the brain send inhibiting information to the SG, which serves as a gate for control of pain.
 3. Central control theory of pain
  a. Some neuropeptides (e.g., substance P) present in the SG seem to be pain-specific neurotransmittors that facilitate pain transmission.
  b. Endogenous molecular neuropeptides called brain opiates (endorphins, enkephalins and others) are opiumlike compounds that have profound analgesic properties.
  c. Specific neuroceptors bind with morphine and brain opiates.
  d. Certain events or situations cause release of brain opiates (e.g., cutaneous stimulation such as massage, electrical stimulation, pain itself, tissue injury, placebos, acupuncture, transcutaneous electric nerve stimulation [TENS]).
 4. *Note:* The gate control model and the central control theory overlap somewhat in current thought; although the central control theory is now the most universally accepted, both are useful.

5. Specificity theory
   a. This theory posits that pain originates in specific pain receptors, not in free nerve endings.
   b. This theory does not explain pain modulation by variables such as social and cultural factors.
   c. It also does not account for pain syndromes such as causalgia and phantom pain.
6. Pattern theory
   a. This theory has been proposed because of the inadequacies of the specificity theory.
   b. However, it does not explain psychologic factors related to pain.
7. Psychologic theories
   a. In many cases, pain results from emotion, hostility, guilt, or depression.
   b. Persons with pain-prone personalities use pain as means to communicate.
   c. According to the psychogenic theory, pain arises from a perceived threat to self.

II. Overview of pain

A. Description

1. Characteristics of the pain experience include:
   a. Subjective and personal; exists wherever and whenever a patient says it does
   b. A physiologic hurt, sometimes broadened to encompass emotional hurts
   c. A symptom, not a disease entity
   d. A valuable diagnostic indicator; usually, but not always, indicative of tissue damage or pathology
   e. Usually considered unpleasant or distressing
2. Components of pain include:
   a. Stimulus; may be mechanical, chemical, thermal, or mental
   b. Sensation of hurt; relies on intact reception, transmission, perception, and interpretation
   c. Reaction: musculoskeletal, autonomic, psychologic responses
3. An intact nervous system is essential to the sensation of and reaction to pain.
4. Phases of the pain experience include:
   a. Anticipation of pain: Fear and anxiety affect a person's response to sensation.
   b. Sensation of pain: Affected by how anticipation was managed; pain increases anxiety, which in turn increases pain.
   c. Aftermath of pain: The most neglected phase; response

may indicate fear, embarrassment, or guilt, all of which can affect future experiences with pain.

5. Pain can have certain beneficial effects, including acting as a warning sign of injury and signaling the need for treatment.

6. Detrimental effects of pain include:

   a. Poses a threat to basic needs: interferes with meeting food, fluid, and sleep needs; affects elimination; interferes with breathing and meeting oxygen needs; limits mobility and leads to impaired skin integrity and altered ability for self care

   b. Poses a threat to higher-level needs: interferes with relationships with significant others, communication, sexuality, social involvement, job performance; causes spiritual distress and potential for violence

   c. Delays rehabilitation: Pain itself may become the disability.

B. Types of pain

1. *Acute pain* can be described as:

   a. Rapid onset

   b. Usually temporary, lasting no more than 6 months

   c. Subsides spontaneously, with or without treatment

2. Characteristics of *chronic pain* include:

   a. Gradual onset

   b. Persists longer than 6 months

   c. May recur at intervals

   d. Serves no useful purpose

   e. May become a major complication

3. *Cutaneous and superficial pain* involves:

   a. Abrupt onset

   b. Sharp, stinging quality

4. *Deep pain* is marked by:

   a. Somatic pain from organs in any body cavity

   b. Slower onset

   c. Burning quality

   d. Diffuse and radiating

   e. Possibly causing nausea and vomiting

5. *Referred pain* is pain at one site perceived in another following dermatome and nerve root patterns.

6. *Phantom pain* may follow amputation or mastectomy; the patient feels pain as if it were in the absent part.

7. *Intractable pain* refers to moderate to severe pain that cannot be relieved by any known treatment.

C. Etiology of pain

1. Pain commonly results from an injury or pathology; other physiologic factors may contribute. Common causes include:

   a. Musculoskeletal disorder caused by spasm, rupture, ischemia, or stretching

b. Visceral disorders
c. Cancer
d. Vascular disorders (caused by cold, pulling, displacement, or distention)
e. Inflammation
f. Contagious disease
g. Trauma (surgical or accidental)
h. Diagnostic tests (e.g., biopsy, venipuncture, invasive scanning)
i. Unmet basic needs (e.g., flatus following abdominal surgery)
j. Necessary nursing interventions (e.g., ambulation or coughing after surgery)
k. Pregnancy, labor, and delivery
l. Chemical irritants (e.g., release of histamine, bradykinin, prostaglandins, and leukokinins)
m. Allergic responses
n. Neuralgia, as follows herpes zoster due to scarring and degenerative changes in nerves
o. Causalgia, as follows peripheral nerve injury

2. Pain also may arise from or be augmented by psychologic or emotional factors. Stress or emotion may produce observable physiologic changes (e.g., chronic excessive muscle contractions).

3. Psychologic factors that can cause a person to interpret pain as more severe or less severe include:
    a. Isolation
    b. Anxiety
    c. Fear
    d. Anticipation of pain

4. A person's past experiences with pain influence the meaning he or she attaches to the pain experience and affects his or her expectations of the health care team.

5. Social factors that can affect pain perception include:
    a. Group status
    b. State of involvement at time of pain episode (e.g., an injury sustained during a sporting event may not be perceived as significant until after the event is over)
    c. Role changes in family and social groups

6. Economic factors that can contribute to pain perception include:
    a. Threat to job or work role
    b. Cost of treatment
    c. Cost of caregiver or care for family

7. Cultural factors influencing pain perception may include:
    a. Whether the person's culture encourages or discourages expression of pain
    b. Whether or not the culture teaches that suffering can serve

some higher purpose (such as spiritual cleansing or a test of faith)

   c.   The culture's view of the role of the health care system and of health care providers

D. Responses to pain

   1.   Sympathetic nervous system responses occur with pain of low to moderate intensity or with severe superficial pain of short duration; these responses may include:

      a.   Skin: pallor, coldness, clamminess

      b.   Vital signs: elevated blood pressure, pulse rate, and respiratory rate

      c.   Diaphoresis

      d.   Dilated pupils

   2.   Parasympathetic nervous system responses occur with pain of severe intensity and long duration or deep pain; these may include:

      a.   Skin: pallor

      b.   Vital signs: decreased blood pressure and pulse rate

      c.   Nausea and vomiting

      d.   Weakness, fainting, prostration

      e.   Possible loss of consciousness

   3.   Behavioral and musculoskeletal responses include:

      a.   Reports of pain

      b.   Postures to splint, hold, or protect painful areas

      c.   Muscle spasms

      d.   Skeletal muscle rigidity

      e.   Reflex abnormalities

      f.   Grimacing, clenching of jaws or fists

      g.   Rapid blinking, squinting eyes, or darting glance

      h.   Drawn facial expression, twitching facial muscles

      i.   Moaning, sighing, crying

      j.   Restlessness

      k.   Immobility, becoming quiet and withdrawn when touched

      l.   Anorexia, nausea, and vomiting

   4.   Psychologic responses may include:

      a.   Fear

      b.   Anxiety

      c.   Anger or irritation

      d.   Depression

      e.   Inability to concentrate

      f.   Desire for extra attention from others

   5.   Some persons demonstrate atypical response patterns to pain; variations in adaptation depend on such factors as:

      a.   Personal perception of appropriate behavior

      b.   Ability for self-distraction

      c.   Attempts to adjust to prolonged pain

E. Pain medications

1. Narcotic analgesics (opiates), which act to depress the CNS and inhibit pain impulses, include:
   a. Morphine
   b. Codeine
   c. Meperidine
   d. Pentazocine
   e. Oxycodone
2. Nonnarcotic analgesics, used to produce analgesia, reduce fever (antipyretic), or reduce inflammation (antiinflammatory), include:
   a. Aspirin (salicylate): analgesic, antipyretic, and antiinflammatory
   b. Acetaminophen: analgesic and antipyretic, not antiinflammatory
   c. Phenacetin: analgesic and antipyretic, not antiinflammatory
   d. Propoxyphene: analgesic, not antipyretic or antiinflammatory
3. Skeletal muscle relaxants, used to relieve muscle spasm and spasticity causing pain, include:
   a. Benzodiazepine
   b. Cyclobenzaprine
   c. Methocarbamol
   d. Dantrolene
4. Antiinfective drugs, used to reduce fever or heat, swelling, and inflammation associated with infection, thus reducing pain stimuli, include:
   a. Penicillins
   b. Cephalosporins
   c. Sulfonamides
   d. Urinary tract antiseptics
   e. Tetracyclines
   f. Aminoglycosides
5. Minor tranquilizers, used to reduce stress and anxiety and thus reduce interpretation of pain, include:
   a. Hydroxyzine
   b. Diazepam
6. For cardiac pain (i.e., angina), sublingual nitroglycerin (a fast-acting nitrate) usually is prescribed.

III. Nursing care of a patient in pain

A. Assessment

1. Keep in mind that pain assessment depends mainly on subjective data; objective signs must be confirmed by the patient, except in certain cases when physiologic changes are obvious.

2. Ask the patient about the nature of the pain, including:
   a. Description (e.g., piercing, aching, shooting, burning, stinging, constant, intermittent, sharp, dull)
   b. Onset or time of occurrence: when it began, how often it occurs, what time of day it occurs
   c. Duration: how long it lasts, whether it is constant or intermittent
   d. Location: Have the patient describe or point to the area or areas. (*Note:* When documenting, use the patient's words and give the correct anatomic terms.)
   e. Intensity or severity: mild, moderate, severe, excruciating; have the patient rate the severity of pain on a scale of 1 to 10, with 1 representing the least pain and 10 the most severe pain; or on a color scale, with green representing the least pain and red the most severe
   f. Apparent or suspected cause
   g. Meaning of the pain to the patient
   h. Apparent or suspected precipitating, aggravating, or alleviating factors
3. Listen carefully to how the patient describes the pain and evaluate implied messages about pain.
4. Using all of your senses, observe:
   a. Nonverbal behavior
   b. The painful body part or area
   c. Unusual odors
   d. Position or posture
   e. Environment
   f. Relationships, if others are present
5. Palpate painful areas for:
   a. Heat
   b. Swelling
   c. Masses
6. Assess vital signs.

B. Nursing diagnoses
1. Pain
2. Chronic Pain
3. Associated nursing diagnoses reflecting aggravating factors or consequences of pain; for example:
   a. Activity Intolerance
   b. Ineffective Airway Clearance
   c. Anxiety
   d. Constipation
   e. Fear
   f. Fluid Volume Deficit
   g. High Risk for Injury
   h. Knowledge Deficit

      i.   Impaired Physical Mobility
      j.   Altered Nutrition: Less Than Body Requirements
      k.   Powerlessness
      l.   Altered Role Performance
      m.   Self-Care Deficit
      n.   Sleep Pattern Disturbance
      o.   Urinary Retention

C.   **Planning and implementation**

    1.   Intervene to alter the etiology or physiology of pain:

      a.   Prepare the patient for surgery if scheduled, to remove the cause of pain (e.g., tumor or infection).

      b.   Prepare the patient for radiation therapy, if scheduled, to reduce the size of a tumor and thus reduce pressure on nerves and organs.

      c.   Promote hypnosis if the patient or physician desires. (*Note:* Why hypnosis is effective for some patients remains unclear; it may stimulate brain opiates or produce a purely psychologic effect.)

      d.   Administer medication for pain as ordered.

      e.   As ordered, administer medication for other problems causing pain (e.g., infection, postsurgical flatus).

      f.   Relieve or prevent factors that aggravate pain (e.g., coughing, vomiting, diarrhea, constipation, bladder fullness, infection).

      g.   Reduce or remove noxious stimuli (e.g., cast, ace bandage, or weight; foreign body in eye; wrinkles in sheets; unsupported heavy bedding; excessive noise; too hot or too cold environment; overbright lights).

      h.   As ordered, provide nonpharmacologic pain relief interventions such as cutaneous stimulation, backrubs, biofeedback, acupuncture, transcutaneous electrical stimulation (TENS), dorsal column stimulation, counter irritation, and contralateral stimulation.

      i.   Encourage noninvasive pain management techniques such as guided imagery and relaxation.

      j.   Provide heat and cold application or menthol rubs as ordered; these methods may relieve swelling and may produce an anesthetizing effect.

      k.   Note any age-related effects on the patient's response to pain and medication administration, and adjust interventions accordingly.

      l.   Refer the patient to a pain center or pain clinic, as ordered, for more in-depth diagnosis and treatment of pain that does not respond to therapy.

      m.   Encourage activity or perform passive range-of-motion exercises. Mild activity or assisted activity, although painful, helps relieve stiffness of arthritic joints and sore muscles, thus eventually reducing pain; it may also increase endorphins.

n. Ensure proper body alignment and reposition regularly; although movement may hurt, repositioning and proper alignment relieves muscle strain and joint stiffness and helps relieves pain.

o. Provide distraction (e.g., with music, TV, radio, reading) to reduce focus on pain and increase other impulses, which may help block pain impulses.

p. Use behavior modification techniques as appropriate.

q. Involve family members to help them understand pain control and the patient's response and to enhance their ability to provide comfort and emotional support.

r. Involve other disciplines (e.g., clergy, social worker, counselor, occupational therapist) as necessary.

s. When performing painful procedures, work gently, swiftly, and skillfully to minimize the amount of pain generated and the time required.

t. Provide adequate rest for the patient or the painful body part.

2. Intervene to alter psychosocial, economic, and cultural factors influencing pain:

a. Explain all interventions, treatments, or symptoms that may frighten or worry the patient; anxiety or fear increase a patient's perception of the severity of pain.

b. Discuss with the patient what the pain means to him or her to help decrease the patient's concerns about the cause of pain (e.g., cancer or incurable disease).

c. Stay with the patient during pain episodes, and convey your empathy and concern; this can help decrease stress and anxiety and ease feelings of isolation and loneliness.

d. Establish a trusting relationship with the patient by keeping your promises and providing excellent physical care.

e. Promote the patient's sense of control and participation in pain control by allowing him or her to make choices regarding therapy, as appropriate, and (if applicable) by using patient-controlled analgesia (PCA).

f. When talking with the patient, avoid using words like "complain," "attack," and "victim," which imply helplessness and criticism and may interfere with pain control; instead, use more neutral or positive terms such as "explain," "episode," and "experience."

g. As ordered, administer medication to reduce stress and anxiety that may be contributing to pain.

h. Discuss with the patient the painful experience both before and after episodes to help decrease any fear or shame associated with perceived inability to cope with pain appropriately.

    i.   Discuss with the patient his or her previous experiences with pain, including how it was managed and how he or she wishes to manage this pain.

    j.   Discuss with the patient any situational factors that may be influencing the pain (e.g., loss of job, recent divorce, death in family, serious diagnosis); this may help decrease anxiety and assure him or her that others are there to help, which can combat feelings of isolation and loneliness.

    k.   As necessary, refer the patient to psychologic counseling, occupational therapy, and other resources to help him or her deal with psychosocial problems.

    l.   Teach the patient what he or she needs to learn to meet any knowledge deficit related to the pain or treatment.

D. Evaluation

  1. The patient reports reduced pain after pain relief interventions.

  2. The patient displays a change in responses to pain:

    a.   Sympathetic nervous system responses

    b.   Parasympathetic nervous system responses

    c.   Behavioral and musculoskeletal responses: verbal and nonverbal

    d.   Psychologic responses

Bibliography

Brunner, L., & Suddarth, D. (1988). *Textbook of medical-surgical nursing* (6th ed.). Philadelphia: J. B. Lippincott.

Brunner, L., & Suddarth, D. (1986). *The Lippincott manual of nursing practice* (4th ed.). Philadelphia: J. B. Lippincott.

Carpenito, L. J. (1987). *Handbook of nursing diagnosis* (2nd ed.). Philadelphia: J. B. Lippincott.

Guyton, A. C. (1986). *Textbook of medical physiology.* Philadelphia: W. B. Saunders.

Melzack, R. (1983). *Pain measurement and assessment.* New York: Raven Press.

STUDY QUESTIONS

1. Pain has both a physiologic and a psychosocial component. Assessment of a patient with rheumatoid arthritis reveals inflamed joints. The patient also exhibits difficulty concentrating and becomes quiet and withdrawn when touched. These assessment data reflect all the following responses *except*
   a. behavioral responses
   b. musculoskeletal responses
   c. psychologic responses
   d. sympathetic nervous system responses

2. Assessment of a patient with postoperative abdominal pain reveals no urinary output for 12 hours, with an IV intake of 1000 cc and a distended lower abdomen. Which of the following nursing diagnoses would be made 1 hour after analgesic administration?
   a. Pain related to abdominal surgery
   b. Fear related to urinary catheterization
   c. Pain related to pressure of a full bladder
   d. Anxiety related to past experiences with pain

3. Which of the following interventions should the nurse plan for a patient with arthritis who remains in bed too long because "It hurts to get started"?
   a. Tell the patient to absolutely limit movement of inflamed joints.
   b. Teach significant others to lift the patient into a wheelchair.
   c. Teach the patient the proper way of massaging inflamed joints.
   d. Administer aspirin, and tell the patient to gently perform range-of-motion exercises before rising.

4. Dan Baker, aged 20, is admitted following a motorcycle accident. He has a fractured right femur and spinal cord injuries and is unable to move either leg. Skeletal traction is applied to his right leg. When assessing Mr. Baker, the nurse notes elevated blood pressure and redness around the pain site although he doesn't complain of pain. Which of the following nursing diagnoses would be the most likely explanation for Mr. Baker's failure to report pain to the nurse?
   a. Ineffective Individual Coping
   b. Sensory and Perceptual Alteration: Tactile
   c. Unilateral Neglect
   d. Knowledge Deficit

5. Aaron, aged 5, has had six fractures since age 3 due to a rare bone disease. While riding his bike, he hits a bump and falls. Aaron grabs his leg and cries, "Oh my leg; it hurts. The pain is so sharp. I broke it again." Based on these data, the pain Aaron is experiencing most likely is caused by impulses traveling from receptors to the spinal cord along which type of nerve fibers?
   a. A-alpha
   b. Type C
   c. A-gamma
   d. A-delta

6. When Aaron is brought to the emergency department, he is holding his leg, rocking and crying, and grimacing. Nursing assessment also reveals parasympathetic nervous system responses to pain. Which of the following outcomes would indicate resolution of these responses?
   a. Aaron exhibits a rise in blood pressure and pulse rate within normal range.
   b. Aaron exhibits decreased blood pressure and pulse rate within normal range.
   c. Aaron demonstrates reduced skeletal muscle rigidity.
   d. Aaron exhibits reduced diaphoresis.

7. Of the various theories of pain, which provides the information most useful to the nurse in planning pain reduction interventions?
   a. central control theory

b. gate control theory
c. specificity theory
d. pattern theory

8. Joseph Clifford, aged 38, has extensive burns over much of his trunk and arms. He complains of intense pain during wound cleansing, dressing change, debridement, and physical therapy. This pain most likely is related to
   a. thermal stimulation
   b. mental stimulation
   c. mechanical stimulation
   d. chemical stimulation

9. Mr. Clifford dreads physical therapy and resists activity; he has difficulty sleeping due to pain and fatigue after the treatments. He lacks appetite for food or fluid. Based on this information, his *priority* nursing diagnosis would be
   a. Activity Intolerance related to pain secondary to burns
   b. Altered Nutrition: Less Than Body Requirements related to pain secondary to burns
   c. Sleep Pattern Disturbance related to pain secondary to burns
   d. Pain related to burns

10. Mr. Clifford continues to experience significant pain after his extensive burn wounds have healed—6 months after his injury. He also expresses concern over possible loss of job and disfigurement. At this stage, the nurse can most effectively intervene for his pain by
    a. referring him for counseling and occupational therapy
    b. staying with him as much as possible and building trust
    c. providing cutaneous stimulation and pharmacologic therapy
    d. providing distraction and guided imagery

11. Eventually, Mr. Clifford's chronic pain and anxiety about his appearance did contribute to his losing his job and disrupting his plans for marriage. He finally heeded the nurse's recommendation and sought treatment at a pain center, after which his pain subsided and he permitted his former fiancee to participate in his rehabilitation process, including looking for a new job. Evaluation criteria for Mr. Clifford's successful rehabilitation should include which of the following?
    a. The patient has no aftermath phase of his pain experience.
    b. The patient experiences decreased frequency of acute pain episodes.
    c. The patient continues normal growth and development with his support systems intact.
    d. The patient develops increased tolerance for severe pain in the future.

12. Which of the following statements regarding pain is *incorrect*?
    a. Intractable pain may not be relieved by treatment.
    b. Pain is an objective sign of a more serious problem.
    c. Psychologic factors can contribute to a patient's pain perception.
    d. Pain sensation is affected by a patient's anticipation of pain.

13. Billy Bragg, aged 5, received a small paper cut on his finger. His mother let him wash it and apply a small amount of bacitracin and a Band-aid. She then let him watch TV and eat an apple. Her interventions for pain are examples of:
    a. providing pharmacologic therapy
    b. providing control and distraction
    c. altering Billy's environment
    d. providing cutaneous stimulation

14. Which of the following represents the best rationale for using noninvasive and nonpharmacologic pain control measures in conjunction with other measures?
    a. These measures are more effective than analgesics.
    b. These measures decrease input to large fibers, reducing transmission of pain impulses to the CNS.
    c. These measures help potentiate the effects of analgesics.
    d. These measures help block transmission of impulses from Type C fibers.

15. Mrs. Brewster, aged 61, underwent a cholecystectomy at 2 PM. At 8 AM the next day, she denies pain, saying to the nurse "No ma'am, I'm all right." Her last analgesia was Demerol 75 mg at midnight. She lies in a fetal position, with eyes squinting, skin ashen, hair wet with perspiration, pupils dilated, and vital signs elevated. She does complain of nausea and vomits a small amount. Nursing health history reveals that she is from a very low socioeconomic group, has worked very hard throughout her life, and has had almost no experience with health care professionals. Based on these data, the nurse could conclude that Mrs. Brewster is experiencing all the following responses to pain *except*

   a. parasympathetic nervous system responses
   b. psychologic responses
   c. sympathetic nervous system responses
   d. behavioral and musculoskeletal responses

16. In evaluating a patient's adaptation to pain, which of the following behaviors would indicate appropriate adaptation?
   a. The patient is able to distract himself or herself during pain episodes.
   b. The patient denies pain.
   c. The patient reports no need for family support.
   d. The patient reports pain reduction with decreased activity.

ANSWER KEY

1. **Correct response: d**
   Difficulty concentrating is a psychologic response to pain; becoming quiet, a behavioral response; and withdrawing to touch, a musculoskeletal response.
   a, b, and c. A sympathetic nervous system response would be manifested by physiologic changes such as diaphoresis, pallor, and dilated pupils.
   Knowledge/Psychosocial/Assessment

2. **Correct response: c**
   Data reveal that the patient's bladder is probably full and causing pressure.
   a. Pain related to surgery should have been relieved by the analgesic.
   b and d. There are no data to support a diagnosis of fear or anxiety.
   Comprehension/Physiologic/Analysis (Dx)

3. **Correct response: d**
   Aspirin raises the pain threshold; although range-of-motion will hurt, mild exercise will relieve pain on rising.
   a. Limitation of motion will increase pain.
   b. Lifting the patient into a wheelchair will not increase mobility.
   c. Massaging will increase inflammation.
   Application/Health promotion/Planning

4. **Correct response: b**
   An intact nervous system is essential for a patient to experience or respond to pain. Even though evidence indicates that the patient should be experiencing pain, pain impulse transmission apparently is impaired because of the spinal cord injury.
   a and d. No evidence indicates that either knowledge deficit or poor coping would interfere with reporting the pain.
   c. Unilateral neglect would result from cerebral dysfunction leading to loss of recognition of one side of the body.
   Analysis/Safe care/Analysis (Dx)

5. **Correct response: d**
   Only A-delta fibers transmit sharp, piercing pain.
   a and c. A-alpha and A-gamma fibers transmit touch, pressure, heat, cold, and movement impulses.
   b. C fibers transmit aching and burning pain.
   Application/Physiologic/Assessment

6. **Correct response: a**
   Blood pressure and pulse rate decrease with parasympathetic involvement.
   b. Blood pressure and pulse rate increase with sympathetic involvement.
   c. Skeletal muscle rigidity is a musculoskeletal response.
   d. Diaphoresis indicates sympathetic involvement.
   Analysis/Physiologic/Evaluation

7. **Correct response: a**
   No one theory explains all the factors underlying the pain experience, but the central control theory discusses brain opiates with analgesic properties and how their release can be affected by actions initiated by the patient and caregivers.
   b, c, and d. These theories don't address pain control in the depth included in the central control theory.
   Knowledge/Health promotion/Planning

8. **Correct response: b**
   Even though the original data indicate that mental stimulation may contribute to the pain experience, it is the least likely cause of pain during treatment.
   a, c, and d. Thermal, mechanical, and chemical stimulation all contribute to the patient's pain in this case.
   Comprehension/Safe care/Analysis (Dx)

9. *Correct response: d*
   Pain is the cause of the other diagnoses; they could be resolved if pain could be prevented.
   a, b, and c. These diagnosis are all secondary to the primary diagnosis of pain.
   Application/Physiologic/Analysis (Dx)

10. *Correct response: a*
    Mr. Clifford needs professional help to get on with his life and handle the limitations he faces.
    b, c, and d. These interventions would have been more appropriate in earlier stages of postburn injury, when physical pain was most severe and fewer psychologic factors needed to be addressed.
    Analysis/Health promotion/Implementation

11. *Correct response: c*
    Even though the patient may experience an aftermath phase, he still can make progress and complete effective rehabilitation.
    a. Aftermath may occur but need not interfere with rehabilitation.
    b. Acute pain would not be expected at this stage of recovery.
    d. Conditioning likely will produce less pain tolerance.
    Analysis/Health promotion/Evaluation

12. *Correct response: b*
    Pain is a subjective sensation that cannot be quantified by anyone except the patient experiencing it.
    a, c, and d. These are all true statements.
    Comprehension/Self care/Planning

13. *Correct response: b*
    Involving Billy in care and providing distraction took his mind off the pain.
    a. Pharmacologic agents for pain—analgesics—were not used.
    c. The home environment was not changed.

    d. Cutaneous stimulation was not provided.
    Application/Physiologic/Implementation

14. *Correct response: c*
    Noninvasive measures may result in release of endogenous molecular neuropeptides with analgesic properties.
    a. No evidence indicates that noninvasive and nonpharmacologic measures are more effective than analgesics in relieving pain.
    b. Decreased input over large fibers allows more pain impulses to reach the CNS.
    d. This is simply incorrect.
    Application/Safe care/Implementation

15. *Correct response: b*
    None of the data definitively indicate a psychosocial response; although the nurse possibly could infer it from the health history, it is impossible to tell whether cultural or other factors are preventing Mrs. Brewster from reporting pain.
    a. Nausea and vomiting represent parasympathetic and behavioral and musculoskeletal responses.
    c. Skin changes, diaphoresis, dilated pupils, and elevated vital signs are all sympathetic responses.
    d. Fetal position and eye squinting represent behavioral and musculoskeletal responses.
    Analysis/Psychosocial/Assessment

16. *Correct response: a*
    The use of distraction is an appropriate method of reducing pain.
    b. Not reporting experienced pain is an inappropriate response.
    c. Exclusion of family members and other sources of support represents a maladaptive response.
    d. Range-of-motion exercises and at least mild activity can help reduce pain and are important to prevent complications of immobility.
    Application/Physiologic/Evaluation

Respiratory Disorders

I. **Anatomy and physiology**
   A. Structure
   B. Function

II. **Overview of respiratory disorders**
   A. Assessment
   B. Laboratory studies and diagnostic tests
   C. Psychosocial implications
   D. Medications used to treat respiratory problems

III. **Pneumonia**
   A. Description
   B. Etiology and incidence
   C. Pathophysiology
   D. Assessment findings
   E. Nursing diagnoses
   F. Planning and implementation
   G. Evaluation

IV. **Chronic obstructive pulmonary disease (COPD)**
   A. Description
   B. Etiology and incidence
   C. Pathophysiology
   D. Assessment findings
   E. Nursing diagnoses
   F. Planning and implementation
   G. Evaluation

V. **Occupational lung disease (pneumoconioses)**
   A. Description
   B. Etiology
   C. Pathophysiology
   D. Assessment findings
   E. Nursing diagnoses
   F. Planning and implementation

   G. Evaluation

VI. **Acute respiratory failure (ARF)**
   A. Description
   B. Etiology
   C. Pathophysiology
   D. Assessment findings
   E. Nursing diagnoses
   F. Planning and implementation
   G. Evaluation

VII. **Pulmonary embolism**
   A. Description
   B. Etiology and incidence
   C. Pathophysiology
   D. Assessment findings
   E. Nursing diagnoses
   F. Planning and implementation
   G. Evaluation

VIII. **Lung cancer**
   A. Description
   B. Etiology and incidence
   C. Pathophysiology
   D. Assessment findings
   E. Nursing diagnoses
   F. Planning and implementation
   G. Evaluation

IX. **Chest trauma**
   A. Description
   B. Etiology
   C. Pathophysiology
   D. Assessment findings
   E. Nursing diagnoses
   F. Planning and implementation
   G. Evaluation

I. Anatomy and physiology

A. Structure

1. The *upper airways* consist of the nose and sinuses, pharynx, epiglottis, and larynx; lined with mucous-secreting cells, cilia, and olfactory sensors.
2. The *lower airways* consist of the trachea, right and left mainstream bronchi, segmental bronchi, terminal bronchioles, and alveoli.
3. The *lungs* are situated in the thoracic cavity on either side of heart, bounded by the clavicles, ribs, vertebrae, and diaphragm.
4. The right lung contains three lobes; the left lung, two lobes.
5. The lungs' primary lobules contain millions of alveolar sacs.
6. Blood supply to the lungs is provided by the pulmonary and bronchial arteries.
7. Neurocontrol of ventilation is centered in the *medulla oblongata*, which contains both inspiratory and expiratory centers and controls the rate and depth of respiration to meet the body's metabolic needs.
8. Parietal and visceral pleura surround the lungs; these two layers are separated by the intrapleural space.
9. The *diaphragm*, a dome-shaped muscle separating the thoracic and abdominal cavities, is innervated by the phrenic nerve (a branch of the vagus nerve).

B. Function

1. Upper airway functions include:
   a. Conduct air to lower airways
   b. Protect lungs from foreign matter
   c. Warm, filter, and humidify inspired air
2. The bronchi conduct air to the alveoli.
3. Cilia and mucus help clear particulate matter from inspired air.
4. The alveoli receive air and exchange oxygen (O_2) and carbon

dioxide (CO_2) across the alveolar membrane to pulmonary capillaries.

5. Mechanics of ventilation involve:
   a. The cyclic process of inspiration and expiration
   b. Lung inflation and deflation, causing O_2 and CO_2 gas exchange at the pulmonary capillary–alveolar interface in the lung parenchyma.

6. The lungs provide the body's primary mechanism for altering CO_2 as a buffer to maintain acid–base balance.

7. Diffusion of gases occurs across the alveolar membrane according to pressure gradient from areas of high to low concentration (Table 6–1).

8. The pressure gradient of O_2 is greater in the lung than in pulmonary capillaries, causing O_2 diffusion across the alveolar membrane into the pulmonary capillaries.

9. The pressure gradient of CO_2 is lower in the lung than in pulmonary capillaries, causing O_2 diffusion from pulmonary vessels to the lungs.

10. In normal anatomic shunting, a small amount of blood from bronchial, pleural, and coronary circulation bypasses pulmonary circulation and thus is not oxygenated.

11. In abnormal physiologic shunting, a large amount of unoxygenated venous blood mixes with oxygenated blood in the left heart chambers as a result of adequate pulmonary perfusion with inadequate or absent alveolar ventilation.

12. Inspired air has a high O_2 concentration ($O_2 = 158$ mmHg); expired air, a high CO_2 concentration ($CO_2 = 46$ mmHg).

13. Negative pressure created by the intrapleural space helps effect elastic recoil of lungs.

14. The major muscle of respiration, the diaphragm assists breathing by rising on expiration and lowering on inspiration.

II. Overview of respiratory disorders

A. Assessment

1. Nursing health history should focus on risk factors for respiratory dysfunction, including:
   a. Personal or family history of lung disease
   b. Smoking (the most significant contributing factor in lung disease)

TABLE 6–1.
Pressure Gradients at Sea Level (mmHg)

	LUNGS	ALVEOLI	PULMONARY (SATURATED)	CAPILLARY (UNSATURATED)
O_2	158	100	97	40
CO_2	0.3	40	40	46

      c.   Occupational or avocational exposure to allergens or environmental pollutants

      d.   Age-related changes in lung capacity and respiratory function

      e.   History of upper respiratory infection

      f.   Postoperative changes resulting in diminished respiratory excursion

2. Inspection involves:

      a.   General appearance: body size, age, skin quality and color, posture

      b.   Configuration and movement of the thorax during respiration

      c.   Characteristics of respiration: rate, rhythm, and muscles used for breathing

      d.   Presence of cough, nature and character of sputum (clear, purulent, bloody, tenacious)

      e.   Clubbing of fingers: angle of nailbed greater than 160, distal phalangeal depth greater than interphalangeal depth; softening of nailbeds

3. Palpation of the chest is done to:

      a.   Detect painful areas or masses on the chest surface

      b.   Evaluate chest excursion and the presence or absence of fremitus (vibration)

4. Chest percussion elicits sound to evaluate underlying tissues:

      a.   Resonant sound: indicates air-filled lung (normal)

      b.   Dull or flat sound: suggests presence of firm mass (usually abnormal)

5. Auscultation involves listening to air movement in lungs to detect normal or adventitious breath sounds, including:

      a.   Vesicular sounds: low-pitched rustling sound heard over most of lung field, most prominently on inspiration; indicative of normal, clear lungs

      b.   Bronchial sounds: high-pitched tubular sound with slight pause between inspiration and expiration; normal over large airways

      c.   Bronchovesicular sounds: combination of vesicular and bronchial sounds, normally heard anteriorly to the right or left of the sternum and posteriorly between the scapulae; inspiration and expiration equal

      d.   Adventitious breath sounds: crackles (fine to coarse), wheezes (sibilant, sonorous), pleural friction rub

6. During assessment, the nurse should be alert for cardinal signs and symptoms of respiratory dysfunction, including:

      a.   Dyspnea (labored breathing)

      b.   Orthopnea (difficulty breathing in all positions except upright)

   c. Cough: may be hacking, brassy, wheezing, productive, or nonproductive

   d. Increased sputum production; purulent (yellow or green), rusty, bloody, or mucoid sputum

   e. Chest pain

   f. Wheezing

   g. Clubbing of fingers

   h. Hemoptysis

   i. Cyanosis

B. Laboratory studies and diagnostic tests

   1. Radiographic and scanning studies, done to visualize respiratory system structures, include:

     a. Chest radiograph

     b. Chest tomography

     c. Lung scan

     d. Computed tomography (CT) scan

     e. Positron-emission tomography scan

     f. Fluoroscopy

     g. Barium swallow

   2. Endoscopy studies, invasive techniques performed to visualize pulmonary structures and obtain tissue specimens, include:

     a. Bronchoscopy

     b. Esophogoscopy

     c. Mediastinoscopy

   3. Thoracentesis involves needle aspiration of pleural fluid for diagnostic and therapeutic purposes.

   4. Needle biopsy is an invasive technique involving entering the lung or pleura to obtain tissue for analysis.

   5. Spirometry (pulmonary function testing) is a noninvasive technique used to determine lung volumes, ventilatory function, airway resistance, and distribution of gases.

   6. Sputum culture determines the presence of pathogenic organisms.

TABLE 6–2.
Normal Arterial Blood Gas Values at Sea Level

PARAMETER	NORMAL RANGE
pH (hydrogen ion concentration	7.35 to 7.45
PaO_2 (partial pressure of oxygen)	80 to 100 mmHg
$PaCO_2$ (partial pressure of carbon dioxide)	35 to 45 mmHg
HCO_3	22 to 28 mEq/L
BE (base excess)	−2 to +2 mEq/L
SaO_2 (saturation of hemoglobin)	>95%

7. Arterial blood gas (ABG) studies determine O_2 and CO_2 content and evaluate the body's acid–base balance (Tables 6–2 and 6–3).

C. Psychosocial implications

1. A patient with respiratory dysfunction may experience coping difficulties related to:
   a. Progressive nature of disease
   b. Chronicity of disease
   c. Diminution of respiratory function
   d. Fear of dying
2. The patient also may develop self-concept concerns due to:
   a. Role changes involving increased dependence
   b. Body image changes with the use of breathing apparatus
3. Lifestyle concerns related to respiratory dysfunction may include potential changes in:
   a. Activity tolerance
   b. Physical mobility
   c. Work performance, with potential for job loss
   d. Self-care ability
4. The chronically ill patient may develop concerns about social interaction, leading to feelings of:
   a. Isolation and loneliness
   b. Depression
   c. Hopelessness

D. Medications used to treat respiratory problems

1. Sympathomimetics (also referred to as adrenergic agonists), used to dilate bronchial smooth muscles in patients with asthma or COPD with bronchospasms, include:
   a. Isoetharine
   b. Metaproterenol
   c. Albuterol
   d. Terbutaline
   e. Epinephrine
   f. Isoproterenol

TABLE 6–3.
Acid–Base Disorders

DISORDER	BLOOD GAS CHANGES
Respiratory acidosis	↓ pH, ↑ $PaCO_2$
Respiratory alkalosis	↑ pH, ↓ $PaCO_2$
Metabolic acidosis	↓ pH, ↓ HCO_3, ↓ BE
Metabolic alkalosis	↑ pH, ↑ HCO_3, ↑ BE

    2. Xanthine derivatives produce bronchial smooth muscle relaxation, resulting in dilation, and are indicated for patients with asthma or COPD with bronchospasms; drugs include:
- a. Aminophylline
- b. Anhydrous theophylline
- c. Theophylline
- d. Ephedrine

    3. Anticholinergics are used to prevent or reverse bronchospasms in patients with asthma or COPD; atropine is the most commonly used anticholinergic.

    4. Corticosteroids, which reduce immune or inflammatory reactions, are used as a follow-up treatment after other agents administered for severe immune or inflammatory reactions; drugs include:
- a. Hydrocortisone
- b. Methylprednisolone
- c. Dexamethasone
- d. Prednisone
- e. Prednisolone
- f. Beclomethasone dipropionate

    5. Cromolyn sodium is used as prophylactic treatment for asthma—not for acute attacks.

    6. Mucolytic agents and expectorants, which facilitate sputum expectoration, are indicated primarily for patients with cystic fibrosis or others with thick secretions or with difficulty raising secretions; acetylcysteine is the most commonly used agent.

III. Pneumonia

A. Description

    1. Pneumonia is an inflammatory process involving the respiratory bronchioles, alveolar space and walls, and lobes caused primarily by specific organisms (bacteria, viruses, fungi, parasites, mycoplasma, or chemical irritants).

    2. It can be broadly classified as bacterial or nonbacterial.

B. Etiology and incidence

    1. Causative organisms in bacterial pneumonia include:
- a. *Streptococcus pneumoniae* (hemolytic type A) accounts for 90% of cases
- b. *Staphylococcus aureus*
- c. *Haemophilus influenzae* (type B)
- d. *Klebsiella pneumoniae*, *Pseudomonas aeruginosa*, *Escherichia coli*, *Enterobacter*, and other gram-negative enteric bacilli

    2. Causes of nonbacterial pneumonia include:
- a. *Mycoplasma pneumoniae*
- b. Influenza viruses, parainfluenza viruses, and other viral infections

       c.   *Pneumocystis carinii*

       d.   *Aspergillus fumigatus*

  3.   Pneumonia is the most common cause of death from infectious disease in North America.

C. **Pathophysiology**

  1.   The infecting organisms trigger inflammation of the airways.

  2.   Inflammatory exudate fills the alveolar air spaces, producing lung consolidation.

  3.   Impaired gas exchange in the alveoli leads to varying degrees of hypoxia, depending on the amount of lung tissue affected.

D. **Assessment findings**

  1.   Common clinical manifestations include:

       a.   Dullness on percussion of chest with consolidation

       b.   Bronchial breath sounds auscultated over consolidated lung fields

       c.   Fever: sudden onset over 100°F

       d.   Shaking chills (with bacterial pneumonia)

       e.   Chest pain

       f.   Dyspnea

       g.   Hacking cough

       h.   Anxiety and confusion

  2.   Laboratory and diagnostic studies may reveal:

       a.   Density changes, primarily in lower lung fields, seen on chest radiograph

       b.   Sputum culture and sensitivity positive for specific causative organism

       c.   Elevated WBC count; depressed in pneumonia of mycoplasmal or viral origin

E. **Nursing diagnoses**

  1.   High Risk for Altered Body Temperature

  2.   Ineffective Breathing Patterns

  3.   Fluid Volume Deficit

  4.   Impaired Gas Exchange

  5.   Pain

F. **Planning and implementation**

  1.   Encourage adequate fluid intake with IV administration and oral hydration as appropriate.

  2.   Humidify inspired air.

  3.   Encourage effective coughing.

  4.   Analyze ABG values to determine the need for oxygen and to evaluate the patient's response to oxygen therapy.

  5.   Relieve pain with analgesics, as ordered, monitoring for signs of respiratory depression.

  6.   Administer antibiotics specific for the causative organism as ordered.

7. Provide patient and family teaching, covering:
    a. Disease process, cause, treatments (including medications), expected response
    b. Deep breathing and coughing techniques
    c. The importance of good handwashing to help prevent infection transmission
    d. The need for adequate rest

G. Evaluation

1. The patient demonstrates response to therapy within 48 hours if no complications occur.
2. The patient demonstrates improved respiratory function and ABG values within normal range.
3. The patient exhibits diminished cough and sputum production.
4. The patient demonstrates resolution of disease process on radiograph.

IV. COPD

A. Description: a group of disorders associated with persistent or recurrent obstruction of airflow; includes chronic bronchitis, emphysema, and asthma, often with overlap of these disorders

B. Etiology and incidence

1. Major causes of and contributing factors to chronic bronchitis and emphysema include:
    a. Smoking
    b. Air pollution
    c. Occupational exposure to respiratory irritants
    d. Allergies
    e. Autoimmunity
    f. Infection
    g. Genetic predisposition
    h. Aging
2. Asthma may be extrinsic or intrinsic; possible causes include:
    a. Extrinsic: external agents or specific allergens (e.g., dust, foods, mold spores, insecticides)
    b. Intrinsic: upper respiratory infection, exercise, emotional stress, cold, or other nonspecific factors
3. The most common chronic lung disease, COPD affects an estimated 17 million persons in the United States; incidence is rising.

C. Pathophysiology

1. Basic pathologic changes in COPD include:
    a. Hypertrophy and hypersecretion in goblet cells and bronchial mucous glands leading to increased sputum secretion, bronchial congestion, narrowing of bronchioles, and small bronchi (chronic bronchitis)

      b.   Increased size of air spaces; loss of elastic recoil of lung due to hyperinflation of distal airways; destruction of alveolar walls; and diffuse airway narrowing causing resistance to airflow due to loss of supporting structure and bronchospasm (emphysema)

      c.   Narrowing of the bronchial airways (asthma)

2. These conditions frequently overlap; most commonly, bronchitis and emphysema occur together.

3. These changes cause disruption of airway dynamics, resulting in obstruction of airflow into or out of the lungs.

D. Assessment findings

    1. Health history findings, clinical manifestations, and laboratory and diagnostic study results in *chronic bronchitis* may include:

      a.   Recurrent acute respiratory infections

      b.   Persistent cough

      c.   Persistent sputum production

      d.   Slow development, typically over several years

      e.   History of smoking, air pollution, occupational exposure

      f.   Pulmonary function studies: decreased forced expiratory volume (FEV), decreased forced vital capacity (FVC), increased residual volume (RV)

      g.   Chest radiograph: flattened diaphragm

      h.   ABG values during acute phase: significantly increased $PaCO_2$, decreased PaO_2

      i.   Sputum culture: secondary bacterial infection with gram-negative or gram-positive organisms, such as *Diplococcus pneumoniae* and *Hemophilus influenzae*

    2. Common assessment findings in *emphysema* include:

      a.   History of chronic bronchitis

      b.   Slow onset of symptoms (typically over several years)

      c.   Progressive dyspnea, initially only on exertion and later also at rest

      d.   Progressive cough and increased sputum production, especially during bouts of infection

      e.   Anorexia with weight loss

      f.   Profound weakness

      g.   Pulmonary function studies: decreased FEV, decreased FVC, increased RV

      h.   Chest radiograph: flattened diaphragm, decreased vascular markings with hyperradiolucence, increased anterior–posterior (A–P) diameter

      i.   ABGs: increased $PaCO_2$, decreased PaO_2

    3. Assessment findings in *asthma* typically include:

      a.   Chest tightness

      b.   Cough

    c.   Wheezing

    d.   Expiration more strenuous and prolonged than inspiration

    e.   Use of accessory muscles of respiration

    f.   Hypoxia with cyanosis, weak pulse, diaphoresis

    g.   Can occur alone without triad of bronchitis, emphysema, and asthma; usually associated with allergy

    h.   Commonly triggered by emotional stress, exercise or change in weather, exposure to allergen

    i.   Pulmonary function studies during acute episode: markedly decreased FEV, increased RV, increased TLC, decreased peak flow (PEFR) that improve after treatment

E. Nursing diagnoses

   1.   Activity Intolerance

   2.   Anxiety

   3.   Ineffective Breathing Patterns

   4.   Impaired Communication: Verbal

   5.   Fatigue

   6.   Impaired Gas Exchange

   7.   Altered Health Maintenance

   8.   Health-Seeking Behaviors

   9.   Impaired Home Maintenance Management

  10.   Altered Nutrition: Less Than Body Requirements

  11.   Pain

  12.   Chronic Pain

  13.   Altered Tissue Perfusion: Peripheral

F. Planning and implementation

   1.   For a patient with bronchitis or emphysema:

    a.   Eliminate or minimize exposure to all pulmonary irritants.

    b.   Control bronchospasms with bronchodilators as prescribed.

    c.   Liquify secretions with increased fluid intake or mucolytics as prescribed.

    d.   Clear airways with postural drainage, and clapping or vibrating and suctioning as appropriate.

    e.   Encourage the patient to perform graded physical exercise, deep breathing and coughing, and relaxation techniques.

    f.   Administer low-flow O_2 to help prevent hypoxia due to loss of respiratory drive (2 to 4 L according to ABG values).

    g.   Avoid narcotics, sedatives, and tranquilizers, which can further depress respirations.

    h.   Provide patient and family teaching, covering: disease

process and treatments; breathing retraining exercises; energy conservation; use of inhalers and nebulizers; medication administration and the importance of compliance; prevention of complications and infections by receiving influenza immunizations and taking broad-spectrum antibiotics as prescribed.

2. For a patient with asthma:
   a. Identify and eliminate or minimize exposure to pulmonary irritants.
   b. Control bronchospasms with bronchodilators as prescribed.
   c. Administer theophylline, cromolyn sodium, or steroids as prescribed.
   d. Encourage the patient to perform graded physical, breathing, and relaxation exercises with acute attacks.
   e. Provide patient and family teaching, covering: disease process and triggering factors; breathing retraining exercises; energy conservation; medication administration, including indications, expected responses, potential side effects, importance of compliance, use of inhaler or nebulizer; importance of receiving influenza immunization as prescribed; prevention of complications and infection.

G. Evaluation
1. The patient displays improved ABG values with compensation.
2. The patient exhibits improved pulmonary function studies with compensation.
3. The patient demonstrates resolution of acute processes.
4. The patient reports eased breathing effort.
5. The patient produces sputum that is more liquid and controlled by coughing.
6. The patient reports and exhibits reduced anxiety.
7. The patient reports symptom improvement with use of work modification strategies.
8. The patient verbalizes an understanding of administration and purpose of prescribed medications.
9. The patient verbalizes an understanding of the disease process and measures to prevent complications, including infection.
10. The patient incorporates health maintenance behaviors into his or her lifestyle.

V. Occupational lung disease (pneumoconioses)
A. Description
1. Lung disorders resulting from occupational exposure to organic or inorganic dusts and noxious gases

2. The most common types include:
    a. Silicosis
    b. Asbestosis
    c. Coal workers' pneumoconiosis (CWP, "black lung")

B. Etiology

1. Silicosis results from inhalation of silica dust in such occupations as mineral mining, stone cutting, quarrying, abrasives manufacturing, and ceramic and pottery work.
2. Asbestosis results from inhalation of asbestos dust and particles in occupations related to manufacture, handling, and removal of asbestos-containing materials. (*Note:* There are more than 4000 known uses of asbestos fiber.)
3. CWP results from accumulation of coal dust in the lungs, most commonly from coal mining.

C. Pathophysiology

1. The effects of inhaling dusts, particles, or gases depend on the substance's composition, its antigenic or irritating properties, the amount inhaled, duration of exposure, and the person's overall health status.
2. Chronic inhalation of silica particles produces nodular lesions throughout the lungs. These lesions become fibrotic, enlarge, and fuse, resulting in obstructive and restrictive lung changes.
3. In asbestosis, inhaled asbestos fibers enter the alveoli, which eventually become obliterated by fibrous tissue surrounding the particles. Progressive pleural fibrosis and plaque formation lead to restrictive lung disease, diminished lung volume, impaired gas exchange, hypoxemia, and eventually, cor pulmonale. Asbestosis also is associated with bronchogenic cancer.
4. In CWP, inhaled coal dust is deposited in the alveoli and bronchioles. Eventually, the alveoli and bronchioles become clogged with dust, macrophages, and fibroblasts, leading to the formation of coal macules, the primary lesion of CWP. As these macules enlarge, bronchiolar dilatation and emphysema result.

D. Assessment findings

1. Common clinical manifestations include:
    a. Asymptomatic in early stages
    b. Chronic cough, often nonproductive in silicosis and asbestosis and productive of black fluid in CWP
    c. Progressive dyspnea
    d. Susceptibility to recurrent upper respiratory infections
    e. Impaired diaphragmatic excursion
    f. Diminished breath sounds with decreased chest expansion
    g. Tachypnea

          h.   Clubbing of fingers and toes

    2.   Chest radiograph findings typically include:

        a.   Silicosis: nodular formation to massive fibrosis and densities in lung fields as disease progresses

        b.   Asbestosis: interstitial density in lower lung fields

        c.   CWP: nodular densities in upper lung fields

    3.   Pulmonary function tests commonly reveal decreased FVC, FEV, TLC and diffusing capacity of CO_2 as the disease progresses.

    4.   ABG values demonstrate decreasing PaO_2 and increasing $PaCO_2$ with disease progression.

E. **Nursing diagnoses**

    1.   Activity Intolerance

    2.   Anxiety

    3.   Impaired Communication: Verbal

    4.   Fatigue

    5.   Altered Health Maintenance

    6.   Health-Seeking Behaviors

    7.   Impaired Home Maintenance Management

    8.   Pain

    9.   Altered Tissue Perfusion: Peripheral

F. **Planning and implementation**

    1.   For a patient experiencing acute symptoms:

        a.   Maintain a patent airway by suctioning or endotracheal intubation.

        b.   Provide adequate oxygenation.

        c.   Maintain cardiac output.

        d.   Initiate mechanical ventilation if respiratory failure occurs.

    2.   Interventions for chronic disease include:

        a.   Maintain bronchial hygiene.

        b.   Administer antibiotics, as ordered, to control infection.

        c.   Administer corticosteroids, as ordered, to relieve inflammation.

        d.   See planning and implementation for COPD (Section IV.F) for additional interventions.

G. **Evaluation (see evaluation for COPD, Section IV.G)**

VI. **Acute respiratory failure (ARF)**

    A. **Description: the condition resulting when the exchange of O_2 for CO_2 in the normal lungs cannot match the rate of O_2 consumption and CO_2 production in body cells**

    B. **Etiology: possible causes of ARF include:**

        1.   Airway obstruction

        2.   Restrictive lung disease

        3.   Central nervous system disorder, such as head trauma or cerebrovascular accident

       4. Drug overdose

       5. Anesthesia and surgical procedures

C. **Pathophysiology**

       1. ARF occurs whenever O_2 and CO_2 exchange in normal lungs fails to fulfill oxygen needs of body causing alveolar hypoventilation.

       2. Effects include hypoxia (PaO_2 <60 mmHg) with or without hypercapnia ($PaCO_2$ >50 mmHg).

D. **Assessment findings**

       1. Clinical manifestations of ARF may include:

          a. Dyspnea

          b. Tachypnea

          c. Tachycardia

          d. Headache

          e. Cyanosis

          f. Anxiety, confusion, restlessness

          g. Decreased or absent breath sounds

          h. Adventitious breath sounds: crackles, wheezing

       2. Laboratory and diagnostic studies may reveal:

          a. ABGs: PaO_2 <60 mmHg; $PaCO_2$ >50 mmHg; pH <7.35

          b. EKG: cardiac dysrhythmias

          c. Chest radiograph: various lung field changes depending on causative factors

       3. Evaluation of the precipitating event is important in differentiating ARF from acute lung damage (e.g., adult respiratory distress syndrome [ARDS]) and chronic respiratory conditions with acute changes (e.g., COPD).

E. **Nursing diagnoses**

       1. Activity Intolerance

       2. Ineffective Airway Clearance

       3. Anxiety

       4. Ineffective Breathing Patterns

       5. Decreased Cardiac Output

       6. Impaired Communication: Verbal

       7. Ineffective Individual Coping

       8. Fluid Volume Excess

       9. Impaired Gas Exchange

F. **Planning and implementation**

       1. Restore and maintain a patent airway by suctioning or performing endotracheal intubation as ordered.

       2. Administer oxygen therapy to maintain adequate alveolar ventilation.

       3. Institute mechanical ventilation if the patient's condition deteriorates.

4. Maintain effective tracheobronchial hygiene.
5. Monitor cardiac status.
6. Monitor ABG values.

G. Evaluation
1. The patient maintains ABG values within preillness ranges.
2. The patient demonstrates restoration of adequate pulmonary function.
3. The patient exhibits and reports reduced anxiety and confusion.

VII. Pulmonary embolism

A. Description: obstruction of one or more pulmonary arteries by a thrombus or thrombi, originating somewhere in the venous system or in the right side of the heart

B. Etiology and incidence
1. Thrombus formation may result from:
   a. Venous stasis, as may result from prolonged immobilization, sitting, or standing
   b. Vessel wall injury
   c. Hypercoagulability of the blood
2. Predisposing factors to pulmonary embolism include:
   a. Prolonged immobility
   b. Chronic lung disease
   c. Congestive heart failure
   d. Thrombophlebitis
   e. Hematologic disorders
   f. Lower extremity fractures or surgery
   g. Pregnancy or oral contraceptive use
3. Pulmonary embolism affects an estimated 6 million adult Americans yearly, resulting in about 100,000 deaths.

C. Pathophysiology
1. Thrombus formation may occur in the deep veins of the legs (most common site); pelvic, renal, or hepatic veins; right heart; and upper extremities.
2. A dislodged thrombus may travel to the pulmonary arterial bed, where obstruction leads to:
   a. Altered ventilation–perfusion ratio
   b. Increase in alveolar dead space
3. The area of obstruction continues to ventilate but receives little or no blood supply, resulting in:
   a. Decreased pulmonary vascular blood pressure
   b. Increased pulmonary artery pressure
4. Unrelieved obstruction may result in right ventricular heart failure and shock; total occlusion of the main pulmonary artery is rapidly fatal.

D. Assessment findings

1. Clinical manifestations commonly include:
   a. Chest pain: may be sudden, sharp or mild, substernal or pleuritic, depending on the site and extent of obstruction
   b. Tachycardia
   c. Dyspnea
   d. Anxiety and restlessness
   e. Decreased breath sounds on auscultation, usually with plural friction rub
   f. Signs of circulatory collapse (weak, rapid pulse; hypotension)

2. Laboratory and diagnostic studies may reveal:
   a. ABGs: PaO_2 <60 mmHg, indicating hypoxemia
   b. Elevated LDH, bilirubin, and fibrin split products
   c. Deficient perfusion and ventilation lung scans
   d. Pulmonary angiogram (most specific for diagnosis): intraarterial filling defect, obstruction of pulmonary artery branch

E. Nursing diagnoses

1. Activity Intolerance
2. Anxiety
3. Impaired Communication: Verbal
4. Impaired Gas Exchange
5. Pain

F. Planning and implementation

1. Administer prescribed medications, which may include:
   a. Anticoagulant therapy: initial therapy heparin IV followed by coumadin
   b. Thrombolytic therapy (urokinase or streptokinase or t-PA)
2. Monitor for bleeding.
3. Administer pain medication as prescribed to relieve chest pain.
4. Correct hypoxemia with oxygen therapy, as necessary.
5. Help reduce venous stasis in legs by applying antiembolic stockings.
6. Provide patient teaching, covering:
   a. Leg exercises to maintain peripheral circulation
   b. Correct use of anticoagulant therapy and monitoring for bleeding

G. Evaluation

1. The patient maintains gas exchange at preemboli level.
2. The patient maintains normal vital signs, including temperature.
3. The patient demonstrates return of breath sounds to normal, with no evidence of pleural friction rub.

4. The patient demonstrates compliance with prescribed antico-agulant therapy to prevent recurrence of thrombi.

VIII. Lung cancer

A. Description

1. Lung cancer refers to a malignant tumor arising within the wall or epithelial lining of the bronchus or resulting from metastatic spread of cancer arising elsewhere in the body.

2. Types include:
   a. Squamous cell (epidermoid): the most common type
   b. Adenocarcinoma
   c. Small cell undifferentiated (oat cell)
   d. Large cell undifferentiated

B. Etiology and incidence

1. Predisposing factors to lung cancer include:
   a. Smoking (Lung cancer is 10 times more prevalent in smokers than nonsmokers.)
   b. Occupational exposure to carcinogenic substances, such as asbestos, arsenic, chromium, nickel, radioactive substances, coal dust, and iron oxides
   c. Family history of lung cancer

2. The most common cause of cancer death in men, lung cancer, has a 5-year survival rate of only 13%.

C. Pathophysiology

1. Squamous cell carcinomas arise most often in the upper lobes, usually in the main stem lobar segmental bronchi. They grow relatively slowly and tend to metastasize late in their course.

2. Adenocarcinomas tend to arise in more peripheral lung areas and grow even more slowly than squamous cell carcinomas. They metastasize relatively early in their course.

3. Small cell carcinomas arise more peripherally than squamous cell carcinomas and grow rapidly. Metastasis commonly is well established by the time of diagnosis.

4. Large cell carcinomas arise more centrally than small cell carcinomas and tend to metastasize early in their course.

5. Regardless of cell type, lung cancer produces some combination of pulmonary effects (principally, disturbance in ventilation and perfusion of lung fields invaded by the tumor), systemic effects, and effects of metastatic spread.

6. Choice of treatment modalities depends on disease stage, tumor type, and the patient's condition, and may include:
   a. Surgical resection of the tumor or lung tissue
   b. Radiation therapy
   c. Chemotherapy
   d. Immunotherapy

D. Assessment findings

1. Symptoms usually occur relatively late and are related to tumor size and location.

    2. Common clinical manifestations include:
- a. Change in nature of normal cough
- b. Hemoptysis
- c. Dyspnea
- d. Hoarseness and wheezing
- e. Chest pain
- f. Weight loss and fatigue

    3. Test results may reveal:
- a. Radiograph: chest mass
- b. Sputum studies: malignant cells
- c. Bronchoscopy specimen: positive for malignant cells
- d. CT lung scan: positive
- e. Pulmonary function studies: decreased pulmonary reserve

E. **Nursing diagnoses**
1. Activity Intolerance
2. Anxiety
3. Ineffective Individual Coping
4. Altered Health Maintenance
5. Impaired Home Maintenance Management
6. Altered Nutrition: Less Than Body Requirements
7. Pain

F. **Planning and implementation** (*Note:* See Chapter 21, Cancer Nursing, for more detailed nursing interventions applicable to all types of cancer.)
1. Prepare the patient for planned tests and treatments.
2. Maintain adequate nutritional status.
3. Control pain with prescribed analgesics or other measures.
4. Provide emotional support to the patient and family; address concerns and uncertainty that contribute to anxiety and depression.

G. **Evaluation**
1. The patient reports relief or control of dyspnea and chest discomfort.
2. The patient demonstrates improved nutritional status.
3. The patient reports reduced anxiety and depression.
4. The patient and family members report acceptance of the diagnosis and make realistic plans.

IX. Chest trauma

A. **Description**
1. Injury to the chest wall or lungs can interfere with inspiration, gas exchange, or expiration.
2. Types include:
- a. Hemothorax: blood in the pleural space
- b. Pneumothorax: air in the pleural space
- c. Open pneumothorax: sucking wound of the chest

B. Etiology
  1. Hemothorax results from penetrating or blunt chest injury.
  2. Pneumothorax can result from disease or injury, most commonly from laceration of the lung parenchyma, tracheobronchial tree, or esophagus.
  3. Open pneumothorax most commonly results from penetrating chest injury.

C. Pathophysiology
  1. In hemothorax, blood in the pleural cavity compresses the lungs and can produce blood loss resulting in shock.
  2. In tension pneumothorax—considered a medical emergency—pressure buildup in the pleural space results in compromised ventilation and can lead to collapse of the lung, decreased ventilation in the other lung, and decreased venous return to the heart.
  3. Open pneumothorax, an acutely life-threatening condition, involves an opening in the chest wall large enough to allow air passage into and out of the chest cavity with each attempted respiration; the rush of air produces a characteristic "sucking" sound. Tidal volume diminishes, and ventilation is compromised.

D. Assessment findings
  1. Clinical manifestations may include:
     a. Dyspnea
     b. Tachypnea
     c. Pain on breathing
     d. Rapid development of cyanosis
     e. Asymmetric chest movement
     f. Hypotension progressing to shock
  2. EKG may reveal cardiac dysrhythmias

E. Nursing diagnoses
  1. Ineffective Airway Clearance
  2. Ineffective Breathing Patterns
  3. Decreased Cardiac Output
  4. Impaired Communication: Verbal
  5. Fluid Volume Deficit
  6. Impaired Gas Exchange

F. Planning and implementation
  1. Establish and maintain a patent airway by suctioning and endotracheal intubation as appropriate.
  2. Administer oxygen to correct hypoxemia as necessary.
  3. Control hemorrhage; treat damage to chest and other injured structures.
  4. Stabilize the chest wall if necessary.
  5. As ordered, assist with insertion of chest tube; maintain closed drainage.

      6. Provide emotional support to reduce anxiety and fear.

      7. Prepare the patient for surgery if appropriate, based on the nature of the injury.

  G. **Evaluation**

      1. The patient displays normal cardiopulmonary function.

      2. The patient exhibits healing of penetrating chest wound without infection.

      3. The patient demonstrates resolution of dysrhythmias.

      4. Vital signs remain in normal ranges.

      5. The patient's lungs are clear on auscultation.

X. Thoracic surgery (thoracotomy)

  A. **Description**

      1. Surgical intervention is viewed as deliberate trauma to the chest to correct an underlying problem (e.g., tumor resection, organ repair, transplant).

      2. Surgery disrupts the negative pressure of the chest, requiring controlled ventilation throughout the procedure to maintain ventilation and pulmonary circulation.

  B. **Planning and implementation: preoperative** (*Note:* See Chapter 24, Perioperative Nursing, for information on general preoperative nursing interventions.)

      1. Assess the patient's preoperative status, including physiologic condition (particularly cardiovascular and pulmonary status) and coping abilities.

      2. Prepare the patient for scheduled diagnostic and laboratory tests, such as chest radiograph, pulmonary function studies, lung scan, ECG, hematologic studies, and ABG analysis.

      3. Teach the patient techniques to use postoperatively to improve alveolar ventilation and overall respiratory function, such as deep breathing, coughing, and incentive spirometry.

      4. Prepare the patient for the planned surgical procedure by providing explanations, reassurance and support, and skillful preoperative nursing care.

  C. **Nursing diagnoses: postoperative**

      1. Ineffective Breathing Patterns

      2. High Risk for Disuse Syndrome

      3. Impaired Gas Exchange

      4. High Risk for Infection

      5. Impaired Physical Mobility

      6. Pain

      7. High Risk for Impaired Skin Integrity

  D. **Planning and implementation: postoperative** (*Note:* See Chapter 24, Perioperative Nursing, for information on general postoperative nursing interventions.)

      1. Maintain effective gas exchange by suctioning or mechanical ventilation as appropriate.

2. Encourage the patient to perform incentive spirometry to aid reinflation of the affected lung.
3. Monitor chest tube function, and evaluate the amount and nature of drainage.
4. Assess for pain related to surgical incision and presence of chest tubes. Help relieve pain by:
   a. Instructing the patient to splint the incision when coughing
   b. Maintaining the patient in Fowler's position
   c. Administering analgesics as ordered (in moderation to avoid respiratory depression)
5. Maintain fluid therapy and blood replacement as ordered.
6. Monitor ABG values for hypoxia or hypercapnia.
7. Monitor vital signs.
8. Assess for signs and symptoms of complications, such as:
   a. Hemorrhage
   b. Respiratory failure
   c. Wound infection
   d. Cardiac abnormalities

E. Evaluation
1. The patient maintains effective respiration without assistance.
2. The patient reports pain control or relief.
3. The patient demonstrates restoration of chest and arm mobility.
4. The patient's ABG values remain within normal ranges.

Bibliography

Ayres, S., Schlichtig, R., & Sterling, M. (1988). *Care of the critically ill.* Chicago: Yearbook Medical Publishers.

Bonner, J., & Hall, J. (1985). *Respiratory intensive care of the adult surgical patient.* St. Louis: C. V. Mosby.

Boyda, E. (1985). *Respiratory problems (RN Nursing Assessment Series 5).* Oradell, NJ: Medical Economics Books.

Brunner, L. S., & Suddarth, D. S. (1988). *Textbook of medical-surgical nursing* (6th ed.). Philadelphia: J. B. Lippincott.

Brunner, L. S., & Suddarth, D. S. (1986). *The Lippincott manual of nursing practice* (4th ed.). Philadelphia: J. B. Lippincott.

Carpenito, L. J. (1990). *Nursing diagnosis: Application to clinical practice* (2nd ed.). Philadelphia: J. B. Lippincott.

Luckmann, J., & Sorensen, K. C. (1987). *Medical-surgical nursing: A psychophysiologic approach* (3rd ed.). Philadelphia: W. B. Saunders.

STUDY QUESTIONS

1. Mr. Roberts, a 34-year-old accountant, called the nurse at the outpatient clinic and reported the following: He had a cold last week, but was feeling better today and so went jogging, as is his usual routine. After a short run, however, he became very short of breath and felt tightness in his chest. He reported no sore throat, fever, or productive cough. Based on this information elicited by way of telephone assessment, the nurse could surmise that Mr. Roberts' symptoms are related to
   a. asthma
   b. pneumoconioses
   c. bronchitis
   d. pneumonia

2. An 18-year-old woman came to the physician's office complaining of general malaise, fever, and a hacking cough. In completing a nursing assessment, which of the following would the nurse expect to find with pneumonia?
   a. conjunctivitis and nasal swelling
   b. tonsillar exudate and pain on swallowing
   c. bronchial breath sounds over lung field with consolidation
   d. productive cough with excess mucous production

3. Tom Baker, aged 18, has a penetrating chest wound and fractured left femur from a one-car accident the day before high school graduation. He was hospitalized with a hemothorax and placed in ICU with a chest tube inserted to help his ventilatory function. He complains frequently about the care he is receiving and talks about his inability to do anything right. "I even screw up graduating." In planning care for this patient, in addition to the nursing diagnosis Altered Respiratory Function, which of the following diagnoses would be most appropriate to address?
   a. High Risk for Altered Body Temperature
   b. Anxiety
   c. Low Self-Esteem: Situational
   d. Altered Nutrition: High Risk for More Than Body Requirements

4. At the time of Tom's discharge, all the following criteria would be appropriate *except*
   a. The patient reports absence or control of pain with medication.
   b. The patient displays closure of chest wound without infection.
   c. The patient expresses understanding of use of anticoagulation therapy to prevent thrombus formation.
   d. The patient displays clear lung fields on auscultation.

5. During hospitalization for a pulmonary embolism, Ms. Stone, aged 75, was being prepared for discharge. The nursing diagnosis, Knowledge Deficit, was identified as a primary concern for focus by the nursing staff to increase Ms. Stone's progress at home. This diagnosis would be based on the patient's need to know which of the following self-care activities?
   a. Reduce walking to only necessary activities around the house.
   b. Maintain peripheral circulation with leg exercises.
   c. Soak feet nightly in warm water to increase circulation.
   d. Avoid bending to pick up objects.

6. Mrs. Smith, aged 64, has been diagnosed with COPD. Although she was hospitalized several times in the last year for acute respiratory failure, she is presently in stable condition. The primary focus of care in the long-term nursing care of Mrs. Smith would be to
   a. Decrease activity to conserve functional lung tissue.
   b. Increase the frequency of postural drainage to every 2 hours while awake.
   c. Increase the RV.
   d. Improve and maintain pulmonary ventilation and gas exchange.

7. Mrs. Smith's condition changed over a period of days, and her arterial blood studies now indicate she is again in acute respiratory failure. The primary nursing intervention most commonly required in the care of patients with COPD who are in acute respiratory failure is to
   a. Establish initial stage of activity.
   b. Discourage patient from sitting in Fowler's position in order to reduce work of heart.
   c. Remove bronchial secretions, and manage oxygen therapy.
   d. Plan with family for home care.

8. Mrs. Smith has been treated aggressively for acute respiratory failure and has improved over the past 4 weeks. She experienced anxiety about being prepared for discharge. The nurse who cares for her should help her develop ways to cope with her chronic obstructive lung disease by:
   a. encouraging the family to take increased responsibility for the patient's care
   b. discouraging the patient from performing activities of daily living if they make her tired
   c. teaching the patient relaxation techniques and breathing retraining exercises
   d. protecting the patient from knowing the prognosis of her disease

9. Mr. Bonner, aged 60, is experiencing an episode of acute respiratory failure following an asthma attack. He has a cuffed endotracheal tube in place. For Mr. Bonner, the inflated pressure in the cuff should be checked and maintained at or less than:
   a. 42 cm H_2O
   b. 24 cm H_2O
   c. 20 cm H_2O
   d. 5 cm H_2O

10. Mr. Brown, a 46-year-old man employed in a steel plant, was referred to the outpatient clinic at the local hospital from work with a tentative diagnosis of pneumonia. The nurse who initially examines Mr. Brown should be aware of the clinical manifestations of pneumonia. Nursing diagnoses appropriate to care for this patient would include which of the following?
    a. Fluid Volume Deficit related to vomiting and diarrhea
    b. Pain related to chest pain radiating to the left shoulder and arm
    c. Hyperthermia related to sudden onset of chills with a rising fever and chest pain
    d. Ineffective Breathing Patterns related to slow, shallow respiration with point tenderness at a rib site

11. Mr. Brown was hospitalized for acute bacterial pneumonia and is now recovering after a course of therapy with Penicillin G. In evaluating the outcome of care, the nurse should expect which of the following outcomes?
    a. The patient displays PaO_2 of 85 mmHg or above.
    b. The patient displays $PaCO_2$ of 80 mmHg or above.
    c. The patient demonstrates decreased breath sounds.
    d. The patient demonstrates signs of restlessness and confusion.

12. Mrs. Stone has just undergone chest surgery for a right lower lobectomy. The nurse planning Mrs. Stone's postoperative care should include which of the following?
    a. Encourage coughing to mobilize secretions.
    b. Ensure that the thoracotomy tube is attached to open chest drainage.
    c. Restrict IV fluids for 24 hours.
    d. Prevent coughing to assure incision integrity.

13. Mr. Bond, aged 52, underwent a right lobectomy 1 day ago and is having difficulty handling mucous secretions. The nurse caring for Mr. Bond performs tracheobronchial suctioning on a p.r.n. basis. A potential complication of suctioning is lobar collapse. This can be avoided by:
    a. using a large catheter the same diameter as the trachea

b. applying suction at high pressure to accomplish the procedure as quickly as possible

c. applying suction continuously for 30 seconds of more

d. using a catheter the size that does not occlude the lumen of the airway during application of suction

14. The partial pressure of oxygen in arterial blood (PO_2) is proportional to the concentration of O_2 because it is mixed with other gases. Keeping this fact in mind, at discharge from a Denver hospital that is at an altitude of approximately 5000 feet, which of the following is an expected acceptable discharge criterion for a person without COPD?

   a. pH 7.3
   b. PaO_2 65 to 75 mmHg
   c. PaO_2 45 to 55 mmHg
   d. PaO_2 80 to 100 mmHg

15. The neurocontrol of ventilation rests in several areas of the nervous system. The primary control of inspiration and expiration occurs in the

   a. baroreceptors
   b. medulla oblongata
   c. alveoli
   d. pons

16. Mr. Green is diagnosed as having respiratory insufficiency due to longstanding restrictive lung disease as a result of working in the coal mines for 35 years. He should be advised to prevent or control respiratory infections by:

   a. taking penicillin for the rest of his life as prophylaxis
   b. smoking low-tar cigarettes
   c. taking influenza injections and broad-spectrum antibiotics as prescribed
   d. having periodic blood studies to determine his PO_2

ANSWER KEY

1. *Correct response: a*

The reported symptoms and lack of symptoms are characteristic of asthma. The previous viral infection may have made the patient more prone to bronchial spasms in response to exercise or cold temperatures.

b. The patient's occupation as an accountant would decrease the likelihood of pneumoconioses.

c and d. The patient's lack of productive cough or fever would decrease the probability of either bronchitis or pneumonia.

Application/Physiologic/Assessment

2. *Correct response: c*

Bronchial breath sounds are commonly found over lung fields with infiltration and consolidation in pneumonia.

a. Eyes and nose symptoms aren't typical in pneumonia.

b. Tonsillar exudate and pain on swallowing are cardinal symptoms of streptococcal sore throat caused by infection of the pharynx.

d. Cough associated with pneumonia is typically hacking and nonproductive.

Application/Physiologic/Assessment

3. *Correct response: c*

The healing from these injuries and compliance with rehabilitation will be affected by Tom's emotional response to this crisis. He is demonstrating low self-esteem related to the loss of involvement in an important event in his life.

a and d. Even though alteration in nutrition and body temperature are possibilities, no evidence suggests that they likely will occur or must be addressed at this time.

b. Anxiety is defined as a feeling of uneasiness about an unknown anticipated experience or event.

Analysis/Psychosocial/Analysis (Dx)

4. *Correct response: c*

In the presence of hemothorax, anticoagulant therapy would be used very cautiously if at all.

a, b, and d. These other criteria would be appropriate ICU discharge criteria.

Application/Health promotion/Evaluation

5. *Correct response: b*

Leg exercises are important in reducing the risk of further thrombus development.

a. Reduction of walking is contraindicated.

c. Soaking the feet is not necessary to increase circulation and is inappropriate, especially in an older person because of its drying effect on skin.

d. No physiologic contraindication to bending is associated with this medical diagnosis.

Analysis/Health promotion/Analysis (Dx)

6. *Correct response: d*

The underlying pathology of COPD affects the lungs' ability to ventilate and exchange O_2 and CO_2. Ventilation and gas exchange are directly dependent on each other. An effective relationship between the two parameters is absolutely necessary for effective physiologic and mental functioning.

a. Decreasing activity level will not conserve functional lung tissue. Rather, treatment should aim to increase activity while implementing work modification techniques.

b. Postural drainage performed every 2 hours would be unnecessary since no evidence links her problem to retained secretions.

c. The goal would be to decrease rather than increase RV, which usually is high in COPD.

Application/Health promotion/ Implementation

7. *Correct response: c*

Acute respiratory failure results from inadequate gas exchange in the lungs. Increasing the availability of oxygen and assisting with secretion removal will improve ventilation.

a. A patient experiencing acute respiratory failure should usually not be started on an activity program: conservation of energy is critical at this stage.

b. The patient most likely will find that semi-Fowler's or Fowler's position facilitates breathing.

d. Planning for home care is important—but not at this stage; the patient's level of self-care deficit is unknown at this point.

Knowledge/Safe care/Implementation

8. **Correct response: c**
Relaxation techniques and breathing retraining will help a patient with COPD maximize energy supplies and effectively use available oxygen.

a and b. A COPD patient should be encouraged to be as independent as possible within physiologic capabilities; total care encourages deterioration.

d. Knowledge of the disease process may help the patient better understand how she can make the most of her life.

Application/Psychosocial/Implementation

9. **Correct response: c**
Proper cuff pressure ensures a tracheal seal for air while avoiding necrosis of the tracheal wall. Pressure should be kept at or below 20 cm H_2O.

a. Cuff pressure of 42 cm H_2O will stop all circulation to the tracheal mucosa and cause tracheal necrosis.

b. Research indicates that cuff pressures of 24 cm H_2O can lead to necrosis of tracheal mucosa over time.

d. A pressure of 5 cm H_2O will not ensure a tracheal seal and can result in loss of oxygen around the tube.

Analysis/Safe care/Implementation

10. **Correct response: c**
Chills, fever, and pain result from inflammation of the terminal airways and alveoli caused by bacterial, viral, or fungal infection.

a, b, and d. These signs and symptoms are not associated with pneumonia.

Comprehension/Physiologic/Analysis (Dx)

11. **Correct response: a**
As lung infection progresses, ventilation is interrupted. PO_2 usually decreases, and a degree of respiratory insufficiency occurs. As the infection subsides and lung function returns, PO_2 typically rises to 85 to 100 mmHg.

b. PCO_2 of 80 mmHg indicates respiratory failure.

c. Decreased breath sounds is an abnormal manifestation.

d. Restlessness and confusion would indicate hypoxia rather than improvement.

Analysis/Physiologic/Evaluation

12. **Correct response: a**
The patient should be encouraged to cough to raise and expectorate sputum. Splinting the incision during coughing is recommended to minimize discomfort.

b. Thoracotomy tubes are always attached to closed sealed drainage to reexpand lung tissue and prevent pneumothorax.

c. IV fluid infusion is indicated following surgery because the patient will not be able to tolerate oral fluids for a time. Restricting fluids would encourage dehydration.

d. Coughing is indicated to mobilize secretions.

Analysis/Safe care/Planning

13. **Correct response: d**
Suctioning may produce lobar collapse if the suction catheter diameter is too large for the size of the airway. Lobar collapse occurs when air cannot enter the lung from around the catheter while suction is applied.

a. This catheter is too large in diameter.

b and c. Performing intermittent suctioning for no more than 8 seconds at a time and using low pressure reduce the risk of trauma or hypoxia.

Application/Safe care/Planning

14. *Correct response: c*

    Atmospheric air comprises oxygen, nitrogen, carbon dioxide, and water. Inhaled air is translated into partial pressure of its components. At an altitude of 5000 feet, the partial pressure of arterial O_2 is 65 to 75 mmHg. The pH remains the same regardless of altitude.

Knowledge/Physiologic/Evaluation

15. *Correct response: b*

    The rhythmicity of breathing is controlled by respiratory centers located in the medulla oblongata of the brain. These inspiratory and expiratory centers control the rate and depth of respiration to meet the body's metabolic demands.

    a. Located in the aortic arch and carotid bodies, baroreceptors respond to increase and decrease in arterial blood pressure and cause reflex

    hypoventilation and hyperventilation.

    c. The alveoli contain stretch receptors that mediate overdistension of the lung.

    d. The pons houses the pneumotaxic center, which is thought to stimulate the expiratory medullary center.

Comprehension/Physiologic/Assessment

16. *Correct response: c*

    Broad-spectrum antibiotics are indicated under medical supervision as a prophylactic treatment against lung infections, particularly during winter months. Influenza injections are regularly recommended for patients with chronic chest problems.

    a. Penicillin is not a broad-spectrum antibiotic.

    b. Patients with lung disease should not smoke any substance in any form.

    d. PO_2 studies are indicated only if exacerbation occurs.

Comprehension/Health promotion/Planning

Cardiovascular Disorders

I. **Anatomy and physiology**
   A. Structure
   B. Function
II. **Overview of cardiovascular disorders**
   A. Assessment
   B. Laboratory studies and diagnostic tests
   C. Psychosocial implications
   D. Medications used to treat cardiovascular disorders
III. **Dysrhythmias**
   A. Overview
   B. Sinus tachycardia
   C. Sinus bradycardia
   D. Paroxysmal atrial tachycardia (PAT) or paroxysmal supraventricular tachycardia (PSVT)
   E. Atrial fibrillation
   F. Atrioventricular (AV) blocks
   G. Premature ventricular contractions (PVCs)
   H. Ventricular tachycardia (VT)
   I. Ventricular fibrillation
IV. **Coronary artery disease (coronary atherosclerosis)**
   A. Description
   B. Etiology and incidence
   C. Pathophysiology
   D. Assessment findings
   E. Nursing diagnoses
   F. Planning and implementation
   G. Evaluation
V. **Myocardial infarction (MI)**
   A. Description
   B. Etiology and incidence
   C. Pathophysiology
   D. Assessment findings

E. Nursing diagnoses
F. Planning and implementation
G. Evaluation
VI. **Congestive heart failure (CHF)**
   A. Description
   B. Etiology
   C. Pathophysiology
   D. Assessment findings
   E. Nursing diagnoses
   F. Planning and implementation
   G. Evaluation
VII. **Acute pulmonary edema**
   A. Description
   B. Etiology
   C. Pathophysiology
   D. Assessment findings
   E. Nursing diagnoses
   F. Planning and implementation
   G. Evaluation
VIII. **Cardiac arrest**
   A. Description
   B. Etiology
   C. Pathophysiology
   D. Assessment findings
   E. Nursing diagnoses
   F. Planning and implementation
   G. Evaluation
IX. **Endocarditis**
   A. Description
   B. Etiology and incidence
   C. Pathophysiology
   D. Assessment findings
   E. Nursing diagnoses
   F. Planning and implementation
   G. Evaluation
X. **Pericarditis**

I. Anatomy and physiology

A. Structure

1. A hollow, muscular organ, the heart lies in the mediastinum (the space between the two lungs) and rests on the diaphragm.

2. The heart is encased in the *pericardium*, a thin, membranous sac that has two layers: a *visceral* layer in contact with the heart and an outer *parietal* layer.

3. The space between the pericardial layers contains 20 to 30 mL of serous fluid, which protects the heart from trauma and friction.

4. The heart wall, specialized muscle tissue, consists of three tissue layers:

   a. *Epicardium*, the thin, serous outer layer
   b. *Myocardium*, the thick, muscular middle layer
   c. *Endocardium*, the smooth inner layer that comes in contact with blood

5. A membranous muscular *septum* divides the heart into two distinct sides, each containing two chambers: an atrium and a ventricle.

6. The *right atrium*, a low-pressure chamber, receives systemic venous blood via the superior vena cava, inferior vena cava, and coronary sinus.

7. The *right ventricle*, another low-pressure chamber, receives blood from the right atrium through the tricuspid valve during ventricular diastole, then ejects deoxygenated blood via the

pulmonic valve through the pulmonary artery and into pulmonary circulation during ventricular systole.

8. The *left atrium*, a low-pressure chamber, receives oxygenated blood returning to the heart from the lung via four pulmonary veins.

9. The *left ventricle*, a high-pressure chamber, receives blood from the left atrium through the mitral valve during ventricular diastole and ejects oxygenated blood via the aortic valve through the aorta and into systemic circulation during ventricular systole.

10. Valves connect the chambers and outflow tracts; types include atrioventricular and semilunar valves.

11. *Atrioventricular valves*, separating the atria from the ventricles, include:

    a. The *tricuspid valve* (so called because it contains three cusps, or leaflets) between the right atrium and ventricle

    b. The *mitral valve* (or bicuspid valve, with two cusps) between the left atrium and ventricle

12. Situated between each ventricle and its corresponding artery, *semilunar valves* (each containing three cusps) include:

    a. The *pulmonic valve* between the right ventricle and pulmonary artery

    b. The *aortic valve* between the left ventricle and aorta

13. *Papillary muscles*, muscle bundles on the ventricular walls, and *chordae tendineae*, fibrous bands extending from the papillary muscles to the valve cusps, keep the valves closed during systole, maintaining unidirectional blood flow through the atrioventricular valves and preventing backflow of blood.

14. The *cardiac conduction system* consists of specialized cardiac cells that either initiate or propagate electrical impulses throughout the myocardium as a precursor to cardiac muscle contraction.

15. Located at the junction of the right atrium and the superior vena cava, the *sinoatrial (SA) node* functions as the pacemaker for the myocardium, initiating rhythmic electrical impulses at an intrinsic rate of 60 to 100 impulses per minute.

16. The *AV node*, located in the right atrial wall near the tricuspid valve, receives impulses from the SA node and relays them to the ventricles.

17. These impulses travel through a bundle of specialized muscle fibers in the myocardial septum—the *bundle of His*—that divides into right and left branches:

    a. The *right bundle branch* (RBB), which conducts impulses down the right side of the septum

    b. The *left bundle branch* (LBB), which divides again into right and left fascicles that fan out into the left ventricular muscle

18. The RBB and LBB terminate in the *Purkinje fibers*, which prop-

agate electrical impulses into the endocardium and on to the myocardium.

19. The *coronary arteries* supply the heart with blood from branches that originate in either the right or left sinus of Valsalva of the aortic valve cusps.

20. The *right coronary artery* supplies blood to the right heart wall. The *left main coronary artery*, which divides into two branches—the left anterior descending (LAD) coronary artery and the circumflex artery—supplies most of the blood to the left heart wall.

B. **Function**

1. The heart has electrophysiologic, mechanical, and neurologic properties that coordinate to produce effective myocardial contraction and pumping of blood.

2. Each complete heartbeat, or *cardiac cycle*, consists of two phases in response to electrical stimulation:
   a. *Systole*, the contraction phase
   b. *Diastole*, the relaxation (filling) phase

3. Systole is triggered by *depolarization* of cardiac muscle cells, which involves a transient change in sodium and potassium ion concentration inside and outside the cell.

4. Immediately after depolarization is completed, the process reverses itself, resulting in *repolarization* and a return to the resting state, or diastole.

5. Heart sounds result from vibrations caused by valve closure and ventricular filling; they include:
   a. The *first heart sound* (S1), associated with tricuspid and mitral valve closure
   b. The *second heart sound* (S2), associated with aortic and pulmonic valve closure
   c. The *physiologic third heart sound* (S3), often normal in persons under age 30 but pathologic in older persons (known as *ventricular gallop*), occurring during the rapid ventricular filling stage of diastole
   d. The *fourth heart sound* (S4), or atrial gallop, linked to resistance to ventricular filling, as in hypertrophy or injury of the ventricular wall

6. Cardiac output (CO) is defined as the volume of blood ejected by each ventricle in 1 minute; CO = SV (stroke volume) × HR (heart rate).

7. Several factors influence CO indirectly by affecting SV, including:
   a. *Preload*, the end-diastolic filling volume of the ventricle; increased by increased returning volume to ventricle
   b. *Afterload*, the resistance to left ventricular ejection; increased by increased systemic arterial pressure

8. Various neurologic factors regulate heart function, including:
   a. Sympathetic nervous system stimulation, with release of norepinephrine, which results in arteriolar vasoconstriction, increased heart rate, and a positive inotropic effect
   b. Parasympathetic nervous system stimulation, with release of acetylcholine, resulting in decreased heart rate and slowed AV conduction
   c. Response of chemoreceptors located in carotid and aortic bodies to decrease in O_2 and increase in CO_2, leading to increased heart rate
   d. Response of baroreceptors located in the aortic arch, carotid sinus, vena cava, pulmonary arteries and atria to blood pressure changes; either decrease or increase heart rate, resulting in blood pressure changes

II. Cardiovascular system overview

A. Assessment

1. During the health history, the nurse should elicit a description of symptoms, including onset, course, duration, location, and precipitating and alleviating factors; significant symptoms in cardiovascular dysfunction include:
   a. Pain: character, quality, radiation, associated symptoms; may be an indicator of myocardial ischemia
   b. Palpitations, characterized by rapid irregular or pounding heart beat; may be associated with dysrhythmias or ischemia
   c. Intermittent claudication, characterized by extremity pain with exercise; indicative of peripheral vascular disease
   d. Dyspnea, characterized by difficult breathing or shortness of breath with activity (dyspnea on exertion), in the supine position (orthopnea), or sudden onset at night (paroxysmal nocturnal dyspnea); commonly associated with compromised cardiac function
   e. Fatigue with or without activity; may be associated with decreased cardiac output
   f. Syncope with or without dizziness; can result from sudden decrease in cardiac output
   g. Diaphoresis with associated clamminess and cyanosis; reflects decreased cardiac output and poor peripheral perfusion
   h. Edema or weight gain (> 3 lb in 24 hours); may indicate heart failure

2. The nurse also should explore the patient's health history for risk factors associated with cardiovascular disease, including:
   a. Positive family history for cardiovascular disease
   b. Age (Incidence increases after age 40.)

    c.   Sex (Mortality from cardiovascular disease is greater in men than in women; difference decreases after menopause.)

    d.   Race (Mortality is greater in nonwhites than in whites.)

    e.   Smoking (The risk of cardiovascular disease is 2 to 4 times greater in cigarette smokers than in nonsmokers.)

    f.   Hypertension, particularly elevated systolic pressure

    g.   Hyperlipidemia (The ratio of HDL to LDL is the best predictor.)

    h.   Obesity, which contributes to the severity of other risk factors

    i.   Physical inactivity (sedentary lifestyle)

    j.   Diabetes (Uncontrolled elevated blood glucose increases risk.)

    k.   Stress, which may contribute to the development of coronary artery disease (CAD).

    l.   Use of oral contraceptives

3.   Physical assessment should include the following:

    a.   Assess the patient's general appearance for signs of distress, anxiety, and altered level of consciousness.

    b.   Assess vital signs, particularly pulse, blood pressure, and respirations.

    c.   Assess peripheral pulses.

    d.   Inspect the lips, earlobes, and buccal mucosa for central cyanosis, reflecting hypoxia.

    e.   Inspect and palpate the carotid arteries.

    f.   Assess jugular venous pressure, and observe for venous distention.

    g.   Inspect and palpate the precordium to locate the point of maximal impulse (PMI) or the apical impulse.

    h.   Systematically auscultate the heart for normal and abnormal heart sounds, murmurs, and friction rub, covering four main areas: aortic area, pulmonary area, mitral area, and tricuspid area.

    i.   Perform a respiratory assessment (see Chapter 6, Section II.A, for more information). Findings pointing to cardiovascular problems may include cough (possibly reflecting pulmonary congestion); rales, crackles, or wheezing (reflecting airway narrowing, atelectasis or left ventricular failure); hemoptysis (possibly pointing to acute pulmonary edema); Cheyne-Stokes respiration (possibly associated with severe left ventricular failure).

    j.   Perform an abdominal assessment (see Chapter 9, Section II.A, for more information), noting particularly liver enlargement and ascites (indicating decreased venous return secondary to right ventricular failure); bladder distention (possibly pointing to decreased cardiac output); and bruits just above the umbilicus (may reflect abdominal aortic obstruction or aneurysm).

B. **Laboratory studies and diagnostic tests**

   1. Important laboratory studies in cardiovascular evaluation include:
      a. Leukocyte count
      b. Lipid profile: cholesterol (LDL and HDL), triglycerides
      c. Cardiac enzymes: lactic dehydrogenase (LDH), creatinine phosphokinase (CPK), and their isoenzymes
      d. Blood coagulation: prothrombin time (PT), partial thromboplastin time (PTT)

   2. Noninvasive diagnostic studies include:
      a. Chest radiograph, to determine heart size and silhouette and visualize the pulmonary system
      b. Electrocardiography (ECG), to evaluate the heart's electrical activity
      c. Ambulatory ECG, to allow 24-hour continuous measurement of the heart's electrical activity
      d. Exercise ECG (graded exercise test), to evaluate electrical activity during physical stress
      e. Vectorcardiography, which provides a graphic representation of the direction and magnitude of the heart's electrical activity
      f. Echocardiography, which yields information about cardiac structures (especially valvular) and function
      g. Radionuclide testing, which evaluates ventricular function, and myocardial blood flow and detects areas of myocardial damage

   3. Invasive diagnostic studies include:
      a. Cardiac catheterization, which enables measurement of chamber pressures and oxygen saturation
      b. Arteriography, done to visualize coronary arteries with injections of radiopaque contrast media
      c. Ventriculography, to visualize ventricles with injection of radiopaque contrast media
      d. Central venous pressure (CVP), which reflects filling pressure of the right ventricle and helps assess cardiac function and intravascular volume status
      e. Pulmonary artery (PA) pressure and pulmonary artery wedge pressure (PAWP), which measure left heart pressures
      f. Arterial line, which allows continuous monitoring of peripheral arterial pressures

C. **Psychosocial implications**

   1. A patient with cardiovascular dysfunction commonly experi-

ences problems in coping with the disease process, related to such factors as:

    a. Sense of loss of control

    b. Perception of the heart as a center of emotion and personality

    c. Uncertain prognosis

    d. Fear of rejection and isolation

    e. Fear of dying

2. The patient also may experience self-concept changes related to fear of:

    a. Sexual dysfunction

    b. Role change toward increased dependence

    c. Body image changes if surgery or an adjunctive device (such as a pacemaker) is needed

3. The patient may have concerns associated with changes in lifestyle due to alterations in:

    a. Physical activity

    b. Work performance, with potential for loss of job

D. Medications used to treat cardiovascular disorders

1. *Antiarrhythmic agents*, used to reduce or prevent cardiac dysrhythmias, include:

    a. Amiodarone

    b. Bretylium

    c. Disopyramide phosphate

    d. Lidocaine

    e. Methoxamine

    f. Procainamide

    g. Quinidine

2. *Anticoagulant agents*, used to treat or prevent deep vein thrombosis or pulmonary embolism, include:

    a. Heparin sodium

    b. Warfarin sodium

3. *Antilipid agents*, administered to reduce serum lipid levels, include:

    a. Cholestyramine

    b. Clofibrate

    c. Colestipol

    d. Neomycin

    e. Nicotinic acid

    f. Probucol

4. Used to treat stable or unstable angina, dysrhythmias, and hypertension in CAD, *beta-adrenergic blockers* decrease the heart rate and force of contraction and reduce vasoconstriction by antagonizing beta-receptors in the myocardium and vasculature; agents include:

    a. Atenolol

      b.   Metoprolol

      c.   Nadolol

      d.   Propranolol

      e.   Timolol

  5. Used to treat angina and coronary artery spasms, *calcium channel antagonists* inhibit movement of calcium ions across myocardial and vascular smooth muscle, resulting in vasodilation of coronary arteries and collateral vessels, decreased myocardial contractility, and vasodilation of peripheral vessels; agents include:

      a.   Diltiazem

      b.   Nifedipine

      c.   Verapamil

  6. *Cardiac glycosides*, which increase the force of myocardial contractions and slow heart rate and conduction through the AV node and bundle of His, are used to treat CHF and atrial dysrhythmias; agents include:

      a.   Digoxin

      b.   Digitoxin

  7. Used to treat angina and coronary artery spasm, *nitrates* reduce myocardial oxygen demand by promoting vasodilation and by increasing oxygen supply to myocardial tissue; agents include:

      a.   Isosorbide dinitrate

      b.   Nitroglycerin

  8. *Thrombolytic agents*, used in acute management of thrombus formation and to dissolve thrombi or emboli in acute myocardial infarction, include:

      a.   Streptokinase

      b.   t-PA (human tissue plasminogen activator)

      c.   Urokinase

III. Dysrhythmias

A. Overview

  1. Dysrhythmia (or arrhythmia) refers to any cardiac rhythm deviating from normal sinus rhythm.

  2. Normal sinus rhythm has the following characteristics:

      a.   Rate: 60 to 100 beats per minute

      b.   P waves: preceding each QRS complex

      c.   P–R interval: 0.12 to 0.20 seconds

      d.   QRS complex: 0.04 to 0.1 seconds

      e.   Conduction: forward through the conduction system

      f.   Rhythm: regular with no abnormal delay

  3. Dysrhythmias result from altered impulse formation, altered impulse conduction, or both.

  4. Symptomatology varies from asymptomatic to death.

  5. Treatment of choice varies depending on type and severity.

B. **Sinus tachycardia**
1. Description: heart rate greater than 100 beats per minute; originates in the sinus node
2. Characteristics
   a. Rate: 100 to 180 beats per minute
   b. P waves: precede each QRS complex
   c. P–R interval: normal
   d. QRS complex: normal
   e. Conduction: normal
   f. Rhythm: regular
3. Causes include exercise, anxiety, fever, drugs, anemia, heart failure, hypovolemia, shock.
4. Clinical manifestations
   a. Usually asymptomatic
   b. Occasionally palpitations
   c. Hypotension, angina with cardiovascular disease
5. Treatment is directed at the primary cause, which usually is not cardiac related.

C. **Sinus bradycardia**
1. Description: heart rate less than 60 beats per minute; originates in the sinus node
2. Characteristics
   a. Rate: less than 60 beats per minute
   b. P waves: precede each QRS complex
   c. P–R interval: normal
   d. QRS complex: normal
   e. Conduction: normal
   f. Rhythm: regular
3. Causes include drugs, vagal stimulation, hypoendocrine states, anorexia, hypothermia or sinus node involvement in myocardial infarction; may be normal in athletes.
4. Clinical manifestations
   a. Often asymptomatic
   b. Fatigue
   c. Lightheadedness
   d. Syncope
5. Treatment is aimed at maintaining adequate cardiac output through treating the underlying cause and administering atropine or using a pacemaker if necessary.

D. **PAT or PSVT**
1. Description: abrupt onset and cessation of rapid heartbeat (palpitations); originates in atria
2. Characteristics
   a. Rate: 150 to 250 beats per minute
   b. P waves: ectopic, may be found in preceding T waves

      c.   P–R interval: shortened, 0.12 second

      d.   QRS complex: normal, may be distorted due to aberrancy

      e.   Conduction: normal

      f.   Rhythm: regular

3. Causes include emotions, drugs, alcohol, smoking, hormones; usually not associated with heart disease.

4. Clinical manifestations

      a.   Palpitations

      b.   Lightheadedness

      c.   Dyspnea

      d.   Anginal pain

5. Treatment depends on the patient's overall clinical situation and how well he or she tolerates the dysrhythmia; aimed at decreasing heart rate and eliminating the underlying cause and may include:

      a.   Carotid sinus pressure or any vagal maneuver

      b.   Digitalis

      c.   Calcium channel blocker

      d.   Propranolol

      e.   Quinidine

      f.   Cardioversion if rapid rate is not tolerated by the patient

E. **Atrial fibrillation**

1. Description: disorganized and uncoordinated twitching of atrial musculature due to overrapid production of atrial impulses

2. Characteristics

      a.   Rate: atrial rate, 350 to 600 beats per minute; ventricular response rate, 120 to 200 beats per minute

      b.   P wave: none discernible, irregular baseline

      c.   P–R interval: not measurable

      d.   QRS complex: normal

      e.   Conduction: normal through ventricle, irregular through AV junction because of overwhelming number of impulses from atria

      f.   Rhythm: irregularly irregular, usually rapid unless controlled

3. Causes include atherosclerosis, rheumatic mitral valve stenosis, congestive heart failure, congenital; chronic obstructive pulmonary disease; thyrotoxicosis.

4. Clinical manifestations

      a.   Asymptomatic

      b.   Palpitations

      c.   Dyspnea

      d.   Pulmonary edema

      e.   Signs of cerebrovascular insufficiency

5. Treatment is directed at decreasing ventricular response, decreasing atrial irritability, and eliminating the cause and may include:
    a. Digitalis
    b. Cardioversion
    c. Other drugs, such as calcium channel blockers, procainamide, and quinidine

F. AV blocks
1. Description: conduction defect within the AV junction that impairs conduction of atrial impulses to ventricular pathways; three types exist: first degree, second degree, and third degree
2. Characteristics
    a. Rate: first degree—usually 60 to 100 beats per minute or the inherent ventricular rate; second degree—slowed, atrial rate 2 to 4 times faster than the ventricular rate; third degree—slowed, 40 to 60 beats per minute or the inherent ventricular rate
    b. P wave: normal and present in each type of block
    c. P–R intervals: first degree—prolonged, 0.20 second; second degree—may be progressively lengthening, as in Type I (Mobitz I or Wenckebach) or fixed, as in Type II (Mobitz II); third degree—no relationship between P waves and QRS complexes; cannot be measured
    d. QRS complex: first and second degrees—usually normal; third degree—widened (0.10 second) if originating from ventricles, or normal duration if originating from the AV junction below the block
    e. Conduction: first degree—delayed in AV junction; second degree—impulses not regularly conducted through the AV junction; third degree—all sinus impulses blocked, conduction through ventricles abnormal
    f. Rhythm: regular
3. Causes include congenital and atherosclerotic heart disease (most common); certain drugs (digitalis, vagotonic agents, sympatholytic agents, beta-adrenergic blockers); hypokalemia
4. Clinical manifestations
    a. first degree: asymptomatic
    b. second degree: vertigo, weakness, irregular pulse
    c. third degree: hypotension, angina, heart failure
5. Treatment
    a. first degree: no treatment necessary; may need to discontinue causative drug
    b. second degree: increase heart rate with atropine; may need a pacemaker with certain types of myocardial infarction
    c. third degree: support of ventricular escape rhythm

through use of atropine or isoproterenol and a pacemaker

G. PVCs

1. Description: early contraction of ventricle due to increased automaticity of ventricular muscle cells; usually not considered harmful but are of concern when more than six occur in 1 minute, if they occur in pairs or triplets, if they are multifocal, or if they occur on or near a T wave

2. Characteristics
    a. Rate: of underlying rhythm, usually 60 to 100 beats per minute
    b. P wave: of underlying rhythm, normal; of premature beat, no P wave
    c. P–R interval: of underlying rhythm, normal; of premature beat, no P–R interval
    d. QRS complex: of underlying rhythm, normal; of premature beat, wide and bizarre (>0.10 second); may have one focus or variety of foci, resulting in many different configurations (multifocal)
    e. Conduction: retrograde through conduction system
    f. Rhythm: usually irregular when premature beat occurs; may be in a regular pattern, as in bigeminy

3. Causes include factors linked to irritability of ventricular muscle cells, including normal variance, exercise, increased catecholamines, electrolyte imbalance, digitalis toxicity, and hypoxia and myocardial damage.

4. Clinical manifestations
    a. Asymptomatic
    b. Palpitations
    c. Weakness
    d. Lightheadedness

5. Treatment is indicated in the presence of underlying disease due to the danger of precipitating ventricular tachycardia or fibrillation; antiarrhythmic drugs used include:
    a. Lidocaine IV (drug of choice)
    b. Procainamide or bretylium IV (if PVCs are not suppressed with lidocaine)

H. VT

1. Description: defined as three or more consecutive PVCs; considered a medical emergency since cardiac output cannot be maintained because of decreased diastolic filling

2. Characteristics
    a. Rate: 100 to 250 beats per minute
    b. P wave: blurred in QRS, but QRS complexes have no association with P waves

      c.   P–R interval: none

      d.   QRS complex: wide, bizarre, T waves in opposite direction

      e.   Conduction: abnormal through ventricular tissue

      f.   Rhythm: usually regular

3. Causes linked to irritability of ventricular muscle (see Section III.G.3)

4. Clinical manifestations

      a.   Lightheadedness

      b.   Weakness

      c.   Dyspnea

      d.   Unconsciousness

5. Treatment

      a.   If the patient is conscious, lidocaine IV; if lidocaine is not successful, procainamide or bretylium

      b.   If the patient is unconscious or if lidocaine is unsuccessful, cardioversion

      c.   If rhythm deteriorates to ventricular fibrillation, or if the patient is pulseless, defibrillation and cardiopulmonary resuscitation (CPR)

I. Ventricular fibrillation

1. Description: rapid, ineffective quivering of ventricles that may be rapidly fatal

2. Characteristics

      a.   Rate: rapid, uncoordinated, ineffective motions

      b.   P wave: not seen

      c.   P–R interval: not seen

      d.   QRS complex: seen as undulation with no specific pattern

      e.   Conduction: no organized conduction, many foci firing at once

      f.   Rhythm: irregular without pattern

3. Cause is most commonly myocardial ischemia or infarction; also may result from untreated VT, electrolyte imbalances (hypokalemia and alkalosis, hyperkalemia and hypercalcemia), digitalis or quinidine toxicity, or hypothermia.

4. Clinical manifestations

      a.   Loss of consciousness

      b.   Pulselessness

      c.   Loss of blood pressure

      d.   Cessation of respirations

      e.   Possible seizures

      f.   Sudden death

5. Treatment involves defibrillation, CPR, and drugs such as lidocaine, bretylium, or procainamide.

IV. Coronary artery disease (coronary atherosclerosis)

A. Description: focal narrowing of large and medium-sized coronary arteries due to intimal plaque formation; the most common cardiac disorder in the United States

B. Etiology and incidence

1. Causes are variable and may involve a combination of factors such as genetic predisposition, metabolic disturbances, arterial hypertension, and altered platelet function that predisposes to plaque formation.

2. Risk factors for coronary atherosclerosis include:
   a. Advanced age
   b. Male or postmenopausal female
   c. Hyperlipidemia
   d. Smoking
   e. Hypertension
   f. Diabetes mellitus
   g. Obesity
   h. Sedentary lifestyle
   i. Family history
   j. Chronic stress
   k. Oral contraceptive use

3. Incidence increases progressively with age; death rate in white males is 10 per 100,000 between ages 25 and 34, 1000 per 100,000 between ages 55 and 64.

4. Incidence is roughly three times greater in men than in women and is greater in blacks than in whites.

C. Pathophysiology

1. Atherosclerosis begins with formation of fatty, fibrous plaques on the intima of coronary arteries.

2. These plaques narrow the arterial lumen, reducing the volume of blood that can flow through the artery to the heart.

3. Reduced coronary blood flow leads to myocardial ischemia and varying degrees of cell damage.

4. Plaque formation also predisposes to thrombus formation and subsequent embolism.

D. Assessment findings

1. Common clinical manifestations include:
   a. Chest pain (angina), the most characteristic symptom, marked by mild to severe retrosternal pain typically described as burning or squeezing that may radiate to the arm, jaw, neck, or shoulder; usually precipitated by exertion, cold, heavy meal, smoking, or excitement (or may occur at rest because of vasospasm), and relieved by rest and nitrates
   b. Nausea and vomiting

      c.   Dizziness, syncope

      d.   Diaphoresis; cool, clammy skin

      e.   Apprehension, a sense of impending doom

2. The patient's ECG may appear normal when pain-free and may show ischemic changes (ST depression, T-wave inversion) during angina episodes or exercise.

E. Nursing diagnoses

1. Activity Intolerance
2. Altered Family Processes
3. Fear
4. Knowledge Deficit
5. Pain

F. Planning and implementation

1. Reduce activity to a point at which pain does not occur.
2. Assess blood pressure and pulse rate during anginal episodes.
3. Monitor ECG during anginal episodes.
4. Support and reassure the patient during anginal episodes.
5. Administer oxygen therapy as prescribed.
6. Relieve pain immediately with nitrates or other analgesics as prescribed.
7. Prepare the patient for coronary angiography if indicated. This procedure evaluates narrowing of arteries due to atherosclerotic plaques, the usual pathology.
8. Prepare the patient for possible treatment (e.g., t-PA therapy, angioplasty, coronary artery bypass grafting).
9. Provide patient and family teaching, covering:
   a. Basic pathophysiology of coronary atherosclerosis, its effects, and treatments
   b. Recognition and avoidance of events precipitating angina
   c. Proper use of medications: purpose, effects, dosage, side effects; include use and maintenance of nitroglycerin
   d. Lifestyle modifications to reduce risk factors
   e. Signs and symptoms to watch for and report promptly
   f. Appropriate action to take when pain occurs
   g. CPR techniques

G. Evaluation

1. The patient verbalizes factors and events that precipitate pain.
2. The patient reports no pain during normal activities.
3. The patient reports relief of anginal pain with nitrate administration.
4. The patient displays decreased anxiety.
5. The patient and family members or significant others verbalize understanding of the disease process, its effects, and prescribed treatment.

V. MI

A. Description: destruction of myocardial tissue in regions of the heart abruptly deprived of adequate blood supply due to reduced coronary blood flow

B. Etiology and incidence

    1. Causes of MI include:

        a. Coronary artery narrowing due to atherosclerosis, coronary artery spasm, or complete arterial occlusion by embolism or thrombus

        b. Decreased coronary blood flow due to hemorrhage or shock, causing a profound imbalance between myocardial oxygen supply and demand

    2. In the United States, well over 1 million cases of MI are reported annually. Incidence is far greater in men than in women.

C. Pathophysiology

    1. In MI, inadequate coronary blood flow rapidly results in myocardial ischemia in the affected area. The location and extent of the infarct determine the effects on cardiac function.

    2. Ischemia depresses cardiac function and triggers autonomic nervous system responses that exacerbate the imbalance between myocardial oxygen supply and demand.

    3. Persistent ischemia results in tissue necrosis and scar tissue formation, with permanent loss of myocardial contractility in the affected area.

    4. Cardiogenic shock may develop due to inadequate cardiac output secondary to decreased myocardial contractility and pumping capacity.

D. Assessment findings

    1. Common clinical manifestations include:

        a. Chest pain (typically persistent and crushing; located substernally with radiation to the arm, neck, jaw, or back and unrelieved by rest or nitrates); a so-called silent MI may produce no pain

        b. Diaphoresis and cool, clammy, pale skin

        c. Nausea and vomiting

        d. Dyspnea with or without crackles

        e. Palpitations or syncope

        f. Restlessness and anxiety, feeling of impending doom

        g. Tachycardia or bradycardia

        h. Decreased blood pressure

        i. Heart sounds: S4, possibly a systolic murmur

    2. Laboratory studies may reveal:

        a. ECG changes: ST segment and T-wave changes, Q waves; location of changes on the monitoring strip depends on the location of the infarct in the heart

  b. Serum enzyme elevations: CPK and CPK-MB, LDH

  c. Elevated WBC count

E. Nursing diagnoses

 1. Anxiety

 2. Decreased Cardiac Output

 3. Impaired Gas Exchange

 4. Pain

F. Planning and implementation

 1. Monitor the ECG to continually assess heart rate, rhythm, and conduction.

 2. Monitor vital signs: temperature, blood pressure, pulse, respiration.

 3. Administer prescribed analgesics to relieve chest pain.

 4. Establish a patent IV line to enable rapid medication and fluid administration if needed.

 5. Maintain the patient on bedrest in semi-Fowler's position.

 6. Administer oxygen therapy as prescribed.

 7. Monitor hemodynamic parameters as necessary.

 8. Carefully record urine intake and output.

 9. Reassure the patient, and explain procedures as the situation warrants.

 10. Provide a quiet, restful environment to the extent possible.

 11. Assess heart and lung sounds regularly.

 12. Institute a liquid diet; advance to a low-sodium, solid diet as tolerated.

 13. Administer stool softeners, as ordered, to prevent the patient from straining on defecation.

 14. Progress the patient's activity according to protocol and the patient's condition.

 15. Provide patient and family teaching, covering:

  a. Basic pathophysiology of MI, its effects, and treatment

  b. Necessary lifestyle modifications (e.g., diet) to reduce risk factors for another MI

  c. Exercise program to begin during hospitalization and continue after discharge

  d. Signs and symptoms of further heart damage to watch for and report

  e. Protocol to follow in the event of recurrence of chest pain or other symptoms of MI

  f. Resumption of sexual activity

  g. Proper use of medications: purpose, effects, dosage, side effects

G. Evaluation

 1. The patient demonstrates stabilization of cardiac rhythm, vital signs, and hemodynamic parameters.

2. The patient reports no pain during normal activities.
3. The patient enters a cardiac rehabilitation or exercise program.
4. The patient exhibits decreased anxiety.
5. The patient and family members or significant others verbalize an understanding of the disease process, its effects, and treatment.

VI. CHF
A. Description
1. CHF is a syndrome of pulmonary or systemic circulatory congestion due to decreased myocardial contractility, resulting in inadequate cardiac output to meet oxygen requirements of tissues.
2. CHF may be classified as:
   a. Left sided (or left ventricular)
   b. Right sided (or right ventricular)
   c. Biventricular
B. Etiology
1. The primary causes of CHF are disorders producing decreased myocardial contractility (e.g., MI, valvular heart disease, hypertension, cardiomyopathy).
2. Other possible causes include:
   a. Conditions increasing afterload (e.g., acute systemic hypertension)
   b. Conditions causing abnormalities in preload (e.g., severe renal failure, constrictive pericarditis)
C. Pathophysiology
1. Left-sided CHF
   a. Congestion occurs primarily in the lungs from backup of blood into pulmonary veins and capillaries due to left ventricular pump failure.
   b. As blood backs up into the pulmonary bed, increased hydrostatic pressure causes fluid accumulation in the lungs.
   c. Blood flow is consequently decreased to the brain, kidneys, and other tissues.
2. Right-sided CHF
   a. Congestion in systemic circulation results from right ventricular pump failure.
   b. As blood backs up into systemic circulation, increased hydrostatic pressure produces peripheral and dependent pitting edema.
   c. Venous congestion in the kidneys, liver, and GI tract also develops.
D. Assessment findings
1. Clinical manifestations of left-sided CHF may include:

      a.   Dyspnea on exertion, nocturnal dyspnea, orthopnea

      b.   Moist crackles on lung auscultation

      c.   Tachycardia with S3 heart sound

      d.   Easy fatiguability

      e.   Insomnia and restlessness

2. Right-sided CHF may be marked by:
    a. Dependent pitting edema
    b. Weight gain
    c. Nausea, anorexia
    d. Distended neck veins
    e. Liver congestion (hepatomegaly), ascites, weakness

3. Laboratory and diagnostic test results in CHF commonly include:
    a. Cardiomegaly and vascular congestion of lung fields on chest radiograph
    b. ECG findings consistent with hypertrophy or myocardial damage
    c. Arterial blood gas values: decreased PaO_2, increased $PaCO_2$
    d. Hemodynamic changes: elevated pulmonary artery and capillary wedge pressures (left-sided CHF), elevated central venous pressure (right-sided CHF)

E. Nursing diagnoses

1. Activity Intolerance
2. Decreased Cardiac Output
3. Fear
4. Impaired Gas Exchange
5. Knowledge Deficit
6. Sleep Pattern Disturbance
7. Altered Tissue Perfusion: Cardiopulmonary

F. Planning and implementation

1. Promote measures to provide rest for the heart; for example:
    a. Maintain bedrest with limited activity.
    b. Ensure a quiet, relaxed environment.
    c. Cluster necessary nursing care to minimize disruptions.
2. Maintain adequate ventilation:
    a. Monitor respiratory status.
    b. Administer oxygen therapy as prescribed.
    c. Position the patient in semi- or high-Fowler's position.
    d. Monitor ABG values as prescribed.
3. Maintain adequate circulation:
    a. Monitor hemodynamic parameters and heart rate and rhythm.
    b. Administer digitalis and diuretics as prescribed.
4. Weigh the patient daily.

    5. Assess for peripheral and dependent edema.

    6. Keep accurate intake and output records.

    7. Provide a low-sodium diet as prescribed.

    8. Monitor serum electrolyte levels daily.

    9. Instruct the patient in or assist in performing range-of-motion exercises, and apply antiembolism stockings to prevent deep vein thrombosis.

    10. Provide patient and family teaching, covering:

        a. Basic pathophysiology of CHF, its effects, and prescribed treatment

        b. Dietary guidelines, including low-sodium foods and, if applicable, high-potassium foods to replace potassium lost through diuretic therapy

        c. Proper use of medications: purpose, action, dosage, side effects

        d. Signs and symptoms of complications to watch for and report

        e. The need for regular follow-up examinations

        f. The importance of getting adequate rest and avoiding fatigue

G. Evaluation

    1. The patient demonstrates stable cardiac rhythm, vital signs, hemodynamic parameters, and urinary output.

    2. The patient limits activities to a level that permits the heart to rest.

    3. The patient exhibits weight loss, indicating reduced fluid overload.

    4. The patient displays decreased anxiety.

    5. The patient and family members or significant others verbalize an understanding of the disease process, its effects, and treatment.

VII. Acute pulmonary edema

    A. Description: rapid fluid accumulation in the extravascular (alveoli and interstitial) lung spaces; considered a medical emergency

    B. Etiology

        1. Major causes of acute pulmonary edema include:

           a. Left ventricular CHF (most common cause), MI, or other cardiac disorders

           b. Circulatory overload from infusions or transfusions

           c. Lung injury (e.g., smoke inhalation, pulmonary embolism)

           d. Drug hypersensitivity, allergy, poisoning, narcotic overdose

           e. Central nervous system damage (e.g., cerebrovascular accident, head trauma)

        f.   Pulmonary infections (e.g., viral, bacterial, or parasitic pneumonia)

    2.   Acute pulmonary edema also may develop after certain procedures and treatments (e.g., cardioversion, coronary artery bypass grafting, postanesthesia).

C. Pathophysiology

    1.   Engorged with blood, the pulmonary capillaries eventually cannot hold their contents, and fluid leaks into adjacent alveoli or interstitial spaces.

    2.   Fluid accumulation causes the lungs to stiffen and impairs normal expansion, resulting in severe hypoxia.

D. Assessment findings

    1.   Signs and symptoms of acute pulmonary edema include:

        a.   Dyspnea and cough producing copious blood-tinged, frothy sputum

        b.   Crackles and wheezes heard throughout the lung fields on auscultation

        c.   Tachycardia, other dysrhythmias

        d.   Cyanotic, cold, clammy, diaphoretic skin

        e.   Restlessness, anxiety

        f.   Jugular venous distension

    2.   Laboratory and diagnostic test findings may reveal:

        a.   Vascular congestion of lung fields ("butterfly" appearance) on chest radiograph

        b.   Hemodynamic changes: elevated central venous, pulmonary artery, and capillary wedge pressures

        c.   ABG alterations: decreased PaO_2, increased $PaCO_2$

E. Nursing diagnoses

    1.   Activity Intolerance

    2.   Decreased Cardiac Output

    3.   Fear

    4.   Impaired Gas Exchange

    5.   Knowledge Deficit

    6.   Sleep Pattern Disturbance

    7.   Altered Tissue Perfusion: Cardiopulmonary

F. Planning and implementation

    1.   Position the patient upright to decrease venous return and allow maximum lung expansion.

    2.   Administer oxygen therapy, as ordered (usually 40% to 60% concentration via face mask).

    3.   Monitor ventilation; assist with intubation or other measures as necessary.

    4.   Administer morphine IV, as ordered, to decrease peripheral resistance and venous capacitance; monitor for respiratory depression.

5. Administer diuretics, as ordered, to reduce circulating blood volume.
6. Administer digitalis, as ordered, to increase myocardial contractions.
7. Administer aminophylline, as ordered, to relieve bronchospasm, promote diuresis, and provide an inotropic effect.
8. Monitor vital signs and hemodynamic parameters, assessing respiratory and cardiovascular status at least hourly.
9. Apply rotating tourniquets to decrease venous return if necessary.
10. Provide reassurance and support to the patient and family members or significant others.
11. Assess renal status through output and electrolyte monitoring.
12. Provide patient and family teaching, covering:
    a. Importance of daily weight measurement and intake and output monitoring to determine the need for further diuresis
    b. Plan for rest periods, gradually increasing daily activity
    c. Dietary guidelines, including foods low in sodium and high in potassium to replace that lost from diuretic therapy
    d. Proper use of medications: purpose, action, dosage, side effects
    e. Signs and symptoms of heart failure to watch for and report

G. Evaluation

1. The patient demonstrates stable cardiac rhythm, vital signs, hemodynamic parameters, and urine output.
2. The patient limits activities to a level that allows the heart to rest.
3. The patient exhibits weight loss, indicating reduced fluid overload.
4. The patient displays decreased anxiety.
5. The patient and family members or significant others verbalize an understanding of the disease process, its effects, and treatment.

VIII. Cardiac arrest

A. Description: sudden, unexpected cessation of the heart's pumping action and effective circulation

B. Etiology

1. Ventricular fibrillation is the major cause of cardiac arrest; possible precipitating factors include:
    a. MI
    b. Congenital heart disease
    c. Heart failure

      d. Pulmonary embolus
      e. Anesthetics, antiarrhythmic drug overdose
      f. Electrical shock
      g. Electrolyte imbalances
      h. Near drowning
      i. Hypothermia
      j. Ventricular irritation due to cardiac pacing during cardiac catheterization or angiography
      k. Acute hemorrhage
      l. Hypoxia or acidosis
      m. Myocarditis

2. Asystole also may trigger cardiac arrest; precipitating factors include:
      a. Drug overdose
      b. Hemorrhage
      c. Anaphylaxis
      d. Respiratory acidosis or hypercapnia
      e. Left-ventricular heart failure

3. Cardiac arrest also can result from electromechanical dissociation stemming from:
      a. Severe MI
      b. Heart wall rupture
      c. Cardiac tamponade
      d. Hemorrhage

4. Other possible causes of cardiac arrest include:
      a. Cardiac standstill resulting from severe hypoxia
      b. Circulatory collapse with acute hypotension due to vasodilation or hypovolemia

C. Pathophysiology

1. Cardiac arrest typically follows premonitory clues (e.g., hypotension, ECG monitor changes, respiratory failure).
2. It represents a medical emergency requiring immediate cardiopulmonary resuscitation (CPR) to restore heart function and circulation.
3. CPR must restore circulation within approximately 4 minutes after the onset of cardiac arrest to prevent irreversible brain damage or death.

D. Assessment findings

1. Clinical manifestations of cardiac arrest include:
      a. Immediate loss of consciousness
      b. Absence of palpable pulses and heart sounds; absence of carotid pulse is the most reliable sign
      c. Apnea or gasping respirations
      d. Ashen-gray skin color
2. Because of the life-threatening nature of cardiac arrest, prompt

identification and initiation of CPR is essential. The nurse should not waste valuable time assessing blood pressure or listening for a heartbeat.

E. Nursing diagnoses
1. Decreased Cardiac Output
2. Impaired Gas Exchange

F. Planning and implementation
1. Begin resuscitation measures immediately to prevent irreversible brain damage.
2. Summon assistance, and establish a patent airway.
3. Provide artificial ventilation by mouth-to-mouth resuscitation or with an Ambu bag; start oxygen as soon as possible.
4. Provide artificial circulation through external cardiac compression.
5. Defibrillate using direct-current countershock for ventricular fibrillation or tachycardia.
6. Establish a patent IV line if not already in place.
7. Administer emergency drugs as ordered.
8. Provide emotional support to family members or significant others and other patients as necessary.
9. Teach family members or significant others:
   a. Steps of CPR
   b. Basic pathophysiology of the underlying disease process

G. Evaluation
1. The patient responds to resuscitative measures.
2. Family members or significant others verbalize an understanding of CPR and the pathophysiology of underlying disease.
3. The patient and family members or significant others display decreased anxiety.

IX. Endocarditis

A. Description: infection of endocardium or heart valves resulting from invasion of bacteria or other organisms; may be acute, subacute, or chronic

B. Etiology and incidence
1. Causative organisms include:
   a. Bacteria (e.g., *Streptococcus viridans*, *Staphylococcus aureus*, *Enterococci*)
   b. Fungi (e.g., *Candida albicans*, *Aspergillus*)
   c. Rickettsiae
2. Predisposing factors include:
   a. History of valvular heart disease
   b. Prosthetic valve replacement surgery
   c. Debilitation
   d. Indwelling catheter placement
   e. Prolonged IV antibiotic therapy

f. IV drug abuse
g. Dental surgery

C. Pathophysiology
1. Ineffective organisms travel through the bloodstream and are deposited on heart valves or other portions of the endocardium.
2. This triggers fibrin and platelet aggregation, which engulf the organisms, forming friable verrucous vegetations.
3. The vegetations typically form on valves but also may extend to the endocardium.
4. Vegetations covering the valve surface can lead to ulceration and necrosis, with subsequent deformity and dysfunction of the valve leaflets.

D. Assessment findings
1. Signs and symptoms of endocarditis include:
    a. Weakness, fatigue
    b. Weight loss, anorexia
    c. Fever, chills, diaphoresis
    d. Cough
    e. Arthralgia
    f. Splenomegaly
    g. Petechiae of the anterior trunk, conjunctivae, and mucosa
    h. Splinter hemorrhages in nail beds
    i. Roth's spots, Osler's nodes, Janeway's lesions
    j. New heart murmur or a change in an existing murmur, especially in the presence of fever
2. Laboratory and diagnostic studies may reveal:
    a. Blood cultures positive for causative organisms
    b. Elevated WBC count and erythrocyte sedimentation rate (ESR)
    c. Anemia
    d. Valvular damage identified on echocardiogram
    e. ECG changes indicating dysrhythmias, cardiomegaly

E. Nursing diagnoses
1. Activity Intolerance
2. Decreased Cardiac Output
3. Knowledge Deficit
4. Pain

F. Planning and implementation
1. Administer antibiotics as prescribed; observe for side effects or signs and symptoms of allergic reaction.
2. Monitor temperature at regular intervals.
3. Draw serial blood cultures to evaluate the effectiveness of therapy.

4. Monitor ECG for dysrhythmias.
5. Observe for signs and symptoms of congestive heart failure.
6. Prepare the patient for possible valve replacement as ordered.
7. Provide psychosocial and emotional support.
8. Provide patient and family teaching, covering:
    a. The need for prophylactic antibiotics before dental work; childbirth; genitourinary, GI, or gynecologic procedures; or any procedure or event that can cause transient bacteremia
    b. Signs and symptoms of complications to watch for and report
    c. The need for regular temperature monitoring

G. **Evaluation**
1. The patient demonstrates stabilization of the inflammatory process.
2. The patient reports reduced pain.
3. The patient exhibits increased tolerance with activity progression.
4. The patient displays decreased anxiety.
5. The patient and family members or significant others verbalize an understanding of the disease process, its effects, and treatment.

X. Pericarditis

A. **Description: inflammation of the pericardium, the fibroserous sac that surrounds the heart; may be acute or chronic**
B. **Etiology**
1. Pericarditis—particularly the acute form—may be idiopathic.
2. Identified causes include:
    a. Bacterial, fungal, or viral infection
    b. Neoplasms
    c. Connective tissue disorders
    d. Hypersensitivity reactions
    e. Injury to the pericardium (e.g., MI, trauma, cardiac surgery)
    f. Drugs such as hydralazine and procainamide
    g. High-dose radiation therapy to the chest
    h. Uremia
    i. Aortic aneurysm with pericardial leakage
    j. Myxedema with cholesterol deposits in the pericardium
C. **Pathophysiology**
1. Acute pericarditis may be fibrinous or effusive, producing serous or hemorrhagic exudate.
2. Chronic constrictive pericarditis is marked by progressive fibrous pericardial thickening.
3. Prognosis varies depending on the underlying cause and is generally favorable, unless constriction occurs.

D. **Assessment findings**
1. Common clinical manifestations include:
   a. Sharp sudden pain over the precordium, radiating to the neck and left scapular region; may be aggravated by breathing or movement and typically decreases when the patient sits and leans forward
   b. Dyspnea due to decreased cardiac output, orthopnea
   c. Tachycardia
   d. Pericardial friction rub
   e. Distant heart sounds
   f. Increased cardiac dullness on percussion
   g. Absent apical impulse
   h. In the presence of cardiac tamponade: pallor, cool and clammy skin, hypotension, pulsus paradoxus, jugular venous distention
2. Characteristic laboratory and diagnostic study findings include:
   a. Normal or elevated WBC count and ESR
   b. Positive pericardial fluid culture
   c. ECG changes: ST segment elevation, T-wave inversion, diminished QRS voltage with effusion
   d. Echocardiography showing free space echo between the ventricular wall and pericardium

E. **Nursing diagnoses**
1. Decreased Cardiac Output
2. Pain

F. **Planning and implementation**
1. Maintain the patient on bedrest.
2. Administer pain medication as prescribed; provide prompt pain relief.
3. Place the patient in an upright position, and administer oxygen as necessary to help relieve dyspnea.
4. Monitor for signs and symptoms of cardiac tamponade: hypotension, muffled heart sounds, pulsus paradoxus.
5. Prepare the patient for possible pericardiocentesis as ordered.
6. Provide reassurance and emotional support.
7. Provide patient and family teaching, covering:
   a. Basic pathophysiology of pericarditis, its effects, and treatment
   b. Progression of activity, with bedrest if pain, fever, or friction rub occur
   c. Proper use of medications: purpose, action, dosage, side effects

G. **Evaluation**
1. The patient reports pain relief with medication administration.
2. The patient demonstrates increased tolerance with activity progression.

3. The patient displays decreased anxiety.
4. The patient and family members or significant others verbalize an understanding of the disease process, its effects, and treatment.

XI. Pacemaker implantation

A. Description

1. A cardiac pacemaker is an electronic device that provides electrical stimuli to the heart muscle to initiate and maintain cardiac contractions when the heart's natural pacemakers are unable to do so; may be temporary or permanent.
2. Pulses are generated from a battery-operated pacer unit and transmitted to the heart through electrodes placed in direct contact with the heart muscle wall.
3. Universal pacemaker classification involves a three-letter identification code:
   a. The first letter identifies the chamber paced: A (atrium), V (ventricle), D (dual).
   b. The second letter identifies the chamber sensed: A (atrium), V (ventricle), D (dual).
   c. The third letter identifies the mode of response: T (triggered), I (inhibited), D (both).

B. Pacing modes

1. In the *asynchronous* (fixed) mode, the rate and rhythm of pacer beats is unaffected by spontaneous heart beats; the pacing electrode is in a ventricle.
2. In the *demand* (standby) mode, the pacer fires only when the rate of spontaneous beats drops below the preset minimum rate; the sensing and pacing electrodes usually are placed in a ventricle.
3. The *synchronous* mode uses a sensing circuit to detect atrial activity prior to ventricular activity; the sensing electrode is placed in an atrium, the pacing electrode in a ventricle.
4. In the *A–V sequential* mode, sensing and pacing electrodes are placed in both the atria and the ventricles.

C. Indications

1. Temporary pacemaker
   a. Diagnostic testing (hemodynamic assessment, antiarrhythmic drug evaluation)
   b. Acute MI
   c. Acute and chronic AV block
   d. Overdrive suppression of dysrhythmia
   e. Symptomatic bradycardia or tachycardia
2. Permanent pacemaker
   a. Stokes-Adams syncope
   b. Sinus node dysfunction

        c.   AV conduction abnormalities

        d.   Chronic bundle branch block

        e.   Recurrent tachydysrhythmias

D.   **Insertion routes**

    1.   Temporary pacemaker

        a.   Transvenous

        b.   Transthoracic (usually emergency)

    2.   Permanent pacemaker

        a.   Transvenous

        b.   Epicardial

        c.   Generator implantation usually under the skin in the pectoral region

E.   **Nursing diagnoses**

    1.   Anxiety

    2.   Fear

    3.   High Risk for Infection

    4.   Knowledge Deficit

    5.   Impaired Physical Mobility

    6.   Pain

    7.   Chronic Pain

F.   **Planning and implementation**

    1.   For a patient with a temporary pacemaker:

        a.   Place the patient in an electrically safe environment.

        b.   Assess pacemaker function, heart rate, and rhythm frequently; note deviations from settings.

        c.   Ensure that all connections are secure.

        d.   Promote comfort.

        e.   Provide reassurance and emotional support.

        f.   Assess the insertion site daily, and provide site care according to protocol.

    2.   For a patient with a permanent pacemaker:

        a.   Assess pacemaker function, heart rate, and rhythm frequently; note deviations from settings.

        b.   Assess the insertion site for bleeding, hematoma, or infection.

        c.   Note data about model, date and time of insertion, location of pulse generator, stimulus threshold, and pacer rate on the patient's chart and at the head of the bed.

        d.   Provide reassurance and emotional support.

        e.   Teach the patient to carry a card specifying important pacemaker information at all times; monitor pulse daily, and report any deviations to the physician; comply with prescribed physical activity limitations; watch for and promptly report signs and symptoms of complications; keep scheduled appointments for regular pacemaker check-up; avoid electromechanical devices that could interfere with pacing (e.g., microwave oven, metal detector).

3. For all patients, monitor for problems and complications, including:
    a. Failure to pace
    b. Failure to sense
    c. Muscle stimulation due to cardiac perforation
    d. Infection
    e. Electromagnetic interference

G. Evaluation

1. The patient demonstrates stabilization of cardiac rhythm with proper pacemaker pacing and sensing.
2. The patient and family members or significant others verbalize understanding of pacemaker function and proper care and pulse monitoring techniques.
3. The patient displays decreased anxiety.
4. The patient reports reduced pain.
5. The patient remains free from infection at the insertion site, as evidenced by normal body temperature and no local redness or drainage.

XII. Heart surgery

A. Description: surgery performed on the heart either with (open-heart surgery) or without (closed-heart surgery) cardiopulmonary bypass or extracorporeal circulation

B. Types

1. Coronary artery bypass grafting (CABG)
2. Aneurysm excision
3. Valvular repair or replacement
4. Septal closure
5. Heart transplantation

C. Indications

1. CAD
2. Acute MI
3. CHF
4. Rheumatic valvular dysfunction
5. Congenital abnormalities
6. Incompetent cardiac muscle

D. Assessment

1. Health history should focus on:
    a. Cardiac history, particularly dysrhythmias
    b. Pulmonary history
    c. The patient's emotional state and knowledge level
2. Physical assessment techniques depend on the underlying cardiac disorder but should always include:

   a.   Vital signs
   b.   ECG for cardiac rate and rhythm
   c.   Monitoring of cardiovascular status, evidence of MI, effects of drugs

E.   Nursing diagnoses: postoperative
   1.   Anxiety
   2.   Decreased Cardiac Output
   3.   Fear
   4.   Impaired Gas Exchange
   5.   High Risk for Infection
   6.   Knowledge Deficit
   7.   Pain

F.   Planning and implementation (*Note:* See Chapter 24, Perioperative Nursing, for more details on general nursing interventions.)
   1.   Preoperative
      a.   Reinforce the surgeon's explanation of the procedure; go over expected events on the day of surgery.
      b.   Provide reassurance and emotional support, and encourage the patient and family members or significant others to express feelings and concerns.
      c.   Obtain baseline laboratory data as requested.
      d.   Orient the patient and family members or significant others to the critical care unit.
      e.   Administer sedatives as prescribed.
      f.   Demonstrate and have the patient practice postoperative activities: coughing, deep breathing, incision splinting, and turning in bed.
   2.   Postoperative
      a.   Secure the endotracheal tube, and maintain an adequate airway.
      b.   Suction as necessary to ensure optimal ventilation.
      c.   Ensure proper connection and functioning of all lines and tubes.
      d.   Monitor physiologic parameters frequently.
      e.   Administer pain medication as prescribed.
      f.   Monitor for and take measures to prevent complications.
      g.   Provide patient and family teaching, covering guidelines for activity limitations and progression of activity; proper use of medications (purpose, action, dosage, side effects); dietary restrictions; wound hygiene; resumption of sexual activity; signs and symptoms of complications to watch for and report; referral to an outpatient rehabilitation program.

G.   Evaluation
   1.   The patient demonstrates stabilization of cardiac rhythm, vital signs, and hemodynamic parameters.

2. The patient displays decreased anxiety, as evidenced by freedom in expressing feelings.

3. The patient and family members or significant others verbalize an understanding of the condition and postoperative care.
4. The patient displays increased tolerance to activity progression.
5. The patient remains free of infection at the incision site, as evidenced by normal body temperature and proper healing at site with no unusual redness or drainage.
6. The patient reports decreased pain.

Bibliography

Alspach, J. G., & Williams, S. (1985). *Core curriculum for critical care nursing*. Philadelphia: W. B. Saunders.

Andreoli, K. G., Zipes, D. P., Wallace, A. G., Kinney, M. R., & Fowkes, V. K. (Eds.). (1987). *Comprehensive cardiac care*. St. Louis: C. V. Mosby.

Brunner, L. S., & Suddarth, D. S. (1988). *Textbook of medical-surgical nursing* (6th ed.). Philadelphia: J. B. Lippincott.

Brunner, L. S., & Suddarth, D. S (1986). *The Lippincott manual of nursing practice* (4th ed.). Philadelphia: J. B. Lippincott.

Darovic, G.O. (Ed.). (1987). *Hemodynamic monitoring*. Philadelphia: W.B. Saunders.

Emanuelson, K. L., & Rosenlicht, J. K. (Eds.). (1986). *Handbook of critical care nursing*. New York: Wiley Medical.

Ford, R. D. (Ed.). (1986). *Cardiovascular care handbook*. Springhouse, PA: Springhouse Corp.

Lamb, J. I., & Carlson, V. R. (Eds.). (1986). *Handbook of cardiovascular nursing*. Philadelphia: J. B. Lippincott.

Luckmann, J., & Sorenson, K.S. (1987). *Medical-surgical nursing: A psychophysiologic approach* (3rd ed.). Philadelphia: W.B. Saunders.

Weeks, L. C. (Ed.). (1986). *Advanced cardiovascular nursing*. Boston: Blackwell Scientific.

STUDY QUESTIONS

1. In assessing a patient with angina, which of the following would *not* be considered a precipitating factor for pain?
   a. exposure to cold
   b. smoking
   c. leaning forward
   d. eating a heavy meal

2. Ms. Smith experienced cardiac arrest while in the CCU with a diagnosis of acute inferior myocardial infarction. After a successful code and stabilization of her heart rhythm and vital signs, she is more agitated and uses her call light more frequently. Which of the following actions would be the best first step to address Ms. Smith's needs?
   a. Assess Ms. Smith's blood pressure more frequently.
   b. Explain to Ms. Smith that another episode is unlikely.
   c. Encourage Ms. Smith to discuss her feelings about the episode.
   d. Tell Ms. Smith not to worry; reassure her that she is being closely monitored.

3. Mr. Carter has been hospitalized several times for congestive heart failure. While discussing his diet and medications, the nurse discovers that he doesn't seem to understand the importance of restricting salt intake and complying with the prescribed medication schedule. Based on these findings, the nurse deduces that a different approach is needed to prevent further acute failure episodes and refers Mr. Carter to a local cardiac rehabilitation program. Which of the following findings would indicate Mr. Carter's compliance with the various aspects of this rehabilitation program?
   a. He demonstrates better nutrition habits by gaining 10 pounds.
   b. He returns to the hospital as an inpatient less frequently.
   c. He significantly improves his activity level.
   d. He attends all the classes.

4. Ms. Robertson is scheduled for transvenous temporary pacemaker implantation. To ensure an electrically safe environment for Ms. Robertson, the nurse should:
   a. Remove all electrical equipment from the room.
   b. Remind staff not to touch the bed rail when adjusting pacemaker settings.
   c. Plug no more than one electrical cord into each two-plug outlet.
   d. Make sure that all electrical equipment is properly grounded.

5. Admitted 3 days ago with an anterior MI, Mr. Jonas has an order for oxygen p.r.n. and has been receiving digitalis and diuretics to treat early signs of CHF. Nursing assessment reveals moderate dyspnea; cool, clammy, very pale skin; and cough producing frothy, blood-tinged sputum. Based on these findings, the nurse would suspect that Mr. Jonas is experiencing:
   a. angina
   b. early congestive heart failure
   c. pulmonary edema
   d. cardiac tamponade

6. Recognizing the seriousness of Mr. Jonas's situation, the nurse should first take which of the following steps?
   a. Call the physician.
   b. Assess airway patency, and administer oxygen via face mask.
   c. Prepare rotating tourniquets in case they are needed to decrease venous return.
   d. Administer an extra dose of digitalis to increase myocardial contractility.

7. Mr. Nelson, a 57-year-old truck driver, underwent CABG surgery 4 days ago. After transfer from the CCU, he becomes withdrawn and expresses anger and hostility toward his family, criticizing everything that they do. The family members, very distraught, ask the nurse for help. Which of the following nursing

diagnoses likely would be most appropriate to address Mr. Nelson's behavior?
a. Impaired Adjustment
b. Ineffective Denial
c. High Risk for Violence
d. Fear

8. During discharge planning, the nurse needs to ascertain how much the patient knows about his or her condition in order to develop a teaching plan. Knowledge of which of the following is *not* important for a patient with chronic congestive heart failure?
a. medication use
b. dietary restrictions
c. signs and symptoms of progressing CHF
d. possible surgical procedures

9. Mr. Rogers, aged 63, has been hospitalized following an anterior MI. This morning, assessment revealed first-degree AV block although he was asymptomatic. Now, in the afternoon, ECG shows second-degree AV block of the Mobitz II type. He remains asymptomatic. Based on these findings, the nurse would call the physician and anticipate which of the following interventions?
a. assisting with pacemaker implantation
b. administering digitalis
c. administering lidocaine by way of IV bolus
d. increasing IV fluid infusion to 175 mL/hr

10. After insertion of a temporary transvenous pacemaker, the nurse should record all the following information *except*
a. the patient's cardiovascular response to the pacemaker
b. pacemaker information (e.g., type, settings)
c. status of the insertion site
d. the patient's activity level

11. Transient bacteremia can cause endocarditis in patients with prosthetic heart valves. Based on the nursing diagnosis Knowledge Deficit, it would be impor-

tant for a such a patient to learn all the following *except*
a. the need to promptly report any unexplained fever
b. using antibiotic prophylaxis for certain procedures that may cause a transient bacteremia (e.g., dental procedures)
c. recognizing signs and symptoms of endocarditis
d. maintaining bedrest for any chest pain

12. Mr. Peters, aged 71, has end-stage congestive heart failure and exhibits signs of impending cardiac arrest. He understands the seriousness of his illness and has made all necessary arrangements for his family in anticipation of his death. Mr. Peters has told the nurse that he wants everything possible done for him even though he knows it probably won't save his life. His physician explains that there is no reason to code him because he has no viable heart muscle left. What would be the nurse's most appropriate course of action in this situation?
a. Do what the physician requests and not call a code.
b. Follow through with a code if cardiac arrest occurs.
c. Intervene on behalf of the patient and persuade the physician to code him.
d. Ignore the situation.

13. In assessing a patient's radial pulses, the nurse finds them to be irregular, with the apical pulse rate about 10 beats faster than the radial pulse rate. These findings point to which of the following cardiac dysrhythmias?
a. atrial fibrillation
b. second-degree AV block
c. ventricular tachycardia
d. sinus bradycardia

14. Ms. Taylor, aged 55, underwent CABG surgery 3 days ago. She has become disoriented and combative and is experiencing hallucinations. Assessment re-

veals increased pulse rate and blood pressure. Her husband is very upset and confused about his wife's status, stating that she has always prided herself on her ability to remain in control of herself. Based on the nursing diagnosis Sensory and Perceptual Alterations, the nurse would conclude that Ms. Taylor likely is experiencing:

a. ICU psychosis
b. repressed emotional problems
c. acute CVA tenderness
d. memory loss

15. The nurse has been assigned to do discharge teaching for Mr. Ramirez, a 46 year old with coronary artery disease. This is Mr. Ramirez's third hospitalization in 3 months for treatment of CHF, and assessment reveals noncompliance with his medication regimen. Which of the following would be the nurse's best course of action for this patient?

a. Reteach him about his medication schedule, and give him pamphlets to read.
b. Collect more data to help identify reasons for his noncompliance.
c. Teach his wife about the medication schedule and the importance of compliance.
d. Arrange for outpatient follow-up to ensure compliance.

16. During recovery from MI, a patient should demonstrate gradual progression of activity. Before discharge, the nurse would expect the patient to do all the following *except*

a. Sit in a chair as desired.
b. Walk the hallway twice daily.
c. Perform isometric exercises.
d. Walk down one flight of stairs and return by elevator.

ANSWER KEY

1. **Correct response: c**
   Leaning forward usually relieves the pain of pericarditis.
   a, b, and d. Exposure to cold, smoking, and heavy meals all can precipitate anginal pain.
   Knowledge/Physiologic/Assessment

2. **Correct response: c**
   Because her vital signs are stable, Ms. Smith likely is exhibiting anxiety related to the ventricular fibrillation episode. Encouraging expression of feelings is an appropriate first step in decreasing anxiety.
   a. Checking blood pressure more frequently will tend to increase anxiety rather than reassure the patient.
   b and d. False or empty reassurances do not meet the patient's needs.
   Comprehension/Psychosocial/Implementation

3. **Correct response: b**
   No need for hospitalization indicates that the patient is maintaining better heart function.
   a. Weight gain may indicate fluid gain and noncompliance with the regimen.
   c. A patient with CHF usually cannot significantly increase activity level.
   d. Merely attending sessions does not necessarily signal compliance with the regimen.
   Analysis/Health promotion/Evaluation

4. **Correct response: d**
   If electrical equipment is not grounded, the patient could receive a shock directly to the heart.
   a, b, and c. These actions are not necessary to ensure electrical safety for the pacemaker patient.
   Application/Safe care/Planning

5. **Correct response: c**
   Frothy, blood-tinged sputum is an indicator of pulmonary edema with interstitial fluid overload in the lungs due to left ventricular failure.
   a, b, and d. These conditions do not produce such sputum.
   Knowledge/Physiologic/Assessment

6. **Correct response: b**
   The first priority is to relieve respiratory difficulties. After ensuring a patent airway, the physician can be called.
   a, c, and d. These interventions would be performed later, and only if ordered by the physician.
   Application/Physiologic/Implementation

7. **Correct response: d**
   A patient's psychoemotional status is typically fragile after surgery; anger often represents an attempt to mask fear.
   a, b, and c. These other diagnoses are not supported by this scenario.
   Analysis/Psychosocial/Analysis (Dx)

8. **Correct response: d**
   Potential surgical procedures would not be appropriate in a teaching plan for a patient with CHF.
   a, b, and c. Medications, dietary restrictions, and abnormal signs and symptoms all are appropriate topics.
   Comprehension/Health promotion/Evaluation

9. **Correct response: a**
   Progression of AV block in the presence of an anterior MI is indication for a pacemaker.
   b. Digitalis possibly would potentiate the AV block.
   c. Lidocaine is indicated for treatment of ventricular arrhythmias.
   d. Increasing IV fluid infusion in the presence of an MI could precipitate heart failure.
   Application/Physiologic/Planning

10. **Correct response: d**
    The patient's activity level is irrelevant

to pacemaker implantation; most likely, the patient will be on bedrest.

a, b, and c. All this information should be documented.

Application/Safe care/Implementation

11. *Correct response: d*

The need for bedrest usually is associated with pericarditis.

a, b, and c. These are important considerations for patients who have undergone valve replacement surgery.

Application/Health promotion/Analysis (Dx)

12. *Correct response: c*

Every patient has a right to receive his choice of care. As the patient advocate in this situation, the nurse should work to ensure that the patient's needs and wishes are met whenever possible.

a, b, and d. These actions would not be appropriate for this patient.

Application/Safe care/Planning

13. *Correct response: a*

The rhythm of atrial fibrillation is irregular, with up to a 10-beat difference between apical and radial pulse.

b, c, and d. The findings do not point to any of these dysrhythmias.

Comprehension/Physiologic/Assessment

14. *Correct response: a*

These signs and symptoms are indicative of ICU psychosis. The etiology is not known.

b, c, and d. These manifestations do not point to any of these disorders.

Analysis/Safe care/Analysis (Dx)

15. *Correct response: b*

The patient may have a valid reason for noncompliance that can be identified and addressed.

a. Reteaching probably would not be effective for a patient with a history of noncompliance.

c and d. Teaching his wife and ensuring outpatient follow-up might work but may cause the patient to lose a sense of control over his condition and its management.

Analysis/Health promotion/Implementation

16. *Correct response: c*

Isometric exercises are not appropriate for a cardiac patient because breath-holding during these exercises causes a sharp rise, then a fall, in cardiac output, precipitating dysrhythmias.

a, b, and d These activities all are appropriate for cardiac rehabilitation.

Analysis/Physiologic/Evaluation

Peripheral Vascular Disorders

I. Anatomy and physiology
A. Structure
B. Functions

II. Overview of peripheral vascular disorders
A. Assessment
B. Laboratory studies and diagnostic tests
C. Psychosocial implications
D. Medications used to treat peripheral vascular disorders

III. Peripheral arterial occlusive disease
A. Description
B. Etiology and incidence
C. Pathophysiology
D. Assessment findings
E. Nursing diagnoses
F. Planning and implementation
G. Evaluation

IV. Deep venous thrombosis (DVT)
A. Description
B. Etiology and incidence
C. Pathophysiology
D. Assessment findings
E. Nursing diagnoses
F. Planning and implementation
G. Evaluation

V. Venous stasis ulcers
A. Description
B. Etiology and incidence
C. Pathophysiology
D. Assessment findings
E. Nursing diagnoses

F. Planning and implementation
G. Evaluation

VI. Varicose veins
A. Description
B. Etiology and incidence
C. Pathophysiology
D. Assessment findings
E. Nursing diagnoses
F. Planning and implementation
G. Evaluation

VII. Lymphedema
A. Description
B. Etiology and incidence
C. Pathophysiology
D. Assessment findings
E. Nursing diagnoses
F. Planning and implementation
G. Evaluation

VIII. Lymphadenitis
A. Description
B. Etiology
C. Pathophysiology
D. Assessment findings
E. Nursing diagnoses
F. Planning and implementation
G. Evaluation

IX. Extremity amputation
A. Description
B. Indications
C. Types of amputation
D. Types of prostheses
E. Complications
F. Psychosocial and rehabilitation considerations

I. Anatomy and physiology

A. Structure

    1. Arteries

        a. The aorta, the first vessel carrying blood out of the heart, branches into arteries, then into arterioles, to distribute blood to the body.

        b. Arterioles end in microcirculation, or capillaries.

        c. Capillaries, thin-walled vessels through which nutrients and waste products pass, consist of a layer of endothelial cells and basement membrane surrounded by a pericapillary sheath of connective tissue.

        d. All other blood vessels (including veins) consist of an outer layer of connective tissue (tunica adventitia), a middle layer of muscle (tunica media), and an inner layer of endothelial cells (tunica intima).

        e. The thick arterial muscle layer can withstand higher pressures than can veins and can dilate or constrict depending on messages sent to it.

    2. Veins

        a. Blood travels from microcirculation into a system of collecting vessels known as veins.

        b. Small veins join to form progressively larger veins until they reach the right atrium of heart as the superior and inferior vena cavae.

        c. Valves in veins (except for the vena cavae and the portal, cerebral, intraabdominal, and pulmonary veins) break the hydrostatic column of blood into smaller units, facilitating movement of blood in one direction and with reduced pressures.

3. Lymphatics
   a. Lymphatics are small, thin, veinlike vessels that conduct lymph through the body; they tend to lie near veins.
   b. Valves and smooth muscle contractions act to direct lymph in one direction by way of the right lymphatic duct (draining the right side of the head, neck, thorax, and upper arms) and thoracic duct (draining most of the rest of the body) to the right and left brachiocephalic veins.
   c. Lymph nodes are small, oval bodies through which lymph flows on its way to veins.
   d. Lymphoid tissue also is located in walls of the intestinal tract and in the spleen and thymus.

B. Function
1. Arteries
   a. Arteries supply nutrients and oxygen to tissues.
   b. An adequate supply of arterial blood to extremities produces normal-appearing skin and nails and good tissue healing.
   c. Regulatory mechanisms from the nervous system and local tissues provide for vasodilation and vasoconstriction as needed.
2. Veins
   a. Veins carry deoxygenated blood and waste products of cellular metabolism to the heart.
   b. Normal venous pressure is much lower than arterial pressure and is lower in the right atrium than in the feet.
   c. This pressure gradient enables veins to channel blood from capillaries to the heart's right side.
   d. Venous volume and pressure are regulated actively by neurogenic venoconstriction caused by alpha-adrenergic nerves, and passively by elastic recoil of the vein wall after distending pressure falls below the level necessary to hold the vein in a rounded shape.
   e. Inspiration creates an intrathoracic vacuum and facilitates blood flow to the right atrium.
3. Lymphatics
   a. The lymphatics collect lymph from tissues and return it to the blood.
   b. This system helps protect the body from infection by microorganisms.

II. Overview of peripheral vascular disorders
A. Assessment
1. The nurse should explore the patient's health history for risk factors for atherosclerosis, a primary cause of peripheral vascular disorders (see Chapter 7, Section II.A.1).

2. Physical assessment should focus on:
   a. Skin color and temperature changes: coolness, possibly indicating deficient blood supply; pallor, also associated with diminished blood supply; blanching, which may indicate diminished arterial pressure in a body part; rubor, which may occur with chronic ischemia; cyanosis, resulting from insufficient blood oxygen and, if localized, indicating poor circulation in that area
   b. Pain due to tissue ischemia
   c. Necrosis and ulceration, which can occur in both arterial and venous disorders, with symptoms depending on cause
   d. Muscle atrophy, loss of strength and joint mobility, which occurs in chronic ischemia
   e. Exercise tolerance (especially important in arterial disorders)
   f. Pulse volume; peripheral pulse grading: 0 = absent, 1+ = weak and thready, 2+ = normal, 3+ = full and bounding
   g. Bruits: heard most easily during systole; pitch correlates with degree of stenosis
   h. Capillary refill time, indicating peripheral perfusion and cardiac output; acceptable time, less than 3 seconds
   i. Blood pressure, both standard arm pressure measurement and ankle arm index (ankle systolic pressure divided by arm systolic pressure): normal ankle arm index is greater than 1.0; 0.5 to 0.7 indices found in patients with claudication, 0.4 to 0 indices in patients with resting pain

B. **Laboratory studies and diagnostic tests**
   1. Noninvasive procedures include:
      a. Doppler ultrasound, a simple, inexpensive, highly reliable procedure used to electronically obtain qualitative and quantitative information about blood flow in arteries or veins
      b. Plethysmography, involving measuring changes in calf volume corresponding to changes in blood volume used to assess changes in venous volume and carotid artery blood flow
      c. Treadmill test, an exercise test done to evaluate total extremity blood flow after exercise and to detect pain occurring with exercise or signs of activity intolerance, such as shortness of breath
      d. Digital subtraction angiography (DSA) or digital intravenous angiography, a radiologic technique that uses image-intensifier video system to display vessels on a television monitor

2. Invasive procedures include:
   a. Phlebography (venography), involving radiograph visualization of veins after injection of contrast medium
   b. Angiography, involving radiograph visualization of arteries after injection of contrast medium
   c. ^{125}I-fibrinogen uptake test, a sensitive, though costly and time consuming, screening for acute calf vein thrombosis; involves injection of radioactive iodine molecules

C. Psychosocial implications

1. A patient with a peripheral vascular disorder may experience problems in coping related to:
   a. The chronic and debilitating nature of the disorder
   b. Fear of loss of body part or function
2. The patient also may have self-concept concerns related to fear of:
   a. Role changes toward increasing dependence
   b. Rejection
   c. Body image changes with disease progression
3. Concerns related to lifestyle changes may be associated with potential changes in:
   a. Physical ability and activity level
   b. Work performance and potential job loss
   c. Economic security
4. The patient also may be concerned about changes in social interaction leading to:
   a. Isolation
   b. Depression

D. Medications used to treat peripheral vascular disorders

1. *Vasodilators*, which dilate vessels and improve blood flow by relaxing vascular smooth muscle and decreasing peripheral vascular resistance, include:
   a. Hydralazine hydrochloride
   b. Minoxidil
2. *Anticoagulants*, used to treat or prevent deep venous thrombosis or pulmonary embolism, include:
   a. Heparin sodium
   b. Coumarin derivatives, such as warfarin sodium
3. *Thrombolytics*, used in acute management of thrombus formation to dissolve thrombi or emboli, include:
   a. Streptokinase
   b. t-PA (human tissue plasminogen activator)
   c. Urokinase
4. Used to treat hypertension, *adrenergic inhibitors* block response to sympathetic nerve impulses or circulating catecholamines,

dilate peripheral vessels, and depress adrenergic activity; agents include:
- a. Methyldopa
- b. Propranolol
- c. Metoprolol
- d. Clonidine hydrochloride
- e. Prazosin hydrochloride
- f. Nadolol

III. Peripheral arterial occlusive disease

- **A.** Description: a form of arteriosclerosis involving occlusion of arteries, most commonly in the lower extremities; may be acute or chronic
- **B.** Etiology and incidence
  1. Acute occlusion may result from trauma, thrombosis, or embolism; 90% occur in the lower extremities.
  2. Possible causes of chronic occlusion include:
     - a. Atherosclerosis
     - b. Inflammation
     - c. Thrombosis
     - d. Embolism
     - e. Trauma
     - f. Autoimmune response
- **C.** Pathophysiology
  1. Narrowing of the arterial lumen or damage to the endothelial lining can result from such factors as:
     - a. Atherosclerotic buildup of lipid deposits
     - b. Arteriosclerosis obliterans, causing arterial occlusion
  2. This leads to reduced or absent peripheral blood flow and, if unchecked, tissue ischemia and eventual necrosis.
  3. Acute arterial occlusion results in immediate decrease in arterial flow distal to the occlusion with a resultant decrease in nutrient and oxygen supply to perfused tissue.
  4. In chronic arterial occlusion, gradual onset allows for some development of collateral circulation around areas of occlusion; chronic nutrient and oxygen deficit causes more trophic changes than with acute occlusion.
  5. Effects of arterial occlusion in the lower extremities may include:
     - a. Aortoiliac arterial stenosis and occlusion
     - b. Femoropopliteal arterial stenosis and occlusion
     - c. Arterial ulcers of distal toes, anterior tibia, and lateral malleolus
     - d. Distal arterial embolization of large or small vessels of the feet
  6. Effects in the upper extremities may include:

      a.   Subclavian steal syndrome, resulting in arm ischemia from blockage of the subclavian artery with subsequent incomplete perfusion from the carotid artery

      b.   Thoracic outlet syndrome, resulting from pinching of the subclavian artery by muscle, the first rib, or the clavicle

D. **Assessment findings**

    1.   Clinical manifestations of acute arterial occlusion are commonly termed the "six P's":

        a.   Pain or loss of sensory nerves secondary to ischemia

        b.   Paresthesias and loss of position sense

        c.   Poikilothermia or coldness

        d.   Paralysis

        e.   Pallor due to empty superficial vessels (can progress to mottled, cyanotic, cadaverous cold leg)

        f.   Pulselessness

    2.   The most important clinical manifestations of chronic arterial occlusion are:

        a.   Intermittent claudication (calf muscle pain occurring when muscle is forced to contract without adequate blood supply, such as after walking a certain measurable distance; alleviated with rest)

        b.   Resting pain (pain at rest when limited blood flow cannot meet even very low tissue requirements)

        c.   Trophic changes in skin and nails: dryness, scaling, and thinning of skin; decreased or absent hair growth; and brittle and thickened nails

    3.   Chronic arterial occlusion also may produce:

        a.   Decreased or absent peripheral pulses

        b.   Coldness, pallor, rubor, or cyanosis

        c.   Arterial ulcers and cellulitis

        d.   Gangrenous changes marking death and decay of tissues

E. **Nursing diagnoses**

    1.   Activity Intolerance

    2.   Altered Nutrition: More Than Body Requirements

    3.   Pain

    4.   Chronic Pain

    5.   Impaired Skin Integrity

    6.   Altered Tissue Perfusion: Peripheral

F. **Planning and implementation**

    1.   Provide proper positioning:

        a.   Place the patient's legs in a dependent position in relationship to the heart to improve peripheral blood flow.

        b.   Avoid raising the patient's feet above heart level unless specifically ordered by the physician (e.g., as part of Burger-Allen exercises).

    c.   Keep the patient in a neutral, flat, supine position if in doubt about nature of peripheral vascular problems.

2. Promote vasodilation:

    a.   Provide insulating warmth with gloves, socks, and other outer wear as appropriate.

    b.   Keep room temperatures comfortably warm.

    c.   Instruct the patient to warm himself or herself with warm drinks or warm baths.

    d.   Never apply a direct heat source to the extremities; limited blood flow combined with possible paresthesias can lead to tissue damage from heat earlier than would occur in a patient with normal circulation.

    e.   Teach the patient about the vasoconstrictive effects of nicotine and caffeine, emotional stress, and chilling; discuss ways to avoid or minimize these risk factors.

    f.   Teach the patient to avoid constricting clothes such as garters, knee-high stockings, and belts.

3. Promote comfort:

    a.   Use measures to increase circulation to extremities to help alleviate pain.

    b.   Administer analgesics as ordered, preferably nonnarcotics to prevent dependency in chronic occlusive disorders.

4. Promote and teach skin and foot care:

    a.   Teach the patient with chronic disease the need for scrupulous daily foot care.

    b.   Provide gentle daily washing and drying of feet with mild soap and warm water.

    c.   Inspect affected limbs (such as feet) daily for areas of injury, broken skin, trophic changes, pulselessness.

    d.   Trim nails with clippers, not scissors.

    e.   Apply lanolin to dry areas.

    f.   Use lamb's wool between overlapping toes.

    g.   Trim nails straight across with clippers, not scissors.

    h.   Use cotton or wool socks to absorb moisture.

    i.   Avoid injury to affected extremity from scratching, home treatment of corns and blisters and injury sites, improper nail cutting, and walking without properly fitting shoes.

    j.   Never use razor blades or harsh commercial products.

    k.   Warn against going barefoot or wearing high heels, tight shoes, shoes with pointed toes, and shoes that cause feet to sweat, such as canvas shoes.

    l.   Do not use heating pads to warm cold feet.

    m.   Seek medical help for treatment of corns, calluses, and ingrown toenails.

     n.   Notify the physician of the first signs of injury.

5. Promote activity and mobility:

     a.   Prevent hazards of immobility with proper turning, positioning, deep breathing, and isometric and range-of-motion exercises.

     b.   Use an orthoframe, a trapeze, a foot cradle, or a padded foot board to promote healing and protect skin.

     c.   For a patient with decreased arterial function but without activity-limiting tissue damage, encourage a program of balanced exercise and rest to promote development of collateral circulation.

     d.   Instruct the patient to use pain or intermittent claudication as a guide to limiting activity during exercise (i.e., view onset of pain as a signal to stop and rest).

6. Provide patient and family teaching, covering:

     a.   The nature of the disorder and its treatment

     b.   Proper foot care

     c.   Risk factors and the importance of complying with the therapeutic regimen

     d.   Prevention of circulatory complications by avoiding injury

     e.   The need for ongoing follow-up care

7. Administer prescribed medications, which may include:

     a.   Vasodilators, anticoagulants, or agents to lower serum cholesterol

     b.   Fibrinolytics

8. Provide care for a patient undergoing angiography or percutaneous transluminal angioplasty (PTA):

     a.   Preprocedure, provide information related to the procedure; validate that informed consent has been obtained; mark peripheral pulses; obtain diagnostic data as ordered; and withhold food and fluids as prescribed.

     b.   Postprocedure, maintain bedrest as ordered, keeping the involved extremity extended; monitor vital signs and assess peripheral pulses and circulation every 15 minutes for 2 hours then every hour for 4 hours; assess for bleeding, hematoma, or swelling at catheter insertion site; encourage oral fluids; and monitor urine output.

9. Provide care for a patient receiving an autogenous saphenous vein or a synthetic (expanded polytetrafluoroethylene [PTFE] or Gore-Tex) bypass graft:

     a.   Prepare the patient for surgery, and mark peripheral pulses.

     b.   Monitor carefully after procedure for signs of graft occlusion (especially for first 24 hours) as manifested by decreased arterial perfusion.

   c. Position the involved extremity in the position prescribed by the physician to prevent constricted arterial flow and edema.

   d. Monitor for development of compartment syndrome (swelling of calf muscles), which can impede circulation and necessitate fasciotomy (incision in fascia to relieve pressure on vessels).

   e. Monitor for embolization with ischemia of foot and lower leg.

   f. Monitor for and take steps to prevent complications of any surgical procedure involving general anesthesia, particularly respiratory problems and infection.

 10. Provide care for a patient who has received axillofemoral or axillobifemoral bypass graft:

   a. Avoid positioning the patient on the side of the graft following the procedure.

   b. Warn the patient not to wear tight clothing, which can lead to graft occlusion.

 11. Provide care for a patient undergoing endarterectomy, sympathectomy, or amputation.

G. **Evaluation**

 1. The patient demonstrates increased arterial blood supply to extremities, as evidenced by:

   a. Warm skin

   b. Improved skin color

   c. Decreased muscle pain with exercise

   d. Palpable peripheral pulses

 2. The patient maintains proper positioning.

 3. The patient exhibits decreased venous congestion, as evidenced by decreased edema in extremities.

 4. The patient complies with measures to promote vasodilation and prevent vasoconstriction, including:

   a. Protecting extremities from cold

   b. Avoiding smoking, constricting clothing and appliances, and crossing the legs

   c. Participating in a stress management program

 5. The patient reports freedom from pain and increased activity tolerance.

 6. The patient exhibits good tissue integrity and adheres to the foot care regimen.

 7. The patient performs self-care activities.

IV. **DVT**

 A. **Description: blood clot formation in the deep veins of the lower extremities or in the pelvic veins**

 B. **Etiology and incidence**

  1. Thrombus formation occurs when two of three conditions of Virchow's triad are present:

      a. Venous stasis
      b. Hypercoagulability
      c. Injury to the venous wall
  2. Conditions contributing to venous stasis include:
      a. Surgery
      b. Obesity
      c. Pregnancy
      d. Congestive heart failure
  3. Conditions associated with hypercoagulability include:
      a. Malignant neoplasms
      b. Dehydration
      c. Blood dyscrasias
      d. Oral contraceptive use
  4. Vein wall trauma may result from:
      a. IV injection
      b. Thromboangiitis obliterans (Buerger's disease)
      c. Fractures and dislocations
      d. Chemical injury from sclerosing agents
      e. Injection of radiopaque media for imaging studies
      f. Use of certain antibiotics (e.g., chlortetracycline)

C. Pathophysiology

  1. A clot forms when platelets adhere to the vein lining or endothelium, release adenosine diphosphate (ADP), and begin the process of platelet aggregation, platelet plug, and clot formation.

  2. As a clot enlarges, it may block blood flow through the vein and thus obstruct venous drainage from the area distal to the clot.

  3. Within 24 to 48 hours after formation, the clot may dislodge and travel to the pulmonary artery (pulmonary embolism), a life-threatening emergency.

  4. Chronic venous insufficiency, or postphlebotic syndrome (PPS), results from dysfunctional valves that reduce venous return, increase venous pressure, and cause venous stasis; it follows most severe cases of DVT and may take 5 to 10 years to develop.

D. Assessment findings

  1. DVT may be asymptomatic, or may produce some or all of the following clinical manifestations:
      a. Swelling (usually unilateral), erythema, and warmth of calf or thigh associated with inflammation of phlebitis
      b. Pain in calf muscle on dorsiflexion (Homans' sign) due to stretching of inflamed vein
      c. Tenderness in calf or thigh
      d. Low-grade fever

      2. Hallmarks of PPS include:
- a. Chronic swollen limbs
- b. Thick, coarse, brownish skin around the ankles
- c. Venous stasis ulcers

E. Nursing diagnoses
1. Fear
2. Impaired Physical Mobility
3. Pain
4. Chronic Pain
5. Impaired Tissue Integrity
6. Altered Tissue Perfusion: Peripheral

F. Planning and implementation
1. Provide proper positioning:
   - a. Elevate the patient's legs above the level of the heart and have the patient avoid prolonged standing or sitting to promote venous return.
   - b. Instruct the patient to avoid activities or positions that produce pressure on leg muscles.
   - c. Maintain the patient in a flat, supine position (bedrest may be used to facilitate healing) if in doubt regarding positioning.
2. Promote venous return in the unaffected leg:
   - a. Instruct the patient to maximize the effects of the calf muscle pump to augment venous return by walking with a heel–toe gait and doing similar exercises if confined to bed.
   - b. Postsurgery, encourage deep breathing exercises and early ambulation to promote venous return and help prevent DVT.
   - c. Elevate the foot of the bed 6 inches while the patient is sleeping.
3. Maximize comfort:
   - a. Decrease discomfort through measures that promote venous return.
   - b. Apply warm packs to the legs to reduce pain.
   - c. Administer mild sedatives or analgesics as needed; avoid certain antiinflammatory agents (such as aspirin or ibuprofen) for a patient receiving anticoagulant therapy.
4. Provide care associated with medical and surgical interventions as appropriate:
   - a. Assess postoperative patients and patients with decreased activity and a history of DVT for signs of thrombophlebitis.
   - b. Observe the lower extremities for skin changes.
   - c. Monitor prothrombin time (PT) for a patient receiving

coumarin derivative therapy, and partial thromboplastin time (PTT) for a patient on heparin therapy.

d. Avoid intramuscular injections, invasive procedures, and minor types of trauma for a patient receiving anticoagulant therapy.

e. Never give aspirin to a patient receiving heparin or coumarin derivative therapy; it may induce bleeding.

f. Be aware that heparin acts almost immediately to interfere with blood clotting, whereas the effects of coumarin derivatives don't begin for 24 to 48 hours.

g. Keep antidotes for heparin (protamine sulfate) and coumarin derivative (vitamin K) overdose on hand.

h. Monitor a patient receiving fibrinolytic therapy (e.g., streptokinase) for bleeding from body orifices or into any body organ or cavity.

i. Carefully monitor venous and arterial function in the affected extremity following an invasive vein procedure such as phlebography, thrombectomy, embolectomy, vein ligation or stripping, or interruption of the vena cava with a filter or other device to prevent emboli.

j. Assess for hemorrhage, infection, nerve damage, and DVT after surgical removal of varicose veins.

5. Provide patient and family teaching, covering:

a. Avoiding sources of pressure above the knees (e.g., crossing the legs, sitting in chairs that are too high, wearing garters and knee-high stockings)

b. Proper positioning and exercises to promote venous return

c. The use of pneumonic vascular compression leggings

d. Signs and symptoms of DVT and chronic venous insufficiency and the need to report them promptly

e. Necessary precautions during anticoagulant therapy

G. Evaluation

1. The patient demonstrates restored skin integrity.

2. The patient verbalizes understanding of measures to avoid trauma to legs.

3. The patient demonstrates knowledge of proper positioning to promote circulation.

4. The patient increases physical mobility with gradual progression to an optimal level of activity and control of pain-inducing activity.

V. Venous stasis ulcers

A. Description: excavation of the skin surface resulting from sloughing of inflamed necrotic tissue, usually in the lower extremities

B. Etiology and incidence

1. Causes of venous stasis ulcers include:
   a. Postphlebotic syndrome and venous stasis (the most common cause)
   b. Deep venous obstruction due to abdominal tumor or pregnancy
   c. Valvular incompetency in the ileofemoral vein
   d. Major burns
   e. Sickle cell anemia
   f. Neurogenic disorders
   g. Hereditary factors
2. Incidence is increasing, especially in the elderly population.

C. Pathophysiology

1. Over time, incompetent valves in veins result in excessive venous pressure and subsequent rupture of small skin veins and venules.
2. Chronic changes of subcutaneous fibrosis, cutaneous atrophy, and lymphatic obstruction associated with stasis contribute to tissue breakdown and infection in local tissues.
3. Once the skin breaks and venous ulcers develop, healing is prolonged, difficult, and probably lifelong.

D. Assessment findings

1. Common clinical manifestations include:
   a. Visible skin ulcers
   b. Dark pigmentation
   c. Eczema or stasis dermatitis
   d. Normal arterial pulses
2. The patient may report varying degrees of pain, ranging from mild discomfort to dull, aching pain; typically relieved by leg elevation.

E. Nursing diagnoses

1. High Risk for Infection
2. Impaired Physical Mobility
3. Pain
4. Chronic Pain
5. Impaired Skin Integrity

F. Planning and implementation

1. Provide for ulcer debridement and healing:
   a. Remove dead or damaged material from the wound, using wet-to-dry dressings with saline solution and coarse-mesh gauze filled with cotton.
   b. Use whirlpool therapy to debride the ulcer bed.
   c. Consider using an enzymatic debrider, such as Debrisan or Elase, to aid removal of debris.
   d. Prepare for surgical debridement if necessary.
   e. Assist in application of Unna boot (dressing of medicated gauze covered with ace wrap) as ordered.

2. See Deep venous thrombosis, Section IV.F, for additional nursing interventions related to promoting venous return, maximizing comfort, promoting healing, and providing patient education.

G. Evaluation (see Deep venous thrombosis, Section IV.G)

VI. Varicose veins

A. Description: abnormally dilated veins with incompetent valves occurring most commonly in the lower extremities and lower trunk, usually in the great and small saphenous veins

B. Etiology and incidence

1. Common causative factors include:
    a. Congenital valve or vein wall defects
    b. Valve damage from trauma, obstruction, DVT, or inflammation
    c. Chronic venous distention associated with occupations requiring prolonged standing, obesity, or pregnancy
    d. Systemic conditions that interfere with venous return
    e. Loss of vein wall elasticity with aging
2. Varicose veins are fairly common, affecting about 15% of the adult population; incidence is about three times greater in women than in men.

C. Pathophysiology

1. Weakened vein walls cannot withstand normal pressure and dilate with pooling of blood.
2. Vein dilation prevents the valve cusps from meeting, resulting in increased backup pressure in lower vein segments.
3. Increased dilation increases valve stretching and worsens the condition.
4. Problems associated with varicose veins include:
    a. Unsightly appearance
    b. Concomitant venous insufficiency of deep veins
    c. Rarely, hemorrhage with abrasion of a vein surface
5. Treatment of mild cases may involve teaching the patient to take measures to promote venous return (see Section VI.F).
6. Severe cases may require surgical ligation and removal of varicose veins.

D. Assessment findings

1. The most obvious manifestation is dilated, tortuous, discolored veins, usually of the legs but possibly on the lower trunk.
2. Many people experience few symptoms beyond dilated leg veins and mild leg aching following prolonged standing.
3. Others experience more serious effects, such as:
    a. Easy leg fatigue
    b. Cramping (especially nocturnal) and a feeling of heaviness in the legs

      c.   Ankle edema

      d.   Signs and symptoms of deep venous insufficiency

      e.   Rarely, bleeding with abrasion of a vein surface

E. **Nursing diagnoses**

    1.   Activity Intolerance

    2.   Chronic Pain

    3.   Altered Tissue Perfusion: Peripheral

F. **Planning and implementation**

    1.   Promote venous return in the unaffected leg:

      a.   Instruct the patient to maximize the action of the calf muscle pump in augmenting venous return by walking with a heel–toe gait or doing similar exercises if confined to bed.

      b.   Encourage deep breathing exercises and early ambulation in postsurgical patients as a means of promoting venous return and preventing DVT.

      c.   Elevate the foot of the bed 6 inches while the patient is sleeping.

    2.   Provide care associated with medical and surgical interventions as appropriate:

      a.   Prepare the patient for surgery, if scheduled.

      b.   Postoperatively, observe for skin changes; monitor venous and arterial function carefully; and assess for hemorrhage, infection, nerve damage, and DVT.

    3.   Provide patient and family teaching, covering:

      a.   The need to avoid anything that can increase pressure above the knees (e.g., crossing the legs, sitting in chairs that are too high, wearing garters and knee-high stockings)

      b.   Proper positioning and exercise to promote venous return

G. **Evaluation**

    1.   The patient demonstrates restoration of tissue perfusion.

    2.   The patient verbalizes precautions to avoid trauma to legs.

    3.   The patient practices proper positioning to promote circulation.

    4.   The patient increases physical mobility with gradual progression to optimal level of activity and control of pain-inducing activity.

VII. Lymphedema

A. **Description: tissue swelling caused by obstructed lymph flow in an extremity**

B. **Etiology and incidence**

    1.   Primary lymphedema (also known as lymphedema of unknown origin or idiopathic lymphedema) may be congenital

(present at birth), praecox (developing early in life), or tardia (developing late in life); it may be associated with:

    a.   Aplasia (no lymph vessels)

    b.   Hypoplasia (smaller or fewer lymph vessels than normal)

    c.   Hyperplasia (larger or more numerous lymph vessels)

2. Lymphedema praecox is the most common type, with peak incidence occurring in the second decade of life and most commonly affecting females.

3. Secondary lymphedema results from damage or obstruction of the lymph system by disease or procedure, such as:

    a.   Trauma

    b.   Neoplasms

    c.   Mosquito-transmitted filariasis, caused by the filarial nematode *Wuchereria bancrofti* and others

    d.   Inflammation

    e.   Surgical excision of axillary, inguinal, or iliac lymph nodes

    f.   High-dose radiation therapy

C. **Pathophysiology**

1. Collection of lymph distal to a blocked lymphatic results in increased intralymphatic pressures, causing lymphatic wall dilation and valve incompetency.

2. Resultant backward lymph flow produces lymphatic dilation and valve incompetency in distal lymphatics and, if unchecked, eventually in even the smallest peripheral lymphatics.

3. Increased intralymphatic pressure leads to protein accumulation in the interstitial spaces.

4. Protein accumulation increases colloid osmotic pressures in the tissues, resulting in fluid retention and edema.

5. Chronic lymph congestion leads to fibrosis, formation of dense connective tissue in subcutaneous tissue.

D. **Assessment findings**

1. Clinical manifestations of primary lymphedema commonly include:

    a.   Nonpitting edema

    b.   Dull, heavy sensation

    c.   Absence of pain

    d.   Roughened skin without ulceration of skin or cellulitis

    e.   Marked limb enlargement

2. Secondary lymphedema related to filariasis may produce:

    a.   Intermittent episodes of high fever with chills

    b.   Malaise and fatigue

    c.   Tender regional lymphadenopathy

    d.   Severe muscle pain

    e.   Areas of erythema with increased edema and elephantiasis (severe edema)

      3. Secondary lymphedema related to neoplasms commonly cause:

         a. Nonpainful lymph node enlargement

         b. Edema

E. **Nursing diagnoses**

    1. Body Image Disturbance

    2. High Risk for Altered Body Temperature

    3. Fatigue

    4. Fluid Volume Excess

    5. Anticipatory Grieving

    6. Impaired Physical Mobility

    7. Pain

    8. Chronic Pain

F. **Planning and implementation**

    1. Assess for lymphedema:

        a. Measure and compare extremities for enlargement in all patients at risk.

        b. Assess for coexisting symptoms of lymphedema (initially pitting then brawny and nonpitting edema, no pain, and absence of infection) to rule out venous disorder as cause of edema.

    2. Promote lymph drainage:

        a. Coordinate physical therapy for arm or leg lymphedema: mechanical or manual squeezing of tissue followed by specific active and passive exercises in order to press stagnant lymphatic fluid into the blood stream.

        b. Elevate the affected extremity (e.g., elevate the arm on a pillow with the elbow higher than the shoulder and the hand higher than the elbow).

        c. Apply an elastic sleeve or stocking if prescribed for chronic lymphedema.

        d. Administer diuretic or anticoagulant therapy as prescribed.

        e. Prepare the patient for excisional removal of edematous subcutaneous tissue, if planned.

    3. Instruct the patient and family to observe for and report red streaks, fever and chills, penetrating wounds, and enlarged and tender lymph nodes.

    4. Provide emotional support:

        a. Assist the patient with a diagnosis of neoplastic disease in coping with associated problems.

        b. Encourage the patient to express fears and concerns, such as altered body image; listen actively.

        c. Assist a patient experiencing altered body image in selecting concealing clothing and applying makeup to emphasize positive aspects of body image.

G. **Evaluation**
1. The patient reports reduced pain and discomfort.
2. The patient exhibits reduced edema with proper positioning of extremity.
3. The patient demonstrates increased activity tolerance as edema subsides.
4. The patient demonstrates compliance with prescribed positioning and exercise program and relates the date and time of the next scheduled follow-up appointment.
5. The patient projects an improved self-concept, as evidenced by:
   a. Acknowledgment of changes in body image
   b. Expressions of self as a whole person
   c. Participation in social interaction

VIII. Lymphadenitis

A. **Description: an inflammatory condition of the lymph nodes; can be acute or chronic**

B. **Etiology**
1. Acute lymphadenitis occurs most commonly in the cervical region in association with infections of the teeth or tonsils, or in the axillary or inguinal regions secondary to infection in an extremity.
2. Generalized lymphadenopathy (involving two or three regionally separated lymph node groups) may result from inflammation, neoplasm, or immunologic reactions.
3. Chronic lymphadenitis results from longstanding infection and scarring with fibrous tissue replacement.

C. **Pathophysiology**
1. Lymph nodes act as defensive barriers and are secondarily involved in almost all systemic infections and in many neoplastic disorders.
2. Acute lymphadenitis involves one of two pathologic processes:
   a. Suppuration in lymph nodes due to pyogenic organism infection
   b. Hyperplasia, edema, and leukocyte infiltration of nodes in nonpyogenic organism infection (e.g., spirochetes, rickettsiae, and viruses)

D. **Assessment findings**
1. Clinical manifestations include:
   a. Enlarged, tender, warm, and reddened lymph nodes
   b. Generalized symptoms of infection such as fever and malaise
2. The infectious process also may produce red streaks from wounds or areas of cellulitis toward regional lymph nodes.

E. Nursing diagnoses
   1. Anticipatory Grieving
   2. High Risk for Infection
   3. Pain
F. Planning and implementation
   1. Promote resolution of infectious processes:
      a. Obtain cultures, and administer antibiotics as prescribed.
      b. Provide instruction in proper use of antibiotics for diagnosed infections, emphasizing the need to take the full amount prescribed.
      c. Assess for signs of lymphangiitis (acute inflammation of lymphatic channels) in patients exhibiting signs and symptoms of infections or with penetrating injuries.
   2. See Lymphedema, Section VII.F, for additional interventions related to patient teaching and emotional support.
G. Evaluation
   1. The patient demonstrates resolution of infectious process with use of prescribed medications and absence of signs and symptoms of infection.
   2. The patient reports reduction in or absence of pain.
   3. The patient projects an improved self-concept, as evidenced by:
      a. Acknowledgment of changes in body image
      b. Expressions of self as a whole person
      c. Participation in social interaction

IX. Extremity amputation
A. Description: surgical resection of a limb or a part of a limb
B. Indications
   1. Life-threatening situations; for example:
      a. Severe toxicity due to gangrene, usually secondary to chronic arterial occlusion
      b. Malignant tumors
      c. Severe osteomyelitis
   2. Intractable limb pain from such conditions as:
      a. Chronic infections
      b. Trophic ulcers
   3. Chronic and severe functional impairment due to a damaged extremity, as in:
      a. Injury, including crushing wounds
      b. Congenital deformities
      c. Chronic ischemia from extensive peripheral vascular disease
C. Types of amputation
   1. *Open* or *guillotine* amputation is usually performed on an infected limb since it allows the wound to drain freely; a second

surgery for stump revision and closure is done once infection has been eradicated.

2. *Closed* or *flap* amputation is performed when there is no evidence of infection and no need for draining.

3. In most cases, amputation is performed at as distal a level as possible; the final level is determined during surgery when the adequacy of blood flow can be evaluated.

4. Common leg amputation sites are above-the-knee amputation (AKA) and below-the-knee amputation (BKA).

D. **Types of prostheses**

1. A total-contact rigid dressing sometimes is applied in the operating room (immediate prosthetic fitting) to protect the stump from injury and prevent stump swelling by gently compressing tissue.

2. A permanent leg prosthesis is a rigid dressing that connects to an adjustable pylon and foot-ankle assembly to permit walking. This prosthesis must be changed three to four times before application of a permanent prosthesis since the stump shrinks with healing.

3. In cases when immediate prosthetic fitting is not possible—as after open amputation—fitting may be delayed until stump healing is complete.

E. **Complications**

1. Infection, bleeding, skin breakdown, and pain are common complications of amputation.

2. Immediate prosthetic fitting is thought to reduce problems of infection and bleeding.

F. **Psychosocial and rehabilitation considerations**

1. Amputation affects self-image and may be difficult to accept, particularly by a young person.

2. On the other hand, a person suffering chronic pain—due to chronic ischemia, for example—may welcome amputation.

3. In most cases, a cooperative, committed person with good coordination and energy can attain independent function with the use of a prosthesis.

4. Conditions and factors that can preclude prosthesis fitting and ambulation include:

   a. Severe neurologic disease
   b. Severe renal failure
   c. Altered mentation (e.g., disorientation, senility, psychosis, severe mental retardation)
   d. Severe cardiopulmonary disease
   e. High risk of gangrene in the opposite leg
   f. Poor stump healing
   g. Lack of motivation

G. **Nursing diagnoses**
1. Body Image Disturbance
2. Anticipatory Grieving
3. High Risk for Infection
4. Knowledge Deficit
5. Impaired Physical Mobility
6. Pain
7. Chronic Pain
8. Altered Tissue Perfusion: Peripheral

H. **Planning and implementation**
1. Provide proper positioning, and take measures to prevent contractures; for example:
   a. Avoiding elevating the stump on a pillow for 24 to 48 hours following surgery
   b. Avoiding positioning the stump in an externally rotated, abducted position to prevent contractures
   c. Preventing abduction contractures by adducting the stump on a regularly scheduled basis
   d. Performing ROM exercises (active or passive) at least three times a day
   e. Positioning the patient prone for several hours each day
   f. Placing a footboard on the end of the bed to prevent footdrop in the remaining leg
   g. Initiating exercises to prevent contractures as soon as possible (ideally, on the first or second postoperative day), including active ROM for the remaining leg, strengthening exercises for the arms, and hyperextension of the stump
   h. Having the patient receiving immediate prosthesis fitting walk as early as the first postoperative day to help prevent contractures (using a rigid cast prevents hip and joint contractures)
2. Promote skin integrity by:
   a. Inspecting the stump and all bony prominences daily for evidence of skin breakdown or infection
   b. Providing a high-protein diet with vitamin and mineral supplements
   c. Keeping the patient well hydrated with oral or IV fluids
3. Keep in mind that phantom limb sensation occurs in 1% to 10% of all patients with amputations, especially in above-knee amputations, for up to 3 months after amputation. Keep the patient active to help decrease phantom limb pain.
4. Administer analgesics as needed. Narcotics may be needed to control severe incisional and phantom pain; Darvon is usually

sufficient to control pain in a patient who received immediate prosthesis fitting.

5. Monitor for excessive bleeding. Mark blood stains on dressings with a pen and observe every 10 minutes for 24 hours for increase in size; report excessive bleeding at once.

6. Keep a large tourniquet at the bedside in case of massive hemorrhage.

7. Assess for hematoma formation, which will delay wound healing and provide a culture medium for bacterial growth. Assist the surgeon with hematoma aspiration as necessary.

8. Take steps to prevent stump edema, including:
   a. Elevating the stump on a pillow for 24 to 48 hours to improve venous return, prevent edema, and promote comfort (*Note:* Do not elevate the stump for more than 48 hours, which could lead to hip contracture.)
   b. Applying a plaster cast sock or elastic compression stocking to the stump immediately after surgery

9. Encourage self-care and independent mobility, and promote a positive self-concept; observe carefully for signs of depression or despondency.

10. Assess for and intervene as necessary to prevent or control general postoperative complications that prolong healing and delay a return to self-care, such as:
    a. Respiratory compromise
    b. Fluid and electrolyte imbalance
    c. Vascular problems
    d. Pulmonary embolism
    e. Nutritional deficits
    f. Elimination problems

11. Assess the patient's and family's adaptation to the amputation.

12. Provide patient and family teaching, covering:
    a. Stump care: washing with mild soap, rinsing carefully, and drying thoroughly, and performing careful daily inspection with a mirror for redness, blistering, or abrasions
    b. The need to avoid putting Band-aids or tape on the stump; they may irritate the skin and cause sores and infection when pulled off
    c. The need to avoid applying any creams or lotions (softens skin excessively) or alcohol (dries the skin, leading to cracking) to the stump
    d. The importance of wearing a woolen stump sock without holes or darned areas and washed in cool water and mild soap to prevent shrinkage
    e. Proper prosthesis use: putting it on immediately on arising and keeping it on all day to prevent stump swelling

    f.   Prosthesis care: cleaning the prosthesis socket daily with a damp cloth—being careful never to pour water into the socket, which may damage leather parts and cause metal parts to rust—and drying it thoroughly to prevent skin irritation

    g.   The importance of never adjusting or mechanically altering the prosthesis without professional help

    h.   The advisability of scheduling a yearly appointment with a prosthetist for follow-up evaluation of the prosthesis and any necessary adjustments

I. Evaluation

1. The patient demonstrates reduced pain.
2. The patient participates in self-care and rehabilitative activities.
3. The patient maintains skin integrity with no evidence of infection.
4. The patient projects good self-esteem and a positive self-concept.
5. The patient demonstrates resolution of the grieving process.
6. The patient achieves independence in self-care; for example:
   a. Balance during transfers and position changes
   b. Safe transfer ability
   c. Proper use of assistive devices
   d. Verbalized satisfaction with ability to perform ADLs
7. The patient achieves the maximum level of independent mobility possible.

X. Hypertensive vascular disease

A. Description: intermittent or sustained elevation in systolic or diastolic blood pressure; occurs as two major types: primary (essential) hypertension and secondary hypertension

B. Etiology and incidence

1. About 20% of the adult population develops hypertension; more than 90% of these cases have no identifiable medical cause (primary hypertension).
2. Identified risk factors for primary hypertension include:
   a. Family history
   b. Stress
   c. Obesity
   d. High dietary intake of sodium or saturated fats
   e. Excessive caffeine, alcohol, or tobacco use
   f. Oral contraceptive use
   g. Sedentary lifestyle
   h. Aging
3. Incidence of primary hypertension is higher in men than in women and is twice as high in blacks as in whites.
4. In about 10% of cases, hypertension is secondary to an identifiable medical diagnosis (secondary hypertension).

5. Conditions associated with secondary hypertension include:
   a. Renal vascular disease
   b. Renal parenchymal disease
   c. Primary hyperaldosteronism
   d. Cushing's syndrome
   e. Pheochromocytoma
   f. Coarctation of the aorta
   g. Thyroid, parathyroid, or pituitary dysfunction
   h. Pregnancy

C. Pathophysiology

1. Onset of primary hypertension typically begins as a labile (intermittent) process in the late 30s to early 50s that gradually becomes permanent.
2. Occasionally, severe hypertension develops abruptly and takes an accelerated or "malignant" course with rapid deterioration; acute elevation (diastolic pressure usually over 130 mmHg), known as *hypertensive crisis*, can rapidly produce irreversible neurologic, cardiac, and renal damage.
3. In hypertension, sensitivity to norepinephrine released at postganglionic nerve fibers of the sympathetic nervous system results in vasoconstriction, as does adrenal medulla.
4. Cortisol and other steroids from the adrenal cortex contribute to this vasoconstrictive response.
5. Vasoconstriction results in reduced blood flow to the kidney, triggering release of renin and leading to formation of angiotensin, a potent vasoconstrictor, secretion of aldosterone by the adrenal cortex, and retention of sodium and water by the renal tubules.
6. The combination of vasoconstriction and sodium and water retention results in elevated blood pressure.
7. Uncontrolled hypertension increases the risk of various complications, including stroke, coronary artery disease, congestive heart failure, renal failure, and eye changes.

D. Assessment findings

1. Hypertension usually produces no symptoms until vascular changes occur in the heart, brain, or kidneys.
2. Diagnosis of hypertension is confirmed by serial blood pressure readings above 140/90 mmHg in persons under age 50 or 160/90 mmHg in persons over age 50.
3. Because many people experience transient blood pressure elevations during examination (so-called white coat hypertension), remeasurement after about 10 minutes is recommended to obtain a more accurate reading.
4. Diagnostic studies associated with hypertension are those that evaluate cardiac, cerebral, and renal function; for example:

        a.   Urinalysis
        b.   Intravenous pyelography
        c.   Serum potassium, BUN, and creatinine
        d.   ECG
        e.   Chest radiograph

E. **Nursing diagnoses**
1. Knowledge Deficit
2. Noncompliance

F. **Planning and implementation**
1. Instruct the patient in and supervise use of prescribed anti-hypertensive medications. (*Note:* Not all persons with primary hypertension need medication to achieve and maintain blood pressure control.) Drugs used in the "stepped-care" approach for primary hypertension include:
   a. Thiazide diuretics (e.g., chlorthalidone, hydrochlorothiazide)
   b. Loop diuretics (e.g., furosemide)
   c. Potassium-sparing diuretics (e.g., spironolactone, triamterene)
   d. Adrenergic inhibitors (e.g., reserpine, methyldopa, propranolol, prazosin hydrochloride, clonidine hydrochloride, metoprolol, nadolol, guanethidine)
   e. Vasodilators (e.g., hydralazine, minoxidil)
2. Discuss side effects specific to each agent, which may include fluid and electrolyte imbalances, orthostatic hypotension and dizziness, mental confusion, depression, drowsiness, congestive heart failure, bradycardia, and changes in sexual function. Instruct the patient to report any unusual effects.
3. Advise the patient to always take medications on time, not to skip doses, and never to take larger dose of medication than prescribed without first consulting the physician.
4. Warn the patient never to suddenly discontinue medications without the primary health care provider's permission; severe hypertension may develop.
5. Provide dietary instruction, focusing on:
   a. Calorie restrictions for weight reduction
   b. Mild to moderate sodium restriction
   c. Restriction of cholesterol and saturated fats
   d. Increased intake of calcium and potassium, based on individual need for a patient receiving a potassium-wasting diuretic
6. Enlist the aid of a dietitian to provide detailed dietary instructions, if possible.
7. Discuss the beneficial role of regular exercise in heightening a sense of well-being, providing an outlet for emotional ten-

sions, raising serum levels of high-density lipoproteins (HDL), and aiding weight control—all of which can help control hypertension.

8. Assist the patient in developing an appropriate exercise program. Recommend a gradually progressive program of aerobic activity such as walking, jogging, or swimming (under medical supervision if the patient has a history of cardiovascular or pulmonary disease); discourage heavy weight lifting and isometric exercises, which can cause significant transient blood pressure elevation.

9. Refer the patient to a holistic health care practitioner for training in relaxation techniques, including progressive relaxation, meditation, autogenic training, biofeedback, and yoga.

10. Encourage the patient to seek regular follow-up evaluation; explain that primary hypertension is a lifelong condition that carries an increased risk of severe organ damage.

11. Evaluate the patient's compliance with the prescribed therapeutic regimen; refer as necessary to promote compliance.

12. Intervene in hypertensive crisis:
    a. Monitor IV drug administration, and assess blood pressure and heart rate often.
    b. Assess for target organ damage as manifested by restlessness, confusion, somnolence, coma, seizures, blurred vision, headache, nausea, vomiting (signs of hypertensive encephalopathy); signs of left ventricular failure and myocardial ischemia; and azotemia, oliguria, protein, sediment, and red blood cells in urine in renal damage.

G. Evaluation

1. The patient exhibits no signs or symptoms of progressive vascular changes.

2. The patient verbalizes understanding of the disease process, potential complications, and treatments.

3. The patient demonstrates compliance with the prescribed therapeutic regimen, including scheduled follow-up evaluations.

Bibliography

Bates, B. (1987). *A guide to physical examination* (4th ed.). Philadelphia: J. B. Lippincott.

Brunner, L. S., & Suddarth, D. S. (1986). *The Lippincott manual of nursing practice* (4th ed.). Philadelphia: J. B. Lippincott.

Brunner, L. S., & Suddarth, D. S. (1988). *Textbook of medical-surgical nursing* (6th ed.). Philadelphia: J. B. Lippincott.

Doyle, J. E. (1986). Treatment modalities in peripheral vascular disease. *Nursing Clinics of North America, 21*(2), 241-253.

Herman, J. A. (1989). Nursing assessment and nursing diagnosis in patients with peripheral vascular disease. *Nursing Clinics of North America, 21*(2), 219-231.

Luckmann, J., & Sorenson, K. C. (1987). *Medical-surgical nursing: A psychophysiologic approach* (3rd ed.). Philadelphia: W. B. Saunders.

Turner, J. A. (1986). Nursing intervention in patients with peripheral vascular disease. *Nursing Clinics of North America, 21*(2), 233-240.

Warbinek, E., & Wyness, M. A. (1986). Peripheral arterial occlusive disease (Part II): Nursing assessment and standard care plans. *Cardiovascular Nurse, 22*(2), 6-10.

STUDY QUESTIONS

1. Mr. White, aged 44, has undergone a right femoral angiogram. Immediately after the procedure, his right foot was warm, pink, and had palpable pedal pulses. About 4 hours later, he reports severe right leg pain. The nurse notes that the right leg and foot are cool and pale, and no pulses are palpable in the foot. Which of the following nursing actions would be *inappropriate*?
   a. Reassure Mr. White that this is a common complication after angiography and it will improve within 24 hours.
   b. Notify Mr. White's physician immediately with the findings.
   c. Elevate the leg, and give Mr. White an analgesic.
   d. Ambulate Mr. White to restore circulation to the foot.

2. Amy Burkholder, aged 17, has been admitted for evaluation of severe right leg lymphedema of idiopathic origin. Included in the nurse's plan of care will be addressing Amy's reaction to the problem. Why is this important?
   a. Lymphedema signals cancer.
   b. The infection results from inadequate bathing.
   c. Leg swelling can cause severe limb disfigurement.
   d. Altered circulation may necessitate leg amputation.

3. Mr. Kayais, aged 76, has just undergone a closed below-the-knee amputation of his right leg due to gangrene of the right foot. As the nurse prepares for Mr. Kayais's return from surgery, he or she should anticipate doing which of the following?
   a. carefully monitoring for bleeding and wound healing
   b. explaining the need for a second surgery in several weeks to prepare the stump for prosthesis fitting
   c. placing the stump in a dependent position immediately after surgery to enhance blood flow and healing

   d. positioning the stump in an externally rotated, abducted position to prevent contractures

4. At a blood pressure screening clinic, Mr. Ableman, aged 73, exhibits a reading of 169/94 mmHg. Which of the following statements by the clinic nurse would be most appropriate?
   a. "Your blood pressure is normal. Please have it checked again in 1 year."
   b. "Your blood pressure is elevated a little above normal. Please have it checked again within 6 months."
   c. "Your blood pressure is elevated a little above normal. Please make an appointment to see your doctor within the next 2 months."
   d. "Your blood pressure is dangerously elevated. Please have it evaluated by your doctor immediately, within 1 week or less."

5. On which of the following areas should the nurse focus during assessment of a patient with calf leg pain associated with exercise?
   a. leg color, temperature, pulses, pain description
   b. smoking history, deep vein thrombosis history, presence of edema
   c. allergy and medication history, usual activity pattern
   d. menopausal state, occupation, and socioeconomic status

6. For a patient with chronic arterial occlusive disease of the lower extremities, placing the legs lower than the heart is an intervention associated with which of the following nursing diagnoses?
   a. Activity Intolerance
   b. Altered Tissue Perfusion: Peripheral
   c. Pain
   d. High Risk for Disuse Syndrome

7. Ms. Mays, aged 63, is admitted to the hospital for a cholecystectomy. Which of the following assessment data indicates that this patient is at increased risk

of developing deep venous thrombosis following surgery?
a. She is 5'7" tall and weighs 125 lb.
b. She walks 2 miles daily for exercise.
c. She has had three pregnancies.
d. She will be immobile during and for a short time after the surgery.

8. Mrs. Adams, aged 58, has been diagnosed as having arteriosclerosis obliterans with decreased circulation to her legs and is admitted to the hospital for surgery. Knowing that arterial leg ulcers and gangrene can develop, the nurse should plan Mrs. Adams's care to include
a. providing and teaching about proper foot care
b. warning against alcohol ingestion
c. promoting a low-residue diet
d. encouraging the use of heavy support stockings

9. Following surgery, Mrs. Adams complains of pain in her right leg. Assessment data reveal a positive Homan's sign, with no edema, redness, or excessive warmth of the skin of the calf; temperature 99.2°F; pulse 92 beats per minute; respirations 24 breaths per minute; and blood pressure 132/84 mmHg. Which of the following statements evaluating these data is most appropriate?
a. A positive Homan's sign indicates the presence of acute arterial insufficiency.
b. Deep venous thrombosis is unlikely without calf swelling.
c. Deep venous thrombosis is highly possible, and physician assessment is indicated.
d. Calf muscle cramping associated with ambulation is probable, and bedrest is indicated.

10. The physician determines that Mrs. Adams has a deep venous thrombosis in her right leg and prescribes heparin infusion. About 12 hours after the infusion is begun, Mrs. Adams reports that her gums are bleeding when she brushes her teeth. The nurse's most appropriate initial action would be to

a. Discontinue the heparin infusion immediately.
b. Notify the physician of the patient's symptoms.
c. Administer a coumarin derivative to reverse the effects of heparin.
d. Reassure the patient that this is a normal response to heparin.

11. Mr. Tolley, aged 54, was admitted to the hospital for a below-the-knee amputation necessitated by gangrene of his right foot related to arteriosclerosis obliterans. Mr. Tolley returns from surgery with a rigid (castlike) dressing in place. Which of the following postoperative nursing diagnoses would *less* likely apply following application of a rigid dressing instead of a soft dressing?
a. Decreased Cardiac Output
b. Self-Esteem Disturbance
c. High Risk for Fluid Volume Deficit
d. Pain

12. Three days after his surgery, Mr. Tolley is in tears as the nurse enters his room. He says his foot that was amputated is "killing me," and he can't understand why it should hurt him so much. The nurse's most appropriate response would be to
a. Assess the stump for bleeding, and administer analgesic medication.
b. Reassure Mr. Tolley that phantom pain commonly occurs and eventually will disappear, and administer an analgesic.
c. Reassure Mr. Tolley that phantom pain is common and will soon disappear, and administer a sedative medication.
d. Monitor Mr. Tolley carefully for infection in the stump, and elevate the stump for 72 hours.

13. On the day of discharge to the rehabilitation unit, Mr. Tolley's outcome criteria is as follows: temperature 97.4°F, pulse 88, respiration 24, and blood pressure 126/88 mmHg; Tylenol with codeine 30 mg, administered once every 4 to 6 hours for pain; no drainage on

dressing; oral fluid intake of 2600 cc/day, good appetite, urinary output 1800 cc over the past 14 hours; bowel movement the previous day; and intact skin. Which of the following data would best meet the expected outcome of absence of infection?

a. The patient demonstrates urinary output within normal limits.
b. The patient reports pain relief from pain medication.
c. The patient demonstrates respiratory rate within normal limits.
d. The patient exhibits body temperature within normal range.

14. Mrs. Randolph, aged 42, has been admitted to the hospital for management of severe diabetes mellitus and hypertension. Admission assessment revealed the following data: blood pressure 184/108, pulse 90, respirations 28, and fasting blood sugar 284. Mrs. Randolph reports that she usually follows her diabetic diet and never eats salt but doesn't like to take her pills because they "make me dizzy." She says she has had the flu for several days and just feels "lousy" now. Based on this information, which of the following nursing diagnoses would be most appropriate for Mrs. Randolph?

a. Noncompliance with the self-care program related to negative effects of prescribed therapy
b. Knowledge Deficit related to the relationship between the treatment regimen and control of the disease process
c. Noncompliance with the self-care program related to recent short-term memory loss
d. Knowledge Deficit related to relationship of medication side effect to therapeutic effects

15. The physician prescribes a regimen for Mrs. Randolph that includes IV fluid therapy, oral hypertensive therapy, regular insulin injections, and education in diabetic and hypertensive self-care. At 9 PM on the day of admission, her blood pressure was 224/118 mmHg, pulse 74, and respirations 22. Knowing what complications can result from high blood pressure, what additional assessment data should the nurse collect before notifying the physician of the findings?

a. most recent blood glucose level
b. most recent bowel movement
c. presence of chest pain
d. presence of leg cramps

16. Mrs. Randolph's physical problems stabilize, and she is eagerly participating in her education program. Which of the following would be the most important indicator that Mrs. Randolph understands and can comply with her regimen to achieve long-term control of her hypertension?

a. She states an understanding of the need to take antihypertensive medications for the rest of her life.
b. She relates the importance of never discontinuing a prescribed medication without the physician's permission.
c. She independently adjusts the dose of her antihypertensive medication.
d. She states the need to continue taking her prescribed antihypertensive medication even if side effects develop.

ANSWER KEY

1. **Correct response: b**
   The findings indicate an acute occlusion of the arterial circulation, possibly by an embolus or thrombus following angiography, necessitating immediate intervention to restore circulation to the leg.
   a. This is not a usual or a normal response.
   c. Although pain medication would be appropriate, elevating the leg would further impede arterial circulation to the foot.
   d. Ambulation and calf muscle exercise would cause further tissue ischemia.
   Analysis/Physiologic/Implementation

2. **Correct response: c**
   Lymphedema praecox is the most common group of idiopathic lymphedema types and results in nonpitting edema with mild to severe enlargement of the limb.
   a. Cancer is not a cause of idiopathic lymphedema; however, lymphedema can be associated with neoplasms.
   b. Lymphedema is not an infection although it may result from one.
   d. Extremity amputation would not be indicated in this case.
   Knowledge/Psychosocial/Planning

3. **Correct response: a**
   Bleeding and infection are common postoperative complications following amputation.
   b. A second surgery is done for open or guillotine amputations, not for closed amputations.
   c. The stump should be elevated for 24 to 48 hours postoperatively to control edema.
   d. External rotation and abduction of the stump can cause contractures.
   Comprehension/Safe care/Planning

4. **Correct response: c**
   Although elevated, it is not a dangerous elevation, but follow-up evaluation by the patient's physician should take place within 2 months.
   a and b. These answers are incorrect; physician evaluation should occur earlier.
   d. This is not an urgent problem necessitating physician evaluation.
   Application/Health promotion/Implementation

5. **Correct response: a**
   Calf leg pain associated with exercise or intermittent claudication is symptomatic of ischemia caused by arterial occlusive disorders of the legs. These parameters can be used to ascertain clinical symptoms of arterial problems.
   b. Nicotine can cause vasoconstriction, but edema and deep venous thrombosis typically do not cause intermittent claudication.
   c and d. These answers are incorrect because the listed parameters are not considered urgent in assessment of a patient experiencing claudication.
   Knowledge/Physiologic/Assessment

6. **Correct response: b**
   Altered tissue perfusion is enhanced as blood flows to the extremities in a dependent position in relationship to the heart.
   a, c, and d. These other diagnoses do not address the basic problem of chronic arterial occlusive disease.
   Comprehension/Health promotion/Analysis (Dx)

7. **Correct response: d**
   The immobility and resultant venous stasis associated with surgery and a general anesthetic represent one of the three conditions necessary for thrombus formation.
   a and c. Although obesity and pregnancy are associated with hypercoagulability (another of the three conditions), the

patient is neither obese nor pregnant.

   b. A history of regular exercise is not identified as either a preventive or risk factor for thrombus formation associated with surgery.

Analysis/Health promotion/Assessment

8. **Correct response: a**
   The hallmark of peripheral vascular nursing, proper foot care, is necessary to prevent further tissue injury and possible amputation.
   b. Alcohol is a vasodilator and not specifically prohibited in arterial occlusive disease.
   c. A controlled-calorie, low-fat diet is appropriate, not a low-residue diet.
   d. Tight garments can inhibit arterial circulation; support stockings are indicated for venous, not arterial, insufficiency.

Application/Safe care/Planning

9. **Correct response: c**
   Because of the risk of pulmonary embolism, calf pain or tenderness in a postoperative patient must be considered a sign of thrombophlebitis until ruled out by physician analysis.
   a. A positive Homans' sign is not associated with assessment for acute arterial insufficiency.
   b. Early thrombophlebitis may not have resulted in obvious tissue swelling.
   d. Before assuming another cause for the pain, thrombophlebitis must be ruled out.

Analysis/Physiologic/Evaluation

10. **Correct response: b**
    Bleeding from body orifices is a side effect of heparin that could indicate excessive anticoagulation, necessitating further physician evaluation, including partial thromboplastin time (PTT) monitoring.
    a. The prescribed dose of heparin might be therapeutic and not excessive. A drug may be discontinued

only following physician's order to do so.
    c. Protamine sulfate, not coumarin derivative, is the reversal agent for heparin.
    d. PTT evaluation and assessment of other potential sources of bleeding must be done before concluding that the symptom is not serious.

Application/Safe care/Implementation

11. **Correct response: c**
    A rigid dressing (immediate prosthetic fitting) is thought to reduce the problems of infection and bleeding.
    a, b, and d. These answers are incorrect because these problems can occur in all patients with amputation regardless of the type of prosthesis, and are based on individual differences.

Comprehension/Safe care/Analysis (Dx)

12. **Correct response: b**
    Phantom pain occurs in up to 10% of all patients who have undergone amputation; it may persist for 2 to 3 months. It is real pain, and analgesic medication is needed for pain control.
    a. Bleeding is not considered the cause for the pain.
    c. Sedation will not alleviate the pain and may interfere with mobility and rehabilitation.
    d. Infection is not considered a cause for phantom pain, and elevation is contraindicated postoperatively because it can promote development of contractures.

Application/Physiologic/Implementation

13. **Correct response: d**
    Body temperature combined with improving wound pain and absence of drainage or induration of the wound are data to support the expected outcome of absence of infection.
    a and c. Good urinary output and normal respiratory rate are not specific indicators point-

ing to absence of wound infection.

b. Pain medication requirement is not the most specific listed indicator of wound infection.

Analysis/Physiologic/Evaluation

14. Correct response: a

Medication side effects are keeping her from taking the pills, resulting in uncontrolled hypertension.

b and c. The data do not reflect lack of knowledge of the treatment regimen or a short-term memory loss problem.

d. This answer is incorrect because it implies the need to tolerate side effects to achieve therapeutic effects, which is not now considered necessary in most cases.

Analysis/Psychosocial/Analysis (Dx)

15. Correct response: c

Cardiac changes, including angina, can result from hypertension.

a, b, and d. These answers are incorrect; none are considered complications of hypertension although they may have an effect on the degree of blood pressure elevation.

Application/Physiologic/Assessment

16. Correct response: b

Life-threatening hypertensive crisis can result from sudden withdrawal from medication in an unsupervised setting.

a. Antihypertensive agents constitute a cornerstone of intervention, yet some patients achieve control with other means.

c. Independent adjustment of antihypertensive medications is not a recognized self-care principle.

d. The available antihypertensive agents and blood pressure management regimens are so varied that individualized treatment regimens can be devised to minimize or eliminate discomforting side effects.

Application/Health promotion/Evaluation

Gastrointestinal Disorders

9

I. **Anatomy and physiology**
   A. Structure
   B. Function
II. **Overview of gastrointestinal disorders**
   A. Assessment
   B. Laboratory studies and diagnostic tests
   C. Psychosocial implications
   D. Medications used to treat gastrointestinal (GI) problems
III. **Stomatitis**
   A. Description
   B. Etiology
   C. Assessment findings
   D. Nursing diagnoses
   E. Planning and implementation
   F. Evaluation
IV. **Achalasia (megaesophagus, aperistalsis, cardiospasm)**
   A. Description
   B. Etiology and incidence
   C. Pathophysiology
   D. Assessment findings
   E. Nursing diagnoses
   F. Planning and implementation
   G. Evaluation
V. **Esophagitis**
   A. Description
   B. Etiology
   C. Pathophysiology
   D. Assessment findings
   E. Nursing diagnoses
   F. Planning and implementation

   G. Evaluation
VI. **Hiatal hernia (diaphragmatic hernia)**
   A. Description
   B. Etiology and incidence
   C. Pathophysiology
   D. Assessment findings
   E. Nursing diagnoses
   F. Planning and implementation
   G. Evaluation
VII. **Peptic ulcer disease**
   A. Description
   B. Etiology and incidence
   C. Pathophysiology
   D. Assessment findings
   E. Nursing diagnoses
   F. Planning and implementation
   G. Evaluation
VIII. **Appendicitis**
   A. Description
   B. Etiology and incidence
   C. Pathophysiology
   D. Assessment findings
   E. Nursing diagnoses
   F. Planning and implementation
   G. Evaluation
IX. **Diverticulitis**
   A. Description
   B. Etiology and incidence
   C. Pathophysiology
   D. Assessment findings
   E. Nursing diagnoses
   F. Planning and implementation
   G. Evaluation

I. Anatomy and physiology
A. Structure

1. The GI system consists of the mouth, esophagus, stomach, small intestine, large intestine, and associated structures.
2. *Mouth* structures include:
   a. Lips
   b. Teeth
   c. Gingivae and oral mucosa
   d. Tongue
   e. Hard palate
   f. Soft palate
   g. Pharynx

3. A muscular tube extending from the pharynx to stomach, the *esophagus* consists of several layers:
   a. External layer: fibrous tissue
   b. Muscular layer: striated muscle in the upper esophagus, smooth muscle in the remainder
   c. Submucosal layer: loose connective tissue, blood and lymphatic vessels, and nerves
   d. Mucosal layer (innermost layer): mucus-secreting glands that lubricate the food bolus to facilitate passage
4. Esophageal openings include the upper esophageal sphincter (UES) at the cricopharyngeal muscle, and the lower esophageal sphincter (LES), or cardiac sphincter, which normally remains closed and opens only to pass food into the stomach.
5. A muscular pouch situated in the upper abdomen under the liver and diaphragm, the *stomach* consists of three anatomic areas:
   a. Fundus
   b. Body (or corpus)
   c. Antrum (or pylorus)
6. The stomach wall has four tissue layers:
   a. Fibroserous coat: outer layer
   b. Muscular coat: produces peristaltic activity
   c. Submucosal coat: contains blood and lymph vessels and nerves
   d. Mucosal lining: epithelial lining of stomach in longitudinal folds (rugae), which allow distention and increase surface area; contains many glands that secrete gastric juice
7. The LES or cardiac sphincter allows food to enter the stomach and prevents reflux into the esophagus. The pyloric sphincter regulates flow of stomach contents (chyme) into the duodenum.
8. The *small intestine*, a coiled tube approximately 22 ft long and 1 in in diameter, extends from the pyloric sphincter to the ileocecal valve at the large intestine; sections include:
   a. Duodenum
   b. Jejunum
   c. Ileum
9. Tissue layers are similar to those of the stomach. Numerous villi—tiny, fingerlike projections in the mucosal layer—provide a vast surface area for secretion, digestion, and absorption.
10. A shorter, wider tube (5 to 6 ft long, 2 to 2½ in in diameter) beginning at the ileocecal valve and ending at the anus, the *large intestine* consists of three sections:
    a. Cecum: a 2- to 3-in blind pouch, extending from the ileocecal valve to the vermiform appendix
    b. Colon: the main portion of the large intestine, divided

into four anatomic sections: ascending, transverse, descending, and sigmoid

    c.   Rectum: 7 to 8 in long, extending from the sigmoid colon to the anus

B. **Function**

    1.   The GI system performs two major body functions:

        a.   Digestion of food and fluid, with absorption of nutrients into the blood stream

        b.   Elimination of waste products through defecation (Fig. 9–1)

    2.   Digestion begins in the mouth with chewing and the action of ptyalin, an enzyme contained in saliva that breaks down starch.

    3.   After food is swallowed, it passes through the esophagus to the stomach, where digestion continues through several processes:

        a.   Secretion of gastric juice, containing hydrochloric acid and the enzymes pepsin and lipase (and, in infants, renin)

        b.   Mixing and churning through peristaltic action

    4.   From the pylorus, the mixed stomach contents (chyme) pass into the duodenum through the pyloric valve.

    5.   In the small intestine, food digestion is completed and most nutrient absorption occurs. Digestion results from the action of numerous pancreatic and intestinal enzymes (e.g., trypsin, lipase, amylase, lactase, maltase, sucrase) and bile.

    6.   In the large intestine, the cecum and ascending colon absorb water and electrolytes from the now completely digested material; the rectum stores feces for elimination.

II. Overview of gastrointestinal disorders

    A.   Assessment

        1.   Health history should focus on:

            a.   History of present illness, which can provide sufficient information for diagnosis in about 80% of patients

            b.   Appetite and food intolerance; usual food intake with 24-hour recall

            c.   Pain: character, location, timing (e.g., before meals or after meals), alleviating measures

            d.   Bowel elimination patterns: frequency, color, consistency, laxative use

            e.   Presence of any of following: dark urine, jaundice, weight loss, nausea and vomiting

            f.   Previous GI tract surgery

        2.   Physical assessment should reveal the following normal findings:

            a.   Mouth: mucosa of mouth smooth, pink, moist; symmetric movement of all structures

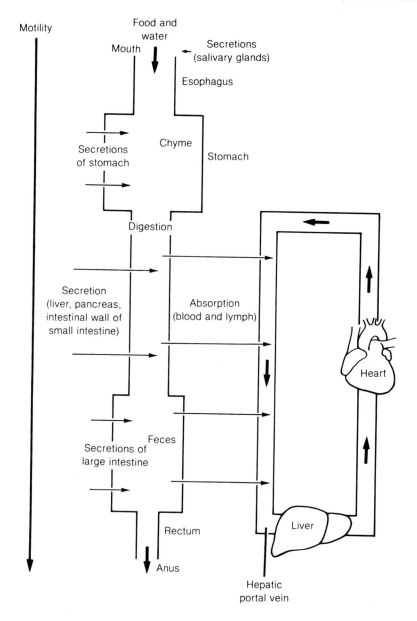

FIGURE 9–1.
Summary of gastrointestinal activity.

   b.   Teeth and gingivae: natural teeth present with dental caries filled or well-fitting dentures; no gingival redness or swelling
   c.   Tongue: pink and velvety
   d.   Throat: no redness or swelling
   e.   Abdomen: see Chapter 1, Nursing Process and Health Assessment, Section IV.B

B.   Laboratory studies and diagnostic tests

1.   Blood and serum studies to evaluate GI function include:
   a.   Albumin–globulin ratio and total protein: responsible for oncotic pressure; decreased in malabsorption and malnutrition
   b.   Alkaline phosphatase: measures enzyme activity in bone, intestine, liver, biliary systems; elevated in liver disorders
   c.   Bilirubin: both unconjugated (direct), liberated from RBCs, and conjugated (indirect) not yet passed through the liver; elevated with impaired biliary excretion or increased RBC production
   d.   Cholesterol: measures circulating free cholesterol; provides information on liver metabolism and synthesis
   e.   Miscellaneous tests to evaluate absorptive activity of GI tract (e.g., iron, calcium, cholesterol, prothrombin time, carotenes, vitamin A)

2.   Urine and fecal studies include:
   a.   Urine urobilinogen: normally present in small amounts; increased when liver fails to reabsorb, decreased in malabsorption
   b.   Fecal urobilinogen: normally present in feces, providing normal color to feces; decreased in biliary obstruction
   c.   Fecal fat (two different evaluations): qualitative evaluation measures fat content as either neutral (such as ingested mineral oil) or fatty acid (such as lipids); in quantitative evaluation, the patient eats a diet with a prescribed amount of fat, and stool is collected for 72 hours
   d.   Stool guaiac: detects occult blood in stool, indicating GI bleeding

3.   Important radiographic studies of the GI system include:
   a.   Upper GI or barium swallow: visualization via fluoroscopy of esophagus and stomach after patient swallows barium; serial radiographs show outline of structures
   b.   Lower GI or barium enema: instillation of barium into the large intestine, with fluoroscopy and filming to visualize structures and determine the efficiency of emptying
   c.   Cholecystogram: radiopaque dye taken by mouth on

evening before radiograph examination; drug excreted in bile

4. Motility studies use manometric catheters to measure intraluminal pressure in GI structures. Esophageal manometry evaluates peristaltic contractions and sphincter integrity; rectal manometry measures internal and external sphincter pressures.

5. Endoscopic studies provide direct visualization of internal GI structures (and a means to obtain biopsy samples) using a long, flexible tube containing a fiberoptic light source; types include esophagoscopy, gastroscopy, colonoscopy, sigmoidoscopy, and esophagogastroduodenoscopy.

6. Other useful studies include:
   a. Ultrasonography
   b. Computed tomography (CT) scanning
   c. Magnetic resonance imaging (MRI)
   d. Scintigraphy, to detect bleeding when endoscopy is not possible
   e. Gastric analysis, to determine the nature of secretions

C. Psychosocial implications

1. Patients with GI disorders may experience coping difficulties related to:
   a. Fear of rejection
   b. Uncertainty about the disease process and prognosis

2. Self-concept concerns commonly related to GI disorders include:
   a. Rejection by others
   b. Body image changes

3. Changes in social interaction related to GI disorders can lead to such problems as:
   a. Isolation
   b. Depression

4. GI disorders also can entail lifestyle concerns related to potential changes in:
   a. Physical abilities
   b. Activity level
   c. Work performance and the potential loss of job

D. Medications used to treat GI problems

1. *Antacids* are administered to treat symptoms of hyperacidity by neutralizing gastric acidity; types include:
   a. Aluminum hydroxide (e.g., Amphojel)
   b. Calcium carbonate (e.g., Tums)
   c. Dihydroxyaluminum sodium carbonate (e.g., Rolaids)
   d. Magaldrate (e.g., Riopan)
   e. Magnesium hydroxide (Milk of Magnesia)

2. *Antiemetics* are given to relieve nausea and vomiting; the choice of drug depends on the cause of vomiting; types include:

   a. Scopolamine (e.g., Transdermscop)
   b. Dimenhydrinate (e.g., Dramamine)
   c. Diphenhydramine hydrochloride (e.g., Benadryl)
   d. Promethazine hydrochloride (e.g., Phenergan)
   e. Chlorpromazine hydrochloride (e.g., Thorazine)
   f. Metoclopramide hydrochloride (e.g., Reglan)
   g. Benzquinamide hydrochloride (e.g., Emete-Con)

3. *Emetic* agents, used to induce vomiting in treatment of some poisonings and drug overdoses, include Ipecac syrup.

4. Used in the treatment of peptic ulcers, *cytoprotective agents* produce an ulcer-adherent complex that hastens healing. The most commonly used cytoprotective agent is sucralfate (Carafate).

5. Used to treat active duodenal ulcers by decreasing the stimulus for hydrochloric acid production, *histamine (H_2) receptor antagonists* include:
   a. Cimetidine (Tagamet)
   b. Famotidine (Pepcid)

6. Given to induce defecation, *laxatives* exert different effects depending on type:
   a. Bulk laxative: absorb water and increase fecal bulk; agents include psyllium (e.g., Metamucil)
   b. Stimulant laxatives: stimulate peristalsis through mucosal irritation; examples include bisacodyl (e.g., Dulcolax), cascara sagrada (e.g., Cas-Evac), and castor oil (e.g., Alphamul)
   c. Stool softeners: facilitate mixing of water in the fecal mass, easing passage of stool; agents include docusate sodium (e.g., Colace)
   d. Saline (osmotic) laxatives: retain and increase water content of feces; examples include magnesium hydroxide (Milk of Magnesia)

III. Stomatitis
A. Description: inflammation of the oral mucosa from various causes
B. Etiology
   1. Stomatitis may be caused by infection, trauma, excessive dryness, chemical irritants and toxic agents, or hypersensitivity.
   2. Infectious agents that can produce stomatitis include:
      a. Viruses (e.g., the herpes simplex virus, which causes acute herpetic stomatitis)
      b. Fungi (e.g., *Candida albicans*, which causes candidiasis, or thrush)
   3. Damage from mechanical trauma (e.g., irritation from jagged teeth, cheek-biting, mouth-breathing, use of a too-stiff tooth brush) can cause characteristic lesions.

   4. Irritants that can produce stomatitis include strong mouth-washes or dentifrices, tobacco, and chemotherapeutic agents.
   5. Causes of aphthous ulcer ("canker sore") remain unclear; suspected predisposing factors include stress, allergy, vitamin deficiency, and viral infection.

C. Assessment findings
   1. Clinical manifestations vary with the type of stomatitis.
   2. Acute herpetic stomatitis is marked by small, clear vesicles in single or multiple eruptions, commonly preceded by sore throat, headache, nausea and vomiting, and malaise; usually lasts about 1 week.
   3. Candidiasis produces characteristic raised white patches and ulcers; infection may spread to other areas of the GI tract, the skin, or the respiratory system.
   4. Manifestations of mechanical trauma vary with the cause; small lacerations or abrasions with bleeding or exudate are common.
   5. Chemical irritation typically produces generalized redness and swelling; chemotherapy may cause swollen, easily bruised mucosa and possibly ulcerations with exudate.
   6. Aphthous ulcer appears as a well-circumscribed lesion with a white center and a reddish ring around the periphery.

D. Nursing diagnoses
   1. High Risk for Fluid Volume Deficit
   2. High Risk for Infection
   3. Altered Nutrition: Less Than Body Requirements
   4. Altered Oral Mucous Membrane
   5. Pain

E. Planning and implementation
   1. Promote meticulous oral hygiene, instructing the patient to:
       a. Brush and floss teeth and massage gums several times daily
       b. When pain prevents use of a toothbrush, use gauze or a sponge toothette to cleanse the oral mucosa
       c. Use saline, water, or diluted solution hydrogen peroxide instead of dentifrice or mouthwash
   2. To treat fungal infection, encourage the use of an antifungal agent (e.g., Nystatin), and "swish and swallow" to coat the oral mucosa.
   3. Promote adequate food and fluid intake; suggest:
       a. A bland diet, avoiding spicy and acidic foods
       b. Use of topical or systemic analgesics
       c. Eating food and fluids served lukewarm or cold, which may minimize discomfort and result in increased intake

F. Evaluation
   1. The patient displays intact oral mucosa with no evidence of inflammation.

2. The patient demonstrates appropriate oral hygiene.
3. The patient is free of pain and discomfort.
4. The patient maintains a nutritionally balanced diet.
5. The patient remains free of systemic infection.

IV. Achalasia (megaesophagus, aperistalsis, cardiospasm)

A. **Description: a condition marked by absence of esophageal peristalsis and the inability of the LES to relax**

B. **Etiology and incidence**
   1. The cause of achalasia is unclear, but it probably results from some disruption of normal neuromuscular mechanisms.
   2. Achalasia occurs in about 1 in 100,000 persons in the United States and equally in both sexes. Peak incidence is between ages 30 and 50.

C. **Pathophysiology**
   1. Onset is typically insidious and progression gradual over many months or years.
   2. Increased pressure on the LES produces obstruction with secondary esophageal dilation and a tendency toward regurgitation, especially when the patient lies down.
   3. Over time, the muscular esophageal wall may hypertrophy, contributing to obstruction.
   4. Possible complications include esophagitis and ulceration, and atelectasis from aspiration of esophageal contents.

D. **Assessment findings**
   1. Common clinical manifestations include:
      a. Dysphagia (may have more difficulty swallowing fluids than solids)
      b. Substernal pain
      c. Regurgitation of undigested food several hours after eating
      d. Weight loss
   2. Diagnostic tests—esophagoscopy, esophageal manometry, and barium swallow—demonstrate a dilated esophagus above a constricted LES, along with absence of normal esophageal peristalsis.

E. **Nursing diagnoses**
   1. High Risk for Fluid Volume Deficit
   2. Knowledge Deficit
   3. Altered Nutrition: Less Than Body Requirements
   4. Pain

F. **Planning and implementation**
   1. Promote adequate nutrition, instructing the patient to:
      a. Drink liquids with meals
      b. Eat small, frequent meals rather than large meals
      c. Chew food thoroughly

2. Instruct the patient to avoid lying down immediately after meals, which can promote regurgitation.
3. Encourage the patient to sleep with the head of the bed elevated slightly.

G. Evaluation

1. The patient maintains adequate nutritional intake.
2. The patient maintains adequate fluid intake.
3. The patient remains free of pain or reports successful control of pain.
4. The patient verbalizes measures to help prevent regurgitation.

V. Esophagitis

A. Description: inflammations of the esophageal mucosa; may be acute or chronic

B. Etiology

1. Esophagitis most commonly results from recurrent reflux of gastric contents into the distal esophagus.
2. Reflux can occur due to:
   a. Incompetent LES
   b. Gastric or duodenal ulcers
   c. Prolonged nasogastric intubation

C. Pathophysiology

1. Normally, the LES blocks reflux of gastric juice into the esophagus. Defects in the LES mechanism (e.g., decreased resting LES pressure, LES relaxation, transient increase in intraabdominal pressure) can lead to reflux.
2. Persistent reflux can lead to esophageal ulcer formation, bleeding, and scarring.

D. Assessment findings

1. Common clinical manifestations include:
   a. Heartburn, acid regurgitation, belching
   b. Dysphagia
   c. Esophageal pain possibly radiating to the arms, neck, back, jaw, and substernal area; may be precipitated by increased abdominal pressure as can occur from bending, straining, obesity, or pregnancy
2. Diagnostic tests may include:
   a. Esophagoscopy, barium swallow
   b. Bernstein acid-perfusion test
   c. Acid-reflux test
   d. Esophageal manometry

E. Nursing diagnoses

1. Knowledge Deficit
2. Altered Nutrition: Less Than Body Requirements
3. Pain

F. **Planning and implementation**
1. Promote adequate nutritional intake; instruct the patient to:
   a. Eat small, frequent meals of mostly bland foods.
   b. Chew food thoroughly before swallowing.
   c. Drink fluids to aid swallowing and food passage down the esophagus.
   d. Avoid irritants such as spicy or acidic foods, alcohol, caffeine, and tobacco.
   e. Do not lie down after eating, and avoid eating within 3 hours of bedtime.
2. Elevate the head of the patient's bed with blocks to help minimize reflux.

G. **Evaluation**
1. The patient verbalizes measures to promote good nutrition.
2. The patient verbalizes understanding of the causes and treatment of esophagitis.
3. The patient reports reduced regurgitation and pain.

VI. **Hiatal hernia (diaphragmatic hernia)**

A. **Description: protrusion of an upper portion of the stomach through an area of weakness in the diaphragm**

B. **Etiology and incidence**
1. Hiatal hernia usually results from diaphragmatic muscle weakening or diaphragm malformations; predisposing factors include:
   a. Aging
   b. Trauma
   c. Surgery
   d. Disorders such as esophageal cancer and kyphoscoliosis
2. The disorder may occur in 10% to 20% of the population; approximately one half of those affected experience no symptoms.
3. Incidence is higher in women than in men and increases with age.

C. **Pathophysiology**
1. Hiatal hernia develops when the muscular collar around the esophageal–diaphragmatic junction weakens and loosens.
2. This loosening allows the upper portion of the stomach to protrude into the chest when intraabdominal pressure increases, as may result from obesity, ascites, pregnancy, bending, straining, coughing, constrictive clothing, or extreme physical exertion.

D. **Assessment findings**
1. Signs and symptoms of hiatal hernia may include:
   a. Heartburn occurring 30 to 60 minutes following a meal
   b. Substernal pain due to reflux; worsens when lying down
   c. Belching, regurgitation of sour-tasting secretions

          d.   Feeling of abdominal fullness
    2.   Important diagnostic tests include:
          a.   Esophagoscopy
          b.   Barium swallow

E. Nursing diagnoses
    1.   Knowledge Deficit
    2.   Pain

F. Planning and implementation
    1.   Teach the patient measures to prevent hiatal hernia or minimize symptoms:
          a.   Avoid bending, lifting heavy objects, straining (Valsalva's maneuver), reclining after meals, tight clothing.
          b.   Avoid spicy and acidic foods, alcohol, and tobacco.
          c.   Eat small, frequent, bland meals.
          d.   Eat a high-fiber diet to help prevent constipation and thus minimize straining on defecation.
          e.   Take antacids as needed.
    2.   If symptoms persist, prepare the patient for surgical repair; possible procedures include:
          a.   Nissen fundoplication
          b.   Hill operation
          c.   Belsey Mark IV operation

G. Evaluation
    1.   The patient verbalizes factors that precipitate symptoms and means of avoiding or minimizing these factors.
    2.   The patient reports decreased pain and other symptoms.

VII. Peptic ulcer disease
    A. Description: ulcers—circumscribed breaks in the mucosa—occurring in the stomach, the duodenum, and less commonly, the distal esophagus and the jejunum

    B. Etiology and incidence
        1.   The exact cause of peptic ulcer disease is not known; possible contributing factors include:
            a.   Altered gastric acid and serum gastrin levels
            b.   Tobacco smoking and alcohol use
            c.   Use of aspirin, other nonsteroidal antiinflammatory drugs, and steroids
            d.   Genetic predisposition
            e.   Psychosomatic factors (e.g., chronic anxiety, Type A personality)
        2.   Peptic ulcer disease occurs in 5% to 10% of the population; only about one half of the cases are diagnosed. Duodenal ulcers are three times more common than gastric ulcers.
        3.   Peak incidence for duodenal ulcers is between ages 25 and 50; it affects four times as many men as women.

4. Peak incidence for gastric ulcers is over age 50; incidence is about equal in men and women.

C. **Pathophysiology**

1. The basic problem in peptic ulcer disease is excessive secretion of hydrochloric acid in relation to the protective effects of mucus secretion and acid neutralization.

2. Normally, tightly packed epithelial cells protect the gastric mucosa from irritation. Back-diffusion of acid through damaged mucosa may cause gastric ulcers.

3. Hypersecretion of acid, possibly related to overactive vagal stimulation, contributes to duodenal ulcer formation.

4. Possible complications of peptic ulcer disease include perforation, hemorrhage, and pyloric obstruction.

D. **Assessment findings**

1. Peptic ulcer disease may be asymptomatic in up to 50% of persons affected.

2. Gastric ulcers may produce:

   a. Pain, commonly described as burning, aching, or gnawing in the upper epigastrium; occurring 30 minutes to 1 hour following meals (rarely at night); and unrelieved by eating

   b. Epigastric tenderness

3. Signs and symptoms of duodenal ulcers may include:

   a. Pain, described as burning, aching, or gnawing in the right epigastrium; occurring 2 to 3 hours after meals, possibly causing the patient to awaken at night; and relieved by eating

   b. Belching, nausea, and vomiting

   c. GI bleeding, either a slow oozing manifested by melena or a sudden rapid loss of large amounts of blood through hematemesis

   d. Epigastric tenderness

4. Important diagnostic tests include:

   a. Barium swallow

   b. Gastroscopy

E. **Nursing diagnoses**

1. Knowledge Deficit

2. Altered Nutrition: Less Than Body Requirements

3. Pain

F. **Planning and implementation**

1. Teach the patient methods to minimize symptoms while still maintaining adequate nutrition, such as:

   a. Avoiding caffeine, alcohol, and spicy and acidic foods

   b. Avoiding other foods that previously have caused pain; specific dietary restrictions will vary from patient to patient

        c.   Eating small, frequent, bland meals
- **2.** Administer medications as prescribed, which may include:
  - a. Antacids
  - b. Anticholinergics
  - c. Histamine (H_2 receptor) antagonists
  - d. Cytoprotective agents
- **3.** Teach the patient about necessary lifestyle changes aimed at decreasing stress and maximizing effectiveness of coping mechanisms.
- **4.** Prepare the patient for surgery if indicated; possible procedures include:
  - a. Vagotomy and pyloroplasty
  - b. Distal subtotal gastrectomy

G. Evaluation
- **1.** The patient reports reduced pain.
- **2.** The patient verbalizes appropriate diet modifications.
- **3.** The patient demonstrates compliance with the prescribed medication regimen.

VIII. Appendicitis

A. Description: inflammation of the vermiform appendix

B. Etiology and incidence
- **1.** The precipitating event in appendicitis is obstruction of the appendix lumen, as can result from:
  - a. Fecalith
  - b. Kinking of appendix
  - c. Inflammation
  - d. Neoplasm
- **2.** Appendicitis occurs in about 7% of the population and affects males more often than females; peak incidence is between ages 10 and 30.

C. Pathophysiology
- **1.** Obstruction of the appendix lumen causes increased intraluminal pressure and triggers an inflammatory process that can lead to infection, necrosis, and perforation.
- **2.** Perforation and rupture can cause peritonitis, a life-threatening complication.

D. Assessment findings
- **1.** Common clinical manifestations include:
  - a. Acute abdominal pain, usually in the right lower quadrant (McBurney's point); rebound tenderness
  - b. Nausea and vomiting
  - c. Low-grade fever
- **2.** Laboratory evaluation may reveal leukocytosis.

E. Nursing diagnoses
- **1.** Fluid Volume Deficit

2. High Risk for Infection
3. Altered Nutrition: Less Than Body Requirements
4. Pain

F. Planning and implementation: prompt surgery is indicated to prevent perforation; provide general preoperative and postoperative care (see Chapter 24, Perioperative Nursing, for details)

G. Evaluation
1. The patient reports reduced pain.
2. The patient remains free of infection.
3. The patient exhibits adequate fluid status; drinks six to eight glasses of water daily.
4. The patient demonstrates appropriate choices in dietary intake.

IX. Diverticulitis

A. Description: a condition involving inflammation of diverticula, small saccular herniations in the colonic wall

B. Etiology and incidence
1. Formation of diverticula is associated with increased intraluminal pressure due to such factors as low-fiber diet, chronic constipation, and obesity.
2. Diverticula develop in about 50% of persons over age 60 in the United States; incidence is greatest in men.
3. Diverticulitis occurs in about 25% of persons with diverticula.

C. Pathophysiology
1. Diverticula form as the colonic mucosa pushes through the muscular coat at weak points; increased intraluminar pressure is the apparent precipitating factor.
2. The diverticula gradually fill with undigested food matter and bacteria; as they enlarge, they become more susceptible to irritation and inflammation.
3. Even a minute perforation of an inflamed diverticulum can lead to bacterial or fecal contamination of pericolic tissues.
4. Inflamed bowel tissue may adhere to the bladder or another pelvic organ; fistula formation may occur.
5. Repeated inflammation causes the colonic wall to thicken, narrowing the lumen and possibly causing acute obstruction.
6. Other dangerous complications include peritonitis and hemorrhage.

D. Assessment findings
1. Clinical manifestations may include:
   a. Change in bowel habits
   b. Dull, steady or episodic pain in the left lower abdominal quadrant or the epigastrium (depending on location of the diverticulitis)
   c. Rectal bleeding
   d. Anorexia

e. Low-grade fever
2. Laboratory evaluation may reveal leukocytosis.
3. Studies performed to aid differential diagnosis may include:
    a. Colonoscopy
    b. Proctoscopy
    c. Barium enema

E. Nursing diagnoses
  1. Constipation
  2. Knowledge Deficit
  3. Altered Nutrition: Less Than Body Requirements
  4. Pain
  5. Chronic Pain

F. Planning and implementation
  1. Provide measures designed to allow the colon to rest (e.g., keep the patient NPO, and administer IV fluids).
  2. Administer antibiotics as prescribed.
  3. Instruct the patient in home care management (e.g., eating a high-fiber diet [controversial], taking stool softeners, drinking six to eight glasses of water daily).
  4. If surgical bowel resection is indicated, provide appropriate preoperative and postoperative care (see Chapter 24, Perioperative Nursing, for more information).

G. Evaluation
  1. The patient reports absence of pain.
  2. The patient exhibits return to normal elimination pattern, marked by:
     a. No abdominal cramping
     b. Passage of soft formed stool
  3. The patient demonstrates appropriate choices in dietary intake.

X. Peritonitis

A. Description: acute or chronic inflammation of the peritoneum, the membrane lining the abdominal cavity and covering the viscera

B. Etiology
  1. Peritonitis usually results from bacterial (commonly, *Escherichia coli* or *Streptococcus faecalis*) invasion of the peritoneum due to such causes as:
     a. Ruptured appendix
     b. Diverticulitis
     c. Perforated gastric or duodenal ulcer
     d. Mesenteric thrombosis
     e. Peptic ulcer disease
     f. Neoplasm
     g. Bowel strangulation
     h. Ulcerative colitis

        i.   Penetrating abdominal wound

   2.   Other possible causes include:

       a.   Chemical irritation, as can result from ruptured bladder, ovary, or fallopian tube

       b.   Bile spillage into the peritoneal cavity, as can result from ruptured gallbladder or gangrenous cholecystitis

       c.   Contamination of the peritoneal cavity with surgical glove powder, talc, particles of suture material, or lint from surgical drapes

C.   **Pathophysiology**

   1.   Peritoneal contamination may be localized in an abscess or diffused throughout the peritoneum, depending on its origin and on the effectiveness of the patient's defenses.

   2.   The infectious process shunts blood to the inflamed area, leading to fluid shifts.

   3.   Paralytic ileus develops in early stages; as ileus and fluid shifting progress, dehydration and, possibly, acidosis occur.

   4.   Life-threatening complications of peritonitis include bowel obstruction, renal failure, respiratory insufficiency, shock, and in some cases, liver failure.

D.   **Assessment findings**

   1.   Onset of peritonitis typically is marked by severe localized or diffuse abdominal pain, with or without guarding and rebound tenderness.

   2.   Paralytic ileus produces abdominal distension, usually with nausea and vomiting and possibly with diarrhea; bowel sounds are decreased or absent.

   3.   Fever, tachycardia, and chills point to sepsis.

   4.   Shallow, guarded respirations suggest diaphragmatic involvement.

   5.   Late manifestations include signs of dehydration and acidosis.

   6.   Laboratory analysis indicates leukocytosis, possibly leukopenia in severe cases.

   7.   Diagnostic tests include:

       a.   Paracentesis, to identify the causative organism

       b.   Abdominal radiograph, which may reveal the location of the perforation

E.   **Nursing diagnoses**

   1.   Ineffective Breathing Pattern

   2.   High Risk for Altered Body Temperature

   3.   High Risk for Fluid Volume Deficit

   4.   High Risk for Infection

   5.   Pain

F.   **Planning and implementation**

   1.   Monitor respiratory status closely.

2. Position the patient to maximize comfort; assess pain frequently.

3. Take steps to reduce and prevent the spread of infection.

4. Monitor fluid and electrolyte balance.

5. Administer analgesics and antibiotics as prescribed.

6. If surgery is indicated, provide general preoperative and postoperative care (see Chapter 24, Perioperative Nursing, for more information).

G. Evaluation

1. The patient remains free of infection.

2. The patient reports absence of pain or control of pain with analgesics.

3. The patient exhibits normal breathing pattern.

4. The patient maintains adequate fluid status; drinks six to eight glasses of water daily.

5. The patient registers normal body temperature.

6. The patient exhibits normal bowel sounds.

XI. Gastroenteritis

A. Description: inflammation of the stomach and small intestine

B. Etiology

1. Gastroenteritis is a generic term for various common specific and nonspecific intestinal disorders.

2. Among the many possible causes of gastroenteritis are:

   a. Bacterial food poisoning (e.g., *Staphylococcus aureus*, *Salmonella*, *Shigella*)

   b. Amebae (e.g., *Entamoeba histolytica*)

   c. Adenoviruses, enteroviruses, and coxsackieviruses

   d. Parasites (e.g., *Ascaris*, *Enterobius*)

   e. Nonbacterial food poisoning from toxins in plants (e.g., mushrooms), seafood, or contaminated food

   f. Side effects of certain drugs (e.g., antibiotics)

C. Pathophysiology

1. In healthy adults, gastroenteritis usually is a self-limiting problem producing minor GI symptoms that are more inconvenient than dangerous.

2. In young children, elderly adults, and debilitated persons, however, these GI symptoms can produce serious—possibly even life-threatening—fluid and electrolyte losses.

D. Assessment findings

1. Clinical manifestations vary with the cause and the level of the GI tract involved; common signs and symptoms include:

   a. Abdominal cramping

   b. Nausea and vomiting

   c. Diarrhea

2. Other possible findings include fever, malaise, and borborygmi.

        3.   Stool culture or blood culture may identify causative organisms.

E. **Nursing diagnoses**
1. Fluid Volume Deficit
2. Pain
3. High Risk for Impaired Skin Integrity

F. **Planning and implementation**
1. Provide measures designed to allow the GI tract to rest (e.g., keep the patient NPO and maintain bedrest).
2. As symptoms subside, gradually provide clear liquids.
3. Closely monitor intake, output, and fluid and electrolyte status; increase fluid intake with IV infusion if necessary.
4. Provide additional perianal skin care for a patient with severe diarrhea.

G. **Evaluation**
1. The patient demonstrates return to normal elimination pattern, marked by:
   a. No abdominal cramping
   b. Passage of soft formed stool
2. The patient maintains intact skin integrity.
3. The patient maintains adequate fluid status; drinks six to eight glasses of water daily.

XII. Malabsorption syndromes

A. **Description: various disorders resulting from impaired absorption of nutrients in the small intestine**

B. **Etiology and incidence**
1. The many possible causes of malabsorption can be divided into two categories: impaired digestion and impaired absorption.
2. Impaired digestion can result from:
   a. Postgastrectomy (especially with gastrojejunostomy), causing decreased pancreatic stimulation due to bypass of the duodenum, decreased mixing of food with digestive enzymes, and decreased intrinsic factor
   b. Impaired function of the liver and biliary tract or pancreas, resulting in lack of digestive enzymes
3. Impaired absorption can result from inadequate absorptive surface due to:
   a. Massive intestinal resection following vascular insult or inflammatory bowel disease (short bowel syndrome)
   b. Jejunal bypass for morbid obesity
   c. Inflammation of the bowel wall causing decreased surface for absorption
4. Postgastrectomy, stagnation of contents in the proximal small bowel can lead to bacterial overgrowth, which breaks down bile salts and impairs fat absorption

5. Impaired absorption also can result from excessively rapid transit time due to:
   a. Lactase deficiency
   b. Mucosal disruption
   c. Crohn's disease
   d. Infections that alter intestinal villi
   e. Gluten intolerance
6. Radiation exposure can affect rapidly proliferating cells in the GI mucosa, leading to inflammation, edema, and ischemic changes through the entire thickness of the bowel wall (radiation enteritis); may appear within days (acute) or months to years (chronic) following radiation treatment.

C. Pathophysiology: pathology varies depending on the cause (Table 9–1).

D. Assessment findings
1. Clinical manifestations vary widely depending on cause (see Table 9–1).
2. Common symptoms in many malabsorption syndromes include:
   a. Diarrhea
   b. Steatorrhea—pale, soft, bulky, malodorous stools
   c. Abdominal distention and cramping
   d. Weakness
   e. Dry skin and hair
   f. Weight loss
3. Laboratory studies and diagnostic test results also vary but may include:
   a. Decreased serum albumin and total protein
   b. Decreased hemoglobin and RBC count
   c. Altered electrolyte levels
   d. Decreased serum carotene level
   e. Thickened intestinal mucosa, demonstrated on barium swallow or barium enema

E. Nursing diagnoses
1. Diarrhea
2. High Risk for Fluid Volume Deficit
3. Altered Nutrition: Less Than Body Requirements
4. High Risk for Impaired Skin Integrity

F. Planning and implementation
1. Assist with initiation and maintenance of total parenteral nutrition, if indicated.
2. Instruct the patient in general nutritional concepts, including:
   a. Basic four food groups
   b. Foods to be avoided—depends on cause of malabsorption (e.g., grain products in gluten intolerance, lactose in lactase deficiency)

TABLE 9-1.
Comparison of Normal Absorption with Malabsoprtion States

NORMAL ABSORPTION			MALABSORPTION	
SMALL BOWEL	NUTRIENT	ALSO REQUIRES	CAUSE	CLINICAL S AND S
Duodenum	Iron	Gastric acid	Lack of gastric acid (gastrectomy)	Pallor, anemia
	Calcium	Vitamin D parathyroid	↓Vitamin D ↓fat digestion	Chvostek, Trousseau tetany, bone pain pathologic fracture
Jejunum	Protein	Pancreatic secretions	↓amt. panc. sec. or inadequate absorptive surface (SBS)	Weakness, fatigue, edema, cachexia
	Carbohydrate	Pancreatic secretions	↓amt. panc. sec (SBS)	Diarrhea, flatulence, abd. distention
	Fat	Pancreatic lipase bile	↓amt. panc. sec.	Steatorrhea, diarrhea, weight loss
			↓bile acid ↓synthesis-liver ↓amt. to duodenum ↓ileal absorption	Jaundice, pruritis
	Vitamin A	Bile salts	Lack of bile salts	Night blindness, dry skin and conjunctiva
	Vitamin D	Bile salts	Lack of bile salts	Osteomalacia, bone pain
	Vitamin E	Bile salts	Lack of bile salts	Rare to have S and S
	Vitamin K	Bile salts	Lack of bile salts	Easy bruisability, bleeding
	Folic acid		Impaired mucosal absorption	Diarrhea, weight loss, irritability, forgetfulness
Ileum	Vitamin B_{12}	Intrinsic factor	Gastric resection, ↓amt. panc. sec. ileal resection	Neuropathy, glossitis anorexia
Colon	Water		↓length of colon →↓absorption →↑excretion	Watery diarrhea

3. Encourage meticulous perianal skin care; clean and dry skin thoroughly after each episode of diarrhea.

G. Evaluation

1. The patient maintains adequate nutritional and hydration status.

2. The patient maintains intact perianal skin integrity.

XIII. Regional enteritis (Crohn's disease)

A. Description: a slowly progressive, persistent granulomatous disease anywhere in the GI tract (but most commonly in the terminal ileum) that extends through the entire thickness of the mucosal wall

B. Etiology and incidence

1. The exact cause is unknown; contributing factors may include:

       a.   Allergies and other immune disorders
       b.   Lymph disorders
       c.   Infection
       d.   Genetic predisposition

  2. Crohn's disease is most prevalent between age 20 and 40, and occurs equally in both sexes. Incidence is highest in Jews and lowest in blacks.

C. **Pathophysiology**

  1. Pathology typically includes:
       a.   Marked thickening and inflammation of the intestinal wall
       b.   Swollen mesenteric lymph nodes
       c.   Focal granulomas
       d.   Cobblestone patches of edematous, reddish-purple tissue interspersed with patches of normal tissue
       e.   Strictures secondary to scarring

  2. Possible complications include intestinal obstruction, abscess and fistula formation, and perforation.

D. **Assessment findings**

  1. Clinical effects vary; the most prominent manifestations commonly include:
       a.   Abdominal tenderness and pain; typically colicky and increasing after meals
       b.   Diarrhea, flatulence, steatorrhea
       c.   Signs of nutritional deficits (e.g., poor skin turgor, weight loss, anemia)
       d.   Perianal fistulas and abscesses
       e.   Systemic effects (e.g., fever, malaise, anorexia)

  2. Other manifestations can affect the liver, kidneys, skin, joints, and eyes.

  3. Important laboratory studies and diagnostic tests include:
       a.   Barium enema
       b.   Proctosigmoidoscopy
       c.   Colonoscopy
       d.   Stool analysis
       e.   Hemoglobin and hematocrit

E. **Nursing diagnoses**

  1. Diarrhea
  2. Fluid Volume Deficit
  3. Knowledge Deficit
  4. Altered Nutrition: Less Than Body Requirements
  5. Pain
  6. High Risk for Impaired Skin Integrity
  7. Impaired Social Interactions

F. **Planning and implementation**

  1. For a patient experiencing diarrhea, provide an easily accessible bedpan or commode.

2.   Provide meticulous skin care to the perianal area.
3.   Administer medications for symptomatic relief of diarrhea.
4.   Monitor intake and output, and weigh the patient daily.
5.   Assess for fluid and electrolyte imbalance, particularly for dehydration; administer IV fluids and electrolytes as indicated.
6.   Promote good nutrition by:
     a.   Offering bland, easily digested foods
     b.   Providing small, frequent meals
7.   Assist the patient with pain management; administer analgesics as needed.
8.   Provide patient teaching, covering:
     a.   The importance of good nutrition and adequate fluid intake
     b.   Stress management techniques
     c.   Perianal skin care
     d.   The need for follow-up visits to the physician
9.   If surgery is indicated, provide appropriate preoperative and postoperative care (see Chapter 24, Perioperative Nursing, for more information).

G.   Evaluation
1.   The patient maintains adequate nutrition and fluid status.
2.   The patient reports relief of pain.
3.   The patient exhibits manageable bowel elimination patterns.
4.   The patient verbalizes appropriate self-care practices (e.g., medications, diet).

XIV.   Ulcerative colitis

A.   Description: an inflammatory disorder affecting the colonic mucosa and submucosa

B.   Etiology and incidence
1.   Etiology is unclear; possible predisposing factors include:
     a.   Family history
     b.   Bacterial infection
     c.   Allergic reaction
     d.   Autoimmune disorder
     e.   Emotional stress
2.   Ulcerative colitis occurs primarily between ages 15 and 40, and affects both sexes about equally. A higher-than-average incidence has been reported in the Jewish population.

C.   Pathophysiology
1.   Ulcerative colitis is characterized by inflammation and ulceration involving the mucosal and submucosal layers only.
2.   It typically begins in the rectum or sigmoid colon and spreads upward, possibly extending throughout the entire colon.
3.   Inflammation produces congestion, edema, and ulcerations that develop into abscesses.

    4. Mild ulcerative colitis may produce only localized symptoms; however, a severe, fulminant case can result in perforated colon, leading to life-threatening peritonitis.

D. **Assessment findings**

    1. The cardinal sign of ulcerative colitis is diarrhea containing pus, blood, and mucus; may or may not contain liquid feces.

    2. Other common symptoms include:

        a. Abdominal cramping and tenderness

        b. Anorexia and weight loss

        c. Fever

    3. Laboratory studies and diagnostic tests are the same as for Crohn's disease (see Section XIII.D).

E. **Nursing diagnoses**

    1. Diarrhea

    2. Fluid Volume Deficit

    3. Knowledge Deficit

    4. Altered Nutrition: Less Than Body Requirements

    5. Pain

    6. High Risk for Impaired Skin Integrity

    7. Impaired Social Interaction

F. **Planning and implementation: nursing interventions similar to those for Crohn's disease (see Section XIII.F)**

G. **Evaluation: refer to evaluation criteria for Crohn's disease (see Section XIII.G)**

XV. **IBS**

A. **Description: a common functional disorder of GI motility not associated with anatomic changes; also known as spastic colon or irritable colon**

B. **Etiology and incidence**

    1. IBS is generally associated with such factors as:

        a. Psychologic stress

        b. Prediverticular disease with changes in the bowel wall

        c. Low-residue diet

    2. It accounts for approximately half of all cases of GI illness in the United States; incidence is greater in women than in men.

C. **Pathophysiology**

    1. IBS develops in the absence of organic disease or anatomic abnormality.

    2. Emotional stress may disturb autonomic nervous system function, leading to disrupted intestinal motility and transit time.

D. **Assessment findings**

    1. The typical triad of findings in IBS includes:

        a. Abdominal pain with tenderness on palpation

        b. Altered bowel habits: diarrhea or constipation

        c. Absence of detectable disease

2. Abdominal pain may be localized in the lower left quadrant, constant or intermittent, and relieved by passing gas or stool.
3. Diarrhea often alternates with constipation; stools may contain increased mucus but seldom blood.
4. Symptoms often mimic those of other conditions, hindering differential diagnosis. Diagnosis must first rule out any organic GI disease or abnormality.
5. The patient may report recent emotional disturbance.
6. Dietary history may reveal a low-residue diet.
7. Laboratory studies and diagnostic tests commonly reveal:
   a. Normal sigmoidoscopy findings
   b. Normal complete blood count
   c. Normal stool analysis

E. Nursing diagnoses
   1. Ineffective Individual Coping
   2. Diarrhea or Constipation
   3. Knowledge Deficit
   4. Pain

F. Planning and implementation
   1. Teach the patient measures to reduce symptoms, such as:
      a. Eating a high-fiber diet and avoiding gas-forming foods
      b. Adhering to a schedule of regular work and rest periods
      c. Avoiding or minimizing stress-producing situations
      d. Drinking six to eight glasses of water daily to prevent constipation
   2. Encourage the patient to comply with any prescribed medication regimen, which may include antispasmodics, anticholinergics, or bulk-producing laxatives.
   3. Provide the patient with reassurance and emotional support to help decrease anxiety and increase his or her sense of control over the situation and its management.

G. Evaluation
   1. The patient remains symptom-free.
   2. The patient complies with prescribed dietary and scheduling modifications.

Bibliography

Brunner, L. S., & Suddarth, D. S. (1988). *Textbook of medical-surgical nursing* (6th ed.). Philadelphia: J. B. Lippincott.

Brunner, L. S., & Suddarth, D. S. (1986). *The Lippincott manual of nursing practice* (4th ed.). Philadelphia: J. B. Lippincott.

Given, B. A., & Simmons, S. J. (1984). *Gastroenterology in clinical nursing* (4th ed.). St. Louis: C. V. Mosby.

Luckmann, J., & Sorenson, K. C. (1987). *Medical-surgical nursing: A psychophysiologic approach* (3rd ed.). Philadelphia: W. B. Saunders.

Phipps, W. J., Long, B. C., & Woods, N. F. (1987). *Medical-surgical nursing: Concepts and practice* (3rd ed.). St. Louis: C. V. Mosby.

Price, S. A., & Wilson, L. M. (1986). *Pathophysiology and clinical concepts of disease process* (3rd ed.). New York: McGraw-Hill.

Vander, A. J., Sherman, J. H., & Luciano, D. S. (1980). *Human physiology: The mechanism of body function* (3rd ed.). New York: McGraw-Hill.

STUDY QUESTIONS

1. Steatorrhea may occur in which of the following conditions?
   a. malabsorption syndromes
   b. gastritis
   c. irritable bowel syndrome
   d. duodenal ulcer

2. Ms. Marley, aged 42, has been hospitalized with weight loss and substernal pain. She has a long history of complications from achalasia and refuses to eat because "last night I almost died" while trying to eat dinner. The nurse adds a new nursing diagnosis—Fear—to Ms. Marley's problem list, based on which of the following nursing diagnoses?
   a. Self-Care Deficit: Feeding
   b. High Risk for Aspiration
   c. Personal Identity Disturbance
   d. Ineffective Denial

3. Symptoms of malabsorption and irritable bowel syndrome are often similar. Mr. Nabokov, aged 30, comes to the clinic complaining of abdominal pain and cramping and diarrhea. He reports a history of frequent GI upsets and a high level of anxiety related to his inability to get relief. The nursing diagnosis that would most appropriately reflect the difference between irritable bowel syndrome and malabsorption would be
   a. Diarrhea
   b. Pain
   c. Ineffective Individual Coping
   d. Altered Nutrition: Less Than Body Requirements

4. When assessing a patient admitted with a bleeding gastric ulcer, the nurse would expect to find which of the following stool characteristics?
   a. coffee-ground color
   b. clay colored
   c. black, tarry
   d. bright red

5. When developing a patient teaching plan for a patient with a hiatal hernia, the nurse should be sure to include instructions to

   a. Eat three large meals per day with no restrictions.
   b. Lay down immediately following a meal.
   c. Gradually increase the amount of lifting done.
   d. Eat frequent, small, bland meals with high-fiber content.

6. When evaluating a patient with dysphagia, the nurse would look for which of the following outcome criteria?
   a. The patient does not display rectal tenesmus.
   b. The patient is free of esophagitis and achalasia.
   c. The patient demonstrates reduced gastric or duodenal inflammation.
   d. The patient has normal gastric architecture.

7. Tom Pringle received radiation therapy to the head, neck, and abdomen 6 months ago. He has developed a malabsorption problem over the last month. For Tom, patient teaching about the cause and ways to decrease symptoms should focus on which of the following areas?
   a. teeth and tongue
   b. sigmoid and rectum
   c. small intestine
   d. large intestine

8. Which of the following actions would be an *inappropriate* outcome criterion for interventions aimed at preventing or minimizing constipation?
   a. The patient eats a high-fiber diet.
   b. The patient avoids physical exercise.
   c. The patient drinks six to eight glasses of water per day.
   d. The patient maintains a physically active lifestyle.

9. For planning at-home reporting criteria for a patient with malabsorption syndrome, which of the following stool characteristics would be most valuable in identifying diarrhea?
   a. quantity

b. constituents
c. color
d. consistency

10. Which of the following statements best describes regional enteritis (Crohn's disease)?
    a. It involves continuous lesions, ultimately spreading throughout the entire large intestine.
    b. It typically appears as patches of normal colon between areas of inflammation.
    c. It involves only the mucosa and submucosa of the bowel wall.
    d. Its cardinal sign is malabsorption.

11. Irritable bowel syndrome can best be described as
    a. an inflammatory process
    b. the result of longstanding GI disease
    c. a functional disorder
    d. an inherited trait

12. Nursing care of a patient with gastroenteritis should include which of the following interventions?
    a. Encourage optimal nutritional intake.
    b. Alleviate abdominal pain and cramping.

c. Administer an oral antiemetic every 2 hours.
d. Monitor intake and output and electrolyte levels.

13. Mr. Baker, aged 56, has developed alopecia and stomatitis as a result of chemotherapy. He has expressed embarrassment at his loss of hair and frustration at not being included in activities. He complains of inability to eat because of the "sores in his mouth." Based on these data, which of the following nursing diagnoses would *least* likely impair this patient's healthy progression during this difficult time?
    a. Impaired Tissue Integrity
    b. Social Isolation
    c. Grieving
    d. Altered Nutrition: Less Than Body Requirements

14. Which of the following nursing actions demonstrates the nurse's understanding of one of the primary complications for peritonitis?
    a. Provide small, frequent meals.
    b. Frequently assess respiratory status.
    c. Assess skin integrity regularly.
    d. Evaluate stools for color and consistency.

ANSWER KEY

242

1. **Correct response: a**
   Steatorrhea—bulky, fatty stools—indicates decreased fat absorption.
   b, c, and d. Steatorrhea is not associated with any of these disorders.
   Comprehension/Physiologic/Assessment

2. **Correct response: b**
   Aspiration poses a risk due to the failure of the esophageal sphincter or absence of esophageal peristalsis.
   a and c. No evidence suggests that this patient has an identity disturbance or is unable to feed herself.
   d. The patient's fear is based on an actual risk and so does not reflect denial.
   Analysis/Psychosocial/Analysis (Dx)

3. **Correct response: c**
   A patient with irritable bowel syndrome will often display signs of psychologic stress and report recent emotional disturbance. Precipitating factors for malabsorption do not include emotional stress.
   a, b, and d. These three nursing diagnoses could be appropriate to either medical diagnosis.
   Analysis/Psychosocial/Analysis (Dx)

4. **Correct response: c**
   Melena, or black, tarry stools, is a sign of bleeding high in the GI tract. The action of the digestive enzymes turns the bright red blood to black and tarry before defecation occurs.
   a, b, and d. Clay-colored stools would be expected with biliary obstruction; bright red blood would indicate bleeding from low in the GI tract.
   Comprehension/Physiologic/Evaluation

5. **Correct response: d**
   The eating of small bland meals with high fiber helps diminish reflux and decrease constipation (to prevent straining).
   a, b, and c. The patient with hiatal hernia should avoid bending, lifting heavy objects, reclining after meals, eating spicy foods, and using alcohol and tobacco.
   Comprehension/Health promotion/Implementation

6. **Correct response: b**
   Dysphagia is commonly associated with esophagitis or achalasia and may be the symptom that prompts the patient to seek medical assistance.
   a, c, and d. Altered gastric structure, gastric or duodenal inflammation, and tenesmus usually are not associated with dysphagia.
   Application/Physiologic/Evaluation

7. **Correct response: c**
   The small bowel (duodenum, jejunum, and ileum) are responsible for the absorption of most of the major nutrients.
   a, b, and d. Although an abnormality of the large bowel could affect water reabsorption, and abnormalities of the teeth and tongue could alter the ability to ingest food, it is the small intestine that supports nutrient absorption.
   Analysis/Health promotion/Implementation

8. **Correct response: b**
   Sedentary lifestyle is a predisposing factor in constipation.
   a, c, and d. Regular physical exercise, a high-fiber diet, and plenty of water all contribute to regular elimination.
   Knowledge/Health promotion/Evaluation

9. *Correct response: d*
   Increased fecal fluid content is most descriptive for diarrhea.
   a, b, and c. It also is important to assess stool color and presence of mucus. The quantity becomes important only when it represents a change from the person's usual elimination pattern.

Application/Safe care/Planning

10. *Correct response: b*
    Crohn's disease generally exhibits a characteristic "cobblestone" appearance involving the entire bowel wall, with patches of normal colon between areas of inflammation.
    a, c, and d. None of these statements is characteristic of Crohn's disease.

Analysis/Physiologic/Planning

11. *Correct response: c*
    Irritable bowel syndrome is a functional disorder of motility (i.e., no anatomic changes are present).
    a, b, and d. None of these responses describes IBS.

Knowledge/Physiologic/Assessment

12. *Correct response: d*
    Vomiting and diarrhea put the patient at risk for fluid volume deficit and electrolyte imbalance.
    a, b, and c. Usually, the GI tract is allowed to rest by omitting all oral intake. The cause of pain cannot be alleviated.

Application/Safe care/Implementation

13. *Correct response: c*
    Grief is an important process in the progression toward healthy resolution.
    a, b, and d. These diagnoses all would have an impact on the patient's physical or emotional health.

Analysis/Health promotion/Analysis (Dx)

14. *Correct response: b*
    The infectious process can progress to respiratory complications.
    a and d. Paralytic ileus commonly occurs, so feeding this patient is inappropriate—as is assuming that diarrhea will occur.
    c. Impaired skin integrity is not a primary potential complication specific to this disease; rather, it can occur in any patient on bedrest.

Application/Safe care/Implementation

Endocrine and Metabolic Disorders

I. Anatomy and physiology

A. Hormones

1. Hormones are chemical substances secreted by endocrine glands directly into the blood stream to act on specific target cells; types include:

   a. Protein or peptide hormones (e.g., insulin, vasopressin, growth hormone (GH), adrenocorticotropic hormone [ACTH]): generally act on cell membranes by binding to receptors

   b. Amine and amino acid derivatives (e.g., epinephrine, norepinephrines): act on cell membranes

   c. Steroids (e.g., cortisol, estrogen, testosterone): act intracellularly to modify protein synthesis

2. Hormones regulate growth and development, fluid and electrolyte balance, reproduction, adaptation to stress, and metabolism.

3. Hormone secretion is regulated through feedback mechanisms (i.e., increased levels of a specific hormone or its cations or metabolites inhibit secretion, and decreased levels stimulate secretion).

B. Pituitary gland

1. Located at the inferior aspect of the brain within the sella tur-

cica (a small recess in the sphenoid bone), the pituitary consists of anterior and posterior lobes.

2. The anterior lobe synthesizes and releases hormones, including:
    a. GH: affects growth of bones and muscles; influences protein, lipid, carbohydrate and calcium metabolism
    b. Prolactin (PRL): affects mammary glands to stimulate milk production
    c. Thyroid-stimulating hormone (THS): stimulates thyroid hormone production
    d. ACTH: stimulates the adrenal cortex to produce steroids (primarily cortisol)
    e. Follicle-stimulating hormone (FSH): stimulates ovaries to develop follicles and secrete estrogen; stimulates testes to develop seminiferous tubules and perform spermatogenesis
    f. Luteinizing (or interstitial cell-stimulating) hormone (LH): stimulates ovaries to form corpus luteum, initiate ovulation, and produce progesterone; stimulates testes to secrete testosterone

3. Anterior pituitary hormone release is regulated by the hypothalamus, which secretes releasing and inhibiting hormones.

4. The posterior lobe stores and releases hormones synthesized in the hypothalamus, including:
    a. Oxytocin: stimulates uterine and mammary gland contractions
    b. Antidiuretic hormone (ADH, vasopressin): acts on the distal renal tubule to increase water reabsorption; rate of release is regulated by plasma osmolality

C. Thyroid gland

1. A butterfly-shaped gland located in the neck behind the trachea, the thyroid produces three hormones:
    a. Thyroxine (T_4) and triiodothyronine (T_3)—produced predominantly from peripheral conversion of T_4 to T_3: regulate cellular metabolic activity; secretion is under the control of TSH
    b. Thyrocalcitonin: secreted in response to high blood calcium levels; lowers blood calcium levels by inhibiting bone resorption

D. Parathyroid glands

1. These small glands, usually four, surround the posterior thyroid tissue; they are often difficult to locate and may be removed accidentally during thyroid or other neck surgery.

2. In response to low blood calcium level, the parathyroids produce parathormone (PTH), which raises blood calcium levels by increasing calcium resorption from kidneys, intestines, and bones.

248

E. Adrenal glands

1. Located at the upper poles of both kidneys, the adrenals contain two distinct types of endocrine tissue.

2. The adrenal medulla, in the center of the gland, reacts to autonomic nervous system signals to release catecholamines:

   a. Epinephrine (80%): prepares the body for the fight or flight response by converting liver glycogen to glucose and increasing cardiac output

   b. Norepinephrine (20%): exerts effects similar to epinephrine and produces extensive vasoconstriction

3. The outer portion, the adrenal cortex, is stimulated by ACTH to produce corticosteroids:

   a. Mineralocorticoids (primarily aldosterone): released in response to angiotensin II and ACTH; increase sodium reabsorption and potassium loss primarily through the renal tubules

   b. Glucocorticoids (primarily cortisol): released in response to ACTH; increase blood glucose by stimulating gluconeogenesis and lipolysis and decrease protein synthesis; suppress the inflammatory response; promote sodium retention and potassium loss

   c. Adrenal sex hormones (androgens and estrogen): govern development of certain secondary sex characteristics

F. Pancreas

1. A slender, elongated organ lying horizontally in the posterior abdomen behind the stomach, the pancreas functions as both an endocrine and an exocrine gland.

2. Exocrine functions involve secretion of pancreatic digestive enzymes by specialized cells.

3. Endocrine functions are controlled by the alpha, beta, and delta cells of the islets of Langerhans:

   a. Alpha cells secrete glucagon, which increases blood glucose through gluconeogenesis.

   b. Beta cells secrete insulin, which regulates protein, carbohydrate, and fat metabolism by facilitating glucose, amino acid, and fatty acid transport; also promotes glycogen, protein, and triglyceride synthesis.

   c. Delta cells secrete somatostatin (inhibitory hormone) and gastrin.

G. Gonads

1. The gonads consist of the ovaries and testes.

2. Although the gonads exert some systemic metabolic effects, their primary function is in reproduction (see Chapter 11, Reproductive and Sexual Disorders, for more information).

II. Overview of endocrine and metabolic disorders

A. Assessment

1. Nursing health history should focus on:

    a. Changes in the patient's usual health patterns and behavior (e.g., mental status, sensory function, nutrition, elimination, activity tolerance, and sleep patterns)

    b. Family history of endocrine disorders

    c. Any past or present health problems, procedures, or treatments that can put the patient at risk for developing an endocrine disorder (e.g., radiation therapy to the head or neck)

2. Important physical assessment aspects include:

    a. Stature, fat distribution, shape of face

    b. Color, texture, and turgor of skin; surgical scars; unusual bruising

    c. Protruding or sunken eyes, lid lag or retraction

    d. Hair distribution

    e. Presence of goiter

    f. Vital signs

    g. Heart sounds

    h. Lung sounds

    i. Body weight

    j. Bowel sounds

B. Laboratory studies and diagnostic tests

1. Measurement of hormones in blood and urine reflects production and activity of hormones related to specific endocrine and metabolic disorders. Specific tests are discussed under the appropriate disorder in this chapter; types of testing include:

    a. Static (present time) measurement: detects elevated or depressed hormone levels; diagnostic for certain disorders

    b. Dynamic testing: involves administration of a stimulating or suppressing agent, followed by measurement of hormone response; requires close collaboration with laboratory personnel to ensure correct sequence of timed specimens

2. Imaging tests assist in identifying causative factors; studies include:

    a. Scans

    b. Computed tomography (CT scan)

    c. Magnetic resonance imaging (MRI)

    d. Bone mineral densitometry

3. Other important studies include:

    a. Visual field testing

    b. Selective venous sampling

C. Psychosocial implications

1. A person with an endocrine or metabolic disorder may experience difficulty coping with the disease process related to such factors as:

        a.   Chronic nature of the disorder

        b.   Sense of loss of control

        c.   Fear of complications or death

2. Common self-concept concerns are related to fears of:
   a. Body image changes
   b. Rejection
   c. Sexual dysfunction
   d. Emotional instability
3. Endocrine and metabolic disorders commonly produce lifestyle concerns related to potential changes in:
   a. Physical and mental functioning (elderly persons at increased risk because declines in physical and mental functioning may be erroneously attributed to aging)
   b. Work performance, with potential for loss of job
4. A patient with an endocrine or metabolic disorder also may experience changes in social interaction due to:
   a. Isolation
   b. Depression

D. Medications used to treat endocrine and metabolic problems

1. Treatment of many endocrine and metabolic disorders involves pharmacologic agents that alter endocrine function either by stimulating or inhibiting hormone release or by interfering with hormone action on target tissues.
2. *Bromocriptine* (Parlodel) is used to decrease the size of prolactinoma and suppress PRL production; it also affects GH production.
3. *Octreotide acetate* (Sandostatin), a somatostatin analogue, is administered via subcutaneous injection to decrease GH production.
4. *ADH replacement agents*, used to conserve renal water in diabetes insipidus (DI), include:
   a. Desmopressin acetate (e.g., DDAVP)
   b. Aqueous pitressin
   c. Lysine vasopressin
   d. Vasopressin tannate
5. *Phenytoin* (Dilantin) is administered to inhibit ADH release; results in free water loss.
6. Used to correct hyperthyroidism by blocking thyroid hormone synthesis; *antithyroid agents* include:
   a. Propylthiouracil (PTU)
   b. Methimazole (Tapazole)
7. *Beta adrenergic blockers* are used to relieve sympathomimetic symptoms of hyperthyroidism by regulating sympathetic nervous system activity; agents include:
   a. Propranolol (Inderal)
   b. Reserpine (e.g., Sandril)

8. *Iodine-containing agents*, given to inhibit release of stored thyroid hormone and retard hormone synthesis in hyperthyroidism, include:
   a. Saturated solution of potassium iodide (SSKI)
   b. Lugol's solution
9. *Glucocorticoids* are administered short term to block conversion of T_4 to more potent T_3 and in replacement therapy; types include:
   a. Hydrocortisone sodium succinate (e.g., Solu-Cortef)
   b. Cortisone acetate (e.g., Cortone)
   c. Methylprednisolone (e.g., Delta-Cortef)
   d. Dexamethasone (e.g., Decadron)
   e. Prednisone (e.g., Deltasone)
10. *Thyroid hormone*, such as levothyroxine (e.g., Synthroid), is used to correct thyroid hormone deficiency in hypothyroidism and in replacement therapy.
11. Used in the treatment of Cushing's syndrome, *adrenocortical steroid inhibitors* such as aminoglutethimide (Cytadren) decrease cortisol production.
12. *Mineralocorticoids*, used in replacement therapy, include:
    a. Fludrocortisone acetate (Florinef)
    b. Desoxycorticosterone (e.g., Doca Acetate)
13. Administered to reduce blood glucose levels by stimulating pancreatic insulin production and increasing cellular sensitivity to insulin, *oral hypoglycemic agents* include:
    a. Tolbutamide (e.g., Orinase)
    b. Acetohexamide (Dymelor)
    c. Chlorpropamide (e.g., Diabinese)
    d. Glipizide (Glucotrol)
    e. Glyburide (e.g., Diabeta)
14. *Insulins* are given to maintain blood glucose levels by regulating protein, carbohydrate, and fat metabolism; types include:
    a. Ultralente/U, PZI: long acting
    b. NPH/N, Lente/L: intermediate acting
    c. Regular/R, Semilente/S: fast acting
    d. 70/30 (70% NDH and 30% R): combination agent

III. Anterior pituitary dysfunction

A. Description: undersecretion or oversecretion of anterior pituitary hormones (ACTH, TSH, GH, LH, PRL)

B. Etiology

1. Causes of undersecretion (hypopituitarism) include:
   a. Pituitary gland infarction
   b. Surgical removal of the pituitary
   c. Genetic disorders or replacement with tumor tissue
2. Oversecretion (hyperpituitarism) commonly results from a se-

cretory adenoma, which stimulates the target gland (adrenal, thyroid) or tissue (GH and PRL).

C.   Pathophysiology

1.   Hypopituitarism affects thyroid, adrenal, and gonadal function (see Section VI, Hypothyroidism, and Section XI, Adrenal hypofunction, for more information).

2.   Hyperpituitarism commonly results in altered ACTH or GH secretion, leading to Cushing's syndrome or acromegaly (see Section X, Cushing's syndrome for more information).

D.   Assessment findings

1.   Clinical manifestations of excessive GH secretion (acromegaly in adults) may include:

a.   Coarse features (e.g., broad skull, protruding jaw, prognathism, broadening of hands and feet)

b.   Thickened heel pads

c.   Thick tongue

d.   Change in ring and shoe size

e.   Dental changes

f.   Hypertension

g.   Diabetes mellitus

h.   Headache, visual disturbances

i.   Lethargy

j.   Sinus congestion

k.   Decreased libido

2.   Diagnostic tests for excessive GH secretion may reveal:

a.   Elevated GH and somatomedin-C levels

b.   Diminished visual fields

c.   Tumor visualized on radiologic examination, such as CT scans

3.   Signs and symptoms of excessive PRL secretion include:

a.   Breast discharge

b.   Decreased libido

c.   Amenorrhea

d.   Impotence

e.   Headache, visual disturbances

f.   Lethargy

4.   In excessive PRL secretion, diagnostic tests may reveal:

a.   Elevated serum PRL level

b.   Decreased visual fields

c.   Tumor visualized on radiologic examination, including CT scans

E.   Nursing diagnoses

1.   High Risk for Injury

2.   Knowledge Deficit

3.   Self-Concept Disturbance

    4. Sexual Dysfunction

F. **Planning and implementation**

    1. Encourage the patient to verbalize feelings about the disorder and its effects on his or her body.

    2. Discuss the disorder's effects on sexual functioning with the patient and partner.

    3. Administer prescribed medications, which may include:

        a. Bromocriptine (Parlodel) to decrease the size of a prolactinoma and decrease PRL production; also affects GH production

        b. Octreotide acetate (Sandostatin) via SQ injection to decrease GH production

    4. If pituitary irradiation is indicated, prepare the patient for therapy.

    5. If surgical removal of a pituitary tumor is indicated, reinforce the surgeon's explanation of the procedure.

    6. Monitor a postsurgical patient for signs of complications, such as:

        a. Hemorrhage

        b. Transient DI

        c. Rhinorrhea, which may indicate cerebrospinal leak

        d. Adrenal insufficiency (see Section XI) and thyroid insufficiency (see Section VI)

        e. Infection, particularly meningitis (marked by fever, nuchal rigidity, headache)

        f. Visual disturbances, particularly decreased visual fields

G. **Evaluation**

    1. The patient verbalizes a sense of well-being.

    2. The patient resumes usual sexual practices.

    3. The patient verbalizes understanding of the treatment regimen.

    4. The patient takes medications as prescribed.

    5. The patient remains free of surgical complications.

    6. The patient demonstrates restoration of normal endocrine function.

    7. The patient exhibits no visual deficits.

IV. **Posterior pituitary dysfunction**

A. **Description**

    1. Dysfunction of the posterior pituitary involves either oversecretion or undersecretion of ADH.

    2. Specific disorders include:

        a. DI, caused by undersecretion of ADH, resulting in excessive dilute urine production

        b. Syndrome of inappropriate ADH (SIADH), involving oversecretion of ADH and resulting in excessive water conservation

B. **Etiology**
1. Possible causes of DI include:
   a. Posterior pituitary destruction from tumors
   b. Vascular accidents
   c. Surgery or hypothalamic damage
   d. Certain drugs that can interfere with ADH secretion or action (e.g., phenytoin, alcohol, lithium carbonate)
2. Nephrogenic DI, either familial or arising from various renal disorders, occurs when the distal renal tubules do not respond to ADH.
3. SIADH can result from:
   a. Central nervous system disorders
   b. Stimulation due to hypoxia or decreased left atrial filling pressure
   c. Pharmacologic agents (e.g., chemotherapy, chlorpropamide)
   d. Overuse of vasopressin therapy
   e. Ectopic ADH production associated with some cancers
   f. Nausea or narcotic use, which can stimulate ADH secretion

C. **Assessment findings**
1. Clinical manifestations of DI include:
   a. Profoundly increased urine output (5 to 20 L/day) of dilute urine
   b. Nocturia
   c. Extreme thirst
   d. Weight loss
   e. Possible tachycardia and hypotension
   f. Weakness
2. Laboratory and diagnostic tests for DI may reveal:
   a. Elevated plasma osmolality and serum sodium level
   b. Water deprivation test demonstrating inability of the kidneys to concentrate urine despite increased plasma osmolality and low plasma vasopressin level
   c. Vasopressin test demonstrating that the kidneys can concentrate urine after administration of ADH; differentiates central (pituitary or hypothalamic) DI from nephrogenic DI
3. Signs and symptoms of SIADH include:
   a. Decreased urine output
   b. Weight gain
   c. Altered mental status (e.g., headache, confusion, lethargy, seizures and coma in severe hyponatremia)
   d. Delayed deep tendon reflexes
4. In SIADH, laboratory study results may include:
   a. Decreased serum sodium and osmolality
   b. Elevated urine sodium and osmolality

   c. Elevated ADH level
 D. **Nursing diagnoses**
   1. Fluid Volume Deficit (DI)
   2. Fluid Volume Excess (SIADH)
   3. High Risk for Injury
   4. Knowledge Deficit
   5. Sleep Pattern Disturbance
 E. **Planning and implementation**
   1. For both DI and SIADH:
    a. Monitor intake and output, and weigh the patient daily.
    b. Monitor vital signs.
    c. Assess skin turgor and mucous membranes.
    d. Provide meticulous skin and mouth care.
   2. For DI:
    a. Replace fluids as indicated; assess for and report any illness, injury, or other problem that could prevent adequate fluid intake.
    b. Encourage the patient to drink fluids in response to thirst.
    c. Administer ADH replacement agents as prescribed (see Section II.D.4 for more information).
   3. For SIADH:
    a. Restrict fluid intake as indicated.
    b. Regularly assess mental status.
    c. Modify the patient's environment as necessary to help reduce the risk of injury.
    d. Administer medications as prescribed, which may include:
     (1) Lithium or demeclocycline, to increase free water loss
     (2) Phenytoin, to inhibit ADH release
 F. **Evaluation**
   1. The patient exhibits restoration of fluid balance.
   2. The patient verbalizes understanding of the treatment regimen.
   3. The patient demonstrates compliance with the prescribed medication regimen.
   4. The patient reports absence of nocturia (in DI).
   5. The patient demonstrates return to previous level of mental functioning (in SIADH).
   6. The patient remains injury-free (in SIADH).

V. Hyperthyroidism
 A. **Description: a metabolic imbalance resulting from excessive thyroid hormone production; Graves' disease the most common form**
 B. **Etiology and incidence**
   1. Autoimmune dysfunction is the most common cause of

Graves' disease; autoantibodies apparently mimic TSH, leading to hypersecretion of thyroid hormones.

2. Genetic factors seem to play a role.

3. Other possible causes include:

    a. Toxic nodular goiter

    b. Exposure to iodine

    c. TSH-secreting pituitary tumor (rare)

    d. Thyroiditis

4. Incidence is greatest between ages 30 and 40 and is higher in women than in men.

C. Pathophysiology

1. Excessive secretion of thyroid hormone leads to increased metabolic rate, excessive heat production, and increased responsiveness to catecholamines.

2. These actions lead to profound changes in many organ systems.

3. Effective treatment usually can control symptoms.

4. However, severe acute exacerbation—thyroid storm—may be a life-threatening emergency.

D. Assessment findings

1. Clinical manifestations of hyperthyroidism may include:

    a. Nervousness, irritability, hyperactivity, emotional lability, and decreased attention span

    b. Weakness, easy fatigability, exercise intolerance

    c. Heat intolerance

    d. Weight change (loss or gain), increased appetite

    e. Insomnia, interrupted sleep

    f. Frequent stools, diarrhea

    g. Menstrual irregularities, decreased libido

    h. Warm, sweaty, flushed skin with a velvety-smooth texture, spider telangiectasias

    i. Tremor, hyperkinesia, hyperreflexia

    j. Exophthalmos, retracted eye lids, staring gaze

    k. Hair loss

    l. Goiter

    m. Bruits over the thyroid gland

    n. Elevated systolic blood pressure, widened pulse pressure, S3 heart sound

2. Laboratory findings may include:

    a. Increased T_4 and T_3 levels

    b. Nondetectable TSH

    c. Presence of antithyroid antibodies and thyroid-stimulating immunoglobulins (TSI), increased radioactive iodine uptake

3. Thyroid storm is marked by hyperthermia, hypertension, delirium, vomiting, abdominal pain, and tachydysrhythmias.

    4. Elderly persons with hyperthyroidism often present with heart failure, atrial fibrillation and few, if any, of the classic symptoms listed above.

E. Nursing diagnoses

    1. Activity Intolerance

    2. Decreased Cardiac Output

    3. Hyperthermia (in thyroid storm)

    4. High Risk for Injury

    5. Knowledge Deficit

    6. Altered Nutrition: Less Than Body Requirements

F. Planning and implementation

    1. Assist the patient and family members or significant others in exploring treatment options. (Include family members or significant others because the patient's attention span deficit may impair his or her retention of information.) Options include:

        a. Pharmacotherapy with drugs that interfere with thyroid hormone synthesis or release (see Section F.2)

        b. Radioactive iodine therapy, which permanently limits thyroid hormone secretion by destroying thyroid tissue. (Hypothyroidism, requiring lifelong replacement therapy, usually develops at some point after this treatment.)

        c. Surgery (thyroidectomy), which is seldom done; thyroid levels must be lowered preoperatively to prevent thyroid storm

    2. Administer antithyroid drugs as ordered, which may include:

        a. PTU or methimazole (Tapazole), to block thyroid hormone synthesis

        b. Beta-adrenergic blockers, to treat sympathomimetic symptoms

        c. Iodine-containing medications, to inhibit release of stored thyroid hormone and retard hormone synthesis

        d. Glucocorticoids, to block conversion of T_4 to more potent T_3

    3. Promote a calm environment conducive to rest and relaxation.

    4. Minimize the patient's energy expenditure by assisting with activities as necessary and encouraging the patient to alternate periods of activity with rest.

    5. Monitor nutritional status; provide increased calories and other nutritional support as needed.

    6. Assess the patient's mental status and decision-making ability; intervene as needed to ensure safety.

    7. Provide eye protection for a patient with exophthalmos: patches, drops, artificial tears; instruct regarding use.

    8. Monitor vital signs and hemodynamic parameters (for an acutely ill patient) for signs of heart failure.

9. Reduce body temperature with a cooling mattress and acetaminophen; avoid aspirin, which may displace thyroid hormone from its carrier protein and increase hormone levels.
10. Supply sufficient fluids to offset losses from diaphoresis.
11. Provide appropriate comfort measures for the febrile patient.
12. Recognize that drug turnover rates may be greatly accelerated in hyperthyroid states.
13. Emphasize the importance of complying with the medication regimen and long-term medical follow-up plans.
14. Reassure the family that any abrupt changes in the patient's behavior likely are disease related and should subside with antithyroid therapy.

G. **Evaluation**
1. The patient reports adequate energy to perform ADLs.
2. The patient maintains adequate nutritional intake to meet metabolic demands.
3. The patient demonstrates stable vital signs, including body temperature.
4. The patient verbalizes understanding of the prescribed medication regimen and of long-term treatment options.
5. The patient verbalizes understanding of the importance of long-term health care follow-up.

VI. Hypothyroidism

A. **Description: a state of insufficient serum thyroid hormone**
B. **Etiology and incidence**
1. Primary hypothyroidism results from pathologic changes in the thyroid gland due to:
   a. Autoimmune thyroiditis (Hashimoto's disease)
   b. Thyroidectomy
   c. Radioactive iodine therapy
   d. Antithyroid medication therapy
2. Secondary hypothyroidism results from failure of the pituitary gland to secrete adequate TSH, possibly due to tumor, surgical removal, or irradiation.
3. Hypothyroidism is most prevalent in persons aged 40 to 50 and is more common in women than in men.

C. **Pathophysiology**
1. Inability of the thyroid gland to secrete sufficient amounts of thyroid hormone leads to decreased cellular metabolic activities, decreased oxygen consumption, and decreased heat production.
2. These actions produce mild to marked effects in all organ systems.
3. A person with hypothyroidism is at risk for life-threatening myxedema coma, which can develop gradually over years or

acutely in response to precipitating factors such as infection, cold exposure, or sedative use.

D. **Assessment findings**
1. Signs and symptoms of hypothyroidism include:
    a. Sluggishness, lethargy, depression, apathy, fatigue, exercise intolerance
    b. Memory impairment
    c. Muscle aches, numbness and tingling in hands
    d. Cold intolerance
    e. Constipation
    f. Weight gain, decreased appetite
    g. Menstrual irregularities, infertility, decreased libido
    h. Dry skin, brittle nails, dry hair
    i. Edema—nonpitting and periorbital
    j. Husky voice, hoarseness
    k. Possible goiter
    l. Possible neck scar from previous thyroid surgery
    m. Delay in muscle contraction and relaxation of tendon reflexes
    n. Diastolic hypertension
    o. Bradycardia
2. Laboratory studies may reveal:
    a. Decreased T_4 and T_3 levels
    b. Increased TSH (primary)
    c. Presence of antithyroid antibodies (autoimmune)
    d. Elevated cholesterol and CPK
3. Affected elderly persons may display few, if any, symptoms of hypothyroidism.
4. Myxedema coma is marked by:
    a. Hypotension
    b. Hypoventilation
    c. Hypothermia
    d. Stupor possibly progressing to coma

E. **Nursing diagnoses**
1. Activity Intolerance
2. Decreased Cardiac Output
3. Constipation
4. Hypothermia (in myxedema coma)
5. Knowledge Deficit

F. **Planning and implementation**
1. Administer thyroid hormone, preferably synthetic levothyroxine, as prescribed; monitor cardiac response to resulting increase in metabolic rate and oxygen requirements.
2. Recognize that thyroid hormone administration may precipitate adrenal insufficiency in a previously undiagnosed patient, possibly necessitating glucocorticoid administration.

3. Keep in mind that a hypothyroid patient is very sensitive to narcotics, anesthetics, and sedatives; drug degradation is delayed, and respiratory depression can develop.
4. Encourage the patient to alternate periods of activity with rest.
5. Administer fluids cautiously—the patient may not be able to excrete a heavy water load. If the patient has hypoglycemia, infuse a concentrated source of glucose.
6. Provide relief of constipation as indicated.
7. Refrain from aggressively rewarming a hypothermic patient, to prevent vascular collapse.
8. Institute respiratory assistance when necessary.
9. Implement infection-prevention measures.
10. Instruct the patient (and family members or significant others, when applicable) in the prescribed medication regimen, including purpose, dosage schedule, and signs of over- and under-replacement.

G. **Evaluation**
1. The patient reports adequate energy to perform ADLs.
2. The patient exhibits stable vital signs, including body temperature.
3. The patient reports restoration of normal bowel function.
4. The patient and family members or significant others verbalize understanding of the prescribed medication regimen and of health care follow-up plans.

VII. **Other thyroid dysfunctions**
A. **Description**
1. Subacute thyroiditis: self-limiting thyroid inflammation
2. Autoimmune (Hashimoto's) thyroiditis: chronic inflammatory disorder
3. Simple goiter: thyroid enlargement not associated with inflammation or neoplasm
4. Thyroid cancer: papillary, follicular, medullary, and anaplastic carcinomas

B. **Etiology**
1. Associated with viral infection, subacute thyroiditis commonly follows mumps, influenza, or coxsackievirus or adenovirus infection.
2. The most common form of thyroiditis, autoimmune thyroiditis, results from antibodies to thyroid antigens in the blood.
3. Simple goiter may result from:
   a. Compensation for dietary iodine deficiency (rare in the United States)
   b. Use of certain drugs (e.g., iodine-containing agents, lithium) in susceptible patients
   c. Compensatory response to excessive TSH secretion, such as results from thyroid hormone hyposecretion

4. Thyroid cancer may be associated with history of exposure to external head and neck radiation.

C. Pathophysiology

1. Subacute thyroiditis may be accompanied by transient hyperthyroidism; inflammation and hyperthyroidism usually resolve spontaneously with no residual effects.

2. In autoimmune thyroiditis, chronic thyroid inflammation leads to lymphocytic infiltration with fibrosis and diminished hormone secretion. These changes produce thyroid enlargement and, in some cases, hypothyroidism.

3. Goiters may be diffuse and symmetric or nodular. Depending on the cause and degree of enlargement, treatment may not be necessary.

4. In thyroid cancer, prognosis depends on cell type. Papillary and follicular adenocarcinoma generally are associated with good prognoses and medullary carcinoma with a less favorable prognosis. Anaplastic carcinoma, most common in older adults, carries a very poor prognosis.

D. Assessment findings

1. Subacute thyroiditis may produce moderate thyroid enlargement, some pain, and mild dysphagia.

2. Autoimmune thyroiditis typically produces painless thyroid enlargement. Diagnosis is confirmed by needle biopsy demonstrating antithyroid antibodies.

3. In goiter, thyroid enlargement ranges from slight to gross. Massive goiter can produce respiratory difficulty and dysphagia due to compression of the trachea and esophagus.

4. Manifestations of thyroid cancer may include:
   a. Reports of respiratory distress, sensation of lump in throat, dysphagia
   b. Palpable, hard, painless nodule in the thyroid
   c. Needle biopsy positive for cancer
   d. Thyroid scan showing area of decreased uptake

E. Nursing diagnoses

1. Anxiety
2. Ineffective Breathing Pattern
3. High Risk for Injury
4. Knowledge Deficit
5. Pain
6. Impaired Swallowing

F. Planning and implementation

1. For subacute thyroiditis, provide symptomatic treatment directed at reducing inflammation.

2. For autoimmune thyroiditis, administer L-thyroxine sodium as prescribed.

3. Treatment for goiter may not be indicated. If appropriate, assist with thyroid suppression therapy or prepare the patient for surgery.

4. Support the patient and family members or significant others as they explore the nature and prognosis of thyroid cancer. Reinforce the importance of long-term follow-up to ensure the most favorable prognosis possible.

5. If surgery is indicated for thyroid cancer, plan interventions for subtotal or total thyroidectomy, including:

   a. Providing preoperative instruction and emotional support

   b. Providing postoperative comfort measures (e.g., analgesics, adequate head support, semi-Fowler's position, humidification)

   c. Monitoring for complications (e.g., respiratory obstruction, hemorrhage, tetany)

   d. Ensuring adequate fluid intake as tolerated

   e. Preparing the patient for total body scan to detect any remaining thyroid tissue; radioactive iodine may be given to eradicate tissue after total thyroidectomy

   f. Reinforcing the importance of taking thyroid hormone replacement exactly as prescribed

G. Evaluation

1. The patient and family members or significant others verbalize knowledge of diagnosis, prognosis, and treatment plan.

2. The patient exhibits stable vital signs, with absence of respiratory difficulty and dysphagia.

3. The patient reports absence of pain.

4. The patient verbalizes the importance of complying with the prescribed medication regimen and plans for long-term follow-up care.

VIII. Hyperparathyroidism

A. Description: overproduction of parathyroid hormone (PTH); results in high blood calcium levels and bone demineralization

B. Etiology and incidence

1. Primary hyperparathyroidism is a common condition usually occurring after age 60 and affecting women more often than men. About 80% of cases are linked to a single adenoma of the parathyroid gland; remaining cases are due to parathyroid hyperplasia. (*Note:* The following sections apply to patients with primary hyperparathyroidism.)

2. Secondary hyperparathyroidism results from an adaptive increase in PTH secretion associated with problems involving chronic hypocalcemia.

C. Pathophysiology

1. PTH is critical to normal calcium homeostasis. Insufficient circulating calcium level stimulates PTH production, which acts

to raise calcium level; when calcium level rises to normal, PTH secretion is inhibited.

2. A parathyroid adenoma or other problem can produce excessive PTH despite normal serum calcium, causing the abnormalities of primary hyperparathyroidism.

D. Assessment findings

1. Hyperparathyroidism may be asymptomatic or may produce such clinical manifestations as:
   a. Fatigue, muscular weakness, listlessness
   b. Height loss and frequent fractures
   c. Renal calculi
   d. Anorexia, nausea, abdominal discomfort, constipation
   e. Memory impairment
   f. Polyuria, polydipsia
   g. Back and joint pain
   h. Hypertension
2. Laboratory and diagnostic studies may reveal:
   a. Elevated total and ionized serum calcium levels
   b. Decreased serum phosphate level
   c. Hypercalciuria and hyperphosphaturia
   d. Bone demineralization on radiograph or bone mineral densitometry
   e. Elevated PTH level
   f. Possible abnormal parathyroid scan
   g. Possible uremia secondary to nephrocalcinosis

E. Nursing diagnoses

1. Activity Intolerance
2. Constipation
3. High Risk for Injury
4. Altered Nutrition: Less Than Body Requirements
5. Pain
6. Altered Patterns of Urinary Elimination

F. Planning and implementation

1. Prepare the patient for surgical treatment of primary hyperparathyroidism: adenoma removal, hyperplastic gland resection. Care is similar to that for thyroidectomy (see Section VII.F).
2. Provide preoperative care, including:
   a. Forcing fluids to prevent dehydration, constipation, and kidney stone formation
   b. Reducing added calcium by eliminating over-the-counter antacids, which may contain calcium; thiazide diuretics, which interfere with renal calcium excretion; and excessive intake of dairy products
   c. Administering furosemide as a diuretic, if necessary
3. As indicated, provide aggressive calcium supplementation after surgery to compensate for "hungry bone" syndrome.

    4.   Assess for renal calculi; report hematuria or flank pain as necessary.

    5.   Take measures to protect the patient from injury, including:
       a.   Assisting with ADLs and ambulation as necessary
       b.   Encouraging weight-bearing to reduce calcium loss from bones
       c.   Instructing about strategies to minimize falls, which may lead to fractures

    6.   Provide relief of constipation as indicated.

    7.   Monitor nutritional status and intervene as necessary.

    8.   Provide comfort measures and analgesics as needed.

    9.   Administer digitalis preparations with caution in hypercalcemic patients; observe for toxicity.

   10.   Instruct nonsurgical candidates in phosphate or estrogen therapy as indicated.

   11.   Instruct the patient in postoperative calcium carbonate supplementation, if ordered.

   12.   Reinforce the health care follow-up schedule.

G.   **Evaluation**

    1.   The patient reports adequate energy to perform ADLs.

    2.   The patient maintains normal bowel function.

    3.   The patient remains injury-free and displays normal surgical wound healing, if applicable.

    4.   The patient reports absence of pain or adequate pain control with oral analgesics.

    5.   The patient displays no evidence of tetany.

    6.   The patient maintains adequate food and fluid intake.

    7.   The patient verbalizes the importance of complying with the prescribed medication regimen and plans for follow-up care.

IX.   Hypoparathyroidism

A.   **Description: PTH deficiency characterized by hypocalcemia, hyperphosphatemia, and neuromuscular hyperexcitability**

B.   **Etiology and incidence**

    1.   Hypoparathyroidism may be iatrogenic, caused by accidental removal of or trauma to parathyroid glands during thyroidectomy, parathyroidectomy, or radical head or neck surgery.

    2.   It also can result from an autoimmune genetic dysfunction (affects women more often than men).

    3.   A reversible form may be associated with hypomagnesemia, which interferes with PTH secretion.

C.   **Pathophysiology**

    1.   Reduced PTH production slows bone resorption, increases neuromuscular irritability, decreases serum calcium level, and increases serum phosphate level.

    2.   In chronic hypoparathyroidism, calcification can occur in some

organs (e.g., the eyes [cataracts] and basal ganglia [possibly causing permanent brain damage]).

D. Assessment findings
1. Clinical manifestations include:
    a. Anxiety, irritability
    b. Numbness, tingling, cramps in extremities
    c. Dysphagia
    d. Photophobia
    e. Evidence of neuromuscular hyperexcitability: positive Chvostek's and Trousseau's signs, carpopedal spasms, bronchospasms, laryngeal spasms, dysrhythmias, convulsion
    f. Paradoxical calcification in eyes
2. Laboratory studies may reveal:
    a. Low ionized and total calcium levels
    b. Elevated blood phosphate level
    c. Low PTH level

E. Nursing diagnoses
1. High Risk for Injury
2. Knowledge Deficit

F. Planning and implementation
1. Intervene for life-threatening tetany as indicated:
    a. Administer IV calcium gluconate.
    b. Expect to administer oral calcium and vitamin D supplementation after the crisis resolves.
    c. Be alert for possible laryngeal spasm and resulting respiratory obstruction; keep a tracheostomy set available.
    d. Institute seizure precautions.
    e. Minimize environmental stimuli.
    f. After the crisis resolves, closely monitor calcium levels; keep IV calcium gluconate in the patient's room.
2. For chronic hypoparathyroidism, administer prescribed medication therapy, which may include:
    a. IV calcium carbonate
    b. Vitamin D and often magnesium supplementation
    c. Thiazide diuretics, to decrease renal calcium loss
3. Teach the patient about the medication regimen, including purpose, dosage schedule, and signs and symptoms of hypocalcemia and hypercalcemia. Inform the patient that dosage will be adjusted periodically based on laboratory findings.
4. Emphasize the importance of regular follow-up evaluation and care.

G. Evaluation
1. The patient exhibits no signs of tetany.
2. Serum calcium level is within normal range.

3. The patient verbalizes understanding of the medication schedule and follow-up plans.
4. The patient verbalizes signs and symptoms of hypocalcemia and hypercalcemia to watch for and report.

X. Cushing's syndrome

A. **Description: a syndrome involving excessive production of adrenocortical hormones, primarily cortisol but also androgens and mineralocorticoids**

B. **Etiology and incidence**
   1. The most common cause of Cushing's syndrome is bilateral adrenal hyperplasia (Cushing's disease).
   2. Other causes include:
      a. Adrenal adenomas and carcinomas
      b. Ectopic ACTH production by tumors in other organs, such as the lungs and pancreas
      c. Glucocorticoid therapy
   3. Incidence is higher in women than in men.

C. **Pathophysiology**
   1. Regardless of etiology, impaired regulation of adrenocortical hormones results in excessive hormone levels.
   2. Manifestations of Cushing's syndrome result from the effects of excessive adrenocortical hormone levels on various body systems and functions.

D. **Assessment findings**
   1. Clinical manifestations depend on the adrenocortical hormones involved and may include:
      a. Weight gain and altered fat distribution (e.g., central obesity with round [moon] face and buffalo hump)
      b. Muscle weakness, proximal muscle wasting, fatigue
      c. Frequent infections and poor wound healing
      d. Symptoms of hyperglycemia
      e. Mental status changes, mood swings
      f. Menstrual disturbances (amenorrhea)
      g. Diminished libido
      h. Skin changes: striae, bruises, acne, thinning of scalp hair
      i. Hypertension
      j. Hirsutism
      k. Susceptibility to compression fractures
      l. Edema
   2. Laboratory studies may reveal:
      a. Hypokalemia or hyperglycemia
      b. Depressed eosinophil and lymphocyte counts
      c. Elevated plasma cortisol and 24-hour urine cortisol
      d. Abnormal dexamethasone suppression test (morning cortisol level above 5 g/dL after administration of 1.0 mg of dexamethasone the night before)

      e.   Elevated ACTH (indicative of ACTH-mediated Cushing's syndrome)

3. Selective venous sampling can differentiate between pituitary and ectopic ACTH production. In this procedure, catheters are inserted into each petrosal sinus draining the pituitary gland and peripheral vein, then ACTH levels are measured after administration of corticotropin-releasing hormone (CRH).

4. Selected radiographic and computerized axial tomography (CAT) studies may be done to determine the site of ectopic ACTH production (e.g., bronchogenic oat cell carcinoma).

E. **Nursing diagnoses**

    1. Activity Intolerance
    2. Ineffective Individual Coping
    3. High Risk for Injury
    4. Knowledge Deficit
    5. Self-Concept Disturbance

F. **Planning and implementation**

    1. Teach the patient and family members or significant others about disease pathology and its influence on the patient's body habitus and mental status.

    2. Encourage them to ask questions and verbalize any concerns.

    3. Take measures to protect the patient from injury and infection, including:

        a. Assessing skin integrity regularly
        b. Avoiding agents that can damage skin (e.g., tape, strong soaps)
        c. Promoting good hygiene
        d. Modifying the environment to remove or minimize hazards

    4. Monitor vital signs, and weigh the patient daily.

    5. Schedule activities to allow adequate rest periods, helping prevent fatigue.

    6. If surgery is indicated, prepare the patient for the scheduled procedure, which may include:

        a. Adrenalectomy, if the cause is adrenal adenoma
        b. Transsphenoidal hypophysectomy, if the cause is pituitary adenoma
        c. Tumor resection

    7. If surgery is not indicated, instruct the patient and family members in prescribed pharmacologic therapy, which may involve:

        a. Ketoconazole (Nizoral)
        b. Aminoglutethimide (Cytadren)
        c. Metyrapone

d.   OP'DDD' (Mitotane)

8.   Keep in mind that any treatment modality will cause temporary (permanent with bilateral adrenalectomy) adrenal insufficiency.

G.   Evaluation

1.   The patient exhibits increased ability to carry out self-care activities.

2.   The patient and family members or significant others verbalize correct understanding of the treatment plan.

3.   The patient remains infection- and injury-free.

4.   The patient openly discusses feelings about the disorder's effects on his or her body image.

5.   The patient decreases or maintains body weight.

6.   The patient verbalizes increased self-esteem.

7.   The patient complies with the prescribed medication regimen.

XI.   Adrenal hypofunction

A.   Description: deficiency of adrenocortical hormones; either primary (Addison's disease) or secondary to another problem

B.   Etiology and incidence

1.   Addison's disease can result from:

a.   An autoimmune process

b.   Hemorrhage into the adrenal gland

c.   Adrenalectomy

d.   Neoplasm

e.   Fungal infection

f.   Tuberculosis

2.   Secondary adrenal insufficiency is associated with:

a.   Suppression of the hypothalamic–pituitary axis secondary to exogenous steroid use

b.   Pituitary destruction or removal

c.   Inadequate cortisol replacement, especially during times of stress

3.   Adrenal hypofunction occurs in all age groups and affects both sexes about equally.

C.   Pathophysiology

1.   Any problem causing adrenal cortex hypofunction results in deficiencies of adrenocortical hormones.

2.   Hormone deficiency produces various fluid, electrolyte, and metabolic disturbances.

D.   Assessment findings

1.   Common clinical manifestations include:

a.   GI complaints (anorexia, nausea, vomiting, abdominal pain, diarrhea)

b.   Fatigue, muscle weakness, arthralgias

c.   Decreased alertness, confusion

        d.   Weight loss

        e.   Dry skin, decreased body hair; possible increased skin pigmentation in excessive ACTH stimulation

        f.   Hypotension

        g.   Hyperthermia

        h.   Tachycardia

  2. Suggestive laboratory findings include:

        a.   Low blood glucose and serum sodium levels

        b.   Increased serum potassium level

        c.   Low 24-hour urinary 17-ketosteroids

        d.   Increased eosinophils

  3. Definitive laboratory findings include:

        a.   Low cortisol and high ACTH levels in primary adrenal failure; low to normal levels in secondary (pituitary) failure

        b.   On the ACTH stimulation test, low to normal cortisol response in secondary failure and flat or absent response in primary failure

        c.   Low plasma aldosterone in primary failure

E. **Nursing diagnoses**

  1. Fluid Volume Deficit

  2. Knowledge Deficit

F. **Planning and implementation**

  1. Monitor vital signs, daily weight, and intake and output.

  2. Assess skin turgor and mucous membrane hydration.

  3. Administer IV fluids to correct fluid deficiency as indicated.

  4. Administer replacement glucocorticoids as prescribed, possibly including:

        a.   Hydrocortisone

        b.   Cortisone acetate

        c.   Methylprednisolone

        d.   Prednisolone

        e.   Dexamethasone

        f.   Prednisone

  5. Administer mineralocorticoids as prescribed, possibly:

        a.   Fludrocortisone acetate

        b.   Deoxycorticosterone (DOCA-A)

  6. Instruct the patient regarding physiologic replacement of glucocorticoids to correct deficiencies, covering:

        a.   Purpose and possible side effects

        b.   The importance of lifelong daily replacement

        c.   Management of acute illnesses or stresses

        d.   Need for medical identification

        e.   Symptoms of over- or under-replacement

        f.   Appropriate times to communicate with health care team

g. The need to inform all health care providers about the steroid replacement therapy

7. If overreplacement of glucocorticoids is indicated, inform the patient of the purpose of therapy and possible side effects—Cushingoid appearance, weight gain, acne, hirsutism, peptic ulcer, diabetes mellitus, osteoporosis, infection, muscular weakness, mood swings, cataracts, hypertension.

8. Help prevent adrenal crisis by ensuring that hospitalized, acutely ill patients on long-term glucocorticoid therapy receive additional doses to compensate for stress.

G. Evaluation

1. The patient exhibits restoration of fluid and electrolyte balance.

2. The patient demonstrates absence of orthostasis.

3. The patient and family members or significant others verbalize understanding of the treatment plan.

4. The patient and family members or significant others verbalize appropriate actions to take during periods of increased stress.

XII. Diabetes mellitus

A. Description

1. Diabetes mellitus is a disorder of carbohydrate metabolism resulting from deficiency of or resistance to available insulin and characterized by hyperglycemia.

2. It is classified as:

    a. Type I, or insulin-dependent diabetes mellitus (IDDM): accounting for 5% to 10% of cases and characterized by insulin deficiency and risk of ketosis

    b. Type II, or noninsulin-dependent diabetes mellitus (NIDDM): accounting for 90% of cases and characterized by defects in insulin release and use, insulin resistance, and little risk of ketosis

    c. Impaired glucose tolerance: an asymptomatic, subclinical stage characterized by blood glucose level that is abnormal but does not meet the diagnostic criterion for diabetes

    d. Gestational diabetes: a transitory glucose intolerance during pregnancy that resolves after delivery; associated with increased risk of developing overt diabetes later in life

    e. Diabetes mellitus associated with other conditions: glucose intolerance caused by other diseases, drugs, or agents

B. Etiology and incidence

1. Type I typically occurs in persons under age 25; its exact cause is unknown, but it may result from an autoimmune process possibly triggered by virus, with genetic factors playing a part.

2. Type II most commonly affects persons over age 40; causative factors include obesity and genetic susceptibility.
3. Diabetes mellitus affects approximately 6% of the U.S. population (about 11 million people) and is the third-leading cause of death from disease.

C. Pathophysiology

1. In diabetes mellitus, insulin secretion is disproportionate to blood glucose levels as a result of:
   a. Deficient insulin production by beta cells
   b. Lack of adequate insulin secretion in response to high blood glucose level
   c. Inactivation of insulin in circulation
2. Defective regulation of alpha and beta cell hormone release causes gluconeogenesis, resulting in mobilization rather than storage of proteins and fats.
3. Lack of adequate number of insulin receptors on cell surfaces impairs glucose absorption by cells, resulting in excessive blood glucose level.
4. Acute complications of diabetes mellitus include:
   a. Diabetic ketoacidosis (DKA): severe hyperglycemia and acidosis resulting from a combination of insulin deficiency (relative or absolute) and increased levels of insulin antagonistic hormones (glucagon, cortisol, GH, epinephrine), associated with failure to take insulin as prescribed, new diagnosis of Type I diabetes, or increased physical stress (e.g., infection, surgery)
   b. Hyperglycemic hyperosmolar nonketotic coma (HHNK): a combination of severe hyperglycemia and hyperosmolality with little or no acidosis, occurring most often in older adults with undiagnosed or mild diabetes and associated with stress (e.g., infection, surgery, hyperalimentation) or ingestion of certain drugs (e.g., thiazide diuretics, glucocorticoids, phenytoin, sympathomimetics)
   c. Hypoglycemia: excessive insulin to blood glucose ratio linked to excessive use of hypoglycemic agents (insulin, oral agents), decreased food intake, increased physical activity, excessive alcohol consumption, or renal failure (secondary to decreased insulin degradation)
5. Diabetes mellitus also can produce chronic complications, including:
   a. Microangiopathy: thickening of capillary basement membrane, most prominently in the retina and glomerulus
   b. Macroangiopathy: atherosclerotic changes accelerated by

lipid abnormalities exacerbated by elevated blood glucose level

    c.   Neuropathy: abnormal nerve function possibly caused by alteration in enzyme system affecting nerve sheaths or neural cell function

    d.   Increased susceptibility to infection resulting from impaired ability of granulocytes to respond to infectious agents

D.   **Assessment findings**

    1.   Common clinical manifestations of diabetes mellitus include:

        a.   Polyuria, polydipsia, and polyphagia

        b.   Weight loss

        c.   Fatigue and weakness

        d.   Visual disturbances

        e.   Recurrent skin, vulva, and urinary tract infections

    2.   Diagnosis is based on fasting blood glucose level above 140 mg/dL or postprandial blood glucose level above 200 mg/dL measured on more than one occasion; oral glucose tolerance tests are rarely recommended for diagnosis.

    3.   Other useful laboratory tests include:

        a.   Glycosylated hemoglobin (includes hemoglobin A1C), to assess average blood glucose level over the previous 2 to 4 months

        b.   Other glycosylated proteins (glycated albumins and serum fructosamine), which assesses blood glucose control over the previous 1 to 3 weeks

        c.   Urine tests for sugar (random, 24-hour) and ketones

    4.   Clinical manifestations and laboratory findings in DKA include:

        a.   Dehydration

        b.   Tachycardia

        c.   Kussmaul's respirations

        d.   Acetone breath

        e.   Decreased level of consciousness (LOC)

        f.   GI disturbances (nausea, vomiting, abdominal pain)

        g.   Elevated serum potassium level

        h.   ABG values indicating acidosis

    5.   HHNK is marked by:

        a.   Dehydration

        b.   Decreased LOC

        c.   Tachycardia

        d.   Hypotension

        e.   Blood glucose >700 mg/dL

        f.   Blood osmolality >330 mOsm/kg

        g.   Absence of ketosis, but possible mild lactic acidosis

        h.   Azotemia

      i.   Electrolyte disturbances (hypernatremia, hypokalemia)

6. Manifestations of hypoglycemia include:
  a. Blood glucose 70 mg/dL
  b. Cool, moist skin or pallor
  c. Tachycardia
  d. Tremor
  e. Paresthesias
  f. Confusion
  g. Headache progressing to loss of consciousness or seizures

E. Nursing diagnoses
  1. Ineffective Individual Coping
  2. Knowledge Deficit
  3. Noncompliance

F. Planning and implementation
  1. Assess the patient's and family members' or significant others' knowledge of diabetes and its management, and develop an individualized teaching plan that covers (as appropriate):
    a. Possible causes and basic pathophysiologic concepts
    b. Use of oral hypoglycemic agents, including purpose, action, dosage schedule, and possible side effects—hypoglycemia, allergy, incompatibility with ingested alcohol
    c. Insulin use, including purpose, action, dosage schedule, preparation and administration techniques (subcutaneous via syringe, jet injector or insulin pump), injection site selection and rotation, insulin storage and equipment care (expiration dates, refrigeration, disposal methods), and possible complications (e.g., allergy, lipodystrophy)
    d. Techniques for prescribed monitoring methods: blood glucose, urine glucose or ketones, including frequency, care and disposal of equipment, record keeping, and reporting of results
    e. Prescribed dietary modifications: typically low fat, low cholesterol, low sodium, and high fiber, based on the food exchange system developed by the American Diabetes Association or some other structured meal plan and with an emphasis on consistent timing and amounts of meals and snacks
    f. Appropriate exercise program
    g. Hygiene and safety measures: foot care and protection, care of minor wounds, the importance of medical identification cards and jewelry, avoidance of noxious substances (e.g., alcohol, smoking), annual ophthalmologic follow-up

  h. Management of acute illness: continuing taking insulin or oral hypoglycemics as prescribed, increasing self-monitoring frequency, testing urine ketones, notifying the physician, maintaining adequate fluid and caloric intake

  i. Signs and symptoms of acute and chronic complications to watch for and report

2. Assess and promote the patient's compliance with the prescribed therapeutic and monitoring regimens. Monitor indicators of glycemic control: glycosylated hemoglobin and other proteins, blood glucose level, and presence of complications.

3. Enhance the patient's and family members' or significant others' coping skills by:

  a. Encouraging open discussion of feelings and concerns

  b. Encouraging questions and answering them honestly

  c. Involving family members or significant others in teaching and planning

  d. Making referrals to support persons or groups as appropriate

4. Intervene as indicated for a patient exhibiting signs and symptoms of DKA:

  a. Restore fluid and electrolyte balance by administering IV fluids and electrolytes (Na, Cl, K, phosphorus).

  b. Reverse acidosis; administer sodium bicarbonate for severe acidosis (pH <7.0).

  c. Monitor urine ketones.

  d. Restore carbohydrate, protein, and fat metabolism by administering regular insulin (usually continuous low-dose IV).

  e. Monitor vital signs.

  f. Monitor blood glucose levels.

  g. Maintain accurate intake and output records.

  h. Prevent complications (e.g., hypokalemia or hypoglycemia [add glucose when blood glucose 300 mg/dL], cerebral edema [monitor LOC]).

  i. Assess for precipitating factors.

5. Intervene as indicated to manage HHNK:

  a. Restore fluid volume, usually with isotonic IV solutions.

  b. Restore electrolyte balance; administer potassium replacement when urine output is adequate.

  c. Prevent complications (e.g., hypoglycemia [add glucose to IV solutions when blood glucose drops], hypokalemia, thrombus formation).

  d. Assess for precipitating factors.

6. For a patient experiencing hypoglycemia:

  a. Monitor blood glucose level.

  b. Replace glucose through oral (15 g carbohydrate) or IV

glucose (50% dextrose) or glucagon (IM or SQ); *do not force oral fluids in a patient with impaired consciousness.*

    c. Protect the patient from injury, and observe closely until he or she is fully recovered.

    d. Administer a source of long-acting carbohydrate to prevent subsequent episodes.

    e. Assess for precipitating factors.

    f. Keep in mind that a person with longstanding diabetes may develop a defect in counterregulatory hormones, which impairs awareness of hypoglycemic symptoms and puts the person at increased risk for brain damage due to prolonged, untreated hypoglycemia.

    g. Recognize that beta-blocker therapy also can blunt sympathetic symptoms of hypoglycemia, interfering with detection.

   7. Monitor for signs and symptoms of chronic complications, and intervene as indicated.

G. Evaluation

   1. The patient and family members or significant others verbalize understanding of the disorder and the therapeutic regimen.

   2. The patient complies with the prescribed medication regimen.

   3. The patient exhibits adequate glycemic control.

   4. The patient achieves or maintains body weight goals.

   5. The patient participates in a regular exercise program, as tolerated.

   6. The patient and family members or significant others openly discuss their feelings and concerns regarding diabetes and its management.

   7. The patient practices precautions aimed at preventing acute and chronic complications.

   8. The patient exhibits no signs of acute or chronic complications.

Bibliography

American Diabetes Association (1989). Standards of medical care for patients with diabetes mellitus. *Diabetes Care,* 12(5), 365–368.

American Diabetes Association (1986). National standards and American Diabetes Association review criteria for diabetes patient education programs. *Diabetes Care,* 9(4), XXXVI–XLIII.

Brunner, L. S., & Suddarth, D. S. (1988). *Textbook of medical-surgical nursing* (6th ed.). Philadelphia: J. B. Lippincott.

Brunner, L. S., & Suddarth, D. S. (1986). *The Lippincott manual of nursing practice* (4th ed.). Philadelphia: J. B. Lippincott.

Greenspan F. S., & Forsham, P. H. (Eds.). (1986). *Basic and clinical endocrinology* (2nd ed). Los Altos, CA: Lange Medical Publications.

Kurtz, S. S. (1990). Adherence to diabetes regimens: Empirical status and clinical applications. *Diabetes Educator,* 16(1), 50–56.

Luckman, J., & Sorenson, K. C. (1987). *Medical-surgical nursing: A psychophysiologic approach* (3rd ed.). Philadelphia: W. B. Saunders.

STUDY QUESTIONS

1. Which of the following assessments would *not* help detect transient diabetes insipidus in a patient who underwent transsphenoidal surgery?
   a. urine output
   b. signs of dehydration
   c. pupillary size
   d. urine specific gravity

2. Fluid management in the patient with SIADH should include
   a. rapid IV fluid infusion
   b. fluid restriction
   c. increasing oral fluid intake
   d. administering glucose-containing IV fluids

3. The patient receiving PTU should be instructed to immediately stop the medication and call the physician if which of the following occurs?
   a. diarrhea
   b. palpitations
   c. fever
   d. weight gain

4. Which of the following statements regarding analgesic therapy for a hypothyroid patient is correct?
   a. Increased dosages will be needed because the patient is overweight.
   b. Analgesics are not needed because the patient already is lethargic.
   c. Decreased dosages will be needed due to prolonged drug degradation rates.
   d. Increased dosages will be needed because of the hypermetabolic state.

5. In the postoperative parathyroidectomy patient, "hungry bone" syndrome is manifested by
   a. carpopedal spasms
   b. weakness
   c. back pain
   d. polyuria

6. Discharge instructions for the hypoparathyroid patient should include which of the following?
   a. Avoid diuretics in order to minimize calcium loss.
   b. Use any over-the-counter vitamin D preparation.
   c. Supplement calcium intake.
   d. Avoid strenuous exercise because of fracture risk.

7. The nursing diagnosis Body Image Disturbance would most likely be associated with which of the following medical conditions?
   a. Addison's disease
   b. thyroiditis
   c. diabetes insipidus
   d. Cushing's syndrome

8. Preoperative care for a patient receiving long-term glucocorticoid therapy should include:
   a. holding the glucocorticoid because the patient is NPO
   b. administering an increased dose parenterally
   c. administering the usual dose intramuscularly
   d. administering the usual dose with a sip of water

9. Which of the following would be the *least* reliable evaluation outcome criterion demonstrating compliance with a therapeutic regimen for diabetes?
   a. The patient has glycosylated hemoglobin drawn every 3 months.
   b. The patient displays puncture marks on his or her fingertips.
   c. The patient maintains weight within 5 lb of his or her ideal weight.
   d. The patient's blood glucose values measured during office visits remain within an acceptable range.

10. Which of the following represents the best indication of good overall diabetes control?
    a. The patient reports urine glucose levels indicating no glucosuria.
    b. The patient displays glycosylated hemoglobin level within control range.
    c. The patient reports urine ketone levels reflecting no ketonuria.

d. The patient records home glucose tests daily.

11. Which of the following represents the best advice to give a diabetic patient about eye examinations?
   a. Examinations should be scheduled every year.
   b. Examinations should be scheduled every 2 years.
   c. Changes in vision do not necessitate immediate medical attention.
   d. Examinations should be performed by an optometrist.

12. Knowledge Deficit is a common nursing diagnosis for the patient with diabetes mellitus. Which of the following patient behaviors would best support this diagnosis?
   a. recent weight gain of 15 lb
   b. failure to monitor blood glucose level
   c. skipping insulin doses when feeling ill
   d. crying whenever diabetes is mentioned

13. Joe McFarland, aged 36, is taking NPH and regular insulins before breakfast and before supper. Urine glucose testing reveals that he is hyperglycemic before breakfast. Which of the following insulin adjustments would indicate that Joe has a good understanding of the effects of both NPH and regular insulin?
   a. Joe increases the morning dose of regular insulin.
   b. Joe increases the evening dose of NPH insulin.
   c. Joe increases the morning dose of NPH insulin.
   d. Joe increases the evening dose of regular insulin.

14. When planning care for a diabetic patient with end-stage renal disease, the nurse should expect that the patient's insulin requirements most likely would:
   a. increase
   b. remain the same
   c. decrease
   d. fluctuate greatly

15. Which of the following situations would *not* interfere with sympathetic nervous system responses to hypoglycemia?
   a. administration of a beta blocker
   b. use of a continuous insulin infusion device
   c. longstanding (15 years' duration) Type I diabetes mellitus
   d. administration of a calcium channel blocker

16. Altered LOC commonly accompanies hyperglycemic hyperosmolar nonketotic coma (HHNC). Which of the following nursing diagnoses reflects the pathophysiologic process accounting for this complication?
   a. Altered Nutrition: Less Than Body Requirements
   b. Impaired Gas Exchange
   c. Fluid Volume Deficit
   d. Fluid Volume Excess

ANSWER KEY

1. **Correct response: c**
Pupil size is not affected by changes in fluid balance.
   a, b, and d. Increased urine output, signs of dehydration, and a low specific gravity all are indicators of ADH deficiency.

Knowledge/Physiologic/Assessment

2. **Correct response: b**
Treatment is geared toward reducing water retention.
   a, c, and d. Administration of fluids only increases water intoxication.

Application/Physiologic/Implementation

3. **Correct response: c**
Fever may be indicative of infection, and infection may be caused by agranulocytosis.
   a and b. Diarrhea and palpitations are symptoms of hyperthyroidism.
   d. Weight gain is a common consequence of decreasing thyroid hormone levels.

Application/Safe care/Planning

4. **Correct response: c**
A hypothyroid patient has increased sensitivity to all drugs because of altered metabolism and excretion, depressed metabolic rate and respiratory status.
   a. Weight is not a factor.
   b. Failure to administer analgesics when appropriate may cause unnecessary suffering.
   d. Increased dosages may lead to overdose.

Analysis/Safe care/Planning

5. **Correct response: a**
In "hungry bone" syndrome, the bones take up calcium at an accelerated rate, leading to hypocalcemia. Carpopedal spasm is a symptom of hypocalcemia caused by neuromuscular irritability.
   b and c. Weakness and back pain are unrelated to calcium balance.

   d. Polyuria is a symptom of hypercalcemia.

Application/Safe care/Assessment

6. **Correct response: c**
Chronic hypoparathyroidism requires calcium supplementation.
   a. Diuretic use is not necessarily discouraged—in fact, thiazide diuretics promote calcium resorption.
   b. Vitamin D is necessary for calcium absorption, but special prescription preparations may be needed.
   d. There is no contraindication to exercise since osteoporosis is rare in this group.

Application/Safe care/Implementation

7. **Correct response: d**
In Cushing's syndrome, excessive cortisol level causes fat redistribution with truncal obesity, moon facies, and buffalo hump; excessive androgen levels cause hirsutism.
   a. In Addison's disease, the only body appearance alteration is excessive skin pigmentation.
   b and c. Thyroiditis and diabetes insipidus do not affect body habitus.

Comprehension/Psychosocial/Analysis (Dx)

8. **Correct response: b**
During periods of stress, such as surgery, glucocorticoid dosages must be increased.
   a, c, and d. Decreased or usual doses may cause adrenal insufficiency.

Application/Physiologic/Implementation

9. **Correct response: d**
The office-measured blood glucose value indicates the level at only one point in time and is influenced by many factors.
   a. Glycosylated hemoglobins are influenced by medications, diet, and lifestyle.
   b. Puncture marks on fingers indicate performance of SMBG.

c. Rapid weight change can be caused by missed insulin doses or excessive caloric intake.

Analysis/Physiologic/Evaluation

10. **Correct response: b**
Glycosylated hemoglobin values reflect the average blood glucose level over a 2-month period.
   a and c. Urine tests (glucose and ketones) reflect blood glucose control over only the past few hours.
   d. Reports of home blood glucose tests may be helpful, but studies have shown that they often are fabricated.

Application/Health promotion/Evaluation

11. **Correct response: a**
The current standards of care published by the American Diabetes Association recommend annual eye examinations by an ophthalmologist. The standards also recommend immediate evaluation of any visual changes.
   b. Annual examinations are recommended.
   c. Any visual change merits immediate evaluation.
   d. An ophthalmologist, not an optometrist, is the appropriate health-care professional for this eye examination.

Knowledge/Health promotion/Implementation

12. **Correct response: c**
During periods of illness, insulin injections should be continued even if food intake is decreased since physical stress increases blood glucose levels.
   a and b. Weight gain and failure to monitor blood glucose level represent noncompliant behavior.
   d. Crying demonstrates ineffective coping.

Comprehension/Health promotion/Analysis (Dx)

13. **Correct response: b**
The NPH insulin taken at supper exerts

its greatest effect during the night and at breakfast. The peak action of regular insulin occurs at 3 to 4 hours, so it could not affect breakfast blood glucose level. The morning dose of NPH will have dissipated long before breakfast.
   a, c, and d. These dosage adjustments would be inappropriate.

Analysis/Health promotion/Evaluation

14. **Correct response: c**
Renal failure prevents the kidneys from degrading insulin normally; as a result, insulin is available longer.
   a and b. This increased availability means that an increased or same dose of insulin may cause hypoglycemia.
   d. Renal failure, by itself, does not cause increased fluctuation of insulin doses.

Analysis/Physiologic/Planning

15. **Correct response: d.**
Calcium channel blockers do not affect sympathetic nervous system (SNS) activity.
   a. Beta blockers block SNS activity.
   b. Anyone using a continuous insulin infusion device has continuous insulin available, which may blunt SNS activity.
   c. A person with a long history of diabetes may have autonomic SNS neuropathy.

Comprehension/Physiologic/Assessment

16. **Correct response: c**
Plasma hyperosmolality resulting from Fluid Volume Deficit causes decreased LOC.
   a and b. Neither Impaired Gas Exchange nor Altered Nutrition is linked directly to altered LOC although they both may be involved in the progression of this syndrome.
   d. Fluid Volume Excess is not implicated in this complication.

Analysis/Physiologic/Analysis (Dx)

Reproductive and Sexual

Disorders

I. **Anatomy and physiology**
   A. Sexual development
   B. Structure
   C. Function

II. **Overview of reproductive and sexual disorders**
   A. Assessment
   B. Laboratory studies and diagnostic tests
   C. Psychosocial implications
   D. Medications used to treat reproductive disorders

III. **Sexually transmitted diseases (STDs)**
   A. Description
   B. Etiology and incidence
   C. Pathophysiology
   D. Assessment findings
   E. Nursing diagnoses
   F. Planning and implementation
   G. Evaluation

IV. **Menstrual disorders**
   A. Description
   B. Etiology and incidence
   C. Pathophysiology
   D. Assessment findings
   E. Nursing diagnoses
   F. Planning and implementation
   G. Evaluation

V. **Gynecologic infections**
   A. Description
   B. Etiology and incidence
   C. Pathophysiology
   D. Assessment findings
   E. Nursing diagnoses

   F. Planning and implementation
   G. Evaluation

VI. **Gynecologic tumors**
   A. Description
   B. Etiology and incidence
   C. Pathophysiology
   D. Assessment findings
   E. Nursing diagnoses
   F. Planning and implementation
   G. Evaluation

VII. **Structural disorders of the uterus and vagina**
   A. Description
   B. Etiology and incidence
   C. Pathophysiology
   D. Assessment findings
   E. Nursing diagnoses
   F. Planning and implementation
   G. Evaluation

VIII. **Breast tumors**
   A. Description
   B. Etiology and incidence
   C. Pathophysiology
   D. Assessment findings
   E. Nursing diagnoses
   F. Planning and implementation
   G. Evaluation

IX. **Infertility (male and female)**
   A. Description
   B. Etiology and incidence
   C. Pathophysiology
   D. Assessment findings
   E. Nursing diagnoses

I. Anatomy and physiology
A. Sexual development
   1. Development begins at conception.
   2. Sex is determined by the male XY chromosome and female XX chromosome; XX chromosome combination with XY chromosome can equal either X from each parent (girl) or X from mother and Y from father (boy).
   3. Gender development also involves psychosocial and behavioral factors.

B. Structure
   1. Female
      a. The external genitalia include the mons pubis, clitoris, labia majora, labia minora, Bartholin's glands, Skene's glands, and urethral meatus.
      b. The internal genitalia include the vagina, uterus, ovaries, and fallopian tubes.

    c.   The perineum is an area of muscle, fascia, and ligaments between the vulva and rectum.

    d.   The vagina is a muscular tube about 2½ inches (6 cm) long anteriorly and 3½ inches (9 cm) long posteriorly.

    e.   The uterus is a pear-shaped organ separated from the vagina by the cervix and usually lying at a 90-degree angle to the vagina. The endometrium lines the uterus; the myometrium is the muscular uterine layer.

    f.   The fallopian tubes terminate in fimbriae that surround the ovaries.

    g.   Each almond-shaped ovary normally measures approximately 1½ inches (3.5 cm) by ¾ inch (2 cm).

    h.   The breasts contain mammary glands organized into lobules with collecting ducts that terminate in the nipples.

2. Male

    a.   The penis contains three columns of erectile tissue and the urethra, which terminates at the glans.

    b.   The scrotum is divided by a septum; each scrotal sac contains a testis, epididymis, and vas deferens.

    c.   Each testis measures about 2 inches (5 cm) by 1 inch (2.5 cm); it contains seminiferous tubules, in which spermatogenesis occurs, and interstitial cells, which produce testosterone.

    d.   The vas deferens enters the ejaculatory duct in the prostate gland, which lies under the bladder and surrounds the urethra.

    e.   A bundle of blood vessels, nerves, muscle fibers, and the vas deferens and muscle fibers, the spermatic cord extends from the testis through the inguinal canal to the abdominal cavity.

C. **Function**

    1. Female

        a.   Hormonally controlled, the menstrual cycle normally ranges from 22 to 34 days (with an average of 28 days).

        b.   During the menstrual phase, comprising the first 5 days of the cycle, low estrogen and progesterone levels stimulate hypothalamic GnRH and pituitary FSH and LH secretion.

        c.   Estrogen secretion causes endometrial buildup during the proliferative phase. Ovulation occurs at midcycle due to a LH surge.

        d.   During the luteal phase, the corpus luteum secretes estrogen and progesterone to maintain the endometrium. When conception does not occur, the corpus luteum degenerates, hormone levels decrease, and the cycle begins again.

        e.   Fertilization of the ovum by a sperm usually occurs in the distal third of the fallopian tube. About 5 days later, the zygote implants into the uterine endometrium.

 f. Menopause occurs when menses has ceased (for at least 1 year); in most women, this happens between age 40 and 55.

 g. After menopause, the ovaries atrophy, estrogen levels fall, and changes occur in the vagina, cardiovascular system, skeletal system, and integumentary system.

 h. Important hormones of the female reproductive system include:

  (1) Gonadotropin releasing hormone (GnRH), secreted by the hypothalamus: stimulates anterior pituitary secretion of FSH and LH

  (2) Follicle stimulating hormone (FSH), secreted by the anterior pituitary: acts on an ovarian follicle to cause it to mature

  (3) Luteinizing hormone (LH), secreted by anterior pituitary: acts on ovarian follicle to secrete estrogen; surges at midcycle to produce ovulation; controls secretion of estrogen and progesterone by the corpus luteum

  (4) Estrogen, secreted by the ovary (follicle, then corpus luteum): causes proliferation of the endometrium

  (5) Progesterone, secreted by the corpus luteum: maintains the endometrium and causes it to become thick and secretory

  (6) Human chorionic gonadotropin (HCG), secreted by chorionic villi in the endometrium of a pregnant female: stimulates the corpus luteum to secrete estrogen and progesterone until the placenta takes over

2. Male

 a. Spermatogenesis begins at puberty and continues throughout life. It occurs in several stages:

  (1) Spermatogonia grow and develop into primary spermatocytes, each containing 44 autosomes and 2 sex chromosomes, X and Y.

  (2) Primary spermatocytes divide to become secondary spermatocytes, each containing 22 autosomes and 1 sex chromosome, either X or Y.

  (3) Secondary spermatocytes divide to form spermatids, each retaining 23 chromosomes.

  (4) Spermatids mature into spermatozoa.

 b. Testosterone, secreted by testicular interstitial (Leydig) cells, is essential for the development and maintenance of male sex organs and secondary sex characteristics.

    c.   Testosterone secretion begins in utero and increases at puberty, controlled by LH and FSH secreted by the anterior pituitary.

    d.   The prostrate gland secretes fluid during sexual activity to add volume to semen, enhance sperm motility, and neutralize male urethral and vaginal acidity to enhance fertility.

3.   Sexual response patterns

    a.   According to Masters and Johnson (1966), both male and female sexual response is characterized by vasocongestion and myotonia.

    b.   Sexual desire is controlled by the limbic system of the brain and is mediated by the ratio of testosterone to estrogen.

    c.   The four phases of sexual response are excitement, plateau phase, orgasmic phase, and resolution phase.

II. Overview of reproductive and sexual disorders

A.   Assessment

    1.   Female

        a.   The nursing health history should focus on obtaining information about:

            (1)   Any pain, unusual discharge, irregular bleeding, fever, or urinary symptoms

            (2)   Menstrual history

            (3)   First day of last menstrual period (LMP)

            (4)   Pregnancy and delivery history

            (5)   Contraceptive use

            (6)   Fertility problems

            (7)   Sexual activity and use of safe sex practices

            (8)   History of STDs

            (9)   Past gynecologic surgery, disorders, or trauma

            (10)   Medication use

            (11)   Family history of gynecologic problems

            (12)   Self-breast exam (knowledge of, frequency of)

            (13)   Pap smear history

        b.   Physical examination is conducted with the patient in the supine position for breast and abdominal exam and in the lithotomy position for a pelvic exam.

        c.   Inspection and palpation of the breasts is done to note any asymmetry, skin dimpling, nipple discharge, tenderness, or masses. Patient teaching for self-examination should be done during assessment.

        d.   The external genitalia are inspected before the internal gynecologic exam is performed. Discharge and lesions should be noted on both external and internal exam.

        e.   The vagina should appear pink with plentiful rugae in the premenopausal woman.

      f.   The cervix is pink to red, firm, with a round or slitlike orifice, nontender, and possibly watery or mucoid discharge.

      g.   Bimanual palpation of the uterus and adnexa should reveal no masses, enlargement, or tenderness.

2.   Male

      a.   The health history should include information about:

         (1)   Pain, discharge, lesions of the genitalia

         (2)   Any difficulty with erection or ejaculation

         (3)   Urinary function

         (4)   Fertility

         (5)   Medication use

         (6)   Family history

         (7)   Previous illnesses, surgery, or trauma of the genitourinary system

         (8)   History of STDs

         (9)   Chronic illnesses that may affect sexual functioning (e.g., diabetes mellitus, cardiovascular or neurologic disease)

        (10) Past and current patterns of sexual activity; safe or unsafe sex practices; contraceptive use

        (11) Testicular self-exam (knowledge of, frequency of)

      b.   Preparation for physical exam involves urination (unless urine sample or urethral discharge specimen will be needed); disrobing from the waist down and draping; and explanation and reassurance and glove donning by the nurse.

      c.   Inspection of the male genitalia involves the penis, scrotum, and inguinal area. The examiner notes skin color and integrity, presence of lesions, discharge from the urethral meatus, retractability of the foreskin in an uncircumcised male, pubic hair distribution, swollen lymph nodes, and bulges that may indicate hernias.

      d.   Palpation of the testes should reveal two nontender, smooth, freely movable oval masses.

      e.   Palpation of the inguinal area is done superficially to detect enlarged or tender lymph nodes, as well as by invaginating the finger through the scrotum into the external inguinal ring to check for hernia while the patient bears down.

      f.   The prostate is palpated during a rectal exam; it should be firm and nontender and not protrude into the rectum.

B. **Laboratory studies and diagnostic tests**

    1.   The Papanicolaou (Pap) test involves cytologic analysis of a sample scraped from the cervis and other tissues to detect infections and malignancy.

2. Tests to detect STDs include:
   a. Culture and sensitivity
   b. Gram staining
   c. Rapid plasma reagin (RPR)
   d. Serologic testing for syphilis
   e. Special enzyme or antibody tests
3. Semen analysis evaluates male fertility by checking sperm motility and quantity.
4. Noninvasive tests to evaluate female internal reproductive organs include hysterosalpingography, computed tomography (CT scan), and pelvic ultrasonography.
5. Invasive female reproductive tract tests include colposcopy and laparoscopy.
6. Diagnostic tests used to detect breast tumors include mammography, thermography, ultrasonography, and tissue biopsy.

C. Psychosocial implications

1. The patient with a reproductive system or sexual disorder may experience self-concept changes related to:
   a. Concern about the ability to perform sexually
   b. Body image changes
   c. Change in role perception as a sexual or reproductive partner
2. Changes in social and interpersonal interaction may include:
   a. Isolation from sexual partner
   b. Depression over loss of or change in function
   c. Inability to alter perception of self as a viable sexual and procreative being
   d. Inability to find alternative and satisfying means of sexual expression
3. The patient may experience difficulty coping with the disease or condition, possibly manifested by:
   a. Fear of rejection
   b. Fear of death
   c. Anxiety about potential dysfunction
   d. Inability to live comfortably with uncertainty of future with altered sexual or reproductive function
4. When caring for a patient with a reproductive or sexual disorder, the nurse should:
   a. Provide a therapeutic environment.
   b. Maintain confidentiality and privacy.
   c. Consider the patient's sensitivity to sexual matters.
   d. Maintain a nonjudgmental attitude to encourage more complete disclosure.

D. **Medications used to treat reproductive disorders**

1. Oral contraceptives prevent conception by hindering FSH secretion from the anterior pituitary, thus preventing ovulation.
2. Progestogens are used to treat abnormal uterine bleeding and amenorrhea; agents include:
   a. Hydroxyprogesterone caproate
   b. Medroxyprogesterone acetate
   c. Norethindrone acetate
   d. Progesterone
3. Estrogens are used to treat menopausal symptoms, abnormal uterine bleeding, and inoperable prostate cancer. Drugs include:
   a. Dienestrol
   b. Diethylstilbestrol
   c. Estrogen, conjugated
   d. Estrogen, esterified
   e. Estrone
   f. Ethinyl estradiol
   g. Quinestrol
4. Clomiphene is a fertility agent used to induce ovulation; it may increase the likelihood of multiple pregnancy.
5. Drugs used to treat STDs include a wide variety of antibiotics and the antiviral agent acyclovir for genital herpes.
6. Danazol, an androgenic steriod that inhibits gonadotropin release, is used to treat endometriosis.

III. STDs

A. **Description**

1. STDs are infections of the genitals and reproductive organs (as well as other body tissues) transmitted through sexual activity.
2. Types include:
   a. Vulvovaginitis
   b. Cervicitis
   c. Urethritis
   d. Pelvic inflammatory disease (PID)
   e. Epididymitis
   f. Genital lesions
   g. Systemic infections

B. **Etiology and incidence**

1. Causative organisms include:
   a. For vulvovaginitis: *Trichomonas vaginalis* (trichomoniasis), a protozoan; *Sarcoptes scabiei* (scabies) and *Phthirus pubis* (pubic lice), two ectoparasites
   b. For cervicitis and urethritis (may ascend to cause PID and epididymitis): *Neisseria gonorrhoeae* (gonorrhea), *Chlamydia trachomatis* (chlamydial infections)

    c.   For genital lesions: herpes simplex virus (genital herpes); human papilloma virus (genital warts, condyloma acuminatum) *Molluscum contagiosum*; *Hemophilus ducreyi* (chancroid); *Chlamydia trachomatis* (lymphogranuloma venereum, or LGV)

    d.   For systemic infection: *Treponema pallidum* (syphilis)

2.   STDs are the most prevalent form of infection in the United States; chlamydia is the most common STD. Incidence of all STDs is rising because of increased sexual activity, more frequent use of nonbarrier contraceptives, and the increasingly high cost of case finding and treatment of partners. Between 400,000 and 500,000 new causes of genital herpes, and over 40,000 cases of syphilis, are reported each year.

C. **Pathophysiology**

    1.   Infectious organisms enter through the skin and mucous membrane of the genital, oral, or anal regions.

    2.   They produce inflammation in surrounding tissue and in some cases ascent the reproductive tract, causing scarring and infertility (gonorrhea and chlamydial infection).

    3.   In syphilis, the organism travels via the bloodstream, and over many years damages remote tissues such as the heart and nervous system.

    4.   In genital herpes, the virus ascends the peripheral nerve to the dorsal root ganglia, where it remains latent until factors such as fever, menses, stress, or pregnancy precipitate recurrent outbreaks.

    5.   Some STDs can be transmitted to the fetus through the placenta or the birth canal, causing spontaneous abortion or congenital infection or the newborn.

D. **Assessment findings**

    1.   History may reveal unprotected sexual activity with a new partner or one who has not been monogamous.

    2.   Vaginitis, cervicitis, and urethritis typically produce complaints of discharge and possibly irritation, itching, or dysuria. On physical exam, the discharge may vary:

        a.   Trichomoniasis: yellow and frothy, with a red, excoriated vulva and vagina (asymptomatic in males)

        b.   Gonorrhea: purulent, yellow

        c.   Chlamydia: watery to mucoid to purulent

    3.   Scabies and pubic lice may produce itching, excoriation, burrows, papules, or visible nits or lice.

    4.   Ascending infections are marked by fever as well as pelvic pain in women and testicular pain and swelling in men.

    5.   Genital lesions may be apparent on inspection of the skin and mucous membranes of the genital, oral, and anal regions;

other symptoms may or may not be present. Examples include:

    a. Syphilis: nonpainful chancre with mild inguinal lymphadenopathy in primary syphilis; generalized rash, fever, and lymphadenopathy in secondary syphilis

    b. Genital herpes: painful vesicles that erode to form ulcers with inguinal lymphadenopathy, possibly headache, milder recurrent outbreaks

    c. Genital warts: nonpainful, soft, fleshy papillary or sessile masses

6. Laboratory findings may include:

    a. Positive RPR or other serologic tests in syphilis

    b. Positive gram stain and culture and sensitivity for *N. gonorrhoeae*

    c. Positive herpes simplex virus tissue culture or antibody test

    d. Positive tissue culture or antibody test for *C. trachomatis*

E. Nursing diagnoses

1. Anxiety
2. Knowledge Deficit
3. High Risk for Infection
4. Noncompliance

F. Planning and implementation

1. Reduce anxiety due to embarrassment and fear by conveying a caring, nonjudgmental attitude; offering reassurance and support; and ensuring confidentiality.
2. Teach the patient about the disorder and its treatment, principles of transmission, possible complications, and safer sex practices.
3. Administer antibiotics, antivirals, antiparasitics, and pain medications as indicated.
4. Explain medication action, side effects, dosage schedule.
5. Teach comfort and hygiene measures, such as sitz baths and saline soaks.
6. Advise sexual abstinence until follow-up has ensured cure.
7. Encourage treatment of sexual partners.

G. Evaluation

1. The patient reports decreased pain and discharge.
2. The patient demonstrates reduced lymphadenopathy and healing of genital lesions.
3. Laboratory tests reveal negative cultures.
4. The patient demonstrates appropriate self-medication.
5. The patient states the intention to abstain from sex for the prescribed period and to use safer sex practices in the future.
6. The patient's sex partner(s) seek(s) treatment.

IV. Menstrual disorders
A. Description
1. Menstrual conditions include:
   a. Premenstrual syndrome (PMS)
   b. Dysmenorrhea
   c. Amenorrhea
   d. Abnormal uterine bleeding
2. PMS is a cluster of symptoms occurring before onset of menstruation in the menstrual cycle.
3. Dysmenorrhea refers to painful menstruation. In primary dysmenorrhea, no pelvic pathology has been identified. In secondary dysmenorrhea, a pelvic condition causes pain.
4. Amenorrhea refers to lack of menstruation; it is either primary (delayed menarche) or secondary (occurring after menarche).
5. Abnormal uterine bleeding involves:
   a. Menorrhagia (excessive bleeding at the usual time of menstrual flow)
   b. Metrorrhagia (bleeding between periods or after menopause)

B. Etiology and incidence
1. Menstrual conditions are caused by hormonal imbalance or pelvic pathology such as tumors or endometriosis.
2. Emotional tension plays a role in many cases.
3. Inadequate nutrition or excessive weight loss may cause amenorrhea.

C. Pathophysiology
1. A disruption in the feedback system between the ovarian, adrenal, thyroid, and pituitary hormonal secretions often occurs.
2. Pelvis pathology such as a uterine tumor or endometriosis may cause abnormal menstruation.
3. In PMS, the estrogen–progesterone ratio is increased during the luteal phase, causing characteristic estrogen-dependent symptoms.
4. In dysmenorrhea, excessive prostaglandin secretion causes uterine hypercontractility and arteriolar spasm.

D. Assessment findings
1. In PMS, the patient relates a history of headache, fatigue, mood swings, irritability, and full, tender breasts approximately 10 days before menses each cycle.
2. In other menstrual conditions, history reveals abnormal menstruation in terms of how often, how long, how heavy, or how painful the menstruation is.
3. Associated history findings may include weight loss, inadequate nutrition, or anorexia or bulimia.
4. Physical exam may reveal a tender abdomen and possibly abdominal masses if underlying pelvic pathology is present.

> 5. Diagnostic tests such as pelvic ultrasonography, hysterosalpingography, and laparoscopy may reveal pelvic pathology contributing to the menstrual problem.
> 6. Complete blood count commonly reveals decreased hemoglobin and hematocrit with menorrhagia.

E. Nursing diagnoses

1. Anxiety
2. Ineffective Individual Coping
3. Knowledge Deficit
4. Pain
5. High Risk for Violence

F. Planning and implementation

1. Offer reassurance and support.
2. Administer pain medications as indicated.
3. Teach self-medication of pain medications and oral contraceptives as indicated, including dosage schedule, side effects, and possible interactions.
4. Advise the patient to keep a diary of the menstrual cycle, including occurrence and heaviness of flow and occurrence of pain and other symptoms.
5. Encourage a well-balanced diet with adequate fluid and vitamin intake.
6. Teach relaxation techniques to promote comfort and relieve tension.

G. Evaluation

1. The patient reports decreased emotional stress and improved pain relief.
2. The patient demonstrates appropriate use of medication.
3. The patient keeps a diary of the menstrual cycle.
4. Hematocrit and hemoglobin remain stable.
5. The patient eats a balanced diet and takes vitamin supplements.

V. Gynecologic infections

A. Description

1. Gynecologic infections include:
    a. Vulvovaginitis
    b. Cervicitis
    c. Bartholinitis and Bartholin abscess
    d. Toxic shock syndrome (TSS)
    e. Pelvic inflammatory disease (PID)
2. They may or may not be sexually transmitted (see Section III).

B. Etiology and incidence

1. Gynecologic infections are caused by microorganisms such as bacteria and fungi. Vulvovaginitis is extremely common in women of all ages.

    a. Vulvovaginitis: *Candida albicans* (fungus) causes candidiasis or yeast vaginitis. *Gardnerella vaginalis* (bacteria) causes gardnerella vaginitis or nonspecific vaginitis; may be sexually transmitted

    b. Cervicitis and PID: *Chlamydia trachomatis* and *Neisseria gonorrhoeae* (sexually transmitted); *Escherichia coli*, streptococci, and staphylococci (not sexually transmitted)

2. Atrophic vaginitis is an inflammatory condition caused by low estrogen levels in a postmenopausal woman that makes the vagina prone to infection by any organism.

3. Bartholinitis and Bartholin abscess formation are caused by *N. gonorrhea* (sexually transmitted) as well as nonsexually transmitted bacteria surrounding the vulva (e.g., *E. coli*, streptococci, and staphylococci).

4. Toxic shock syndrome (TSS) is caused by the toxins released by *Staphylococcus aureus*.

C. Pathophysiology

1. Microorganisms invade the vulva and vaginal mucosa and may colonize and ascend the reproductive tract.

2. Altered vaginal mucosal conditions (e.g., altered pH, disrupted normal vaginal flora, and low estrogen levels) alter resistance to infection.

3. Childbirth, abortion, and some intrauterine procedures allow bacteria to gain intrauterine access by direct invasion and possibly by spreading through the blood and lymphatics.

4. Menstruation provides a growth media for bacteria that may ascend upward to cause salpingitis and parametritis.

5. In TSS, magnesium-absorbing fibers of tampons cause decreased magnesium levels, contributing to toxin production by bacteria in the lower reproductive tract.

D. Assessment findings

1. Signs and symptoms of vulvovaginitis include:

    a. History of recent antibiotic use (may include risk factors for infection such as oral contraceptive use, diabetes mellitus, menopause, pregnancy, poor hygiene, synthetic or tight-fitting undergarments and clothing, frequent douching or use of vulvovaginal products)

    b. Complaint of vulvovaginal itching, irritation, fishy odor, and thick white to creamy grayish discharge

    c. Reddened, swollen vulva and vagina

2. Assessment findings for bartholinitis and abscess formation include:

    a. Possible history of sexual activity with an infected partner

    b. Acute pain between the labia, unilaterally

c. Possible fever
d. Red, swollen vulva unilaterally possibly with drainage or visible abscess

3. Assessment findings for PID include:
   a. History of sexual activity with an infected partner; past episodes of infection; or recent childbirth, abortion, or intrauterine procedure
   b. Complaints of lower abdominal pain, fever, nausea, and vaginal discharge
   c. Unilateral or bilateral lower abdominal tenderness, cervical discharge, cervical motion tenderness, and adnexal tenderness on examination
   d. Elevated WBC level and positive cervical cultures

4. Assessment findings in TSS may include:
   a. History of recent menses and tampon use
   b. Complaints of sudden high fever, headache, vomiting, diarrhea, myalgias
   c. Hypotension, possibly shock
   d. Development of a red, macular rash that desquamates in 7 to 10 days
   e. Possible decreased urine output and respiratory distress
   f. Elevated WBCs, BUN, bilirubin, and CPR levels

E. **Nursing diagnoses**
   1. Anxiety
   2. Hyperthermia
   3. Knowledge Deficit
   4. Pain
   5. Altered Tissue Perfusion

F. **Planning and implementation**
   1. Provide reassurance, confidentiality, and support to allay anxiety.
   2. Administer antimicrobial and pain medications as indicated.
   3. Teach self-administration of vaginal medications or irrigation as indicated.
   4. Explain the action, side effects, and interactions of all prescribed medications.
   5. Maintain hydration for patients with nausea and vomiting, fever, and shock with IV fluids.
   6. Promote comfort measures such as sitz baths and application of warm soaks as needed.
   7. Teach the patient to avoid risk factors for infection, if possible.
   8. Promote safer sex practices and treatment of sex partner(s) as indicated.
   9. Prepare the patient with Bartholin's abscess for surgical drainage as indicated.

   10. Ensure proper follow-up evaluation and care.
 G. **Evaluation**
   1. The patient demonstrates decreased temperature, discharge, and tenderness and exhibits normal blood pressure.
   2. The patient reports adequate pain relief.
   3. The patient verbalizes understanding of the medication dosage schedule, method of administration, and side effects that warrant reporting.
   4. The patient states risk factors and sexual practices that can be altered to help prevent reinfection.
   5. WBC count and other laboratory studies return to normal.

VI. **Gynecologic tumors**
 A. **Description**
   1. Gynecologic tumors include:
    a. Benign conditions such as ovarian cysts, uterine leiomyomas, and endometriosis
    b. Malignant conditions or cancer of the vulva, cervix, uterus, and ovary
   2. Benign conditions usually do not predispose to malignancy.
 B. **Etiology and incidence**
   1. The exact cause of most gynecologic tumors is unknown.
   2. The following factors have been associated with increased incidence of gynecologic tumors:
    a. Multiple sex partners and early sexual activity (cervical cancer)
    b. Estrogen therapy (uterine cancer)
    c. Diethylstilbestrol (DES) therapy by pregnant women (uterine cancer in their female offspring)
    d. Family history of ovarian cancer
   3. Leiomyomas (also called fibroid tumors) occur in 20% of white women and 40% to 50% of black women.
   4. The incidence of endometriosis is increasing, possibly due to delayed childbearing. It is common in nulliparous 25- to 35-year-old women.
   5. The incidence of uterine cancer has been decreasing due to widespread annual Pap testing; however, it still ranks third among all cancers in women.
 C. **Pathophysiology**
   1. Ovarian cysts arise as normal ovarian constituents enlarge during the menstrual cycle (corpus luteal and follicular cysts) or as an ovum abnormally matures (dermoid cysts).
   2. In endometriosis, retrograde menstruation (transplantation theory) or retained remnants of embryonic epithelial tissue (metaplasia theory) causes aberrant proliferation of the endometrium, which bleeds and causes adhesions during menstruation.

    3. Many gynecologic tumors disrupt the normal menstrual cycle as they grow; some also may exert pressure on adjacent abdominal and pelvic structures.

D. **Assessment findings**

    1. The patient with an ovarian cyst may be asymptomatic or may experience such signs and symptoms as:

       a. Lower abdominal and back pain

       b. Dyspareunia

       c. Abnormal uterine bleeding

       d. Palpable ovarian mass

       e. Acute abdominal pain and guarding with rupture

       f. Rebound tenderness with rupture

       g. Ascites

    2. The patient with leiomyomas may be asymptomatic or may exhibit the following findings:

       a. Pelvic pain, backache

       b. Constipation

       c. Urinary retention or urgency

       d. Dysmenorrhea, menorrhagia

       e. Palpable enlarged or irregular uterus

    3. Common assessment findings in endometriosis include:

       a. Dysmenorrhea starting 1 or 2 days before menstruation and persisting for 2 to 3 days

       b. Abnormal uterine bleeding

       c. Dyspareunia

       d. Infertility

       e. Tender palpable masses

    4. Manifestations of cervical cancer may include:

       a. Vaginal discharge (early)

       b. Spotting (early)

       c. Chronic erosions of the cervix (early)

       d. Pain in the back and legs (late)

       e. Abnormal Pap smear findings

    5. Assessment findings for endometrial cancer may include:

       a. Irregular vaginal bleeding and postmenopausal bleeding

       b. Abnormal Pap smear findings (in only 25% of patients)

    6. Cancer of the vulva may be marked by:

       a. Pruritus (early)

       b. Vulvar bleeding, foul-smelling discharge, and pain

       c. Vulvar mass or ulceration

    7. Assessment findings for ovarian cancer may include:

       a. Pelvic pain or backache (early)

       b. Irregular menses

       c. Premenstrual tension

       d. Postmenstrual bleeding

       e. Dyspepsia

f.   Acne

g.   Breast tenderness

E.   Nursing diagnoses

1.   Anxiety

2.   Anticipatory Grieving

3.   Knowledge Deficit

4.   Pain

5.   Self-Care Deficit

6.   Self-Concept Disturbance

7.   Sexual Dysfunction

8.   Altered Tissue Perfusion

F.   Planning and implementation

1.   Relieve pain by administering prescribed pain medications. Monitor respirations and blood pressure if narcotics are given.

2.   Teach the patient about side effects of hormonal therapy, and warn her to notify the doctor if signs of thromboembolism occur.

3.   Prepare the patient for surgery by offering information and re-assurance and performing routine preoperative care.

4.   Provide appropriate postoperative care, monitoring for complications such as infection, urinary retention, paralytic ileus, fluid and electrolyte imbalance, and thromboembolism.

5.   Monitor hemoglobin and hematocrit levels and transfuse blood products, as ordered, for a patient with menorrhagia.

6.   After a vulvectomy, perform vulvar irrigations to promote hygiene, comfort, and healing.

7.   Educate the patient about side effects of radiation therapy, if indicated for treatment of ovarian and some other cancers.

8.   When caring for a patient with a radiation implant, follow safety precautions for appropriate time and distance restrictions, discarding of linens, etc.

9.   Provide emotional support, and encourage the patient to express any concerns about sexual function, body image, fertility, and fear of death. Clear up any misconceptions the patient may have.

G.   Evaluation

1.   The patient reports adequate pain control.

2.   The patient displays reduced signs of anxiety (e.g., tachycardia, poor concentration, irritability, sweating, hyperventilation).

3.   The patient exhibits no fever, purulent wound drainage, wound swelling, or tenderness.

4.   Hemoglobin and hematocrit remain stable.

5.   The patient verbalizes understanding of the effects of the disease process and treatment options.

6.   Postoperatively, the patient voids, bowel sounds return, vital signs stabilize, and ambulation is attained.

VII. Structural disorders of the uterus and vagina

A. Description

1. Structural disorders of the vagina include:
   a. Vesicovaginal fistula
   b. Rectovaginal fistula
   c. Cystocele
   d. Rectocele
2. Structural disorders of the uterus include:
   a. Uterine displacement (retroversion and retroflexion)
   b. Uterine prolapse

B. Etiology and incidence

1. Structural disorders occur congenitally or as a result of pregnancy, delivery, surgery, or radiation therapy.
2. They become more common as aging weakens supporting tissues of the uterus and vagina.

C. Pathophysiology

1. With vaginal fistulas, an abnormal opening is formed through impaired tissue between the bladder or rectum and the vagina, allowing a trickle of urine or feces to flow through the vagina, causing irritation and infection.
2. Cystocele and rectocele develop as the pelvic floor muscles atrophy or weaken, allowing the bladder or rectum to bulge onto the anterior or posterior vaginal walls, interfering with urination and bowel elimination.
3. Normally, the uterus lies at a right angle to the vagina, inclined forward; however, in backward displacement of the uterus, the uterus has weakened supporting structures and thus tilts or is flexed backward.
4. Weakened supporting ligaments allow the uterus to work its way down the vaginal canal (prolapse) or outside the vaginal orifice (procidentia).

D. Assessment findings

1. The patient commonly has a history of childbirth, pelvic surgery, or perineal or pelvic trauma.
2. Clinical manifestations may include:
   a. Pelvic pressure or pain, backache
   b. Urinary frequency, retention, or incontinence
   c. Fecal incontinence, constipation, flatus
   d. Leukorrhea (with fistulas)
   e. Visible uterine prolapse
3. Pelvic examination may reveal the structural disorder.

E. Nursing diagnoses

1. Bowel Incontinence
2. High Risk for Infection
3. Knowledge Deficit

       4. Pain

       5. Impaired Tissue Integrity

F. Planning and implementation

       1. Provide reassurance that structural disorders are not "normal" changes due to aging and that treatment will alleviate symptoms.

       2. Provide and teach good perineal hygiene preoperatively and postoperatively to prevent infection, with perineal irrigations, douches, and sitz baths.

       3. Explain surgical options, including possible postoperative complications (e.g., incisional infection and urinary retention).

       4. Monitor urine output; insert a bladder catheter, if necessary.

       5. Provide prescribed pain medications and ice packs postoperatively.

       6. Teach the patient how to apply and care for a pessary, if indicated.

       7. Teach perineal muscle strengthening exercises to enhance support of pelvic structures and improve urinary continence.

       8. Encourage good nutrition, heat application, and adequate rest to enhance fistula healing.

G. Evaluation

       1. The patient reports relief of discomfort, urinary incontinence, and bowel incontinence.

       2. The patient remains free of urinary tract infection and incisional infection.

       3. The patient demonstrates proper hygiene.

       4. The patient demonstrates proper technique for perineal muscle strengthening exercises.

VIII. Breast tumors

A. Description

       1. Tumors of the breast are:

          a. Benign (e.g., fibrocystic disease, fibroadenoma, and intraductal papilloma)

          b. Malignant, including breast cancer and Paget's disease

       2. Intraductal papilloma and Paget's disease affect the nipple.

B. Etiology and incidence

       1. Although the cause of breast cancer has not been elucidated, the effects of estrogen may play a role.

       2. Risk factors include:

          a. Over age 40

          b. Familial history of breast cancer

          c. Early menarche

          d. Late menopause

          e. Nulliparous or birth of first child after age 34

          f. High-fat diet

   g. Oral contraceptive use

   h. Radiation exposure

   i. Presence of other cancer

  3. Worldwide, breast cancer incidence is estimated at 1 million annually.

C. Pathophysiology

  1. In fibrocystic disease of the breast, small cysts are produced by overgrowth of fibrous tissue around the ducts.

  2. In intraductal papilloma, a wartlike epithelial mass grows in a large collecting duct. It bleeds on trauma, and blood collects in the duct until areolar pressure expresses it out.

  3. Paget's disease starts with an eczematoid condition of the nipple that spreads, erodes and ulcerates, and becomes cancerous.

  4. Breast cancer, a primary carcinoma of breast tissue, attaches to the chest wall, invades surrounding tissue, and metastasizes by way of lymph channels.

D. Assessment findings

  1. Clinical manifestations of benign breast tumors may include:

   a. Breast pain and tenderness

   b. Change in mass size (larger and smaller) with menstrual cycle

   c. Palpable masses—firm, round, and freely movable

  2. Assessment findings for conditions affecting the nipple include:

   a. Bloody nipple discharge (intraductal papilloma)

   b. Eczematous or ulcerated nipple (Paget's disease)

   c. Usually minimal pain

  3. Signs and symptoms of breast cancer may include:

   a. A nontender lump, usually in an upper outer quadrant

   b. Pain (late)

   c. Axillary lymphadenopathy (late)

   d. Fixed, nodular breast mass (late)

E. Nursing diagnoses

  1. Ineffective Coping

  2. Fear

  3. Anticipatory Grieving

  4. High Risk for Infection

  5. Knowledge Deficit

  6. Impaired Physical Mobility

  7. Pain

  8. Self-Care Deficit

  9. Self-Concept Disturbance

  10. Sexual Dysfunction

F. Planning and implementation

  1. Help allay the patient's fears by offering information and support during the diagnostic process.

    2. To minimize discomfort, teach a patient with fibrocystic disease to wear a supportive bra, use analgesics, reduce methylxanthine intake, adhere to a low-salt diet, and apply warm or cool compresses.

    3. Reinforce information the surgeon has told the patient about treatment options, including breast reconstruction and prosthesis use.

    4. After surgery for breast cancer, provide meticulous wound care to prevent infection and promote healing of grafts.

    5. Postsurgery, elevate the arm on the affected side to promote drainage and enhance comfort.

    6. Administer prescribed pain medications to reduce pain; monitor respirations and blood pressure with narcotic use.

    7. Teach the patient to avoid irritation or injury to the incision site or arm of the affected side, to help prevent infection stemming from reduced lymphatic circulation.

    8. As indicated, provide referrals to self-help groups such as "Reach for Recovery," and for prosthesis or special garments.

    9. Teach all women proper breast self-examination (BSE) technique.

G. **Evaluation**

    1. The patient expresses concerns about possible cancer, surgery, and effects on body image and sexuality.

    2. The patient reports pain relief.

    3. The patient participates in self-care activities.

    4. The patient demonstrates good recovery from surgery; ambulates and has improved ROM of affected arm.

    5. The patient displays good wound healing with no signs of incisional infection.

    6. The patient exhibits minimal arm edema.

    7. The patient demonstrates proper BSE technique.

    8. The patient states an intention to seek help from support groups.

IX. **Infertility (male and female)**

A. **Description**

    1. Infertility refers to a couple's failure to achieve pregnancy within 1 to 2 years of unprotected intercourse.

    2. It may be classified as primary or secondary.

B. **Etiology and incidence**

    1. The cause of infertility may lie with the female, the male, or both.

    2. Causes include uterine displacement, tumors, congenital abnormalities, and inflammation.

    3. Causative factors and their approximate incidence include ovarian, 20%; tubal, 30%; cervical, 18%; and seminal, 30%.

C. Pathophysiology

1. Inflammation or structural abnormalities of the fallopian tubes or uterus can prevent the transportation of ovum and sperm or implantation of a fertilized ovum.

2. The ovaries may not produce and release ova regularly or secrete sufficient progesterone to produce an endometrium sufficient for implantation.

3. The pH of semen or vaginal secretions or conditions of cervical mucus may alter reception to sperm and prevent fertilization.

4. Sperm quantity, motility, or morphology may be inadequate for fertilization.

D. Assessment findings

1. The health history of an infertile woman may include STDs, reproductive tract surgery, abortions, PID, endometriosis, adhesions, displaced uterus, or an endocrine disorder.

2. History findings in an infertile man may include STDs, genital trauma, tuberculosis, mumps, orchitis, or cryptorchidism.

3. Pelvic examination may reveal structural disorders (uterine displacement) or inflammation (such as salpingitis).

4. Examination of the male genitalia may reveal structural disorders (cryptorchidism) or inflammation (epididymitis or orchitis).

5. Tubal insufflation may reveal poor tubal patency.

6. Postcoital cervical mucus test may be abnormal.

7. Sperm count or motility may be abnormal (fewer than 20 million).

E. Nursing diagnoses

1. Anxiety
2. Altered Role Performance
3. Sexual Dysfunction

F. Planning and implementation

1. Allay anxiety by providing information about the cause of infertility, diagnostic tests, and possible treatments.

2. Encourage both partners to express feelings related to loss and disappointment, altered roles, and sexual identity.

3. If indicated, assist with artificial insemination, instructing the patient to lie flat for 30 minutes afterward.

4. Provide ongoing reassurance; most patients require repeated procedures, and success rate for infertility is only 25% to 50%.

5. Encourage the couple to explore other options, such as adoption.

G. Evaluation

1. The patient and partner verbalize feelings, understand treatment options, and cope with the outcome.

2. Pregnancy or a satisfactory alternative is achieved.

X. Penile disorders
A. Description
1. Conditions of the penis include:
   a. Phimosis and paraphimosis
   b. Priapism
   c. Penile cancer
2. In phimosis, the foreskin is constricted and cannot be retracted; in paraphimosis, the foreskin is retracted behind the glans and cannot be replaced.
3. Priapism—uncontrolled, persistent erection—is a urologic emergency.

B. Etiology and incidence
1. Poor hygiene of the uncircumcised penis plays a role in the development of phimosis and penile cancer.
2. Priapism results from neural or vascular pathophysiology, such as sickle cell thrombosis, spinal cord tumors, or tumor invasion of the penis and its blood vessels.
3. Cancer of the penis represents about 0.5% of malignancies in the United States and is more common in countries where circumcision is uncommon.

C. Pathophysiology
1. In phimosis, normal secretions of the prepuce accumulate and cause balanitis, with subsequent scarring and calcification preventing foreskin retraction.
2. In paraphimosis, once the foreskin is retracted, edema prevents reduction.
3. In priapism, the corpora cavernosa become engorged with blood, and venous drainage is impaired; ischemia, fibrosis, gangrene, and impotence may result.

D. Assessment findings
1. Phimosis is marked by a constricted, fixed foreskin over the glans.
2. Paraphimosis typically involves sudden restriction of the foreskin behind the glans with edema of the penis distally.
3. Common assessment findings in penile cancer include a painless, wartlike growth or ulcer on the glans or coronal sulcus.
4. Priapism is characterized by persistent, painful erection in the absence of sexual desire.

E. Nursing diagnoses
1. Fear
2. Knowledge Deficit
3. Pain
4. Sexual Dysfunction

F. Planning and implementation
1. Encourage bedrest, elevation of the penis, and ice application to reduce pain and swelling.

2. Administer narcotics for pain relief, monitoring respirations and blood pressure.
3. Prepare the patient for circumcision, penectomy, or a blood shunting procedure as indicated.
4. Postoperatively, monitor bleeding, administer analgesics, and change the petroleum gauze or pressure dressing as indicated.
5. Offer reassurance to the patient with penile cancer. Tell him that he may still be able to participate in sexual intercourse after partial penectomy. Offer referral for counseling.
6. Teach uncircumcised patients proper cleansing of the glans and prepuce.

G. **Evaluation**
1. The patient reports decreased pain.
2. Swelling is relieved, the foreskin is reducible, or erection subsides.
3. The patient demonstrates proper cleansing of the penis.
4. The patient remains free of bleeding or infection postoperatively.
5. The patient expresses concerns about sexual activity and sexuality and seeks counseling as necessary.

XI. Impotence
A. **Description**
1. Impotence refers to the inability to achieve or maintain an erection sufficient to accomplish intercourse.
2. It may be classified as erectile or ejaculatory, and primary or secondary.

B. **Etiology and incidence**
1. Psychogenic causes include anxiety, fatigue, depression, and undue pressure to perform sexually.
2. Possible organic causes include:
    a. Occlusive vascular disease
    b. Endocrine conditions (e.g., diabetes, pituitary tumors, hypogonadism)
    c. Genitourinary conditions (e.g., prostatectomy)
    d. Hematologic disorders (e.g., Hodgkin's disease, leukemia)
    e. Neurologic disorders (e.g., neuropathy, parkinsonism)
    f. Genital trauma
    g. Alcohol and drug abuse
    h. Medication use (e.g., antipsychotics, anticholinergics, antihypertensives)
3. Incidence increases with age.

C. **Pathophysiology**
1. Pathologic processes are diverse but commonly involve decreased blood flood flow to the penis, altered nerve conduction, or decreased hormonal secretion.

2. Impotence may be partial or full, intermittent or constant, transient, selective for partners, and of sudden or gradual onset.

D. Assessment findings
1. The patient history may reveal a chronic disease or condition, emotional or psychologic problem, or use of an implicated medication.
2. Nocturnal penile tumescence monitoring, Doppler studies of penile blood flow, and nerve conduction studies may be abnormal or normal.

E. Nursing diagnoses
1. Anxiety
2. Altered Role Performance
3. Sexual Dysfunction

F. Planning and implementation
1. Help reduce anxiety by maintaining privacy and confidentiality and encouraging the patient to talk about sex- and role-related concerns.
2. Encourage professional sex counseling if impotence is of apparent psychogenic origin.
3. Encourage patients with chronic disease or who are on medications to follow up regularly and follow doctor's orders, to prevent impotence as a complication. Encourage them to discuss any erectile dysfunction with their doctors; medications may be changed or treatment adjusted to promote sexual function.
4. If a penile prosthesis is indicated, instruct the patient on its use, and monitor for bleeding, infection, pain, or displacement after surgery.

G. Evaluation
1. The patient demonstrates and reports reduced anxiety.
2. The patient reports satisfaction in sexual relationships.

XII. Male genitourinary infections

A. Description
1. Male genitourinary infections include:
   a. Prostatitis
   b. Orchitis
   c. Epididymitis
2. Prostatitis may be acute or chronic.

B. Etiology and incidence
1. Microorganisms such as bacteria, viruses, fungi, or parasites cause genitourinary infections.
2. The most common bacterial offenders are gram-negative organisms.
3. Sexually transmitted organisms also can cause these infections (see Section III).

4. Noninfection inflammation of the prostate, epididymis, and testes may also result from trauma or chemical irritation.
5. An estimated 35% of men older than age 50 suffer from chronic prostatitis.
6. The cause of epididymitis in men younger than age 35 is usually *Chlamydia trachomatis*.

C. **Pathophysiology**
1. Microorganisms may be carried up the urethra to infect the prostate, epididymis, and testis, or they may be spread through the bloodstream.
2. Chemical irritation and inflammation of these organs results from extravasation of urine, possibly secondary to urethral stricture or prostatic hyperplasia.
3. Poor diffusion of antimicrobial medications into the prostate gland may cause relapsing infection in chronic prostatitis.

D. **Assessment findings**
1. Signs and symptoms of prostatitis include:
    a. Sudden onset of fever and chills (acute prostatitis)
    b. Dysuria, urgency, frequency
    c. Perineal pain or low back pain
    d. Tender, swollen, warm indurated prostate on palpation
    e. Divided urine sample positive for bacteria and WBCs
2. Assessment findings in epididymitis include:
    a. Inguinal and scrotal pain
    b. Fever
    c. Tender, swollen epididymis
    d. Swollen, warm scrotum
    e. Possibly urine containing bacteria and WBCs
3. Common assessment findings in orchitis include pain and swelling of the testes.

E. **Nursing diagnoses**
1. Hyperthermia
2. Infection, High Risk for Reinfection
3. Pain

F. **Planning and implementation**
1. Promote comfort by administering pain and antiinflammatory medications, baths, ice, bedrest, or scrotal elevation.
2. Administer antimicrobial medications as ordered; encourage the patient to comply with lengthy therapy and follow-up to prevent relapse.
3. Discourage sexual activity until infection is resolved. (However, sex may be beneficial with chronic prostatitis.) Encourage treatment for the patient's sexual partner(s), if indicated.
4. Encourage adequate hydration to ensure adequate diffusion of antimicrobials.

G. Evaluation
   1. Pain, fever, and swelling are resolved.
   2. Urine cultures are negative.
   3. Urine output is adequate.
   4. The patient complies with the treatment regimen and scheduled follow-up.

XIII. **Prostate disorders**
   A. **Description**
      1. Benign prostatic hyperplasia (BPH) is a benign enlargement of the prostate gland.
      2. Prostate cancer is a malignant adenocarcinoma.
   B. **Etiology and incidence**
      1. Although their etiology is unknown, both conditions are hormone dependent.
      2. Prostate cancer is the second most common cancer in men; incidence is greatest after age 50.
   C. **Pathophysiology**
      1. In both conditions, prostatic gland enlargement or the enlarging tumor obstruct urine outflow, leading to urinary retention, stasis, and infection.
      2. Male sex hormones stimulate growth and enlargement.
   D. **Assessment findings**
      1. Clinical manifestations may include:
         a. Symptoms of urinary obstruction (urgency, frequency, hesitancy, decreased urine stream, dribbling)
         b. Hematuria (cancer)
         c. On palpation, an enlarged, firm prostate (BPH) or a hard, fixed nodule (cancer)
      2. Laboratory studies may reveal elevated acid phosphatase level (cancer) or abnormal renal function tests (advanced BPH).
   E. **Nursing diagnoses**
      1. Anxiety
      2. High Risk for Fluid Volume Deficit
      3. High Risk for Infection
      4. Knowledge Deficit
      5. Pain
      6. Urinary Retention
   F. **Planning and implementation**
      1. Reduce anxiety by maintaining privacy, explaining all procedures and treatments, answering questions, and assuring the patient.
      2. Explain treatment options, which may include:
         a. Transurethral resection: suprapubic, perineal, or retropubic prostatectomy
         b. Radical prostatectomy and orchiectomy (for cancer only)

c.   Radiation therapy

d.   Hormonal therapy

3.   Provide preoperative and postoperative teaching, including complications such as bleeding, infection, and thrombosis.

4.   Maintain urinary catheter drainage to prevent urinary retention and infection. Postoperatively, maintain bladder irrigation to prevent hemorrhage. Monitor intake and output, bleeding, and vital signs.

5.   Administer pain medications as prescribed.

6.   Teach the patient perineal muscle exercises to help regain urinary control; warn him to avoid the Valsalva maneuver until healing is complete.

7.   Provide information about sexual function.

G.   Evaluation

1.   The patient verbalizes understanding of treatment, complications, and nursing care he will receive.

2.   The patient exhibits no urinary retention, fever, or hemorrhage.

3.   The patient reports adequate pain control.

4.   The patient maintains urinary control and sexual function.

XIV.   Testicular tumors

A.   Description

1.   Testicular cancers are classified as:

a.   Germinal (seminomas, teratocarcinomas, embryonal carcinomas)

b.   Nongerminal (epitheliomas)

2.   Hydrocele (collection of fluid in the tunica vaginalis of the testis) and varicocele (dilation of veins in the spermatic cord) are noncancerous masses.

B.   Etiology and incidence

1.   Cryptorchidism, systemic infections, epididymitis, endocrine factors, and local trauma may play a role in the development of testicular tumors.

2.   Varicocele is a congenital condition.

3.   Although relatively rare, testicular cancer is the leading cause of cancer deaths in males aged 20 to 35.

C.   Pathophysiology

1.   Testicular cancers arise from germinal or nongerminal cells of the testes as malignant tumors spread to regional lymph nodes and metastasize early.

2.   In hydrocele, fluid accumulates in the tunica vaginitis, possibly compromising testicular circulation, or it may become chronic.

3.   In varicocele, enlargement or the spermatic vein may lead to infertility.

D. **Assessment findings**
1. Signs and symptoms of testicular cancer may include:
   a. Painless enlargement of the scrotum
   b. Feeling of heaviness in the scrotum
   c. Backache, abdominal pain
   d. Weight loss, weakness
   e. Palpable firm, smooth testicular mass
   f. Elevated alpha-fetoprotein and HCG levels
2. Assessment findings in hydrocele and varicocele are minor but may include an enlarged scrotum and, in hydrocele, a testicular mass that transilluminates.

E. **Nursing diagnoses**
1. Anxiety
2. Body Image Disturbance
3. Knowledge Deficit
4. Sexual Dysfunction

F. **Planning and implementation**
1. Provide emotional support during the diagnostic process.
2. Explain treatment options, including:
   a. Orchiectomy, retroperitoneal lymph node dissection (RPLND), radiation therapy, or chemotherapy for testicular cancer
   b. Simple resection for symptomatic hydrocele or varicocele
3. Discuss patient concerns about body image, sexual function, and fertility. Offer information about testicular prosthesis and sperm banking.
4. Administer prescribed pain medications postoperatively.
5. Provide ice and scrotal support postoperatively to reduce pain and swelling.
6. Teach the patient to perform monthly testicular self-examination to aid early detection of testicular masses.

G. **Evaluation**
1. The patient verbalizes understanding of the diagnosis, treatment, and prognosis.
2. The patient reports adequate pain relief postoperatively.
3. The patient verbalizes any concerns about sexuality.
4. The patient demonstrates correct testicular self-examination technique.

Bibliography

Brunner, L. S., & Suddarth, D. S. (1988). *Textbook of medical-surgical nursing* (6th ed.). Philadelphia: J.B. Lippincott.

Brunner, L. S., & Suddarth, D. S. (1986). *The Lippincott manual of nursing practice* (4th ed.). Philadelphia: J.B. Lippincott.

Luckmann, J., & Sorenson, K. C. (1987). *Medical-surgical nursing: A psychophysiologic approach* (3rd ed.). Philadelphia: W.B. Saunders.

Masters, W., & Johnson, V. (1966). *Human sexual response*. Boston: Little, Brown & Company.

STUDY QUESTIONS

1. Sexual development begins at conception when the male zygote unites with the female zygote. Which of the following will result in a female fetus?
   a. XX
   b. XY
   c. XXY
   d. YYX

2. Which uterine layer responds to hormonal stimulation, thickens during the proliferative phase of the menstrual cycle, and sheds during the menstrual phase?
   a. myometrium
   b. endometrium
   c. leiomyoma
   d. mucous membrane

3. The scrotum is divided by a septum into two sacs, each containing
   a. a testis, ejaculatory duct, and vas deferens
   b. a testis, epididymis, and vas deferens
   c. a testis, vas deferens, and prostate gland
   d. a testis, vas deferens, and inguinal gland

4. Ovulation occurs at the midpoint of the menstrual cycle as a direct result of secretion of which hormone?
   a. estrogen
   b. progesterone
   c. GnRH
   d. LH

5. For which of the following functions is testosterone *not* responsible?
   a. spermatogenesis
   b. development of male sex organs
   c. neutralization of urethral and vaginal acidity during intercourse
   d. maintenance of secondary sex characteristics

6. The human sexual response pattern, as described by Masters and Johnson, involves
   a. orgasmic, plateau, resting, and resolution phases
   b. excitement, plateau, orgasmic, and resolution phases
   c. excitement, resting, resolution, and resting phases
   d. excitement, orgasmic, resolution, and resting phases

7. Breast examination through inspection and palpation should reveal any abnormalities. Which of the following findings would most strongly indicate breast cancer?
   a. slight asymmetry of breasts
   b. fixed, nodular breast mass with dimpling of overlying skin
   c. bloody discharge from nipple
   d. multiple firm, round, freely movable masses that change with the menstrual cycle

8. Estrogens are used as oral contraceptives, as postmenopausal replacement therapy, and to treat inoperable prostatic cancer. Which of the following is a possible serious adverse reaction of estrogen therapy?
   a. thromboembolism
   b. weight gain
   c. diarrhea
   d. peptic ulcer disease

9. Which of the following STDs are caused by viruses and therefore will not respond to antibiotics?
   a. trichomoniasis and gonorrhea
   b. LGV and chlamydial cervicitis
   c. condyloma acuminatum (genital warts) and molluscum contagiosum
   d. syphilis and chancroid

10. Patient teaching topics for women with PMS and other menstrual conditions would include all the following *except*
    a. keeping a diary of menstruation and related symptoms
    b. dosage schedule, side effects, and interactions of oral contraceptives
    c. relaxation techniques to relieve pain and tension
    d. complications of radiation therapy

11. When caring for a patient just admitted

with possible PID, the nurse could expect to see all the following assessment findings *except*

a. fever
b. low abdominal pain and tenderness
c. history of sexual activity with an infected partner or recent childbirth, abortion, or intrauterine procedure
d. positive RPR

12. Structural disorders of the uterus and vagina include displacement and prolapsed uterus and cystocele and rectocele. What medical treatment would be appropriate for such a disorder if surgery is contraindicated or refused?

a. radiation therapy
b. insertion of an intrauterine device (IUD)
c. bedrest
d. insertion of a pessary

13. One nursing intervention that can help decrease morbidity from gynecologic cancer is

a. teaching women the importance of yearly Pap smears
b. encouraging women to stop smoking
c. encouraging women to breast-feed
d. teaching women about contraception

14. Common causes of infertility include all the following *except*

a. STDs
b. displaced uterus
c. endometriosis
d. psychogenic causes

15. Although cancer of the penis is rare in the United States, a major etiologic factor in the cases that do occur is

a. frequent urinary tract infections
b. poor hygiene of the uncircumcised penis
c. circumcision
d. lack of sexual intercourse

16. Which of the following nursing interventions would *not* be appropriate for a patient with epididymitis?

a. Apply ice and elevate the scrotum to relieve pain.
b. Administer antibiotics to fight infection.
c. Encourage sexual activity to relieve pressure.
d. Encourage testing of sexual partners for STDs.

ANSWER KEY

1. **Correct response: a**
An X chromosome from each parent results in a female fetus (XX).
   b. An XY chromosome combination produces a male fetus.
   c and d. XXY results in a genetic defect, as does YYX.
Knowledge/Physiologic/NA

2. **Correct response: b**
The endometrium responds to hormonal stimulation, thickens during the proliferative phase, and sheds during the menstrual phase.
   a. The myometrium is the muscular uterine layer.
   c. A leiomyoma is a benign tumor of the myometrium.
   d. There is no mucous membrane in the uterus.
Comprehension/Physiologic/NA

3. **Correct response: b**
Each scrotal sac contains a testis, an epididymus, and a vas deferens.
   a, c, and d. The ejaculatory duct lies internally within the prostate gland, which lies below the bladder and surrounds the urethra. The inguinal canal separates the male pelvis from the abdominal cavity.
Knowledge/Physiologic/NA

4. **Correct response: d**
LH surges at midcycle, after estrogen levels have peaked and stimulated a buildup of the endometrium.
   a. Estrogen levels peak early in the cycle.
   b. Progesterone is secreted in large amounts from the corpus luteum (after ovulation) during the secretory phase.
   c. GnRH secretion increases early in the menstrual cycle as a result of low estrogen and progesterone levels.
Knowledge/Physiologic/NA

5. **Correct response: c**
Neutralization of urethral and vaginal acidity is accomplished through prostatic fluid secretion to enhance sperm performance during intercourse.
   a, b, and d. Testosterone is the primary male sex hormone that is responsible for spermatogenesis, development and maintenance of male sex organs, and secondary sex characteristics.
Comprehension/Physiologic/NA

6. **Correct response: b**
According to Masters and Johnson, the human sexual response pattern consists of the excitement, plateau, orgasmic, and resolution phases.
   a, c, and d. These answers are rearrangements of the phases; "resting" is a coined term.
Comprehension/Physiologic/NA

7. **Correct response: b**
A fixed nodular breast mass with dimpling of the overlying skin is a common late sign of breast cancer.
   a. Slight asymmetry of the breasts is often normal.
   c. Bloody discharge from the nipple occurs in intraductal papilloma, a benign condition.
   d. Multiple firm, round, freely movable masses that change in size with the menstrual cycle typically represent benign fibrocystic disease.
Application/Physiologic/Assessment

8. **Correct response: a**
Thromboembolism may result from prolonged estrogen therapy.
   b. Weight gain is an adverse reaction of estrogen but is not considered serious.
   c and d. Diarrhea and peptic ulcer disease are not caused by estrogen.
Application/Physiologic/Evaluation

314

9. Correct response: c
Genital herpes is also caused by a virus.
  a. Trichomoniasis is caused by a protozoa.
  b and d. Gonorrhea, LGV, chlamydial cervicitis, syphilis, and chancroid are caused by bacteria.
Comprehension/Physiologic/NA

10. Correct response: d
Radiation therapy is not used for PMS or menstrual disorders or their causes.
  a. Keeping a diary of menstruation and symptoms can help with diagnosis and treatment of menstrual disorders.
  b. Oral contraceptives are frequently used to treat menstrual disorders.
  c. Relaxation therapy may be helpful in pain relief.
Application/Health promotion/ Implementation

11. Correct response: d
A positive RPR is not an assessment finding in PID but rather in syphilis.
  a, b, and c. Fever; lower abdominal pain and tenderness; history of sexual activity with an infected partner; and recent child birth, abortion, or intrauterine procedure are all characteristic findings in PID.
Application/Physiologic/Assessment

12. Correct response: d
Insertion of a pessary can provide support to the uterus and vagina.
  a, b, and c. Radiation, insertion of an IUD, and bedrest are not appropriate therapies for structural disorders.
Comprehension/Physiologic/NA

13. Correct response: a
Annual Pap smears aid early detection of gynecologic cancer, enabling prompt treatment.
  b, c, and d. Although these responses are good nursing interventions, they will not result in decreased gynecologic cancer deaths.
Application/Health promotion/ Implementation

14. Correct response: d
Psychogenic causes will not prevent conception if sexual intercourse is taking place. A couple having trouble conceiving should be encouraged to seek medical evaluation.
  a, b, and c. STDs, displaced uterus, and endometriosis all can cause infertility.
Comprehension/Psychosocial/NA

15. Correct response: b
Poor hygiene of the uncircumcised penis is a major contributing factor to penile cancer.
  a, c, and d. Frequent urinary tract infections, circumcision, and lack of sexual intercourse do not lead to penile cancer.
Comprehension/Health promotion/NA

16. Correct response: c
Encouraging sexual activity will not relieve pressure and is not appropriate for epididymitis. It may be helpful with chronic prostatitis, however.
  a, b, and d. These interventions would be appropriate for a patient with epididymitis.
Application/Physiologic/Implementation

Immunologic Disorders

I. Anatomy and physiology

A. Immune system components

1. The *lymphatic system*—lymph nodes and vessels—performs several important functions, including:
   a. Transporting lymph
   b. Filtering and phagocytizing antigens
   c. Generating lymphocytes and monocytes
2. Major functions of the *spleen* include:
   a. Removing worn-out erythrocytes from blood
   b. Storing blood and platelets
   c. Filtering and purifying blood
3. The *liver* is involved in:
   a. Phagocytosis by Kupffer cells (macrophages)
   b. Filtering and purifying blood
4. The *hematopoietic system*—bone marrow and lymphatic tissue—produces blood cells, including those involved in immunologic

defense (leukocytes). Table 12–1 gives more information on types of leukocytes.

B. Immune mechanisms

   1. Defense: resisting infection
   2. Homeostasis: state of equilibrium of internal environment
   3. Surveillance: recognition of self versus nonself
   4. General immune responses include:
       a. Phagocytic: ingestion of foreign particles by white blood cells
       b. Humoral: formation of antibodies by plasma cells in response to foreign proteins
       c. Cellular: attack of microbes by special killer T cells formed from lymphocytes

C. Nonspecific immunologic defense

   1. This defense system provides the body's natural immunity.
   2. External defenses consist of physical and chemical barriers (e.g., intact skin and mucous membranes, enzymes in tears and saliva, acidic gastric juices) that prevent entrance of foreign substances (antigens) or immunogens.

TABLE 12–1.
Types of Leukocytes

CELL TYPE	NORMAL LEVEL	CHARACTERISTICS	FUNCTION
Granulocytes (polymorphonuclear leukocytes)	5000–10,000/mm³	Formed in bone marrow Granular (under microscope)	Immediate response to cellular injury
Neutrophils	50%–70% of all leukocytes	12-hr life span; 2–4 hr life span with infection	Phagocytic First cell to site of cellular injury Contain lysosomes
Eosinophils	2%–4% of all leukocytes		Weak phagocytes
Basophils	<1% of all leukocytes	Granules filled with heparin; histamine	
Agranulocytes		Produced in lymphatic system Nongranular (under microscope)	
Lymphocytes	25%–33% of all leukocytes	Classified as B cells or T cells	Phagocytosis Release of lymphokines Production of gamma globulins Cell-mediated reactions
Monocytes	4%–6% of all leukocytes	Circulate in blood but also settle in tissue where they are transformed into macrophages	Phagocytosis (can ingest larger particles than neutrophils; 5 times as many in 1 ingestion)

3. Internal defense systems, activated when antigens gain access to the internal environment, include phagocytosis by WBCs, inflammatory responses, and internal secretions (e.g., interferon).

D. **Specific immunologic defense**
1. *Active acquired immunity* involves production of antibodies and sensitized lymphocytes in response to an antigen or immunization.
2. Memory cells generated result in rapid immune response (defense) on reexposure to the antigen.
3. Adults require tetanus and diphtheria booster injection IM at least every 10 years; all health care workers should receive the hepatitis B vaccine.
4. *Passive acquired immunity* is a temporary immunity acquired by introduction of antibodies or sensitized lymphocytes from another source (e.g., antibodies through placental circulation to a fetus, gamma globulin, and antiserum from blood plasma of a person with acquired immunity); the body does not generate memory cells.
5. Both active and passive acquired immunity involve humoral (B-lymphocyte) and cellular (T-lymphocyte) immunity.

E. **Humoral immunity**
1. B lymphocytes (bursa derived) are involved in antibody (i.e., immunoglobulin) production.
2. Unsensitized B cells proliferate and mature into plasma cells after exposure to antigen.
3. Plasma cells differentiate into memory cells (which trigger B-cell response on subsequent exposure to same antigen) and antibodies.
4. Five types of antibodies are produced by the body:
   a. IgG (75% of total): activates complement, enhances phagocytosis, crosses placenta (passive immunity), active in second response (reinfection)
   b. IgA (15% of total): present in body fluids (blood, saliva, and tears; pulmonary, GI, prostatic, and vaginal secretions; and breast milk)
   c. IgM (10% of total): first antibody produced in the immune response; activates the complement system
   d. IgD (0.2% of total): role unclear; may be required on B-cell surface for transformation into plasma cells
   e. IgE (0.004% of total): associated with allergic and hypersensitivity reactions

F. **Cellular immunity**
1. T lymphocytes (thymus derived), on exposure to antigen, proliferate and differentiate into one of several types of T cells:

       a.   Helper T cells (T4): assist B cells in humoral response to form antibodies

       b.   Suppressor T cells (T8): suppress B-cell synthesis of antibody production via feedback mechanism

       c.   Memory T cells: store future immune response to some antigen

       d.   Cytotoxic T cells: directly attack antigen, thus altering cell membrane with resultant cells lysis; also release chemical mediators known as lymphokines (i.e., interferon, migration inhibitory factor), which can attract and hold macrophages and lymphocytes to the site of injury

  2. Cellular immunity functions primarily in:

      a.   Delayed hypersensitivity reactions

      b.   Rejection of transplants

      c.   Viral, fungal, and chronic infections

G. **Stages of cellular and humoral immunity**

  1. Recognition: Circulating lymphocytes and macrophages recognize foreign material or antigens as "nonself."

  2. Proliferation: Sensitized lymphocytes proliferate, differentiate, and mature into respective T and B cells.

  3. Response: Antibody is produced with specific T-cell action.

  4. Effector: Antigen is destroyed by antibody produced by B-cell or cytotoxic T-cell action.

H. **Complement**

  1. Complement is a group of at least 20 circulating plasma proteins, made in the liver, that are sequentially activated in the presence of an antigen.

  2. Functions include:

      a.   Cell lysis

      b.   Opsonization: making antigen more susceptible to phagocytosis

      c.   Chemotaxis: inducing phagocytes to antigen

      d.   Agglutination: clumping of antigens

      e.   Neutralization of viruses

      f.   Anaphylatoxin: stimulation of inflammatory response

  3. Activation of complement can occur in one of two basic ways:

      a.   Classical: antigen–antibody complex activates C1 (first of circulating complement proteins)

      b.   Alternate: no antigen–antibody complex required; can be initiated by release of endotoxins; begins with C3

I. **Hypersensitivity reactions**

  1. These reactions represent immune response to allergens that results in tissue destruction.

  2. In Type I (anaphylactic) reactions, mediated by IgE antibody, most cell degranulation occurs, resulting in release of histamine.

3. Commonly involved organs in Type I reactions include GI tract, skin, and lungs. Common causative agents include drugs (penicillin and cephalosporins), insect venoms, blood products, and iodinated contrast dye.

4. Type II (cytotoxic) reactions (e.g., hemolytic anemia) are mediated by IgG and IgM antibodies, which attach to self (usually circulating blood elements) and cause cell lysis.

5. Type III (immune complex) reactions (e.g., rheumatoid arthritis, Goodpasture's disease, serum sickness) are mediated by antigen–antibody complexes that deposit in the lining of blood vessels or on tissue surfaces.

6. Type IV (delayed hypersensitivity) reactions (e.g., contact dermatitis, transplant rejection) are mediated by lymphokines released from sensitized T-cell lymphocytes.

J. **Allergic disorders**

1. Interaction between antigen and antibody typically results in one or more manifestations of tissue injury.

2. Persons experiencing allergies are genetically predisposed to forming IgE antibodies.

3. Histamine and other mediators are released on reexposure to the allergen to which the person is sensitized.

K. **Autoimmune disorders**

1. In autoimmune disorders, the body no longer differentiates self from nonself.

2. Alterations in T cells or B cells produce autoantibodies and autosensitized T cells that cause tissue injury; these changes may involve one organ or many organ systems.

3. The cause remains unknown; many theories exist.

L. **Immune deficiency**

1. Immune deficiency is defined as a deficit in the immune system, either congenital or acquired, that makes the person susceptible to life-threatening opportunistic infection.

2. In congenital, or primary immunodeficiency, the body produces inadequate amounts of one or more immune cells. Deficits can be humoral (B cell), cell-mediated (T cell), or combined.

3. Acquired, or secondary, immunodeficiency is attributed to various etiologies, including:

   a. Immunosuppressive therapy: chemotherapeutic agents, corticosteroids, nonsteroidal antiinflammatory agents, irradiation

   b. Age: deterioration in thymus gland and T-cell functioning; decreased number of suppressor T cells and helper T cells

      c.   Disruption of skin integrity such as with burns and trauma

      d.   Nutritional deficits

      e.   Malignancies such as leukemia, lymphoma

      f.   Infectious processes such as sepsis and AIDS

    4.   Manifestations vary according to the part(s) of the immune system affected. Humoral deficit predisposes to bacterial infections; cell-mediated deficit, to viral, fungal, and protozoan infections.

II. Overview of immune disorders

A. Significant assessment findings

    1.   General

        a.   Overall health status

        b.   Recurrent infections

        c.   Seasonal symptoms

        d.   Weight loss

        e.   Fever

    2.   Integumentary system

        a.   Rashes

        b.   Lesions

    3.   Head

        a.   Eyes: itching, burning, watering, vision problems, infections

        b.   Ears: recurrent infections, drainage

        c.   Nose: rhinitis, sneezing

        d.   Mouth: oral lesions, infections, sore throat

    4.   Neck: adenopathy

    5.   Respiratory

        a.   Cough

        b.   Wheeze

        c.   Dyspnea

        d.   Recurrent infection

    6.   Cardiovascular

        a.   Palpitations

        b.   Pain

        c.   Raynaud's phenomenon

    7.   Gastrointestinal

        a.   Nausea

        b.   Vomiting

        c.   Diarrhea

    8.   Genitourinary

        a.   Recurrent infections

        b.   Dysuria

        c.   Hematuria

    9.   Musculoskeletal

        a.   Weakness

   b. Fatigue

   c. Joint pain

   d. Range of motion (ROM)

   e. Ability to perform activities of daily living (ADLs)

 10. Neurologic

   a. Orientation

   b. Level of consciousness

   c. Sensorium

   d. Paresthesias

 11. Lymphatic and hematologic

   a. Adenopathy

   b. Abnormal bleeding

B. **Important laboratory studies and diagnostic tests**

 1. T- and B-lymphocyte assays

 2. Immunoglobulin assays

 3. Radioallergosorbent test of IgE (RAST)

 4. Serum complement assays

 5. Autoantibody tests

   a. Antinuclear antibodies (ANA)

   b. Rheumatoid factor (RF)

 6. HIV (human immune virus) test

C. **Psychosocial implications**

 1. A patient with an immunologic problem may experience coping difficulties related to:

   a. The chronic, progressive nature of the disorder

   b. Debilitating disease effects

   c. Loss of friends and loved ones from the disease (e.g., from AIDS)

   d. Fear of dying

 2. The patient may express self-concept concerns related to fears of:

   a. Body image changes with disease progression

   b. Rejection

   c. Loss of outlets for sexual expression

   d. Role changes toward increased dependence

 3. The patient may need to adjust to lifestyle changes made necessary by altered:

   a. Physical capacity

   b. Self-care ability

   c. Work performance, with potential for job loss and economic insecurity

 4. Disease-related changes in social interaction patterns can lead to:

   a. Isolation

   b. Depression

        c.   Hopelessness

D. **Medications used to treat immune problems**
1. *Antihistamines* help relieve symptoms of allergic rhinitis and allergic dermatoses by inhibiting further histamine release; types include:
   a. Chlorpheniramine maleate (e.g., Chlor-Trimeton, Teldrin)
   b. Diphenhydramine hydrochloride (e.g., Benadryl)
   c. Terfenadine (Seldane)
2. Used to treat asthma and allergic rhinitis, *sympathomimetics* exert effects on beta 2 receptors, relaxing smooth bronchial muscle and dilating airways; agents include:
   a. Isoetharine hydrochloride (e.g., Bronkosol, Bronkometer)
   b. Metaproterenol sulfate (Alupent, Metaprel)
   c. Albuterol sulfate (e.g., Ventolin, Proventil)
   d. Terbutaline sulfate (Brethine, Bricanyl)
   e. Epinephrine (e.g., Bronkaid)
   f. Isoproterenol (e.g., Isuprel)
3. Used to treat asthma by relaxing bronchial smooth muscle, *xanthine derivatives* include:
   a. Aminophylline (e.g., Amoline)
   b. Anhydrous theophylline (Synophylate)
   c. Theophylline (e.g., Theo-dur, Theolair, Slo-Bid)
   d. Ephedrine (e.g., Bofedrol, Efedron)
4. *Corticosteroids* are used in follow-up treatment of severe immune or inflammatory reactions; agents include:
   a. Hydrocortisone (e.g., Solu-Cortef)
   b. Methylprednisolone (e.g., Solu-Medrol)
   c. Dexamethasone (e.g., Decadron)
   d. Prednisone (e.g., Deltasone)
   e. Prednisolone (e.g., Delta-Cortef)
   f. Beclomethasone dipropionate (e.g., Vanceril, Beclovent)
5. *Cromolyn sodium* (e.g., Intal) is administered as prophylactic therapy for asthma.
6. Used to treat anaphylaxis, *vasopressors* rapidly restore blood pressure; agents include:
   a. Norepinephrine bitartrate (Levophed)
   b. Metaraminol bitartrate (Aramine)
7. *Salicylates* (aspirin) are administered to reduce inflammation and pain in rheumatoid arthritis and LE.
8. *Nonsteroidal antiinflammatory drugs (NSAIDs)* also can reduce inflammation and pain in rheumatoid arthritis and LE; agents include:
   a. Ibuprofen (e.g., Motrin, Advil)

      b.   Indomethacin (e.g., Indocin)

      c.   Meclofenamate (Meclomen)

      d.   Naproxen (Naprosyn)

  9.   Administered to treat primary humoral immunosufficiency, immunoglobulin (Gamimune N) supplies a broad spectrum of IgG antibodies to protect against infection.

  10.   *Antimicrobial* agents used in the treatment of AIDS and AIDS-related infections (e.g., *Pneumocystis* pneumonia) include:

      a.   Azidothymidine (AZT), an antiviral agent that inhibits HIV reproduction in cells

      b.   Trimethoprim-sulfamethoxazole (TMP/SMZ), an antibacterial

III. Allergic rhinitis (hay fever)

A. Description: an allergic reaction to inhaled airborne allergens, characterized by seasonal occurrences

B. Etiology and incidence

  1.   The most common form of respiratory allergy, hay fever most commonly is induced by airborne pollens.

  2.   Common seasonal pollens include:

      a.   Spring: tree pollens (e.g., oak, maple, birch)

      b.   Summer: grass pollens (e.g., sheep sorrel, plantain)

      c.   Fall: weed pollens (e.g., ragweed)

  3.   Incidence occurs in all age groups but is especially high in children and adolescents.

C. Pathophysiology

  1.   Allergic rhinitis occurs when IgE antibodies in the nasal mucosa combine with inhaled allergens on the mucosal surface.

  2.   The resultant cell injury causes typical symptoms—sneezing, itching, and runny nose.

D. Assessment findings

  1.   Common clinical manifestations include:

      a.   Itching, burning nasal mucosa

      b.   Copious mucous secretions causing runny nose

      c.   Red, burning, tearing eyes

      d.   Sneezing

      e.   Pale, boggy nasal mucosa

  2.   The patient may have a family history of allergies.

  3.   Laboratory studies may reveal:

      a.   Eosinophils in nasal secretions

      b.   Lymphocyte count above $1200/\mu L$

      c.   Elevated serum IgE

      d.   Offending allergens identified by skin testing

E. Nursing diagnoses

  1.   Ineffective Airway Clearance

  2.   Knowledge Deficit

3. Sleep Pattern Disturbance

F. Planning and implementation

   1. Obtain a comprehensive patient history to try to determine the causative agent.

   2. Administer antihistamines, sympathomimetics, and antipruritics as prescribed.

   3. Administer immunotherapy as prescribed.

G. Evaluation

   1. The patient exhibits relief of symptoms.

   2. The patient verbalizes understanding of the allergic reaction, its prevention, and treatment.

   3. The patient complies with the prescribed medication regimen.

IV. Allergic dermatoses

A. Description: a group of inflammatory conditions caused by skin reaction to irritating or allergenic materials; includes allergic contact dermatitis and atopic dermatitis

B. Etiology

   1. Many substances can produce allergic contact dermatitis; common causes include exposure to poison ivy, topical medications, cosmetics, soaps, and industrial chemicals.

   2. The cause of atopic dermatitis is unknown, but it appears to be associated with a family history of allergic respiratory disorders (e.g., allergic rhinitis, asthma). Exacerbating factors appear to include irritants, infection, and certain allergens.

C. Pathophysiology

   1. Allergic contact dermatitis involves delayed hypersensitivity and requires a latent period ranging from several days (for strong sensitizers such as poison ivy) to years.

   2. Although atopic dermatitis may appear at any age, it most commonly begins in infancy or early childhood. It may subside spontaneously, to be followed by unpredictable exacerbations throughout life.

D. Assessment findings

   1. Common clinical manifestations include:

      a. Burning, itching, swelling, and erythema of skin

      b. Crusting, weeping lesions

   2. Health history may reveal known or suspected exposure to an allergen.

   3. The extent of rash depends on the type of allergen exposure; may be local or generalized.

   4. Diagnosis may be made on the basis of skin eruptions and history of allergen exposure.

E. Nursing diagnoses

   1. High Risk for Infection

   2. Knowledge Deficit

        3. Pain

        4. Self-Esteem Disturbance

        5. Impaired Skin Integrity

F. Planning and implementation

    1. Provide symptomatic relief with antihistamines, antipruritics, or steroid creams as prescribed.

    2. Provide patient and family teaching, covering:

        a. Basic pathophysiology of allergic reactions

        b. Methods to minimize exposure to offending allergens

        c. Comfort measures for symptomatic relief

        d. Stress-reduction measures

        e. Prescribed medications, including purpose, effects, dosage, administration, and possible side effects

G. Evaluation

    1. The patient displays clear skin free of rash, itching, burning, infection.

    2. The patient verbalizes understanding of the allergic reaction, its prevention, and treatment.

    3. The patient complies with the prescribed therapeutic regimen.

V. Asthma

A. Description: a chronic reactive respiratory disorder producing episodic, reversible airway obstruction

B. Etiology and incidence

    1. Allergic asthma results from an immunologically mediated hypersensitivity to inhaled allergens such as airborne pollens and molds, dust, and animal danders.

    2. Incidence is estimated at 3% to 8% of the population, with more than half the cases occurring in children under age 10.

C. Pathophysiology

    1. Although the pathologic mechanisms of allergic asthma remain somewhat unclear, the fundamental process presumably involves a reaction of sensitized IgE antibodies to an inhaled allergen, with subsequent release of chemical mediators such as histamine, slow-reacting substance of anaphylaxis (SRS-A), and eosinophil chemotactic factor of anaphylaxis (ECF-A).

    2. Obstruction results from constriction of bronchial smooth muscle, swelling of bronchial membranes, and hypersecretion of mucus.

D. Assessment findings

    1. Clinical manifestations of asthma include:

        a. Chest tightness

        b. Prolonged, strenuous expirations

        c. Wheezing on expiration

        d. Cyanosis

        e. Cough, nonproductive at first, followed by violent

coughing that produces thin, gelatinous mucus and is relieved by an aerosol bronchodilator

    f.   Nausea and vomiting

    g.   Anxiety

2.   Health history may reveal exposure to a known or suspected precipitating substance.

3.   Pulmonary function studies reveal airway obstruction and decreased peak expiratory flow rate.

4.   Radiologic or bronchoscopic examination may be needed to rule out other causes of bronchial obstruction.

5.   Arterial blood gas (ABG) analysis typically reveals:

    a.   Decreased PaO_2

    b.   Initially, decreased $PaCO_2$ and increased pH

    c.   Later, increased $PaCO_2$ and decreased pH

E.   Nursing diagnoses

1.   Ineffective Airway Clearance

2.   Fear

3.   Knowledge Deficit

F.   Planning and implementation

1.   Intervene immediately to relieve respiratory distress as needed.

2.   Administer bronchodilators or adrenergics as prescribed.

3.   Administer oxygen as prescribed.

4.   Elevate the head of the bed, and lean the patient forward to provide maximum lung expansion and ease respiratory effort.

5.   Monitor respiratory rate and depth, and auscultate lung sounds.

6.   Monitor ABGs to detect any changes from baseline.

7.   Provide reassurance and emotional support to help relieve anxiety.

8.   Monitor for and take precautions to prevent complications, such as:

    a.   Pneumothorax

    b.   Pulmonary hypertension

    c.   Right heart failure

    d.   Respiratory failure

9.   Provide adequate hydration to decrease viscosity of secretions.

10.   Promote adequate rest to increase respiratory efficiency.

11.   Provide patient and family teaching, covering:

    a.   Basic pathophysiology of disease process, treatment, and prevention of further exacerbations

    b.   Importance of strict compliance with the therapeutic regimen

    c.   Purpose, effects, dosage, administration, side effects, and interactions of all prescribed medications

    d.   Signs and symptoms of complications to watch for and report

  e. The need for increased fluid intake to thin bronchial secretions

  f. Activities allowed and discouraged

  g. Stress reduction methods

  h. The importance of follow-up care to monitor progress

 G. **Evaluation**

  1. The patient displays relief of respiratory distress: absence of chest tightness, wheezing, cyanosis, cough, exaggerated expiratory effort.

  2. The patient uses appropriate coping mechanisms to control anxiety.

  3. The patient and family verbalize understanding of the disease process, prevention of acute asthma attacks, and treatment.

  4. The patient complies with the prescribed therapeutic regimen.

VI. **Anaphylaxis**

 A. **Description: an acute, life-threatening allergic reaction marked by rapidly progressive urticaria and respiratory distress**

 B. **Etiology**

  1. Anaphylaxis results from ingestion or other systemic exposure to allergenic substances.

  2. Possible causative substances include:

   a. Drugs, such as penicillin and other antibiotics, vaccines, hormones, salicylates, and local anesthetics

   b. Foods (e.g., legumes, nuts, berries, seafood, and egg albumin)

   c. Sulfite-containing food additives

   d. Insect venom (e.g., wasp, hornet, honeybee, certain spiders)

 C. **Pathophysiology**

  1. Anaphylactic reaction requires previous sensitization to the triggering allergen, with production of specific IgE antibodies that bind to mast cells and basophils.

  2. On reexposure, IgE reacts immediately with the allergen and triggers release of potent chemical mediators (histamine, ECF-A) from basophils and mast cells.

  3. Concurrently, IgG or IgM activates release of complement fractions, and two other chemical mediators—bradykinin and leukotrienes—trigger profound vascular changes that can lead to vascular collapse.

  4. Anaphylaxis is considered a medical emergency because of the possibility of respiratory obstruction and vascular collapse. In severe cases, death may occur as quickly as 5 to 10 minutes after onset of reaction.

 D. **Assessment findings**

  1. Clinical manifestations depend on whether mediators remain local or are systemic.

      2.   Local effects include wheals with surrounding red flares and urticaria; usually not dangerous.

      3.   Systemic manifestations involve:

          a.   Intense urticaria and edema at the site of injection or injury, rapidly spreading to the face, hands, and other body areas

          b.   Respiratory distress from bronchospasm, coughing, sneezing, wheezing

          c.   Dysrhythmias, tachycardia or bradycardia, hypotension, and signs of circulatory collapse

          d.   Nausea and vomiting, abdominal pain, diarrhea

E. **Nursing diagnoses**

      1.   Altered Cardiac Output: Decreased

      2.   Fear

      3.   Impaired Gas Exchange

F. **Planning and implementation**

      1.   Treat an anaphylactic attack as a medical emergency.

      2.   Maintain an open airway.

      3.   Administer IM epinephrine per protocol.

      4.   Administer oxygen as indicated.

      5.   Prepare to assist with emergency tracheostomy if necessary.

      6.   Monitor vital functions, evaluating:

          a.   Blood pressure, pulse, respirations

          b.   ABG values

          c.   ECG

          d.   Urine output

      7.   Establish a patent IV line for rapid drug and fluid administration.

      8.   Administer antihistamines, epinephrine, corticosteroids, or vasopressors as prescribed.

      9.   Administer fluid replacement and volume expanders as prescribed.

   10.   After an acute episode, promote rest and continue monitoring vital signs.

   11.   Provide patient and family teaching, covering:

          a.   Basic pathophysiology of reaction and preventive measures

          b.   Identification and elimination of offending allergens

          c.   Importance of informing others of allergies, such as by wearing a Medic-alert bracelet

          d.   The use of commercial "antisting" kits, if applicable

G. **Evaluation**

      1.   The patient demonstrates relief of respiratory distress: absence of bronchospasm, wheezing, dyspnea.

      2.   The patient maintains a regular pulse with a rate of 60 to 100 beats per minute.

3. The patient exhibits no edema.
4. The patient verbalizes understanding of anaphylactic allergic reaction, prevention of recurrence, treatment of early signs and symptoms, and when to seek help.

VII. Rheumatoid arthritis

A. **Description: a chronic, progressive disease involving inflammation of synovial joints**

B. **Etiology and incidence**

1. Etiology is unknown although it apparently is an autoimmune disorder; exacerbations may be associated with increased physical or emotional stress.
2. Incidence is three times greater in women than in men. Peak age of onset is between age 30 and 60 although the disease can develop at any age.

C. **Pathophysiology**

1. Pathologic changes begin as inflammation and progress to destruction of joints, producing deformity and loss of motion.
2. The disease may affect only joints or may extend to body organs and blood vessels.

D. **Assessment findings**

1. Common clinical manifestations include:
   a. Swollen, warm, tender joints
   b. Limited ROM in affected joints
   c. Generalized edema or nodules around affected joints
   d. Impaired mobility and ability to perform ADLs
   e. Fatigue, weakness, anorexia
   f. In later stages, weight loss, fever, anemia, muscle atrophy, Sjögren's syndrome
2. Laboratory and diagnostic findings may include:
   a. Radiographic abnormalities: progressive joint damage
   b. Increased immunoglobulin levels, increased complement levels
   c. Increased RF titer
   d. Increased erythrocyte sedimentation rate (ESR)

E. **Nursing diagnoses**

1. Knowledge Deficit
2. Impaired Physical Mobility
3. Altered Nutrition: Less Than Body Requirements
4. Self-Esteem Disturbance

F. **Planning and implementation**

1. Direct care at relieving pain, maintaining function, and preventing deformities.
2. Promote adequate rest; pay attention to maintaining proper body alignment and preventing contractures.

3. Administer salicylates, NSAIDS, or corticosteroids as prescribed

4. Apply hot or cold to affected joints according to the patient's needs.
5. After the acute phase resolves, begin physical therapy.
6. Provide patient teaching, covering:
    a. Basic pathophysiology of disease process and causes of exacerbation
    b. Importance of an activity program for self-care
    c. Principles of joint conservation and energy conservation
    d. Importance of maintaining optimum nutritional status
    e. Purpose, effects, dosage, administration, side effects, and interactions of all prescribed medications
    f. The need for follow-up care to monitor progress

G. Evaluation
1. The patient maintains independence in ADLs.
2. The patient verbalizes relief of joint pain and discomfort.
3. The patient maintains adequate nutrition.
4. The patient maintains adequate muscle strength and ROM.
5. The patient verbalizes understanding of the disease process, measures to prevent further decrease in function and movement, and prescribed medical treatments.
6. The patient complies with the prescribed medical regimen.

VIII. LE

A. Description
1. Systemic lupus erythematosus (SLE): a chronic systemic inflammatory disease affecting multiple body systems
2. Discoid lupus erythematosus (DLE): a form of lupus affecting the skin only

B. Etiology and incidence
1. SLE and DLE are thought to be autoimmune disorders.
2. SLE is the most common of the two; incidence is approximately 75 in 1 million people, with women affected at least 8 times more often than men and women of childbearing age particularly susceptible.

C. Pathophysiology
1. SLE involves markedly increased B-cell activity, hypergammaglobulinemia, autoantibody production, and decreased T-cell functions.
2. Symptoms result from immune complex invasion of body systems.
3. Disease progression is widely variable, characterized by recurring remissions and exacerbations.
4. Approximately 5% of patients with DLE develop SLE.

5. Prognosis is good with early detection and treatment; however, SLE can lead to potentially serious complications, including cardiovascular, renal, and neurologic problems and severe bacterial infections.

D. Assessment findings

1. Clinical manifestations of SLE vary depending on the organs affected.
2. Early signs and symptoms may include:
    a. Fatigue, weakness
    b. Anorexia
    c. Occasional fever
    d. Joint stiffness
    e. Skin rash
3. Disease progression typically produces:
    a. Characteristic "butterfly" rash on face
    b. Skin eruptions on trunk or extremities
    c. Alopecia
    d. Photosensitivity
4. Associated manifestations may include:
    a. Raynaud's phenomenon
    b. Arthritis and deformity
    c. Polymyositis, peripheral vasculitis with hypertension
    d. Pericarditis, pericardial effusion
    e. Renal failure
    f. Nausea, vomiting, abdominal pain
    g. Signs and symptoms of pneumonitis, pleuritis, chronic obstructive pulmonary disease, interstitial fibrosis
    h. Psychosis, convulsions
5. DLE is marked by characteristic raised, red, scaling plaques, most commonly on the face, scalp, ears, neck, and other parts of the body exposed to sunlight.
6. Laboratory studies may reveal:
    a. Anemia, thrombocytopenia, leukocytosis, or leukopenia
    b. LE cells in blood
    c. Positive anti-Sm and anti-DNA cell tests
    d. Proteinuria, cellular casts in urine
    e. False-positive rapid plasma reagin (RPR) test
    f. Increased ANA

E. Nursing diagnoses

1. Body Image Disturbance
2. Ineffective Breathing Pattern
3. Decreased Cardiac Output
4. Ineffective Individual Coping

5. High Risk for Fluid Volume Deficit
6. Altered Nutrition: Less Than Body Requirements
7. Pain
8. Altered Role Performance
9. Self-Esteem Disturbance
10. Sensory and Perceptual Alterations
11. Impaired Skin Integrity

F. Planning and implementation
1. Aim treatment at reducing the inflammatory process.
2. Administer salicylates, NSAIDs, and steroids as prescribed.
3. Keep skin clean and dry; apply topical ointments as prescribed.
4. Inspect the skin for vasculitic lesions.
5. Provide meticulous mouth care.
6. Promote frequent rest periods to decrease fatigue.
7. Convey empathy and reassurance to the patient and support persons.
8. Arrange for a dietary consult to ensure optimal nutrition while meeting the patient's need for soft, easily tolerated foods.
9. Relieve joint pain and stiffness by applying warm packs as needed.
10. Maintain mobility and strength by instituting an appropriate exercise program.
11. Provide patient teaching, covering:
    a. Basic pathophysiology of the disease and its progression
    b. Purpose, effects, dosage, administration, side effects, and interactions of all prescribed medications
    c. Importance of follow-up care and of monitoring for and reporting new symptoms
    d. The need to consult a physician before receiving immunizations or taking birth control pills or over-the-counter drugs
    e. Recommended and prohibited activities
    f. Necessary lifestyle changes, such as avoiding sun and ultraviolet light exposure
    g. Available community support groups

G. Evaluation
1. The patient reports relief from joint pain and discomfort.
2. The patient displays clean, dry skin with little or no itching, scaling, infections, or ulcerations.
3. The patient reports acceptable energy level with minimal weakness and fatigue.
4. The patient demonstrates adequate nutritional status.
5. The patient verbalizes understanding of the disease process, prevention of infection, and treatment of exacerbations.

IX. Progressive systemic sclerosis (PSS)

A. Description: a diffuse connective tissue disorder characterized by fibrotic and degenerative changes of muscles, skin, joints, and viscera

B. Etiology and incidence

1. The etiology of PSS remains unclear although it likely is an autoimmune disorder.

2. PSS is relatively rare; women are affected two to three times more often than men, especially between ages 30 and 50.

C. Pathophysiology

1. The basic process in PSS appears to be vascular endothelial cell injury.

2. Intimal damage in capillaries and small arteries produces increased vascular permeability, tissue edema, and eventually, vessel occlusion and tissue ischemia.

3. Fibroblast proliferation, with resultant increased collagen production, causes fibrotic changes with progressive thickening and hardening of connective tissue throughout the body.

4. Prognosis is poor; approximately 30% of affected persons die within 5 years of diagnosis.

D. Assessment findings

1. Common clinical manifestations include:

a. Joint pain and stiffness, eventually immobility

b. Muscle weakness

c. Tense, wrinkle-free, hard appearing skin

d. Dyspnea, dysphagia

e. Digestive disturbances

f. Raynaud's phenomenon

g. Renal failure

h. Telangiectasis

2. Laboratory studies may reveal:

a. Increased serum ANA

b. Fibrotic changes in major body organs

c. Calcium deposits in tissues

E. Nursing diagnoses: the same as for LE (see Section VIII.E)

F. Planning and implementation

1. See LE, Section VIII.F, for applicable nursing interventions.

2. Avoid administering antiinflammatory agents, which generally are not helpful in a patient with PSS.

G. Evaluation: the same as for LE (see Section VIII.G)

X. Hypogammaglobulinemia

A. Description: primary humoral immunodeficiency marked by inadequate gamma globulin in the blood and associated with decreased resistance to infection

B. Etiology and incidence

1. X-linked hypogammaglobulinemia is a congenital disorder inherited via a gene located on the X chromosome.

2. The disorder affects male infants almost exclusively; incidence is about one in 50,000 to 100,000 births.

3. Unlike the X-linked form, acquired hypogammaglobulinemia is of unknown etiology, typically appears between ages 15 and 35, and affects males and females about equally.

C. Pathophysiology

1. In X-linked infantile hypogammaglobulinemia, B cells and B-cell precursors in the bone marrow and blood fail, for some unknown reason, to mature and secrete immunoglobulin.

2. In acquired hypogammaglobulinemia, most patients have a normal circulating B-cell count but deficient immunoglobulin synthesis or release.

D. Assessment findings

1. Manifestations of hypogammaglobulinemia include:

   a. Severe, recurrent bacterial infections; acute in X linked, chronic in acquired

   b. Possibly signs and symptoms of associated SLE, rheumatoid arthritis, or vasculitis

2. Laboratory and diagnostic tests may reveal:

   a. Low or absent IgG, IgA, IgM, IgE, IgD

   b. Deficiency of B lymphocytes in congenital disease, no plasma cells in acquired disease

   c. Depleted B-cell germinal centers seen on lymph node biopsy

E. Nursing diagnosis: High Risk for Infection

F. Planning and implementation

1. Prevent and treat bacterial infection as indicated.

2. Administer gamma globulin per protocol.

3. Administer antibiotics as prescribed.

4. While the patient is hospitalized, provide protective isolation to guard against nosocomial infections.

5. Provide patient teaching, covering:

   a. Basic pathophysiology of immune deficiency

   b. Recognition and prevention of bacterial infections

   c. Signs and symptoms for which to seek medical assistance

   d. Purpose, effect, dosage, administration, side effects, and interactions of all prescribed medications

   e. The need for continued medical follow-up

G. Evaluation

1. The patient demonstrates decreased incidence of recurrent bacterial infections.

2. The patient verbalizes understanding of the disorder, infection prevention, and treatment.

3. The patient complies with the therapeutic regimen.

XI. Primary IgA deficiency

    A. Description: a primary humoral immunodeficiency of IgA

    B. Etiology and incidence

        1. IgA deficiency seems to involve autosomal dominant or recessive inheritance.

        2. It is the most common immunoglobulin deficiency, with incidence as high as one in 800 persons.

    C. Pathophysiology

        1. The primary mechanism in IgA deficiency appears to be abnormal terminal differentiation of IgA-bearing B cells.

        2. Usually a benign disorder, IgA deficiency has been associated with increased incidence of:

            a. Bacterial infections

            b. Coexisting autoimmune disorders (e.g., SLE, rheumatoid arthritis)

            c. Allergic disorders (e.g., asthma, allergic rhinitis)

            d. Increased susceptibility to cancer

    D. Assessment findings

        1. Many patients remain asymptomatic throughout a normal lifespan.

        2. Possible manifestations include:

            a. Chronic respiratory infection

            b. Respiratory allergy

            c. GI disorders (e.g., celiac disease, ulcerative colitis)

            d. Signs and symptoms of autoimmune disorders

            e. Signs and symptoms of malignant tumors (e.g., squamous cell carcinoma of the lungs, thymoma)

        3. Laboratory tests typically reveal:

            a. Low IgA level (<5 mg/dL)

            b. Normal IgG level

            c. Normal or elevated IgM level

    E. Nursing diagnosis: High Risk for Infection

    F. Planning and implementation

        1. See the sections of this text covering specific allergic disorders or autoimmune disorders as applicable.

        2. Administer antibiotics as prescribed.

        3. Determine any known allergies before administering any medication or applying lotions, soaps, or creams.

        4. Provide patient teaching, covering:

            a. Basic pathophysiology of immune deficiency and associated autoimmune disorders

            b. Ways to avoid exposure to allergens

            c. How to recognize and prevent bacterial infections

            d. Signs and symptoms to watch for and report

            e. Purpose, effects, dosage, method of administration, side effects, and interactions of all prescribed medications

      f.   The importance of follow-up care
      g. The increased susceptibility to anaphylaxis associated with blood transfusions
      h. Early cancer detection measures

G. **Evaluation**
    1. The patient remains free of bacterial infection.
    2. The patient verbalizes understanding of the disorder, infection prevention, and treatment.
    3. The patient complies with the therapeutic regimen.

XII. SCID

A. **Description: a disorder characterized by total or near-total absence of both cellular and humoral immunity**

B. **Etiology and incidence**
    1. SCID usually is transmitted as an autosomal recessive trait although it may be X linked.
    2. Estimated incidence is 1 in 100,000 to 500,000 births; males are affected more often than females.

C. **Pathophysiology**
    1. In SCID, primary T-cell and B-cell immune deficiency results from defects in precursor T- and B-stem cells.
    2. The affected infant is susceptible to infection from all types of microorganisms; most untreated infants die from infection before age 1 year.

D. **Assessment findings**
    1. Clinical manifestations may include:
      a. Recurrent infections
      b. Failure to thrive (many infants die before diagnosis made)
      c. Chronic diarrhea
      d. Recurrent oral yeast infections
      e. Persistent otitis media
      f. Sepsis
      g. Severe reactions to vaccinations
    2. Laboratory findings may reveal:
      a. Very low levels of T and B lymphocytes
      b. Decreased or absent antibodies
      c. Low blood group antigen titers
      d. No response to antigenic stimulation

E. **Nursing diagnoses**
    1. High Risk for Infection
    2. Anticipatory Grieving

F. **Planning and implementation**
    1. Provide comfort measures.
    2. Provide protective isolation to prevent infection.
    3. Monitor vital signs.

4. Administer antimicrobials as prescribed.
5. Provide emotional support to the infant's parents.
6. Refer the parents to support groups or pastoral care as necessary.
7. Prepare the patient and family for possible bone marrow transplantation.
8. Teach the parents about:
    a. Basic pathophysiology and disease process
    b. Purpose, effects, dosage, administration, side effects, and interactions of all prescribed medications
    c. Measures for prevention and early detection of opportunistic infection
    d. The importance of follow-up care
    e. Names and locations of available support groups

   G. **Evaluation**
1. The patient remains free of recurrent infections.
2. The patient attains normal growth milestones.
3. The parents verbalize understanding of the disorder, infection prevention, and treatment.
4. The patient and parents comply with the therapeutic regimen.
5. Parents proceed normally through the grieving process.

XIII. AIDS
   A. **Description: severe immunodeficiency caused by the human immunodeficiency virus (HIV), which allows normally benign organisms to flourish and cause disease**
   B. **Etiology and incidence**
1. HIV is primarily a sexually transmitted virus, but it also can be contracted through direct contact with blood or blood products.
2. Persons at risk for contracting HIV include:
    a. Homosexual or bisexual men
    b. Hemophiliacs and other recipients of transfused blood or blood components
    c. Intravenous drug abusers
    d. Heterosexual partners of persons with AIDS
    e. Children (perinatally) of mothers with HIV

   C. **Pathophysiology**
1. HIV can be isolated from blood, semen, saliva, tears, breast milk, and cerebrospinal fluid.
2. After infection, the incubation period of HIV ranges from 6 months to 5 years, with an average of 2 years.
3. The clinical spectrum of AIDs encompasses:
    a. Persons who are HIV-seropositive and asymptomatic
    b. Persons with AIDS-related complex (ARC)
    c. Persons with AIDS who suffer from opportunistic diseases

4. To date, no cure has been found; approximately 75% of patients die within 2 years of diagnosis.

D. Assessment findings

1. Health history findings may include recurring viral and bacterial infections.
2. Clinical manifestations may include:
   a. Fatigue
   b. Fever, night sweats
   c. Weight loss
   d. Generalized lymphadenopathy
   e. Nonproductive cough, shortness of breath
   f. Skin lesions, dry skin, pallor
   g. GI upset, chronic diarrhea
   h. Edema
   i. Visual impairment
   j. Painful oral lesions
   k. Bruising and bleeding tendencies
   l. Joint pain
3. Laboratory studies may reveal presence of HIV in serum.
4. Associated conditions may include:
   a. Opportunistic infections, such as *Pneumocystis carinii* pneumonia, mycobacterial infections, cryptococcus, toxoplasmosis, histoplasmosis, and cytomegalovirus
   b. Kaposi's sarcoma, AIDS-related lymphoma
   c. Neurologic deficits
   d. HIV wasting syndrome

E. Nursing diagnoses

1. Activity Intolerance
2. Ineffective Airway Clearance
3. Ineffective Individual Coping
4. Ineffective Family Coping
5. Diarrhea
6. Fear
7. High Risk for Fluid Volume Deficit
8. Impaired Gas Exchange
9. Anticipatory Grieving
10. Altered Nutrition: Less Than Body Requirements
11. Pain
12. Self-Care Deficit
13. Self-Esteem Disturbance
14. Impaired Skin Integrity
15. Social Isolation

F. Planning and implementation

1. Direct care toward maintaining optimal health and preventing complications.

2. Use appropriate precautions to protect yourself from exposure to the patient's blood or body fluids.
3. Monitor vital signs, ECG tracings, other vital functions as necessary.
4. Monitor respiratory functions: lung sounds, skin color, respiratory effort, sputum production.
5. Administer oxygen as prescribed.
6. Position the patient to maximize lung expansion.
7. Administer antibiotics, narcotics, antianxiety agents, or antipyretics as prescribed.
8. Monitor and record daily weight and intake and output.
9. Promote increased fluid intake; maintain IV fluid infusion if necessary.
10. Promote good nutrition; provide preferred foods, maintain tube feeding if necessary.
11. Administer antiemetics and antidiarrheals as requested.
12. Keep the patient's skin clean and dry.
13. Turn or reposition the patient every 2 hours; provide an antipressure mattress as necessary.
14. Apply protective barriers to the skin as necessary.
15. Help the patient maintain as normal an environment as possible while hospitalized (e.g., pictures and personal items from home in the room).
16. Allow the patient adequate time to visit with family, friends, and other support persons; encourage open communication of feelings and fears.
17. Promote a balanced schedule of sleep, rest, and activity.
18. Provide for psychologic and spiritual counseling as requested.
19. Support the patient and support persons throughout the grieving process.
20. Teach the patient and support persons about:
    a. Basic pathophysiology and progression of disease
    b. Purpose, effects, dosage, administration method, and side effects of all prescribed medications
    c. Principles of nutrition and the importance of maintaining optimal nutrition high in protein and calories
    d. Good hygiene practices and their importance
    e. Prevention and early detection of opportunistic infection
    f. Methods to prevent spread of HIV to others
    g. Signs and symptoms to report to the physician
    h. The importance of follow-up care
    i. Names and locations of local AIDS support groups

G. Evaluation
1. The patient remains free of opportunistic infection and respiratory problems.

2. The patient exhibits relief of symptoms such as fatigue, fever, night sweats, weight loss, diarrhea.
3. The patient maintains skin and oral mucosa integrity.
4. The patient maintains adequate nutritional status and fluid and electrolyte balance.
5. The patient reports relief of pain and discomfort, joint pain, nausea, abdominal pain.
6. The patient maintains an acceptable activity level without undue fatigue.
7. The patient exhibits decreased anxiety.
8. The patient and family members or significant others verbalize understanding of the disease process, infection prevention measures, and treatments.
9. The patient and family members or significant others progress through the grieving process.
10. The patient and family members or significant others demonstrate appropriate coping mechanisms and use of support systems.
11. The patient and family members or significant others verbalize acceptance of imminent death.
12. The patient complies with the therapeutic regimen, including precautions to prevent disease transmission.

Bibliography

Brunner, L. S., & Suddarth, D. S. (1988). *Textbook of medical-surgical nursing* (6th ed.). Philadelphia: J. B. Lippincott.

Brunner, L. S., & Suddarth D. S. (1986). *The Lippincott manual of nursing practice* (4th ed.). Philadelphia: J. B. Lippincott.

Cotran, R. S., Kumar, V., & Robbins, S. L. (1989). *Robbins pathologic basis of disease* (4th ed.). Philadelphia: W. B. Saunders.

Flaskerud, J. H. (ed.) (1989). *AIDS/HIV infection: A reference guide for nursing professionals*. Philadelphia: W. B. Saunders.

Guyton, A. C. (1986). *Human physiology and mechanisms of disease* (3rd ed.). Philadelphia: W.B. Saunders.

Hood, G. H., & Dincher, J. R. (1988). *Total patient care: Foundations and practice* (7th ed.). St. Louis: C. V. Mosby.

Kinney, M. R., Packa, D. R., & Dunbar, S.B. (eds.) (1988). *AACN's clinical reference for critical-care nursing*. New York: McGraw-Hill.

Kneisl, C. R., & Ames, S. W. (eds.) (1986). *Adult health nursing: A biopsychosocial approach*. Reading, MA: Addison-Wesley.

Lewis, S. M., & Collier, I. C. (eds.) (1987). *Medical-surgical nursing: Assessment and management of clinical problems* (2nd ed.). New York: McGraw-Hill.

Luckman, J., & Sorenson, K. C. (1987). *Medical-surgical nursing: A psychophysiologic approach* (3rd ed.). Philadelphia: W. B. Saunders.

Sodeman, W. A., & Sodeman, T. M. (1985). *Sodeman's pathologic physiology mechanisms of disease* (7th ed.). Philadelphia: W. B. Saunders.

STUDY QUESTIONS

1. Anaphylaxis is mediated by
   a. IgG
   b. IgM
   c. IgA
   d. IgE

2. Mr. Matthews, aged 27, has been diagnosed with AIDS. After a long period of declining health, he is now hospitalized with *Pneumocystis carinii* pneumonia. As the nurse brings his breakfast one morning, Mr. Matthews starts crying, stating that he has lost most of his friends and his family won't talk to him anymore. Which of the following would be the nurse's best action?
   a. Help him with his tray, and tell him not to worry.
   b. Ask the physician for a psychiatric consult to assess Mr. Matthews' mental functioning.
   c. Sit down and listen to him voice his concerns and frustrations.
   d. Tell him that his friends probably weren't true friends anyway if they would abandon him like this.

3. The Dunn's young son, Jason, has primary IgA deficiency. During his appointment for follow-up of bacterial pneumonia, the nurse notices that they have missed three previously scheduled appointments. In talking to them, the nurse discovers that they aren't sure of what is wrong with Jason and what the implications for his care are. The nurse spends extra time with the parents, gives them pamphlets, and plans to speak with them later in the day (since their son must be hospitalized for his infection). After several sessions with them, which of the following actions by the parents would best demonstrate that the nurse's interventions have been successful?
   a. The Dunns state that they have no questions about Jason's care.
   b. The Dunns bring Jason to the clinic the next time he exhibits signs and symptoms of bacterial infection.

   c. The Dunns call at least twice weekly to report on Jason's progress and ask questions.
   d. The Dunns bring Jason to the clinic regularly and, although Jason continues to get infections, they are detected early and he requires no hospitalization.

4. Mrs. Hunt, a 68-year-old woman with rheumatoid arthritis, complains that her joints always hurt and that she "just feels like staying in bed all day." In planning a program for her to maintain as much function as possible, the nurse should include all the following *except*
   a. refraining from exercise since it only aggravates the disease process
   b. applying heat or cold to increase her pain threshold
   c. alternating rest with periods of activity to maintain mobility
   d. promoting in-water exercises to enhance joint mobility

5. When caring for a patient with hypogammaglobulinemia, the nurse should anticipate preparing the patient for which of the following diagnostic tests?
   a. erythrocyte sedimentation rate
   b. antinuclear antibodies (ANA)
   c. lymph node biopsy
   d. skin biopsy for Kaposi's sarcoma

6. Ms. White, aged 19, has just been started on immunotherapy for allergies. Shortly after the first injection, the nurse notes a large red wheal on her arm, coughing, and expiratory wheezing—pointing to an anaphylactic reaction to the injection. What should the nurse do first?
   a. Notify the physician of what is happening.
   b. Administer IM epinephrine per protocol for anaphylaxis.
   c. Begin oxygen by way of nasal cannula.
   d. Start an IV for medication administration.

7. Mr. Lester, aged 34, is hospitalized for AIDS treatment. He has refused visitors for the past week and communicates with staff only when asked a direct question. Conversations with Mr. Lester reveal that his knowledge of AIDS transmission is based on myths and unfounded fears. Accordingly, the nursing care plan is directed at providing accurate information and promoting open communication. Evaluation criteria reflecting successful achievement of these outcomes would include all the following *except*
   a. The patient verbalizes feelings of acceptance and a nonjudgmental attitude from staff.
   b. The patient openly discusses feelings and concerns.
   c. The patient verbalizes the intention of decreasing the risk of AIDS transmission by decreasing contact with others.
   d. The patient verbalizes understanding that AIDS cannot be transmitted through merely touching another person.

8. Mrs. Boyle, aged 56, has been admitted for treatment of complications of SLE. Which of the following nursing diagnoses would most likely apply to Mrs. Boyle?
   a. Functional Incontinence
   b. Impaired Swallowing
   c. Urinary Retention
   d. Altered Tissue Perfusion: Renal

9. When caring for Ms. Summers, a 32-year-old woman with AIDS, the nurse assists the physician with inserting a central line for administration of medications and parenteral nutrition. To protect herself from contaminated blood and body fluids during this procedure, the nurse should
   a. wear mask, gloves, goggles, and a gown or apron
   b. wear gown and gloves
   c. wear mask, gloves, and a gown or apron
   d. wear mask and gloves

10. Ms. Hargrove, aged 39, has hypogammaglobulinemia and is scheduled for elective surgery to repair a ventral hernia. Which of the following would be an important nursing diagnosis for directing this patient's care during hospitalization?
    a. Fatigue
    b. High Risk for Fluid Volume Deficit
    c. High Risk for Infection
    d. Decreased Cardiac Output

11. Amy Sutton, aged 9, was stung by a bee on the hand 1 hour ago and now exhibits redness and swelling in the hand and forearm. When providing care to Amy, the nurse should be sure to explain that
    a. Baking soda is the best treatment for a bee sting.
    b. Amy may be hypersensitive to bee stings, and her parents might consider purchasing a bee sting kit.
    c. She shouldn't worry; people can't develop an allergy to bee stings.
    d. She should have have regular check-ups to determine the status of her allergy to bee stings.

12. The nurse is about to administer cefaclor to Brian, a 2-year-old with primary IgA deficiency who has otitis media. Before administration, the nurse should check
    a. Brian's chest radiograph
    b. Brian's history of previous illness
    c. Brian's history for any known allergies to medications
    d. Brian's chart for any other current infections

13. Mr. Bishop, aged 29, states that he has been suffering from runny nose, itching and burning eyes, and sneezing for the past 3 weeks. Nursing assessment reveals that he had his sister visit him for 8 days about 3 weeks ago and that she brought her cat with her. These findings and his symptoms are consistent with
    a. allergic rhinitis
    b. viral cold
    c. bronchitis
    d. asthma

14. Mr. Rogers, a 24-year-old with AIDS, has been hospitalized with enterocolitis and has had chronic diarrhea for the last year. His weight is 130 lb, and he has lost 18 lb in 6 months. His skin is pale and with poor turgor, his mucous membranes are dry, and he is listless. Although the nurse should be concerned about his weight loss, a more immediate problem would be described by the nursing diagnosis
    a. Fluid Volume Deficit related to diarrhea and abnormal fluid loss
    b. Altered Nutrition: Less Than Body Requirements
    c. Altered Thought Processes related to CNS effects of disease
    d. Diarrhea related to disease process and acute infection

15. Because Mr. Rogers has had chronic diarrhea, anorexia, and a history of oral candidiasis and has lost weight, the nurse will want to include teaching on nutrition in the discharge plan. This dietary teaching should focus on

    a. eating a low-protein, high-carbohydrate diet
    b. eating three large meals per day
    c. eating only unpasteurized dairy products
    d. eating a high-protein, high-calorie diet

16. Jenny Davidson, an 8-month-old infant with severe combined immune deficiency (SCID), was admitted with diarrhea and generalized weakness. On initial assessment, the nurse observes that her perineal area is red and excoriated and her skin and mucous membranes are dry. Criteria to evaluate nursing care for this patient would include all the following *except*
    a. The patient displays no evidence of skin breakdown or infections.
    b. The patient exhibits signs of adequate hydration.
    c. The patient maintains stools of normal pattern, color, and consistency.
    d. The patient reduces fluid intake.

ANSWER KEY

1. **Correct response: d**
   IgE is associated with allergic and hyper-sensitivity reactions.
   a and b. IgG and IgM in Type II are associated with cytotoxic reactions.
   c. IgA is present in body fluids such as blood, saliva, and tears.
   Knowledge/Physiologic/Assessment

2. **Correct response: c**
   Mr. Matthews is beginning to express his concerns to the nurse; active, non-judgmental listening can help build a relationship of trust. The other choices are inappropriate.
   a. Providing false reassurance will not help the patient cope.
   b. Further assessment is needed to determine whether a psychiatric consult should be considered.
   d. Discounting his feelings and giving advice would hinder development of a therapeutic relationship.
   Comprehension/Psychosocial/Implementation

3. **Correct response: d**
   Jason is receiving follow-up care, and his infections are caught early, indicating that his parents understand his disease process.
   a. Not asking questions does not necessarily indicate understanding.
   b. Bringing Jason in only after he develops another bout of pneumonia may indicate that the parents still don't understand the importance of early detection and prevention of infection.
   c. Constant questions could indicate the need for further explanation.
   Analysis/Health promotion/Evaluation

4. **Correct response: a**
   Persons with rheumatoid arthritis should maintain an active exercise program to strengthen and preserve muscle movement.
   b. Heat or cold applications can help relieve pain.

   c. Just as with exercise, adequate rest is essential for the arthritic patient.
   d. Water exercises are excellent because the buoyancy allows for easier joint movement.
   Application/Safe care/Planning

5. **Correct response: c**
   A lymph node biopsy will show depleted B-cell germinal centers in hypo-gammaglobulinemia.
   a. ESR is used to detect inflammatory processes.
   b. ANA are measured to detect autoimmune disease.
   d. Kaposi's sarcoma is usually associated with AIDS.
   Knowledge/Physiologic/Assessment

6. **Correct response: b**
   Immediately give 0.2 to 0.5 mL of 1:1000 epinephrine IM.
   a, c, and d. These other interventions will follow.
   Comprehension/Physiologic/Implementation

7. **Correct response: c**
   From the information given, it would appear that the patient is already socially isolated; decreasing contact is not necessary and would cause further isolation.
   a, b, and d. These criteria would be appropriate.
   Analysis/Psychosocial/Evaluation

8. **Correct response: d**
   Decreased renal perfusion (as well as GI and peripheral perfusion) is often present due to vasculitis.
   a and b. Although problems associated with SLE commonly affect renal function, neither urinary retention nor incontinence typically occurs.
   c. Impaired swallowing is associated with other diseases (e.g., myasthenia gravis), not with SLE.
   Comprehension/Physiologic/Analysis (Dx)

9. **Correct response: c**
   Although this is an invasive procedure,

it is not likely to generate droplets or blood splashes; thus, protective goggles may be advisable but not necessary.

a, b, and d. The other precautions are considered necessary.

Application/Safe care/Implementation

10. **Correct response: c**

A patient with hypogammaglobulinemia is at increased risk for nosocomial infections while hospitalized and therefore should be in protective isolation.

a, b, and d. These other diagnoses would not be expected for this surgery nor specifically for this patient.

Application/Health promotion/Analysis (Dx)

11. **Correct response: b**

This patient has experienced a moderate reaction to the bee sting. She may be hypersensitive and should have access to a bee sting kit in the event she should be stung again.

a, c, and d. These interventions are all inappropriate.

Application/Health promotion/Planning

12. **Correct response: c**

For a patient with primary IgA deficiency, it is important to identify any allergies before administering medications.

a, b, and d. Chest radiograph and history of illness or infection are irrelevant to medication administration.

Application/Safe care/Implementation

13. **Correct response: a**

This patient most likely is suffering from allergic rhinitis triggered by his sister's cat.

b. A cold would not produce such symptoms for 3 weeks.

c and d. Bronchitis and asthma produce symptoms in the lower respiratory tract.

Application/Physiologic/Assessment

14. **Correct response: a**

This patient's most pressing problem is dehydration due to the diarrhea.

b, c, and d. These other problems, although they may occur, are of lower priority than dehydration.

Analysis/Health promotion/Analysis (Dx)

15. **Correct response: d**

Teaching should include this in addition to small, frequent meals and low-microbial foods (e.g., pasteurized dairy products, washed and peeled fruits and vegetables, and well-cooked meats).

a, b, and c. These instructions are all inappropriate for this patient.

Analysis/Physiologic/Planning

16. **Correct response: d**

Major nursing diagnoses for this patient would likely include Diarrhea, Altered Skin Integrity, and Fluid Volume Deficit with outcomes as given. Reducing fluid intake would be contraindicated.

a, b, and c. All of these evaluation criteria would be appropriate for this patient.

Analysis/Safe care/Evaluation

Integumentary Disorders

13

Note: This chapter does not discuss all disorders with significant skin involvement. Refer to the appropriate chapters in this text for information on the following skin disorders:

► Candidiasis: Chapter 20, Infectious Disorders
► Pressure sores: Chapter 22, Gerontologic Nursing

I. Anatomy and physiology

A. Structure

1. The body's largest organ, the skin comprises three layers:
   a. Subcutaneous layer, or hypodermis
   b. Dermis
   c. Epidermis
2. Subcutaneous layer
   a. Consisting of loose connective tissue and fat cells, the hypodermis anchors the skin to bone and muscle.
   b. It also provides shock absorbing and insulating actions.
   c. Anatomic distribution of this layer is a secondary sex characteristic, different in women and men.
3. Dermis
   a. The layer beneath the epidermis, the dermis primarily comprises collagen fibrils, which provide mechanical strength to the skin.
   b. The dermis also contains blood vessels, nerves, lymphatics, hair follicles, and sebaceous and sweat glands.
4. Epidermis
   a. This thin, avascular outermost layer of skin is nourished by diffusion from blood vessels in the dermis.
   b. The epidermis contains two main types of cells: melanocytes and keratinocytes.
   c. Scattered throughout the basal layer of the epidermis, *melanocytes* produce melanin, a pigment that shields deeper skin structures from sunlight. People of all races have basically the same number of melanocytes; differences in skin color are due to differences in the size and distribution of melanosomes produced by melanocytes.
   d. *Keratinocytes* develop from cells in the basal layer, then mature and move to the skin surface (stratum corneum), where they flatten, dehydrate, and become keratinized. Alterations in this process account for many dermatologic problems.
5. Epidermal appendages, formed from epidermal cells anatomically located in both the epidermis and dermis, include:
   a. Hair
   b. Nails

    c.   Glands (apocrine, eccrine, sebaceous)

6. Hair
   a. Hair growth occurs in phases: resting phase (telogen), growth phase (anagen), atrophy phase (catagen).
   b. Scattered patterns of these phases keep the total number of hairs relatively constant.
   c. Chemical, mechanical, or physiologic factors can convert all hair to atrophy phase, resulting in baldness.
   d. Hair follicles are distributed on all skin surfaces except on the palms and soles.
   e. No new hair-producing structures are produced after birth.
   f. Scalp hair grows about 1 cm per month.

7. Nails grow from nail matrix; they comprise a specialized keratin that becomes dry and firm

8. Apocrine glands
   a. Located in the axillae, areolae, groin, perineum, and circumanal and periumbilical regions, these large sweat glands are rudimentary structures with no known useful purpose.
   b. They respond to autonomic, rather than thermal, stimulation to produce odorless, viscous, milklike droplets that cause a distinctive body odor when acted on by the bacteria normally present on the skin surface.

9. Eccrine glands
   a. These small sweat glands, distributed in the skin all over the body, are true secretory glands that produce sweat, which functions in thermoregulation and other processes.
   b. Sweat is a clear aqueous solution containing 99% water and 1% solids. Hypotonic under normal conditions, a high rate of sweating may produce isotonic concentrations.
   c. Sweat moves to the skin surface by way of sweat ducts.
   d. Nerve fibers to sweat glands liberate acetylcholine. Atropine and other anticholinergics block receptor sites from responding, interfering with secretion.
   e. At environmental temperatures above 32°C, sweating occurs over the entire body; at lower environmental temperatures, sweat glands periodically secrete microscopic droplets as part of the body's total insensible water loss.
   f. Sweat provides the skin with an "acid mantle" (average pH 5.7 to 6.4); acidity retards growth of many bacteria that reside in the epidermal layer, glands, and hair follicles.

10. Sebaceous glands
    a. Most prevalent and largest on the face, scalp, upper chest, and back (and absent from the palms and soles), sebaceous glands secrete sebum, a complex lipid mixture that empties into hair shafts.
    b. The male hormone androgen initiates and sustains sebum production.

B. Function
1. Protective functions
    a. The skin forms a barrier between the internal organs and the external environment.
    b. It is continuous with mucous membranes at external openings of the digestive, respiratory, and genitourinary systems.
    c. The normally acidic skin and perspiration protect against invasion by bacteria and foreign matter.
    d. The thickened skin of the palms and soles provides a tough covering to protect from the constant trauma to these areas.
2. Percutaneous absorption
    a. The epidermis is relatively impermeable to most chemical substances although various lipids (fatty substances) may be absorbed through the skin (e.g., vitamins A and D and steroid hormones).
    b. Substances enter through the epidermis (transepidermal route) or through orifices of hair follicles (follicular holes).
    c. Lipid-soluble substances absorb through the skin fairly rapidly and completely; absorption appears to be faster for substances that also are water soluble.
    d. The rate of absorption is comparable to that for substances in the GI tract or injected subcutaneously.
    e. Pharmacologic application of this absorption is currently the subject of intense research and development since certain drugs (e.g., dimethyl sulfoxide) are chemically linked with substances known to penetrate the skin.
3. Sensory functions
    a. Receptor endings of nerves in the skin provide constant monitoring of the immediate environment.
    b. The primary functions of these receptors include sensing coldness, warmth, pain, and touch pressure.
    c. Each type of receptor nerve ending responds to only one kind of cutaneous sensation.
    d. The density of receptors varies in different body areas (e.g., the fingertips and lips are high-density areas compared to the back).

e. The skin contains various types of sensory endings:
    (1) Naked nerve endings, which mediate all four sensory modalities
    (2) Free nonmyelinated nerve endings, which mediate pain sensation
    (3) Expanded tips on sensory nerve terminals, which mediate touch (Merkel's disks) and warmth (Tuffini endings)
    (4) Encapsulated nerve endings, which mediate pressure (Pacinian corpuscles), touch (Meissner's corpuscles), and cold (Krause's end-bulbs)

4. Vitamin D production
    a. Endogenous production of vitamin D, necessary for the synthesis of vitamin D critical to bone metabolism, occurs in the epidermis.
    b. Only a few minutes of sun exposure on a small body area are needed for this production to occur.

5. Barrier function
    a. The skin prevents water and electrolyte loss and moistens subcutaneous tissues.
    b. Small amounts of water—approximately 500 mL/day in adults, varying with body and environmental temperatures—continuously evaporate from the skin surface as insensible perspiration.
    c. During immersion in water, the skin can accumulate up to three to four times its weight in water.
    d. The skin surface normally is covered with microorganisms, especially bacteria such as *Staphylococcus epidermis* and diphtheroids; infection occurs when the balance between host and microorganisms is upset.
    e. Healthy persons can develop bacterial skin infections, but predisposing factors such as moisture, obesity, skin disease, systemic steroids and antibiotics, chronic disease, and diabetes mellitus increase risk.

6. Thermoregulatory functions
    a. The body continuously produces heat as a by-product of cellular metabolism; this heat is dissipated locally, primarily through the skin.
    b. Three primary processes are involved in heat loss from the body to the external environment:
        (1) Radiation: the body's ability to give off its heat to another object of lower temperature situated at a distance
        (2) Conduction: transfer of heat from the body to a cooler object in direct contact
        (3) Convection: heat transferred by conduction to the air surrounding the body removed by bulk

movement of warm air molecules away from the body

c. The body's internal core body temperature normally is maintained at a constant 37.6°C through a balance between heat production and heat loss.

d. The rate of heat loss depends primarily on the skin's surface temperature, which in turn depends on skin blood flow, regulated by neural mechanisms. Increased blood flow results in delivery of more heat to the skin and a greater rate of heat loss from the body; when body temperature falls, the skin's blood vessels constrict to reduce heat loss from the body.

e. Perspiration facilitates heat loss from the body; it is regulated by body temperature, environmental temperature and humidity, and neurologic factors such as response to emotional stress.

7. Immunologic functions

a. Wheal and flare reaction

(1) This reaction involves a combination of swelling (wheal) and diffuse redness due to increased temperature in area from stimulus; dependent on local neurologic mechanisms; dilation of arterioles and venules (flare) constitutes normal reaction to injury

(2) Wheal caused by increased capillary permeability induced by trauma as protein-containing fluid leaks out of capillaries locally to produce edema

(3) Reaction associated with release of histamine, bradykinin

b. Immune complexes

(1) Major deposition sites of immune complexes include the dermal–epidermal junction and dermal vessels of the skin.

(2) Deposition of immune complexes leads to fixation and activation of complement at tissue sites.

(3) Vasodilation and increased permeability result from anaphylatoxin components of C3 and C5; neutrophils and monocytes attracted by complement-generated chemotactic factors result in acute and perhaps chronic inflammation.

8. Circulatory function

a. Changes in the cutaneous vascular system contribute significantly to systemic circulatory status.

b. Skin color depends in part on the quantity of blood in the small vessels; skin temperature depends chiefly on the rate of blood flow through the skin.

       c.   Stimulation of sympathetic fibers supplying the skin causes vasoconstriction of cutaneous vessels; interruption of these fibers results in vasodilation of small arteries and arterioles.

       d.   The cutaneous circulatory system also responds to chemical agents, such as:

          (1)   Acetylcholine, which causes vasodilation

          (2)   Norepinephrine, epinephrine, and vasopressin, which cause vasoconstriction

    9.   Esthetic function

       a.   The skin also contributes to each person's unique appearance and identity.

       b.   Skin defects or problems can have negative effects on a person's body image and self-esteem.

II. Overview of integumentary system disorders

A. Assessment

    1.   Nursing health history should focus on obtaining information about:

       a.   Normal hygienic practices

       b.   Usual patterns of sun exposure

       c.   Exposure to irritants

       d.   Radiation exposure

       e.   Allergies

       f.   Nutritional status, especially intake of protein and vitamins A, B complex, C, and K

    2.   Important aspects of physical examination include:

       a.   Assessing skin color, texture, and turgor

       b.   Inspecting the skin for abnormal growths, lesions, rashes, scars, or discoloration

       c.   Noting any areas of scaliness or dryness

       d.   Inspecting for signs of skin infection

B. Diagnostic procedures

    1.   Skin cultures and microscopic examination can identify infectious organisms.

    2.   Skin biopsy and histologic examination is done for cancer diagnosis.

C. Psychosocial implications

    1.   A person with a serious skin disorder may have coping difficulties related to:

       a.   Short- and long-term skin disruptions

       b.   Chronicity of the disorder (e.g., burns)

       c.   Unknown prognosis (e.g., malignancies)

    2.   The patient may have self-concept concerns related to fear of:

       a.   Body image changes

       b.   Rejection by others

       c.   Loss of a body part

        d.   Role changes toward increased dependence

   3. The patient also may have lifestyle concerns related to potential changes in:

        a.   Physical ability

        b.   Work performance, with possibility of job loss

        c.   Self-care ability

   4. Disease-related changes in social interaction patterns can lead to such problems as:

        a.   Isolation

        b.   Depression

        c.   Hopelessness

D. **Medications used to treat skin problems**

   1. *Systemic antibiotics* used to treat bacterial infections (pyodermas) include penicillin and cloxacillin.

   2. *Acyclovir* (e.g., Zovirax) is used in herpes zoster to reduce pain and slow disease progression.

   3. *Topical antifungals*, used to treat fungal skin infections, include:

        a.   Miconazole (e.g., Monistat-Derm)

        b.   Clotrimazole (e.g., Lotrimin)

        c.   Griseofulvin (e.g., Fulvicin)

        d.   Ketoconazole (e.g., Nizoral)

        e.   Tolnaftate (e.g., Tinactin)

   4. *Scabicides*, such as Lindane (e.g., Kwell), are used to treat scabies and pediculosis; they are absorbed directly into skin parasites.

   5. *Topical agents* used to treat psoriasis include anthralin (e.g., Anthra-Derm).

   6. *Cytotoxic agents* used to treat unresponsive psoriasis include methotrexate.

   7. *Corticosteroids*, such as prednisone (e.g., Deltasone), are administered in pemphigus vulgaris to control disease and reduce skin blisters.

III. Seborrheic dermatitis

A. **Description: a chronic, inflammatory, scaling eruption characterized by periodic remissions and exacerbations**

B. **Etiology and incidence**

   1. Seborrheic dermatitis is associated with genetic predisposition and aggravated by physical or emotional stress.

   2. It most commonly develops in middle-aged or older people as multiple lesions occurring chiefly on the scalp, face, or trunk.

C. **Pathophysiology**

   1. Seborrhea refers to excessive production of sebum by sebaceous glands.

   2. The typical clinical picture involves lifelong recurrences persisting for weeks, months, or even years.

D. Assessment findings
1. Common clinical manifestations include:
   a. Scaling (dry, moist, or greasy), predominantly in areas where glands are normally found in large numbers (e.g., trunk, face, scalp) and in skin folds
   b. Patches of sallow, greasy-appearing skin with or without scaling and slight erythema
   c. Pruritus and pain
2. Diagnosis must rule out psoriasis.

E. Nursing diagnoses
1. Body Image Disturbance
2. Pain
3. Impaired Skin Integrity

F. Planning and implementation
1. Remove any external irritants.
2. Instruct the patient to avoid excessive heat and perspiration.
3. Tell the patient to avoid scratching and rubbing affected areas.

G. Evaluation: Patient demonstrates absence of symptoms.

IV. Noninfectious inflammatory dermatoses

A. Description
1. Psoriasis: a chronic inflammatory disease marked by epidermal proliferation
2. Exfoliative dermatitis: a serious skin disorder characterized by progressive inflammation
3. Pemphigus vulgaris: a serous autoimmune skin disease marked by blisters on the skin and mucous membranes
4. Toxic epidermal necrolysis (TEN): a rare, potentially fatal skin disorder marked by epidermal erythema, necrosis, and skin erosions

B. Etiology and incidence
1. Psoriasis appears to be a hereditary defect. It affects about 2% of the population in the United States; incidence is highest in whites.
2. The many possible causes of exfoliative dermatitis include:
   a. A secondary or reactive response to an underlying skin disease
   b. Lymphoma disease (may accompany or precede lymphoma)
   c. Severe reaction to a wide number of drugs (e.g., sulfonamides, penicillins, anticonvulsants, analgesics)
3. Pemphigus vulgaris is an autoimmune disorder of unknown etiology.
4. The etiology of TEN is unknown but is probably related to immune function, as a reaction to drug ingestion or possibly secondary to viral infection.

C. **Assessment findings**
1. Psoriasis is marked by:
   a. Profuse erythematous scales or plaques, often covering large areas of the body
   b. Pruritus and sometimes pain
   c. Possibly arthritic symptoms (e.g., joint stiffness)
2. Manifestations of exfoliative dermatitis include:
   a. Skin effects: patchy or generalized erythematous eruption (initially), followed by characteristic scaling, possibly with hair loss and nail shedding
   b. Systemic effects: possible severe fluid and electrolyte imbalance, anemia, systemic infections
3. Pemphigus vulgaris produces:
   a. Widespread bullae on the skin and mucous membranes that enlarge and rupture, leaving denuded areas that eventually form crusts
   b. Possible fluid and electrolyte imbalance, systemic infection, or impaired nutrition, which may lead to critical illness requiring frequent hospitalization
4. Manifestations of TEN include:
   a. Formation of large, flaccid bullae in some areas with shedding of large sheets of epidermis (along with toenails, fingernails, eyebrows, and eyelashes) in others
   b. Possibly serious fluid and electrolyte imbalance and systemic infection that may lead to sepsis

D. **Nursing diagnoses**
1. Body Image Disturbance
2. High Risk for Fluid Volume Deficit
3. High Risk for Infection
4. Knowledge Deficit
5. Impaired Actual Skin Integrity

E. **Planning and implementation**
1. Take steps to promote healing and prevent infection.
2. Relieve pain as indicated.
3. Maintain or restore fluid and electrolyte imbalance as appropriate.
4. Teach the patient about:
   a. The nature of the disorder, its treatment, and prognosis
   b. Use of prescribed medications (e.g., topical steroids)
5. Prepare the patient for prescribed treatments, which may include:
   a. Systemic cytotoxic therapy, oral retinoids, or photochemotherapy (psoriasis)
   b. Systemic corticosteroids and antibiotics (exfoliative dermatitis)

c.   Systemic corticosteroids, immunosuppressive agents, plasmapheresis (pemphigus vulgaris)
d.   High-dose systemic corticosteroids, antibiotics, silver nitrate compresses (TEN)

F.   Evaluation
1.   The patient remains free of acute infection.
2.   The patient exhibits intact or only minimally disrupted skin integrity.
3.   The patient experiences fewer episodes of exacerbation.
4.   The patient demonstrates adequate fluid balance.
5.   The patient exhibits healthy adaptation to body image changes.

V.   Acne vulgaris

A.   Description: an inflammatory disease of the sebaceous follicles
B.   Etiology and incidence
1.   Etiology appears to involve multiple factors, including:
   a.   Genetics
   b.   Hormonal factors
   c.   Bacterial infection
2.   Contrary to popular belief, diet does not affect incidence or severity.
3.   Incidence is highest at puberty although it may occur as early as age 8 and persist into adulthood in some people.

C.   Pathophysiology
1.   Acne eruptions are initiated by increased sebum production activated by androgenic hormones.
2.   Sebum is secreted into dilated hair follicles containing normal skin bacteria, such as *Propionibacterium acnes*.
3.   The bacteria secrete the enzyme lipase, which reacts with sebum to produce free fatty acids, which in turn trigger inflammation.
4.   At the same time, keratin produced by the hair follicles combines with sebum to form plugs in dilated follicles.

D.   Assessment findings
1.   Acne lesions may include:
   a.   Closed comedones (whiteheads)
   b.   Open comedones (blackheads)
   c.   Papules
   d.   Pustules
   e.   Nodules
   f.   Cysts
2.   Primary sites include the face, chest, shoulders, and upper back.

E.   Nursing diagnoses
1.   Body Image Disturbance

      2. High Risk for Infection

      3. Impaired Skin Integrity

  F. **Planning and implementation**

      1. Encourage compliance with the prescribed topical therapy, which may include:

         a. Benzoyl peroxide

         b. Vitamin A acid

         c. Topical or systemic antibiotics (e.g. tetracycline)

      2. Advise the patient that heat, humidity, and perspiration exacerbate acne.

  G. **Evaluation**

      1. The patient exhibits resolution of acne lesions.

      2. The patient remains free of infection.

VI. Bacterial infections (pyodermas)

  A. **Description and etiology**

      1. Impetigo: superficial skin infection caused by streptococci, staphylococci, or multiple bacteria; especially common in children living in poor hygienic conditions

      2. Folliculitis: staphylococcal infection arising in hair follicles

      3. Furuncle (boil): acute inflammation arising deep in one or more hair follicles and spreading into surrounding dermis

      4. Carbuncle: abscess of skin and subcutaneous tissue representing extension of a large, deep-seated furuncle that has invaded several follicles

  B. **Assessment findings**

      1. Impetigo begins as small, red maculas and rapidly progresses to discrete, thin-walled vesicles; these vesicles rupture and become covered with a loosely adherent, honey-yellow crust.

      2. Folliculitis produces single or multiple, superficial or deep papules or pustules close to hair follicles.

      3. A furuncle is marked by tenderness, pain, surrounding cellulitis, and after the furuncle localizes, a boggy center with a yellow or white head on the skin surface.

      4. A carbuncle is marked by skin abscess along with such systemic symptoms as fever, pain, prostration, and leukocytosis.

  C. **Nursing diagnoses**

      1. High Risk for Infection

      2. Impaired Skin Integrity

      3. Pain

  D. **Planning and implementation**

      1. Administer systemic antibiotics as prescribed.

      2. Isolate drainage in severe cases of folliculitis, furuncles, or carbuncles.

  E. **Evaluation**

      1. The patient reports reduction of pain.

    2. The patient remains free of infection.

    3. The patient exhibits return to intact skin without inflammation.

VII. Herpes zoster (shingles)

  A. Description: an acute viral infection marked by painful vesicular skin eruptions

  B. Etiology and incidence

    1. Herpes zoster is caused by the varicella-zoster virus (V-Z), which also causes varicella (chicken pox).

    2. Herpes zoster results from reactivation of latent V-Z virus that has lain dormant since a previous episode of varicella. The cause of reactivation is unknown.

    3. Incidence is greatest in adults older than age 50.

  C. Assessment findings

    1. Herpes zoster is marked by painful vesicular eruptions along the route of inflamed nerves from one or more posterior ganglia.

    2. Eruption is preceded and accompanied by pain, which may radiate over entire region supplied by involved nerves.

  D. Nursing diagnoses

    1. Pain

    2. Impaired Skin Integrity

  E. Planning and implementation

    1. Control pain with appropriate medications, and reduce itching with medications and topical lotions.

    2. Administer acyclovir systemically as prescribed.

  F. Evaluation

    1. The patient reports absence of pain.

    2. The patient displays intact skin without vesicular eruption.

VIII. Parasitic skin diseases

  A. Description and etiology

    1. Pediculosis—infestation by lice—involves three different parasites:

      a. *Pediculus humanus capitis* (head louse)

      b. *Pediculus humanus corporis* (body louse)

      c. *Phthirus pubis* (pubic or crab louse)

    2. Scabies involves infestation by the itch mite, *Sarcoptes scabiei*.

  B. Pathophysiology

    1. Lice live on the host's skin surface and depend on the host for nourishment, feeding on human blood approximately five times daily.

    2. They inject their digestive juices and excrement into the host's skin, and lay their eggs (nits) on hair shafts.

    3. Adult itch mites burrow into the superficial layer of skin and lay two to three eggs daily for up to 2 months.

      4.   Eggs hatch in 3 to 4 days; clinical symptoms are related to a sensitivity reaction as larvae emerge to the skin surface.

C. **Assessment findings**

    1.   Manifestations of pediculosis include:

        a.   Itching

        b.   Excoriation from scratching

        c.   Possibly small red papules in infested areas

        d.   Tiny, gray-white nits on hair shafts

    2.   Scabies is marked by:

        a.   Severe itching

        b.   Excoriated lesions possibly appearing as erythematous nodules

        c.   Possibly secondary bacterial infection

D. **Nursing diagnoses**

    1.   Knowledge Deficit

    2.   Pain

    3.   Impaired Skin Integrity

    4.   Social Isolation

E. **Planning and implementation**

    1.   Teach the patient with lice (or a parent if the patient is a child) to shampoo with Kwell soap and remove nits with a fine-tooth comb.

    2.   Instruct in using a scabicide, as prescribed, to kill scabies.

    3.   Teach precautions to help prevent future infestations.

F. **Evaluation**

    1.   The patient exhibits no sign of infestation.

    2.   The patient reports no discomfort.

    3.   The patient verbalizes important preventive measures to avoid reinfestation.

IX. **Skin cancer**

A. **Description and etiology**

    1.   Basal cell carcinoma: localized, slow-growing malignancy accounting for at least 75% of all skin cancers

    2.   Squamous cell carcinoma: a primary lesion commonly surrounded by satellite nodules; more malignant and more clearly defined than basal cell carcinoma; grows rapidly in weeks or months and metastasizes readily

    3.   Sweat gland carcinoma: a rare tumor usually occurring in the sixth and seventh decades of life but also reported in adolescents

    4.   Kaposi's sarcoma: commonly associated with human immunodeficiency virus although etiology and pathogenesis have not been resolved

    5.   Melanoma: a rare malignant lesion originating in melanoblasts of skin

B. **Assessment findings**
1. Features of basal cell carcinoma include:
   a. Waxy, grayish-yellow, darkly pigmented or pink lesions; firm, but not indurated
   b. Lesions occurring in almost any body area, with the head and neck the most common sites
   c. Few signs of inflammation
2. Squamous cell carcinoma, commonly occurring on the lip, in paranasal folds, or in the axilla, typically appears as an ulcerated nodule with an indurated base.
3. A sweat gland carcinoma appears as a soft tissue mass present for many years.
4. Kaposi's sarcoma usually starts on the hands or feet as multiple plaques; reddish to purple in color; and flat, ulcerated, or polypoid in shape. Lymph nodes also may be involved. In terminal stages, tumors extend to the mucous membranes and portions of the GI tract.
5. Melanoma may develop in any area of the skin or pigmented region of the eye and occurs in three types:
   a. Superficial spreading melanoma: small, elevated, multicolored nodules with irregular margins
   b. Nodular melanoma: typically a polypoidal, darkly pigmented nodule somewhat resembling a blackberry
   c. Lentigo meligna melanoma: large, flat, darkly pigmented area with irregular margins and scattered black nodules

C. **Nursing diagnoses**
1. Body Image Disturbance
2. Ineffective Individual Coping
3. Ineffective Family Coping: Compromised
4. Fear
5. Knowledge Deficit
6. Pain
7. Impaired Skin Integrity

D. **Planning and implementation**
1. Review the treatment plan with the patient and family or significant others; as indicated, discuss:
   a. Surgical excision with possible skin grafting
   b. Cryotherapy
   c. Curettage and electrodesiccation
   d. Radiation therapy
   e. Chemotherapy
2. Prepare the patient for scheduled treatments as indicated.
3. Treat pain with analgesics as prescribed.
4. Help reduce anxiety and facilitate coping by providing emo-

tional support and reassurance and encouraging open expression of feelings and concerns.

5. Teach the patient and family or significant others about:
    a. Postoperative wound care as appropriate
    b. The need to limit sun exposure
    c. Photoprotection methods
    d. The importance of regular follow-up assessment to ensure early detection of any recurrence
    e. Early signs of skin cancer to watch for and report

E. **Evaluation**
    1. The patient and family demonstrate positive coping skills.
    2. The patient demonstrates acceptance of altered body image and disease prognosis.
    3. The patient states appropriate self-care measures.
    4. The patient exhibits intact skin with no signs of infection.
    5. The patient reports adequate pain control.

X. **Burns**

A. **Description: skin injury resulting from heat, electric current, chemicals, friction, or excessive sunlight exposure**

B. **Classification: depth of burn**
    1. Based on the standard depth of injury classification, burns are either first-, second-, or third-degree.
    2. Characteristics of *first-degree* burns (e.g., sunburn) include:
        a. Superficial tissue destruction involving the epidermis only
        b. Local pain and erythema; blisters absent for about 24 hours
        c. Mild to absent systemic response
        d. Requiring no treatment except in large burns of infants or elderly persons
        e. Rapid healing (normally 3 to 5 days) without scarring
    3. Characteristics of *second-degree superficial partial-thickness* burns include:
        a. Tissue destruction involving the epidermis and dermis
        b. Skin appearing red to pale ivory and moist
        c. Formation of wet, thin-walled blisters immediately after injury
        d. Intact tactile and pain sensors
        e. Healing in 21 to 28 days with variable amount of scarring
    4. Characteristics of *second-degree deep partial-thickness* burns include:
        a. Tissue destruction involving possibly the entire dermis, leaving only skin appendages
        b. Mottled appearance with large areas of waxy white injury

       c.   Dry surface

       d.   Clinically indistinguishable from full-thickness burns at time of admission

       e.   Healing spontaneously in about 30 days (However, current therapy indicates excision and skin grafting to diminish scarring and achieve early wound closure.)

   5.   Characteristics of *third-degree full-thickness* burns include:

       a.   Involving the epidermis, dermis, and underlying subcutaneous tissue

       b.   Injury appearing white, cherry red, or black; may or may not contain deep blisters or visible thrombosed veins

       c.   Dry, hard leathery appearance due to loss of epidermal elasticity

       d.   Marked edema and decreased elasticity, which may necessitate escharotomies of circumferential burns within first few hours postinjury

       e.   Painless to touch because of destruction of all superficial nerve endings in skin

       f.   Requiring skin grafting with patient's own skin (autograft) because all dermal elements have been destroyed and cannot regenerate

C.   **Classification: extent of burn**

   1.   The severity of burn injury can be classified according to American Burn Association criteria for minor, moderate uncomplicated, or major burn injuries.

   2.   *Minor* burn injuries involve:

       a.   Second-degree burn of <15% total body surface area (TBSA) in adults or <10% TBSA in children

       b.   Third-degree burn of <2% TBSA not involving special care areas (eyes, ears, face, hands, feet, and perineum)

   3.   *Moderate uncomplicated* burn injuries include:

       a.   Second-degree burns of 15% to 25% TBSA in adults or 10% to 20% TBSA in children

       b.   Third-degree burns of <10% TBSA not involving special care areas

   4.   *Major* burn injuries involve:

       a.   Second-degree burns of >25% TBSA in adults or >20% TBSA in children

       b.   All third-degree burns of 10% TBSA or greater

       c.   All burns involving the hands, face, eyes, ears, feet, or perineum

       d.   All inhalation injury, electrical injury, and complicated burn injuries involving fractures or other trauma

       e.   All poor-risk patients with burn injury of any size

D.   **Nursing diagnoses**

   1.   Ineffective Airway Clearance

    2. Body Image Disturbance
    3. Ineffective Breathing Patterns
    4. Decreased Cardiac Output
    5. Constipation
    6. Ineffective Individual Coping
    7. Diarrhea
    8. Fluid Volume Deficit
    9. Impaired Gas Exchange
    10. Impaired Physical Mobility
    11. Altered Nutrition: Less Than Body Requirements
    12. Pain
    13. Sensory and Perceptual Alterations
    14. Sexual Dysfunction
    15. Impaired Skin Integrity
    16. Sleep Pattern Disturbance
    17. Impaired Tissue Integrity
    18. Altered Tissue Perfusion, Peripheral
    19. Altered Patterns of Urinary Elimination

E. Planning and implementation

    1. Eliminate the source of the burn, depending on cause:
        a. Flame: If clothes are smoldering, wet them using any available water; or smother flames using a blanket, rug, coat, etc.
        b. Scald: Pour cool liquid over area, and remove clothing.
        c. Chemicals: Remove clothing from involved areas and dilute chemical by flushing area with copious amounts of water; if eyes are involved, flush each eye with at least 1 L of Ringer's lactate or other solution.
        d. Tar, asphalt, or melted plastic: Cool area by flushing with water; do not attempt to remove material unless the airway is compromised. (Solvents may be used after initial assessment to soften product and facilitate removal.)
        e. Electric current: Do not touch a person still in contact with an electrical source; if safe, move the person away from the electrical source without touching the source.
    2. Ensure a patent airway; administer oxygen, if indicated.
    3. Assess for and treat associated injuries.
    4. Assess for and treat smoke inhalation injury; support pulmonary function through early intubation and volume ventilator-assisted respiration with optimal positive end expiratory pressure, large tidal volume, and lowest possible inspired oxygen concentration.
    5. Assess for and treat carbon monoxide inhalation; administer 100% oxygen as prescribed until arterial blood gas results dem-

onstrate adequate oxygenation, and perform frequent neurologic assessment until hypoxia resolves.

6. Monitor acid–base balance and electrolyte levels; intervene as necessary to correct imbalances.

7. Take special actions for electrical burns, including:
   a. Applying a cervical collar and placing the patient on a spinal board as soon as possible (Severe contractions produced by electrical current passing through body may injure the spinal cord.)
   b. Monitoring for cardiac arrest or dysrhythmias for at least 24 hours postinjury
   c. Assessing for and treating myoglobinuria resulting from massive soft tissue destruction accompanying major electrical injury; administering IV infusion of Ringer's lactate at rate to maintain urine output at 100 mL/hour in adults or 2 mL/kg/hour in children until urine clears
   d. Preparing the patient for early surgical exploration and wound debridement following cardiovascular stabilization, with debridement every 48 to 72 hours until wound closure is complete
   e. Preparing the patient for amputation if indicated (Because of extensive deep damage caused by electrical current, amputation is necessary in more than 90% of electrical injuries.)
   f. Discussing potential late complications of electrical injury (e.g., corneal cataracts, ataxic gait abnormalities, and other associated neurologic problems)

8. Monitor for and treat burn shock, which occurs in all patients with major burn injury; sequence begins within minutes of injury and leads to death from hypovolemic shock unless treated appropriately.

9. Estimate burn size using either the Rule of Nines or the Lund and Browder chart (Fig. 13–1).

10. Provide appropriate fluid resuscitation, based on the Parkland formula (4 mL of Ringer's lactate × % TBSA burn × kg body weight = total fluid requirement for 24 hours postburn), with one half of total given in the first 8 hours postburn, one fourth of total given in second 8 hours postburn, and the last one fourth given in the third 8 hours postburn.

11. Estimate adequacy of fluid resuscitation based on urine output of 30 mL/hour; increase or decrease fluid to maintain hourly urine output.

12. Teach the patient about planned skin grafting procedures as indicated.

13. Promote optimum recovery through such measures as:
    a. Ensuring optimum nutrition

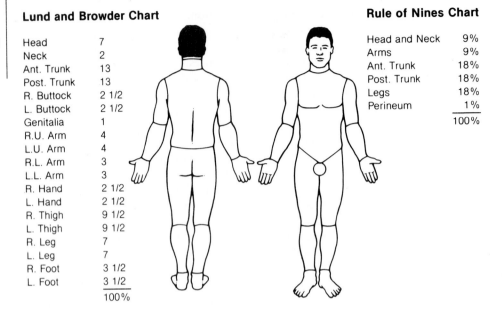

Lund and Browder Chart

Head	7
Neck	2
Ant. Trunk	13
Post. Trunk	13
R. Buttock	2 1/2
L. Buttock	2 1/2
Genitalia	1
R.U. Arm	4
L.U. Arm	4
R.L. Arm	3
L.L. Arm	3
R. Hand	2 1/2
L. Hand	2 1/2
R. Thigh	9 1/2
L. Thigh	9 1/2
R. Leg	7
L. Leg	7
R. Foot	3 1/2
L. Foot	3 1/2
	100%

Rule of Nines Chart

Head and Neck	9%
Arms	9%
Ant. Trunk	18%
Post. Trunk	18%
Legs	18%
Perineum	1%
	100%

FIGURE 13–1.
Two methods of estimating extent of burns.

    b. Providing meticulous wound management to prevent infection and achieve early wound coverage

    c. Initiating physical therapy to regain and maintain optimal range of motion and prevent contractures

    d. Providing psychosocial support to promote mental health

    e. Monitoring carefully to detect problems early and provide appropriate interventions to minimize complications

    f. Providing family-centered care to promote integrity of the family unit as it meets the demands of the rehabilitating burn patient over several years

    g. Encouraging postdischarge follow-up for several years of reconstructive therapy as needed

F. Evaluation

    1. The patient remains free of respiratory complications.

    2. The patient maintains or regains intact skin integrity.

    3. The patient remains free of infection at burn and harvest sites.

    4. The patient maintains optimal nutritional balance to promote healing.

    5. The patient participates in physical therapy to maintain optimal range of motion and function and prevent contractures.

    6. The patient remains free of late complications related to burns.

7. The patient and family maintain an intact family unit.
8. The patient and family make use of support services as needed.

Bibliography

Brunner, L. S., & Suddarth, D. S. (1988). *Textbook of medical-surgical nursing* (6th ed.). Philadelphia: J. B. Lippincott.

Brunner, L. S., & Suddarth, D. S. (1986). *The Lippincott manual of nursing practice* (4th ed.). Philadelphia: J. B. Lippincott.

Groer, M. W., & Shekleton, M. E. (1989). *Basic pathophysiology: A holistic approach* (3rd ed.). St. Louis: C. V. Mosby.

Lewis, S. M, & Collier, I. C. (Eds.) (1992). *Medical-surgical nursing: Assessment and management of clinical problems* (2nd ed.). New York: McGraw-Hill.

Luckmann, J., & Sorenson, K. C. (1987). *Medical-surgical nursing: A psychophysiologic approach* (3rd ed.). Philadelphia: W. B. Saunders.

STUDY QUESTIONS

1. A relationship exists between the wide range of skin colors and the size and distribution of
   a. keratinocytes
   b. melanosomes
   c. stratum corneum
   d. melanin

2. Nursing interventions to prevent death due to fluid and electrolyte imbalances and systemic infection leading to sepsis is necessary in all the following conditions *except*
   a. psoriasis
   b. exfoliative dermatitis
   c. pemphigus vulgaris
   d. toxic epidermal necrolysis

3. The Parkland formula for fluid resuscitation is used to treat the burn shock that occurs as a result of major thermal injury. Although evaluation of the effectiveness of treatment will be based on urine output, evaluation of adequate fluid replacement by the nurse is based on which of the following outcome criteria?
   a. The patient received 2 mL/kg body weight ÷ TBSA burned over the first 24 hours postburn.
   b. The patient received 4 mL/kg body weight ÷ % TBSA burned over the first 24 hours postburn.
   c. The patient received 4 mL/kg body weight ÷ % TBSA burned over the first 36 hours postburn.
   d. The patient received 1 mL/kg body weight ÷ % TBSA burned over the first 24 hours postburn.

4. Which skin layer primarily comprises collagen fibrils to provide the mechanical strength of skin?
   a. dermis
   b. epidermis
   c. hypodermis
   d. stratum corneum

5. Secretion of the apocrine glands would most likely occur in a patient with which of the following nursing diagnoses?

   a. Altered Body Temperature
   b. Fear
   c. Impaired Tissue Integrity
   d. Impaired Physical Mobility

6. Which of the following statements related to administering drugs through the transdermal route is *incorrect*?
   a. Substances enter through the epidermis (transepidermal) route.
   b. The rate of absorption is comparable to that of GI or subcutaneous injection.
   c. Substances enter through orifices of hair follicles (follicular holes).
   d. Lipid-soluble substances are not absorbed through the skin.

7. The sensation of pain is elicited from
   a. free nonmyelinated nerve endings
   b. Merkel's disks
   c. Ruffini's endings
   d. Pacini's corpuscles

8. Some dermatologic conditions disrupt the skin's barrier function. When this occurs, the nurse should observe for all the following *except*
   a. drying and necrosis of underlying subcutaneous tissues
   b. increased fluid and electrolyte losses in the presence of elevated core body temperature
   c. during immersion in water, skin accumulation of up to three to four times its own weight in water
   d. increased amount of water continuously evaporating from the skin surface as insensible perspiration

9. Using tepid sponge bathing to lower elevated core body temperature assists the skin in its thermoregulation function by way of which one of the following principles?
   a. radiation
   b. conduction
   c. convection
   d. dissipation

10. One of the immunologic functions of the skin is the wheal and flare reaction.

When evaluating a patient's response to treatment, which of the following responses would indicate an immunologic rather than an infectious process?
   a. reduced swelling (wheal) and diffuse redness
   b. reduced dilation of arterioles and venules (flare)
   c. resolution of the reaction associated with release of histamine
   d. intact neurologic function

11. When evaluating the effectiveness of patient teaching about health promotion and maintenance behaviors regarding skin care, the nurse would look for all the following *except*
   a. The patient avoids prolonged sun exposure.
   b. The patient avoids repeated exposure to irritants and allergens.
   c. The patient avoids radiation exposure.
   d. The patient avoids excessive sun exposure, if middle aged.

12. For a previously healthy patient presenting with erythema, bullae, and seborrhealike lesions, the nurse would obtain a nutritional history to determine whether symptoms may be associated with a dietary deficiency of the niacin and pyridoxine found in
   a. vitamin B
   b. vitamin C
   c. vitamin K
   d. vitamin A

13. Patient education regarding acne vulgaris should include all the following points *except*
   a. Acne is characterized by closed comedos (whiteheads) and open comedos (blackheads), which can become infected.
   b. Acne occurs commonly at puberty.
   c. Dietary intake affects incidence and severity.
   d. Treatment may include topical or systemic therapy.

14. A furuncle has spread and now is being treated as a carbuncle. The patient's treatment would be based on which of the following nursing diagnoses?
   a. High Risk for Infection
   b. Altered Oral Mucous Membrane
   c. High Risk for Disuse Syndrome
   d. Altered Tissue Perfusion: Peripheral

ANSWER KEY

1. **Correct response: b**
   Melanosomes are produced by melanocytes.
   a. Keratinocytes are epidermal cells that produce keratin.
   c. The stratum corneum is the outermost skin layer.
   d. Melanin is a pigment produced by melanocytes.
   Analysis/Physiologic/Assessment

2. **Correct response: a**
   Psoriasis is the only one of the listed noninfectious inflammatory dermatoses that will not potentially lead to fluid and electrolyte imbalance.
   b, c, and d. These disorders all may lead to fluid and electrolyte imbalance.
   Application/Safe care/Planning

3. **Correct response: b**
   a, c, and d. The other answers are incorrect formulas for fluid replacement.
   Application/Safe care/Evaluation

4. **Correct response: a**
   The dermis lies under the epidermis.
   b. The epidermis is the superficial vascular layer of skin.
   c. Hypodermis refers to below the skin.
   d. The stratum corneum is the horny outermost layer of the epidermis.
   Knowledge/Physiologic/Assessment

5. **Correct response: b**
   The apocrine glands respond to autonomic nervous stimulation.
   a. The apocrine glands do not respond to thermal stimulation.
   c and d. Neither impairment of tissue integrity nor mobility stimulates secretions from these glands.
   Analysis/Physiologic/Analysis (Dx)

6. **Correct response: d**
   Lipid substances may be absorbed through the skin.

   a, b, and c. All the other responses are true in relationship to absorption.
   Comprehension/Safe care/Implementation

7. **Correct response: a**
   Free nonmyelinated nerve endings mediate pain sensation.
   b. Merkel's disks mediate touch.
   c. Ruffini's endings mediate warmth.
   d. Pacini's corpuscles are encapsulated nerve endings that mediate pressure.
   Knowledge/Physiologic/Assessment

8. **Correct response: d**
   There would be an increased insensible loss with loss of barrier function.
   a, b, and c. These other options are correct.
   Knowledge/Physiologic/Assessment

9. **Correct response: b**
   Conduction transfers heat from the body to a cooler object in contact such as tepid water.
   a. Radiation involves the giving off of heat to cooler objects at a distance.
   c. Convection involves bulk removal of warm air away from body to air surrounding body.
   d. Dissipation is not a thermoregulatory function.
   Comprehension/Physiologic/Implementation

10. **Correct response: d**
    An intact nervous system is required for an immunologic response.
    a, b, and c. All these responses can occur with either an immunologic or infectious process.
    Analysis/Physiologic/Evaluation

11. **Correct response: d**
    All the behaviors are correct, but everyone—not just middle-aged persons—should avoid excessive sunlight.
    a, b, and c. All these measures are recommended.
    Application/Health promotion/Evaluation

12. *Correct response: a*
    Vitamin B is essential to complex metabolic functions.
    b and c. Vitamins C and K are essential for connective tissue formation and normal prothrombin synthesis, respectively.
    d. Vitamin A is essential for normal cell structure in the epithelium.
Comprehension/Health promotion/Implementation

13. *Correct response: c*
    Dietary intake does not affect either incidence or severity.

   a. Acne is characterized by both open and closed comedones.
   b. Acne commonly occurs at puberty.
   d. Either topical or systemic therapy may be used.
Application/Health promotion/Planning

14. *Correct response: a*
    Infection is very common, often resulting in abscess.
    b, c, and d. These other diagnoses would not be expected with this bacterial infection.
Analysis/Health promotion/Analysis (Dx)

Neurologic Disorders

14

I. **Anatomy and physiology**
   A. Central nervous system: cranial
   B. Central nervous system: spinal cord
   C. Peripheral nervous system

II. **Overview of neurologic disorders**
   A. Assessment
   B. Laboratory studies and diagnostic tests
   C. Psychosocial implications
   D. Medications used to treat neurologic problems

III. **Head trauma**
   A. Description
   B. Etiology and incidence
   C. Pathophysiology
   D. Assessment findings
   E. Nursing diagnoses
   F. Planning and implementation
   G. Evaluation

IV. **Brain tumors**
   A. Description
   B. Etiology and incidence
   C. Pathophysiology
   D. Assessment findings
   E. Nursing diagnoses
   F. Planning and implementation
   G. Evaluation

V. **Cerebrovascular disorders**
   A. Description
   B. Etiology and incidence
   C. Pathophysiology
   D. Assessment findings
   E. Nursing diagnoses
   F. Planning and implementation
   G. Evaluation

VI. **Epilepsy**
   A. Description
   B. Etiology and incidence
   C. Pathophysiology
   D. Assessment findings
   E. Nursing diagnoses
   F. Planning and implementation
   G. Evaluation

VII. **Spinal cord injuries**
   A. Description
   B. Etiology and incidence
   C. Pathophysiology
   D. Assessment findings
   E. Nursing diagnoses
   F. Planning and implementation
   G. Evaluation

VIII. **Spinal cord tumors**
   A. Description
   B. Etiology and incidence
   C. Pathophysiology
   D. Assessment findings
   E. Nursing diagnoses
   F. Planning and implementation
   G. Evaluation

IX. **Intervertebral disk herniation**
   A. Description
   B. Etiology and incidence
   C. Pathophysiology
   D. Assessment findings
   E. Nursing diagnoses
   F. Planning and implementation
   G. Evaluation

X. **Multiple sclerosis (MS)**
   A. Description
   B. Etiology and incidence
   C. Pathophysiology
   D. Assessment findings
   E. Nursing diagnoses

I.   Anatomy and physiology

A.   Central nervous system: cranial

   1.   Structure

      a.   The brain is enclosed within the bones of the cranium
and covered by three meningeal layers: dura mater
(outer), arachnoid mater, and pia mater (inner).

      b.   Manufactured in the choroid plexus of the ventricular
system, cerebrospinal fluid (CSF) circulates in the subarachnoid space.

      c.   Ventricular structures include the lateral, third, and

fourth ventricles; aqueduct of Sylvius; and the foramina of Luschka and Magendie.

d. The cerebrum is divided into left and right hemispheres by the falx, an indentation of the dura. Each cerebral hemisphere contains frontal, temporal, parietal, occipital, and limbic lobes.

e. The cerebellum also is divided into left and right hemispheres, which are connected by the vermis.

f. Brain stem structures include the medulla, pons, and midbrain.

g. The basal ganglia encompasses the caudate nucleus, putamen, globus pallidus, and substantia nigra.

h. Other structures in the brain include the thalamus, hypothalamus, and pituitary gland.

i. Supratentorial structures (above the dura fold) are known as the tentorium; infratentorial structures lie below the tentorium.

j. Vascular supply to the brain is provided from the basilar artery, formed from the union of two vertebral arteries, and the internal carotids; these two systems join to form the Circle of Willis.

2. Function

a. According to the Monro Kellie principle, an increase in any one of three components (brain tissue, normally 88%; CSF, 9% to 10%; intravascular blood, 2% to 3%) results in increased intracranial pressure (ICP) because the skull bones do not allow for expansion from pressure buildup.

b. The meninges protect the brain from injury and infection.

c. Between 500 and 700 mL of CSF is manufactured daily, but only 150 mL is circulating at any one time; excess CSF is absorbed through the arachnoid villi into the venous system.

d. Interference with CSF flow results in increased ICP.

e. The tentorium helps stabilize cranial structures within the skull.

f. The frontal lobe, prerolandic, is the brain's center of fore sight, abstract thinking, and judgment.

g. The frontal lobe, postrolandic, controls voluntary motor movements.

h. The temporal lobe is the center of memory and contains visual and auditory association areas.

i. The parietal lobe controls sensory functions such as recognition of pain, temperature, and pressure and sense of position of the body and limbs.

    j.   The occipital lobe is the center of visual function.

    k.   The limbic lobe is the center of emotions, drives, and basic survival functions.

    l.   The cerebellum is involved in coordination of muscle movements and maintenance of equilibrium and muscle tone.

    m.   The medulla oblongata contains several vital centers, including those for respiration, heart rate, vomiting, and hiccoughing.

    n.   In the pons, the pneumotaxic system controls respiratory patterns.

    o.   In the brain stem, the reticular activating system (RAS) maintains alertness.

    p.   The basal ganglia is involved in smooth muscle movement and processing of proprioceptive input.

    q.   The thalamus serves as the chief relay station for sensory fibers.

    r.   The hypothalamus helps regulate body temperature, fluid balance, and some endocrine functions.

    s.   The pituitary gland is the chief regulator of endocrine functions.

    t.   The brain uses about 20% of total cardiac output. An autoregulation mechanism maintains blood flow to the brain despite changes in systemic pressure; trauma can disrupt this mechanism.

    u.   The blood–brain barrier prevents many toxic substances in the blood stream from entering the brain.

B. **Central nervous system: spinal cord**

    1.   Structure

        a.   The spinal cord is encased within the vertebral column, which consists of 31 vertebrae in cervical (C), thoracic (T), lumbar (L), sacral (S), and coccygeal segments.

        b.   The cervical, thoracic, and lumbar vertebrae are separated by disks. The disk's outer covering is termed the annulus; the inner part, the nucleus pulposus.

        c.   Like the brain, the spinal cord is covered by meninges (see Section A.1.a).

        d.   Vascular supply is provided from the radicular arteries and posterior and anterior spinal arteries.

        e.   Major descending tracts in the spinal cord include the lateral corticospinal (pyramidal), ventral corticospinal, reticulospinal, and vestibulospinal tracts.

        f.   Major ascending tracts include the lateral spinothalamic and ventral spinothalamic tracts and the posterior columns. Fibers of the lateral spinothalamic tract cross in the brain stem.

2. Function
   a. The vertebral column protects the cord and helps maintain an upright body position.
   b. The lateral corticospinal tract transmits impulses controlling voluntary motor movement.
   c. The lateral spinothalamic tract transmits pain and temperature impulses.
   d. The posterior columns carry tactile and kinesthetic impulses.

3. Neurologic dysfunction associated with cord damage depends on the level of injury:
   a. Below C4: loss of motor and sensory function from the neck down, including independent respiratory function and bowel and bladder control
   b. Below C6: loss of motor and sensory function below the shoulders; loss of bowel and bladder control; impaired intercostal muscle function
   c. Below C8: loss of motor control and sensation to parts of the arms and hands; loss of bowel and bladder control
   d. Below T6: loss of motor control and sensation below the midchest but with motor control and sensation preserved in the arms and hands; loss of bowel and bladder control
   e. Below T12: loss of motor control and sensation below the waist; loss of bowel and bladder control
   f. Below L2: loss of motor control and sensation in the legs and pelvis; loss of bowel and bladder control
   g. Below L4: loss of motor control and sensation in parts of the thighs and legs; loss of bowel and bladder control

C. **Peripheral nervous system**
   1. Structure
      a. The peripheral nervous system contains 12 pairs of cranial nerves and 31 pairs of spinal nerves.
      b. Cranial nerves, which are numbered, include the olfactory (CN I), optic (II), oculomotor (III), trochlear (IV), trigeminal (V), abducens (VI), facial (VII), acoustic (VIII), glossopharyngeal (IX), vagus (X), spinal accessory (XI), and hypoglossal (XII) nerves.
      c. The nuclei of many cranial nerves are located in the brain stem.
      d. Spinal nerves exit through vertebral foramina.
   2. Function
      a. Spinal nerves contain both sensory and motor fibers.
      b. Motor fibers are of two types: *somatic*, which terminate in skeletal muscle, and *autonomic*, which innervate cardiac smooth muscle and glands.

c. CNs III, IV, and VI control eye movement and pupil size.

d. CN VII controls facial movements.

e. CN IX controls the gag reflex.

f. CN X controls many autonomic nervous system functions.

II. Overview of neurologic disorders

A. Assessment

1. Neurologic assessment involves assessing neurologic system intactness, with particular emphasis on sensation, motor ability (including coordination), alertness, and cognition (see Chapter 1, Section X, for details of a complete neurologic assessment).

2. In the presence of specific pathologies or nursing diagnoses, additional assessments or more in-depth assessment of specific areas may be done. The acuity of the patient's condition determines the necessary frequency of neuro checks.

3. Various assessment tools (e.g., the Glasgow coma scale) may be used.

4. The nurse assesses sensory function as follows:
   a. With the patient blindfolded, touch all levels of each extremity, and ask him or her to identify the different pressure points.
   b. Ask if the patient feels numbness, tingling, or other abnormal sensations.
   c. Assess whether the patient with decreased arousal moves the extremities in response to pressure or more intense stimuli.
   d. Evaluate each extremity, and note any deficits.

5. Motor function assessment involves the following:
   a. Ask the patient to grasp the examiner's hands with his or hers and to push against the examiner's palms with his or her feet; evaluate muscle strength.
   b. Have the patient lift each arm and foot.
   c. Evaluate the patient's ability to walk; assess posture, gait, and coordination.
   d. To assess fine motor coordination, have the patient touch the examiner's fingertip, then his or her own nose.
   e. In a patient with decreased arousal, assess movement in response to pressure or more intense stimuli.

6. Assessing alertness (level of arousal and orientation) involves these steps:
   a. Speak the patient's name. If the patient doesn't respond, speak louder, shake him or her, and finally apply a slightly painful stimulus; note whether the patient opens his or her eyes or responds verbally.

b. Ask a responsive patient to state his or her name, where he or she is, and the date, along with other questions that will provide data on level of orientation.

7. The nurse assesses a patient's level of cognition (including judgment) by:
   a. Determining whether the patient can follow commands
   b. Asking questions to evaluate memory (both recent and past)
   c. Determining the patient's ability to calculate numerical problems
8. Pupil examination evaluates pupil size and response to light, along with equality of response.
9. Reflex assessment includes determining the presence or absence of the corneal and gag reflexes.
10. Neurologic assessment also should include vital signs and respiratory pattern.

B. Laboratory studies and diagnostic tests

1. Magnetic resonance imaging (MRI) and computed tomography (CT) identify pathology such as tumors, hematomas, and edema.
2. Angiography detects vascular problems, tumors, and hematomas.
3. Electroencephalography (EEG) evaluates the brain's electrical activity (alpha, beta, theta, and delta waves); used primarily in diagnosis of epilepsy and brain death.
4. Ventriculography allows visualization of the ventricular system through injection of contrast media (usually air) directly into a ventricle; generally used when infratentorial lesions are suspected.
5. Lumbar puncture involves inserting a needle into the subarachnoid space to obtain data on CSF, CSF pressure, and presence of infection. (Normal CSF is clear; contains 15 to 45 mg of protein per 100 mL, 50 to 80 mg glucose per 100 mL, and no red blood cells; and has a specific gravity of 1.007.)
6. In myelography, radiographs taken after injection of contrast media into the spinal column detect tumors, disk abnormalities, or other spinal cord problems.

C. Psychosocial implications

1. A patient with a serious neurologic problem may experience coping difficulties due to such factors as:
   a. Chronic nature of the disorder
   b. Uncertain prognosis
   c. All-encompassing nature of limitations
2. The patient also may have self-concept concerns related to fears of:

a. Increased dependency, loss of independence
b. Body image changes related to neurologic deficits
c. Diminished outlets for sexual expression

3. Lifestyle concerns may be related to potential changes in:
   a. Physical ability
   b. Work performance, with possibility of job loss
   c. Self-care ability
   d. Mental capacity
   e. Economic stability

4. The patient also may be prone to changes in social interaction related to:
   a. Depression
   b. Isolation
   c. Hopelessness

D. Medications used to treat neurologic problems

1. Used in treating head trauma, *osmotic diuretics* (e.g., mannitol) help decrease cerebral edema by promoting extracellular fluid loss.

2. *Corticosteroids* (e.g., dexamethasone) are given to help reduce increased ICP secondary to brain tumor.

3. Used in the treatment of transient ischemic attack (TIA), *anticoagulants* such as warfarin sodium (e.g., Coumadin) help prevent further clot extension by inhibiting synthesis of vitamin K-dependent coagulant factors.

4. *Sedatives* (e.g., phenobarbital) are used to reduce restlessness in patients experiencing cerebral aneurysm.

5. *Antiepileptics*, given to control seizures, include:
   a. Carbamazepine (e.g., Tegretol)
   b. Phenytoin (Dilantin)
   c. Phenobarbital (e.g., Donnatal)

6. Used to treat Parkinson's disease, *anticholinergics* include:
   a. Trihexyphenidyl hydrochloride (e.g., Artane)
   b. Procyclidine hydrochloride (Kemadrin)
   c. Benztropine mesylate

7. *Levodopa* also is used in symptomatic treatment of Parkinson's disease.

8. Used to treat myasthenia gravis by increasing muscle responsiveness to nerve impulses, *anticholinesterase agents* include:
   a. Pyridostigmine bromide (e.g., Mestinon)
   b. Neostigmine bromide (Prostigmin)

III. Head trauma

A. Description

1. Head trauma refers to direct or indirect impact to the head that produces some degree of brain injury.

2. Common types of head trauma include:
   a. Closed head injuries (concussion, contusion, laceration)
   b. Intracranial hemorrhage (epidural, subdural, or intracerebral hematoma)
   c. Skull fractures (open or closed)

B. Etiology and incidence

1. Common causes of head trauma include falls, automobile accidents, and beatings with blunt objects; intracerebral hematoma commonly results from missile injury (e.g., gunshot or stab wound).
2. Head trauma causes between 80,000 and 100,000 deaths each year in the United States; another 700,000 cases require hospitalization.

C. Pathophysiology

1. Whatever the cause of head trauma, the most serious complication is increased ICP.
2. Compensatory mechanisms for maintaining ICP within normal limits include:
   a. Increased CSF absorption
   b. Shunting of blood to the spinal subarachnoid space
   c. Decreased CSF production
3. Failure of these compensatory mechanisms results in the following sequence of events:
   a. Decreased cerebral blood flow with inadequate perfusion
   b. Increased PCO_2 and decreased PO_2, leading to hypoxia
   c. Vasodilation and cerebral edema
   d. Further increases in ICP
4. Management of head trauma involves identifying and correcting the underlying cause of increased ICP and cerebral edema.

D. Assessment findings

1. Clinical manifestations of head trauma depend on the type, site, and extent of injury.
2. A common manifestation is loss of consciousness, ranging from a few minutes to an hour or longer.
3. Signs and symptoms of increasing ICP include:
   a. Altered level of consciousness—particularly restlessness, a common early sign
   b. Pupil changes: fixed, dilated, slowed response, inequality
   c. Increasing systolic blood pressure with stable or falling diastolic pressure
   d. Bradycardia, widening pulse pressure
   e. Bradypnea, irregular breathing pattern
   f. Hyperthermia (late sign)

    g.   Focal neurologic signs: visual changes (blurred or double vision, photophobia), muscle weakness or paralysis, decreased response to pain stimulus, positive Babinski's sign, decerebrate or decorticate posturing

    h.   Headache

    i.   Vomiting

  4. ICP monitoring detects increased ICP (generally >15 mmHg); the catheter can be placed in the ventricles, subdural space, or epidural space.

E. **Nursing diagnoses**

  1. Ineffective Airway Clearance

  2. Hyperthermia

  3. High Risk for Infection

  4. High Risk for Impaired Skin Integrity

  5. Altered Thought Processes

  6. Altered Tissue Perfusion: Cerebral

F. **Planning and implementation**

  1. Monitor neurologic status, including vital signs, level of consciousness, oculomotor nerve function, and motor and sensory status.

  2. Help maintain cerebral perfusion by:

    a.   Administering osmotic diuretics or corticosteroids, as ordered, to reduce edema

    b.   Administering sedatives and analgesics carefully because they may depress respirations and mask decreasing level of consciousness

    c.   Reducing or eliminating noxious stimuli

    d.   Elevating the head of the bed 30 degrees

    e.   Hyperventilating the patient before suctioning

  3. Maintain a patent airway; suction as needed, and position to prevent airway obstruction.

  4. Manage hyperthermia by:

    a.   Providing only minimal bedcoverings and clothing

    b.   Using a hypothermia blanket; avoid rapid cooling

    c.   Administering antipyretics as prescribed

    d.   Forcing fluids unless contraindicated

  5. Prevent infection by using sterile technique for wound care and insertion of the ICP monitoring device and by maintaining the intactness of the monitoring system.

  6. Maintain skin integrity by:

    a.   Turning the patient on regular schedule and protecting pressure points as needed

    b.   Changing moist or wet linens immediately

    c.   Lifting—not pulling—the patient when changing position in bed

  7. Provide passive range-of-motion (ROM) exercise to prevent contractures from prolonged immobility.

       8. Help orient the patient and reduce confusion by:
- a. Reducing external stimuli
- b. Providing for adequate rest
- c. Giving simple directions
- d. Providing familiar objects in the patient's environment

G. **Evaluation**
1. The patient exhibits ICP within normal limits.
2. The patient demonstrates absence of lung infections or infiltrates.
3. The patient's body temperature is within normal range.
4. The patient maintains good skin integrity.

IV. Brain tumors

A. **Description**
1. Brain tumors are localized, space-occupying intracranial neoplasms.
2. Primary tumors (originating from brain tissue) include:
   - a. Gliomas (astrocytomas, glioblastomas, ependymomas, medulloblastomas, oligodendrogliomas), accounting for 50% of primary brain tumors
   - b. Meningiomas, accounting for 13% to 18% of primary brain tumors
   - c. Pituitary adenomas
   - d. Neurinomas, accounting for about 8% of primary brain tumors

B. **Etiology and incidence**
1. The etiology of brain tumors remains unclear.
2. Incidence is approximately 4.5 per 100,000 persons in the United States; periods of peak incidence are before age 1 year, between ages 2 and 12 years, and between ages 40 and 60 years.

C. **Pathophysiology**
1. Arising from glial cells in the brain's connective tissue, gliomas tend to be fast-growing, infiltrative, and difficult to excise completely.
2. Meningiomas arise from the brain's dural covering; they are relatively slow growing and usually benign.
3. Pituitary adenomas may arise from various pituitary tissues and commonly affect endocrine function and vision.
4. Neurinomas arise from the coverings of any of the cranial nerves, most commonly from the acoustic nerve (CN VIII).
5. Metastatic tumors can migrate to the brain from other sites; common primary sites include the lung, breast, and colon.

D. **Assessment findings**
1. Signs and symptoms depend on tumor type, location, and rate of growth.

2. General manifestations include those related to increased ICP, such as headache, vomiting, papilledema, and altered sensorium.

3. Brain tumors also may produce focal neurologic effects, including motor abnormalities (e.g., weakness, paralysis, seizures) and sensory abnormalities (e.g., distorted vision, smell, hearing, touch).

4. CT scan or MRI can locate the tumor; other useful diagnostic studies may include angiography, ventriculography, and radionuclide scanning.

E. Nursing diagnoses

1. Anxiety
2. Body Image Disturbance
3. Hopelessness
4. High Risk for Injury
5. Sensory and Perceptual Alteration: Visual, Auditory, Tactile
6. High Risk for Impaired Skin Integrity
7. Altered Thought Processes
8. Altered Tissue Perfusion: Cerebral

F. Planning and implementation

1. See Chapter 21, Cancer Nursing, for general nursing interventions appropriate to all cancer patients.

2. As applicable, prepare the patient for craniotomy to remove the tumor or a portion of the tumor. Provide preoperative and postoperative care (see Chapter 24, Perioperative Nursing).

3. Carefully monitor for signs of increased ICP and neurologic deficits.

4. Provide information on tests, treatments, and other procedures to the patient and family.

5. Provide eye care if the patient experiences decreased corneal reflex.

6. If the patient is confused, determine whether family members can stay with him or her; use restraints judiciously.

7. If the patient experiences paresis or paralysis, provide needed assistance with mobility.

8. Assist with adaptation to sensory and perceptual changes (e.g., teach the patient to turn or move his or her head to view the entire environment, to place needed items within his or her visual field, to face persons when talking, and to turn his or her head or position self so that he or she can hear well).

9. Assist the patient with grooming and other self-care measures as needed.

10. Provide information on wigs and other items that can improve appearance as appropriate.

11. Teach the patient and family stress management techniques

such as progressive muscle relaxation, breathing techniques, guided imagery, and meditation.

12. Allow time for expression of feelings and concerns; if appropriate, encourage the patient to keep a journal.

13. Refer the patient and family to the chaplain or social services as appropriate.

14. Instruct the patient and family in necessary home care measures.

15. Provide information on appropriate community resources, such as local support groups and the Brain Tumor Association.

G. Evaluation

1. The patient's ICP remains within normal range.
2. The patient remains alert and well oriented.
3. The patient remains injury-free.
4. The patient maintains good skin integrity.
5. The patient and family members demonstrate low levels of anxiety.
6. The patient interacts with others and participates in self-care.
7. The patient and family acknowledge the patient's condition; the patient expresses positive statements of self-worth.

V. Cerebrovascular disorders

A. Description

1. This group of disorders involves disruption of blood supply to the brain.
2. Types include:
   a. Cerebrovascular accident (CVA, stroke)
   b. TIA
   c. Cerebral aneurysm

B. Etiology and incidence

1. Causes of CVA include thrombosis (most common), embolism, and vessel rupture or spasm; the most common site is the middle cerebral artery.

2. CVA strikes more than 500,000 persons each year and is the third leading cause of death in the United States (about 172,000 deaths annually); about half those who survive suffer permanent neurologic deficits.

3. Considered a warning sign of CVA, TIA results from occlusion of an intracranial or extracranial artery, commonly associated with atherosclerosis. The most common site of TIA is at the bifurcation of the common carotid artery.

4. Cerebral aneurysm results from a weakness in a vessel wall due to a congenital defect or a degenerative process, such as hypertension or atherosclerosis. The most common type is berry aneurysm, and the most common site is in the anterior portion of the Circle of Willis, usually at a vessel junction.

C. **Pathophysiology**

1. In CVA, sudden interruption of blood supply to areas of the brain results in cerebral anoxia and impaired cerebral metabolism, which damages brain tissue and produces focal neurologic deficits of varying severity.

2. In a TIA, temporary interruption of blood flow (lasting from seconds to hours) produces transient neurologic deficits that clear completely within 12 to 24 hours.

3. A cerebral aneurysm is prone to rupture, which causes blood to leak into the subarachnoid space (and sometimes into brain tissue, where it forms a clot), resulting in increased ICP and brain tissue damage.

D. **Assessment findings**

1. Clinical manifestations of CVA depend on the artery affected, the severity of damage, and the extent of collateral circulation that develops. Common signs and symptoms include:
   a. Hemiplegia and sensory deficits
   b. Aphasia (Impairment may be in speaking, listening, writing, comprehending; most are mixed expressive and receptive.)
   c. Homonymous hemianopia
   d. Unilateral neglect of paralyzed side
   e. Bladder impairment
   f. Possible respiratory impairment
   g. Impaired mental activity and psychologic effects

2. Manifestations of TIA may include:
   a. Temporary loss of consciousness or dizziness
   b. Paresthesias
   c. Garbled speech

3. A patient with a nonruptured cerebral aneurysm often is asymptomatic or reports nonspecific symptoms such as headache or blurred vision. Aneurysm rupture produces varying manifestations, which may include:
   a. Signs and symptoms of increased ICP (see Section III.C)
   b. Severe headache
   c. Nuchal rigidity and pain on neck movement
   d. Photophobia and possible blurred vision
   e. Irritability and restlessness
   f. Slight temperature elevation

E. **Nursing diagnoses**

1. Impaired Verbal Communication
2. Fatigue
3. Impaired Physical Mobility
4. Pain
5. Altered Role Performance

6. Self-Care Deficit: Feeding, Dressing and Grooming, Bathing and Hygiene
7. High Risk for Impaired Skin Integrity

8. Social Isolation
9. Unilateral Neglect

F. Planning and implementation

1. Enhance communication by:
    a. Using alternative means of communication as appropriate (e.g., gestures, pictures, alphabet board)
    b. Giving simple commands with gestures; pointing to objects as you name them
    c. Eliminating extraneous stimuli when communicating (e.g., turn off the television)
2. Plan the patient's care to allow for adequate periods of uninterrupted rest. Schedule therapy sessions after rest periods.
3. Provide a balanced diet, and assist the patient with eating if necessary. Allow sufficient time for meals, place food so that the patient can see it, and provide foods that are easy to handle.
4. Maximize the patient's opportunities for social interaction.
5. Consider the patient's interests when planning daily activities.
6. Teach the patient how to use a walker, cane, or wheelchair as appropriate.
7. Instruct the patient in the use of assistive devices, such as for putting on stockings.
8. Encourage the patient to wear simplified clothing, such as with front opening snaps, secured.
9. Discuss necessary home adaptations (e.g., wheelchair ramps, shower seat, other bathroom modifications).
10. Assist the patient with personal hygiene as necessary (e.g., hair washing and brushing, makeup application, shaving).
11. Teach and assist with or perform ROM exercises to help maintain muscle tone and prevent contractures.
12. Encourage the patient to touch the paralyzed side and to participate in passive ROM as appropriate.
13. When the patient is in bed, position him or her on side with the hips slightly flexed.
14. Reduce pain by:
    a. Administering analgesics as prescribed
    b. Positioning to decrease discomfort
    c. For a patient with subarachnoid hemorrhage, reducing external stimuli, moving the patient slowly, turning the neck gently
15. Administer medications as prescribed, which may include:
    a. Anticoagulants for a patient experiencing TIA

       b.   Sedatives (phenobarbital) to reduce restlessness in a patient with cerebral aneurysm

       c.   Aminophylline or isoproterenol to control vasospasm after aneurysm rupture

16.   Prepare the patient for surgical intervention as appropriate, which may include:

       a.   Carotid enterectomy for a patient experiencing TIA

       b.   Craniotomy for surgical clipping of aneurysm

17.   Teach the patient's family:

       a.   Effective communication techniques

       b.   New ways of interacting with the patient posthospitalization

       c.   Ways to encourage the patient in self-feeding

       d.   Safety precautions (e.g., removing throw rugs and other potential hazards, keeping the patient's environment clear of obstacles)

G. **Evaluation**

1.   The patient demonstrates decreased frustration and increased ability to make his or her needs known.

2.   The patient exhibits the ability and sufficient energy to carry out necessary activities.

3.   The patient displays skin free of redness and breaks in integrity.

4.   The patient maintains interactions with others and seeks out social situations.

5.   The patient demonstrates the ability to use assistive devices or transfer himself or herself safely.

6.   The patient maintains weight within normal range with no undue weight loss.

7.   The patient exhibits good personal hygiene and grooming and dresses appropriately.

8.   The patient does not have accidents and remains injury-free.

9.   The patient acknowledges his or her entire body and shows no evidence of unilateral neglect.

10.   The patient reflects absence of discomfort by facial expressions, body movements, and vital signs.

VI. Epilepsy

  A. **Description**

1.   Epilepsy refers to paroxysmal, uncontrolled excessive firing of hyperexcitable neurons in the brain; not a disease entity in itself but rather an indicator of underlying pathology.

2.   Types of seizures include:

       a.   tonic–clonic (grand mal)

       b.   Absence (petit mal)

       c.   Complex (temporal lobe; psychomotor)

       d.   Jacksonian

B. **Etiology and incidence**
   1. About 50% of cases of epilepsy are idiopathic, for which no underlying pathology can be identified.
   2. Possible causes include:
      a. Birth trauma
      b. Head trauma
      c. Brain tumor
      d. Meningitis, encephalitis, or brain abscess
      e. Metabolic disorders (e.g., hypoglycemia, phenylketonuria)
      f. Cerebrovascular disorders
   3. Approximately 2 million Americans have some form of epilepsy.

C. **Pathophysiology**
   1. Seizure activity represents excessive, disordered firing of brain neurons.
   2. Seizures are classified as partial (complex, Jacksonian), arising from a localized area of the brain, or generalized (tonic–clonic, absence), marked by widespread electrical abnormality in the brain.
   3. Status epilepticus refers to continued seizure activity, a medical emergency.

D. **Assessment findings**
   1. Tonic–clonic seizures are marked by:
      a. Generalized seizure activity with no focal onset, lasting about 2 minutes
      b. Possible prodrome of a vaguely uneasy feeling
      c. Loss of consciousness, with falling if upright at onset
      d. In the tonic phase, muscle contraction (including jaw clenching), possibly periods of apnea
      e. In the clonic phase, rhythmic, forceful movement of extremities; excessive salivation; rapid pulse
      f. Possible incontinence
      g. Stupor for 5 to 10 minutes following the clonic phase
   2. Features of absence seizures include:
      a. Generalized seizure activity with no focal onset, occurring primarily in children
      b. Momentary (10- to 30-second) loss of consciousness, marked by a glassy stare; usually no falling
      c. Possibly occurring repeatedly over the course of a day
   3. In a complex seizure, the patient exhibits altered behavior (e.g., automatisms, unusual sensations, delusions) but is not aware of what is happening.
   4. A Jacksonian seizure begins in one part of the body (e.g., twitching of one side of the face or abnormal movements of

one hand) and may progress to a generalized tonic–clonic seizure.

E. Nursing diagnoses
1. Anxiety
2. High Risk for Injury
3. Knowledge Deficit
4. Impaired Social Interaction

F. Planning and implementation
1. Observe and record the patient's movements and behavior before, during, and after the seizure.
2. Note the part(s) of the body affected by seizure activity.
3. Note the duration of seizure activity.
4. Administer medications as prescribed, which may include:
   a. Carbamazepine
   b. Phenytoin
   c. Phenobarbital
5. Monitor for medication side effects.
6. Provide patient and family teaching, covering:
   a. Aura or indications of seizure
   b. Care needed during seizure activity: protecting the head and extremities so that they do not hit objects during seizure; avoid restraining the patient
   c. The need to provide for adequate rest after the seizure
   d. Medication regimen, including side effects and signs of toxicity
   e. Necessary lifestyle modifications such as getting adequate sleep, abstaining from alcohol, using relaxation techniques
   f. The need for social interaction opportunities
7. Encourage family and friends not to be overprotective of the patient.
8. Provide information on available community resources, including support groups.

G. Evaluation
1. The patient maintains blood level of medications within the therapeutic range.
2. The patient exhibits no medication side effects, or if side effects do occur, they are detected early.
3. The patient displays no bruises, fractures, or lacerations.
4. The patient reports feeling rested and relaxed.
5. The patient reports feeling good about social interactions and increased interactions.

VII. Spinal cord injuries

A. Description: fractures, contusions, or compression of the vertebral column with damage to the spinal cord

B. Etiology and incidence

1. Causes of spinal cord injury include motor vehicle accidents, diving accidents, falls, sports injuries, and gunshot wounds.
2. Common sites of injury include the cervical spine and the junction of the thoracic and lumbar areas (T-12 and L-1).

C. Pathophysiology

1. Spinal cord injuries can result from flexion, extension, rotation, compression, or a combination of these mechanisms.
2. Injury may directly damage the cord, or vertebral fracture or dislocation can be a potential source of cord injury, in which inappropriate movement can cause permanent damage.
3. Cord injury may be complete, involving total cord transection, or incomplete, with partial transection or other damage.
4. Damage ranges from mild transient cord concussion to immediate and permanent quadriplegia.
5. With cord damage, spinal shock may occur, with loss of motor, sensory, and autonomic activity below the level of injury. This condition may persist for several days to months after injury.

D. Assessment findings

1. Common immediate symptoms of spinal cord injury include pain and paresthesias or, conversely, loss of sensation; altered motor function, ranging from paresis to paralysis; and possibly loss of consciousness.
2. Neurologic damage depends on the level of cord injury (see Section I.B.3); edema may temporarily increase deficits.
3. Spinal radiograph can locate the area of cord damage.

E. Nursing diagnoses

1. Body Image Disturbance
2. Bowel Incontinence
3. Ineffective Individual Coping
4. Dysreflexia
5. Impaired Home Maintenance Management
6. High Risk for Infection
7. High Risk for Injury
8. Impaired Physical Mobility
9. Altered Patterns of Sexuality
10. High Risk for Impaired Skin Integrity
11. Altered Role Performance
12. Reflex Urinary Incontinence

F. Planning and implementation

1. Provide emergency treatment:

a. Do not move the patient until adequate personnel and equipment are available.

b. Keep the neck in alignment.

c. Immobilize the head and neck.

2. Perform frequent neuro checks to evaluate muscle strength, degree and type of movement, sensation, and warmth of all four extremities.

3. Apply skeletal traction as prescribed; may use a Stryker or Circ-O-Lectric bed.

4. Explain all aspects of care and turning to the patient and family.

5. Prepare the patient for surgery, if appropriate—usually in fractures or dislocations to stabilize the spinal column (see Chapter 24, Perioperative Nursing, for more information).

6. Perform passive ROM exercises on paralyzed limbs to maintain joint mobility.

7. Teach the patient active ROM exercises to maintain or increase strength and mobility in the upper extremities.

8. Work with other disciplines in securing needed assistive devices for ambulation and home maintenance management.

9. Teach the patient transfer skills, if appropriate.

10. Provide for adequate rest periods.

11. Teach the patient and family signs and symptoms of impending dysreflexic episodes.

12. Establish a regular bowel routine, and institute other measures to prevent constipation, such as:

    a. Setting a schedule for defecation, preferably 15 to 20 minutes after a meal

    b. Providing a warm liquid before defecation time

    c. Encouraging the patient to ingest sufficient dietary roughage and adequate fluids, and to avoid foods that can cause constipation

    d. Encouraging the patient to attempt defecation in the sitting position, if possible

13. Provide bladder care to prevent urine stasis, including:

    a. Scheduling frequent times for voiding

    b. Maintaining an adequate fluid intake but avoiding fluids before bedtime

    c. Identifying and using triggering mechanisms that can stimulate voiding

    d. Administering anticholinergic medications as prescribed

    e. Performing intermittent bladder catheterization as appropriate

14. Administer antihypertensive medications as prescribed to decrease blood pressure.

15. Collaborate with the patient's family to identify ways to adapt the home environment to the patient's needs.

16.   Evaluate the patient's and family members' coping strategies, and teach new strategies if needed, particularly problem-focused strategies.

17.   As appropriate, provide information on alternative means for achieving sexual satisfaction.

18.   Encourage the patient and family members to verbalize feelings and concerns.

G. Evaluation

1.   If neurologic deficit has resulted from injury, the patient exhibits no increase in deficit.

2.   If no deficit has occurred, the patient develops no deficit.

3.   The patient demonstrates maximum use of remaining abilities in self-care and mobility.

4.   The patient maintains good skin integrity.

5.   The patient expresses positive adaptation to deficits in psychologic and social realms.

6.   The patient verbalizes realistic expectations about the future and expresses feelings about his or her condition and its impact on his or her life.

7.   Family members verbalize understanding of the patient's condition and demonstrate the willingness and ability to assist the patient in functioning at his or her optimum level.

8.   The patient demonstrates adequate bowel and bladder control, with no constipation or urinary tract infections.

9.   The patient reports satisfaction with sexual expression.

VIII. Spinal cord tumors

A. Description: neoplasms of the spinal cord or its nerve roots; tumor types are the same as for intracranial tumors (see Section IV.A)

B. Etiology and incidence

1.   The etiology of spinal cord tumors is unclear.

2.   Incidence is rare compared to intracranial tumors (a ratio of about 1:4).

C. Pathophysiology

1.   Tumors can develop anywhere along the spinal cord or its roots; the most common site is the thoracic area.

2.   Primary cord tumors may be intramedullary (within the cord), extramedullary–intradural (within the subarachnoid space), or extradural (outside the dural membrane).

3.   Effects depend on tumor type, location, and rapidity of growth.

4.   Tumors may invade the vertebral column; erosion of bone may cause collapse of vertebrae with resulting pressure on the spinal nerves and spinal cord.

D. Assessment findings

1.   Common clinical manifestations of spinal cord tumors include:

a. Pain
b. Motor dysfunction (e.g., muscle weakness and spasticity, decreased muscle tone, hyperreflexia, positive Babinski's sign)
c. Sensory deficits (e.g., loss of pain, temperature, and touch sensation; paresthesias)
d. Urinary retention and constipation

2. Neurologic deficits resulting from cord tumors often are similar to those associated with cord injury (see Section VII.D).
3. CT scan, MRI, myelography, and spinal radiographs can determine tumor location and the extent of involvement.

E. Nursing diagnoses
1. Anxiety
2. Bowel Incontinence
3. Constipation
4. Impaired Physical Mobility
5. Pain
6. Sexual Dysfunction
7. High Risk for Impaired Skin Integrity
8. Urinary Incontinence
9. Urinary Retention

F. Planning and implementation
1. Prepare the patient for surgery, if appropriate (see Chapter 24, Perioperative Nursing, for more information).
2. Prepare the patient for radiation therapy, if prescribed (see Chapter 21, Cancer Nursing, for more information).
3. Control pain with analgesics, proper body positioning, relaxation techniques, or transcutaneous electrical nerve stimulation (TENS), as appropriate.
4. Provide other care depending on manifestations (e.g., urinary incontinence or retention, bowel incontinence or constipation, impaired mobility). Care is similar to that for a patient with spinal cord injury (see Section VII.F).
5. Provide reassurance and emotional support as the patient and family cope with the diagnosis and uncertain prognosis (see Chapter 21, Cancer Nursing, for details).

G. Evaluation
1. The patient reports adequate pain control.
2. The patient demonstrates maximum use of remaining abilities in self-care and mobility.
3. The patient maintains good skin integrity.
4. The patient verbalizes realistic expectations about the future and expresses feelings about his or her condition and its impact on his or her life.
5. Family members verbalize understanding of the patient's con-

dition and demonstrate the willingness and ability to assist the patient in functioning at his or her optimum level.

6. The patient reports satisfaction with sexual expression.

7. The patient exhibits no bowel or bladder problems.

IX. Intervertebral disk herniation

A. **Description: a disorder involving impingement of a vertebral disk's nucleus pulposus on spinal nerve roots, causing pain and possible neuromuscular deficit**

B. **Etiology and incidence**
1. Herniated disk can result from:
    a. Degenerative disorders
    b. Trauma
    c. Congenital predisposition
2. A common back problem, herniated disk most commonly affects men younger than age 45.

C. **Pathophysiology**
1. Rupture of the annulus pulposus (the disk's outer ring) allows part of the nucleus pulposus (the soft, gelatinous inner portion) to protrude and press against spinal nerve roots, producing symptoms.
2. Herniation can occur anywhere along the vertebral column but is most common in the lumbar area (more than 90% of cases).
3. Clinical manifestations vary with the location and degree of herniation and the course of its progression. In lumbar disk herniation, pressure on the sciatic nerve can produce severe—sometimes debilitating—pain and if chronic, possible motor and sensory changes.

D. **Assessment findings**
1. Common signs and symptoms of herniated disk include:
    a. Back pain (in lumbar herniation, often with radiation down the posterior thigh and leg), exacerbated by coughing, sneezing, or straining
    b. Varying degrees of motor and sensory impairment (e.g., muscle weakness, diminished deep tendon reflexes in the lower extremities)
    c. Positive straight-leg raising test or LeSegue's test
2. CT scan, MRI, or myelography may reveal the location of herniation.

E. **Nursing diagnoses**
1. Anxiety
2. Impaired Physical Mobility
3. Pain

F. **Planning and implementation**
1. Assess the location, nature, course, and progression of back pain.

2. Monitor motor and sensory status.
3. Provide conservative management, if indicated, including:
   a. Encouraging bedrest
   b. Positioning in Williams position
   c. Applying heat
   d. Instructing in appropriate exercises
4. If laminectomy is ordered to remove protruding disk fragments, provide appropriate perioperative care (see Chapter 24, Perioperative Nursing, for information on general patient care measures).
5. After surgery:
   a. Assess strength, sensation, and movement of extremities.
   b. Keep the patient in proper body alignment when in bed (providing a firm mattress) and when turning (using log-rolling technique).
   c. Encourage the patient to wear good walking shoes when ambulating.
   d. Teach the patient proper body mechanics to help prevent injury.
   e. Teach the patient to avoid slippery surfaces and activities that can involve sudden back movements.

G. **Evaluation**
   1. The patient reports reduced pain; facial expression and body movements reflect increased comfort.
   2. The patient walks with a normal gait.

X. Multiple sclerosis (MS)

A. **Description: a progressively disabling demyelinating disease affecting nerve fibers of the brain and spinal cord and marked by periodic exacerbations and remissions**

B. **Etiology and incidence**
   1. The cause of MS is unknown; theories include a slow-growing virus, an autoimmune process, and an allergic response to an infectious agent.
   2. Incidence is greater in women than in men and is highest in temperate climates; age of onset is typically between age 20 and 40.

C. **Pathophysiology**
   1. MS produces patches of demyelination throughout the central nervous system, impeding transmission of nerve impulses.
   2. The random pattern of demyelination causes widely varying neurologic effects.
   3. The course of MS is marked by periodic and unpredictable exacerbations and remissions.
   4. Prognosis is variable; MS can cause rapid, sometimes fatal, dis-

ability, but about 70% of patients lead active, productive lives with long periods of remission.

D. **Assessment findings**
1. Clinical manifestations of MS vary widely but may include:
   a. Visual problems: diplopia, blurred vision, nystagmus
   b. Motor dysfunction: muscle weakness, paralysis, spasticity, hyperreflexia, tremors, gait ataxia
   c. Fatigue
   d. Bladder or bowel incontinence
   e. Mental changes: mood swings, irritability, depression
2. No single diagnostic test confirms diagnosis. Lumbar puncture and CSF analysis may reveal elevated CSF gamma globulins; MRI may confirm the presence of demyelinating plaques.

E. **Nursing diagnoses**
1. Anxiety
2. Body Image Disturbance
3. Bowel Incontinence
4. Fatigue
5. High Risk for Injury
6. Impaired Physical Mobility
7. Altered Role Performance
8. Functional Urinary Incontinence

F. **Planning and implementation**
1. Assess the nature and degree of neuromuscular deficits and their effect on the patient's lifestyle.
2. Assess the patient's sleep and rest patterns; encourage adequate rest to avoid fatigue.
3. Assist the patient in planning lifestyle modifications to decrease stress and fatigue and maximize functional abilities.
4. Administer adrenocorticotropic hormone (ACTH) or adrenal corticosteroids during exacerbations as prescribed.
5. Provide appropriate care during exacerbations (e.g., help the patient establish bladder and bowel control, prevent skin breakdown, prevent and treat muscle spasticity).

G. **Evaluation**
1. The patient demonstrates positive adjustment to altered lifestyle.
2. The patient exhibits a low anxiety level.

XI. Parkinson's disease

A. **Description: a progressive neurologic disorder secondary to degeneration of basal ganglia in the cerebrum**

B. **Etiology and incidence**
1. The etiology of Parkinson's disease is unknown.
2. Suspected causes include:
   a. Viral infection

      b.   Chemical toxicity

      c.   Cerebrovascular disease

      d.   Effects of such drugs as major tranquilizers and reserpine

  3.   The second most common neurologic disorder in the elderly, Parkinson's disease affects about 1 in 100 persons over age 60; incidence is higher in men than in women.

C.   **Pathophysiology**

  1.   Dopamine, a neurotransmitter secreted by the basal ganglia, is essential to extrapyramidal function; depletion of dopamine results in loss of normal neuromuscular inhibiting mechanisms.

  2.   Characteristic neurologic deficits associated with Parkinsonism include:

      a.   Bradykinesia

      b.   Muscle rigidity

      c.   Resting tremor

  3.   Progressive deterioration progresses for an average of 10 years; death commonly results from pneumonia or another infection.

D.   **Assessment findings**

  1.   Common clinical manifestations include:

      a.   Tremor, an early sign, commonly affecting the hands and more prominent at rest; also known as resting and "pill rolling" tremor

      b.   Bradykinesia (dyskinesia, akinesia): loss of spontaneous movement, slowness in voluntary movement, difficulty initiating movement

      c.   Rigidity: decreased muscle tone and stiffness, with jerky movements ("cogwheel rigidity")

      d.   Fatigue and muscle weakness

      e.   Stooped posture, shuffling gait with marked arm swinging

      f.   Impaired ability to turn in bed and rise from chair

      g.   Masklike facial expression, increased blinking reflex

      h.   Autonomic manifestations, such as oily skin (seborrhea) and excessive perspiration

      i.   Dysphagia, drooling

      j.   Monotone speech, impaired articulation (dysarthria)

      k.   Constipation, due to decreased fluid intake and autonomic dysfunction

      l.   Depression, withdrawal

  2.   No tests are diagnostic for Parkinson's disease; however, urinalysis may reveal increased dopamine levels, supporting diagnosis.

E.   **Nursing diagnoses**

  1.   Impaired Verbal Communication

2. Constipation
3. High Risk for Injury
4. Knowledge Deficit
5. Impaired Physical Mobility
6. Altered Nutrition: Less Than Body Requirements
7. Self-Care Deficits
8. Self-Concept Disturbance
9. Sleep Pattern Disturbance
10. Impaired Social Interaction
11. Altered Role Performance

F. **Planning and implementation**
   1. Administer medications as prescribed, which may include:
      a. Levodopa
      b. Anticholinergics
      c. Antihistamines
   2. If indicated, prepare the patient for stereotaxic surgery to reduce tremors and rigidity.

G. **Evaluation**
   1. The patient demonstrates the ability to perform activities of daily living (ADLs).
   2. The patient exhibits adequate social interaction.

XII. Amyotrophic lateral sclerosis (ALS)

A. **Description: a progressively debilitating and eventually fatal disease involving degeneration of motor neurons**

B. **Etiology and incidence**
   1. The cause of ALS is unknown.
   2. ALS affects 2 to 7 of every 100,000 persons, with men affected about four times more often than women; onset typically occurs between ages 40 and 70.

C. **Pathophysiology**
   1. ALS is marked by progressive destruction of motor cells in the anterior gray horns and pyramidal tract; both upper and lower motor neurons are affected.
   2. As motor neurons die, the muscle cells that they supply undergo atrophic changes. Progressive paralysis typically results.
   3. Prognosis is variable; most patients with ALS die within 3 to 10 years of onset, usually from secondary causes such as pneumonia.

D. **Assessment findings**
   1. Clinical manifestations vary with the location of affected motor neurons and disease stage, and may include:
      a. Progressive weakness, atrophy, spasticity, and tremors of upper extremities, followed by involvement of lower extremities and then respiratory muscles

          b.   Fatigue
          c.   Impaired speech, chewing, and swallowing
          d.   Breathing difficulty
          e.   Depression

    2.   There are no diagnostic studies specific to ALS; diagnosis is based on patient history and neurologic assessment findings.

E. Nursing diagnoses

    1.   Ineffective Airway Clearance
    2.   High Risk for Aspiration
    3.   Body Image Disturbance
    4.   Impaired Verbal Communication
    5.   Ineffective Individual and Family Coping
    6.   Impaired Gas Exchange
    7.   Hopelessness
    8.   Powerlessness
    9.   Altered Role Performance
   10. High Risk for Impaired Skin Integrity
   11. Impaired Swallowing

F. Planning and implementation

    1.   Because no treatment currently is available to slow disease progression, provide supportive care, focusing on:
          a.   Maximizing functional abilities (e.g., mobility, self-care, communication)
          b.   Preventing skin breakdown
          c.   Preventing respiratory complications
          d.   Ensuring adequate nutrition
          e.   Providing intellectually stimulating activities since the patient typically experiences no cognitive deficits
    2.   Provide emotional support as the patient and family deal with the poor prognosis and the grieving process.

G. Evaluation

    1.   The patient demonstrates the ability to perform ADLs to the maximum of his or her functional capacity.
    2.   The patient displays no respiratory complications, skin breakdown, or other untoward problems.
    3.   The patient and family exhibit positive coping with absence of depression.

XIII. Myasthenia gravis

  A. Description: a progressive disorder affecting neuromuscular transmission of impulses in voluntary muscles

  B. Etiology and incidence

    1.   Myasthenia gravis is considered to be an autoimmune response.
    2.   Incidence is one in 25,000 persons and is higher in women than in men; initial symptoms typically occur between ages 20 and 40.

C. Pathophysiology

1. In myasthenia gravis, acetylcholine receptor (AChR) antibodies interfere with impulse transmission across myoneural junctions.
2. This causes abnormal weakness and fatigability of skeletal muscle, particularly of the eyes, face, jaw, and neck; also may involve muscles of upper extremities and respiratory muscles.
3. The disorder follows an unpredictable course of periodic exacerbations and remissions. For most patients, drug therapy allows patients to lead normal lives; however, progressive weakness of respiratory muscles may cause life-threatening respiratory distress or myasthenic crisis.

D. Assessment findings

1. Clinical manifestations typically include:
   a. Abnormal weakness of any striated muscle (particularly of the face, neck, and arms and hands), typically worsening after activity and improving with rest
   b. Severe fatigue
   c. Drooping facial muscles; ptosis
   d. Diplopia
   e. Impaired chewing and swallowing
   f. Breathing difficulty related to weakened respiratory muscles
2. Diagnosis is based on history of weakness of specific muscle groups; positive Tensilon test confirms diagnosis.

E. Nursing diagnoses

1. Ineffective Airway Clearance
2. High Risk for Aspiration
3. Fatigue
4. Impaired Gas Exchange
5. Altered Role Performance

F. Planning and implementation

1. Administer anticholinesterase medications (corticosteroids, neostigmine, or pyridostigmine) as prescribed.
2. If indicated, prepare the patient for other treatments, such as plasmapheresis or thymectomy.
3. Prevent problems associated with swallowing difficulty; provide small, frequent meals, and keep suctioning equipment readily available.
4. Encourage adjustment in lifestyle to prevent fatigue.

G. Evaluation

1. The patient exhibits positive adjustment to lifestyle changes.
2. The patient remains free of respiratory complications.
3. The patient demonstrates adequate ability to perform ADLs.

XIV. **Guillain-Barré syndrome**

   A. Description: an acute, rapidly progressive form of polyneuritis producing muscle weakness and mild sensory disturbances

   B. Etiology and incidence
   1. Guillain-Barré syndrome is a postinfectious polyneuritis of unknown origin that commonly follows febrile illness.
   2. It can develop at any age but is most common between ages 30 and 50; incidence is about equal in men and women.

   C. Pathophysiology
   1. Segmental demyelination of peripheral nerves causes inflammation and degenerative changes in sensory and motor nerve roots.
   2. Most patients experience spontaneous and complete recovery although mild deficits may persist.

   D. Assessment findings
   1. Common signs and symptoms include:
       a. Paresis in the legs (usually the initial manifestation)
       b. Motor weakness progressing to involve the entire peripheral nervous system, including respiratory muscles
       c. Paresthesias
   2. Progression may involve total or partial paralysis.
   3. Lumbar puncture and CSF analysis may reveal elevated CSF proteins.

   E. Nursing diagnoses
   1. Anxiety
   2. Ineffective Gas Exchange
   3. Impaired Physical Mobility

   F. Planning and implementation
   1. Explain all procedures and care measures to help reduce the patient's anxiety.
   2. Monitor respiratory status (if muscles of respiration are involved).
   3. Assist with plasmapheresis, if it is prescribed.

   G. Evaluation
   1. The patient exhibits a low level of anxiety.
   2. The patient remains free of complications.
   3. The patient experiences a complete return of function.

XV. **Meningitis**

   A. Description: infection or inflammation of the meninges covering the brain and spinal cord

   B. Etiology and incidence
   1. Bacterial meningitis most often results from previous infection with *Neisseria meningitidis*, *Streptococcus pneumoniae*, or *Haemophilus influenzae*.

2. Aseptic meningitis may be caused by viral infection or other causes.
3. Children are more prone than adults because of their greater propensity for respiratory infection.

C. Pathophysiology
1. Infective organisms that enter the brain quickly disseminate through the meninges and into the ventricles.
2. This dissemination may result in:
    a. Meningeal congestion
    b. Cerebral edema
    c. Increased ICP
    d. Generalized inflammation with exudate formation
    e. Hydrocephalus if exudate blocks ventricular passages
3. Prognosis is good with early detection and prompt treatment; however, untreated meningitis (or delayed treatment) commonly proves fatal, particularly in children and elderly persons.

D. Assessment findings
1. Clinical manifestations may include:
    a. Headache and fever
    b. Altered level of consciousness
    c. Signs of meningeal irritation: nuchal rigidity, positive Brudzinski's and Kernig's signs, exaggerated deep tendon reflexes, opisthotonos
    d. Signs and symptoms of increased ICP (see Section III.D)
2. Diagnosis is confirmed by isolation and identification of the causative organism in CSF.

E. Nursing diagnoses
1. Hyperthermia
2. Pain
3. Other nursing diagnoses associated with increased ICP (see Section III.E)

F. Planning and implementation
1. Administer prescribed antibiotics to treat bacterial meningitis.
2. Apply a hypothermia blanket, as prescribed, to relieve hyperthermia.
3. Intervene as appropriate to reduce increased ICP (see Section III.F).

G. Evaluation
1. The patient maintains body temperature within normal range.
2. The patient reports or exhibits reduced pain.
3. The patient exhibits no signs and symptoms of increased ICP.

XVI. Bell's palsy
A. Description: a disorder of the facial nerve (CN VII) producing unilateral facial paresis or paralysis
B. Etiology and incidence
1. Bell's palsy results from facial nerve inflammation, most com-

monly due to infection, vascular disorders, or local trauma. In some cases, an autoimmune reaction may be involved.
   2. It affects all age groups but is most prevalent in persons younger than age 60.
 C. Pathophysiology
   1. The inflamed, edematous facial nerve becomes compressed, causing paresis or paralysis of facial muscles.
   2. In most patients, spontaneous recovery occurs within 3 to 5 weeks. Partial recovery may leave the patient with facial contractures.
 D. Assessment findings
   1. Clinical manifestations include:
      a. Drooping mouth on one side, possibly with drooling
      b. Possible pain
      c. Inability to close the eyelid on the affected side
   2. Diagnosis is based on patient history and signs and symptoms.
 E. Nursing diagnoses
   1. Body Image Disturbance
   2. High Risk for Injury
   3. Altered Nutrition: Less Than Body Requirements
 F. Planning and implementation
   1. Administer prednisone, if prescribed, to reduce facial nerve edema.
   2. Provide small, frequent feedings of soft foods.
   3. Provide eye care; teach patient to close lids periodically and to use artificial tears.
   4. Apply a facial sling to support facial muscles.
   5. Massage facial muscles gently and apply heat.
 G. Evaluation: patient exhibits complete return of function

Bibliography

Brunner, L. S., & Suddarth, D. S. (1988). *Textbook of medical-surgical nursing* (6th ed.). Philadelphia: J. B. Lippincott.

Luckmann, J., & Sorensen, K. C. (1988). *Medical-surgical nursing: A psychophysiologic approach* (3rd ed.). Philadelphia: W. B. Saunders.

Mitchell, P. H., Hodges, L. C., Muwaswes, M., & Walleck, C. A. (1988). *AANN's neuroscience nursing*. Norwalk, CT: Appleton and Lange.

STUDY QUESTIONS

1. Mr. Chapman, aged 20, received a severe blow to the head. He was unconscious for several minutes following the trauma but now responds to stimuli. Mr. Chapman has been hospitalized for observation. When monitoring him for signs of increasing ICP, the nurse should be particularly alert for
   a. pupillary changes
   b. difficulty arousing Mr. Chapman
   c. decreasing blood pressure
   d. elevated temperature

2. Appropriate actions for a patient experiencing a tonic–clonic seizure would include which of the following?
   a. placing a tongue blade between the teeth
   b. elevating the head
   c. protecting the head and extremities from hitting objects
   d. restraining the arms and legs

3. Ms. Janus, aged 33, has suffered a subarachnoid hemorrhage and complains of severe pain when moving her head. For this patient, the nursing diagnosis of Pain would be related to
   a. blood causing irritation of the meninges
   b. lack of oxygen to the parietal lobe
   c. increased production of CSF
   d. decrease in neurotransmitters

4. Which of the following parameters should the nurse use in evaluating the effectiveness of interventions to prevent bladder infection?
   a. Cystogram reveals normal findings.
   b. The patient does not complain of pain.
   c. Urine output is 150 mL/day.
   d. Temperature is within normal limits, and urine culture is negative.

5. Ms. Thurlow, aged 39, has undergone craniotomy to excise a glioma-type brain tumor. She responds minimally to stimuli, and her respirations sound very moist. These findings would lead the nurse to make the nursing diagnosis of

   a. Decreased Cardiac Output
   b. Ineffective Airway Clearance
   c. Ineffective Breathing Patterns
   d. Anxiety

6. Mr. Homer, aged 55, is recovering from a severe head injury in which his prefrontal lobe was damaged. When caring for Mr. Homer, the nurse should remain particularly alert for which of the following problems?
   a. visual impairment
   b. swallowing difficulty
   c. impaired judgment
   d. hearing impairment

7. Mrs. Lippett, aged 66, is experiencing sensory and perceptual problems that affect her right visual field (right homonymous hemianopia). When placing a meal tray in front of Mrs. Lippett, the nurse should
   a. Place all the food on the right side of the tray.
   b. Before leaving the room, remind the patient to look over all the tray.
   c. Place food and utensils within the patient's left visual field.
   d. Stay with the patient, and periodically draw her attention to the food on the right side of the tray.

8. The nurse should include which of the following in preprocedure teachings for a patient scheduled for carotid angiography?
   a. "You will be put to sleep before the needle is inserted."
   b. "The test will take several hours."
   c. "You may feel a burning sensation when the dye is injected."
   d. "There will be no complications."

9. What deficits would the nurse expect in a right-handed person experiencing a stroke affecting the left side of the cortex?
   a. expressive aphasia and paralysis on the right side of the body
   b. expressive aphasia and paralysis on the left side of the body

c. dysarthria and paralysis on the right side of the body

d. mixed aphasia and paralysis on the right side of the body

10. Which of the following would be the most important consideration in providing emergency care to a person with a possible cervical spinal injury?
    a. Monitor vital signs every 5 minutes.
    b. Place the neck in a flexed position.
    c. Check to see if the patient can move his or her toes.
    d. Immobilize the head and spine, keeping them in alignment.

11. What would be the most appropriate intervention for a patient with aphasia who states, "I want a . . ." and then stops?
    a. Wait for the patient to complete the sentence.
    b. Immediately begin showing the patient various objects in the environment.
    c. Leave the room and come back later.
    d. Begin naming various objects that the patient could be referring to.

12. Which of the following statements would be most appropriate when assisting a patient who has the nursing diagnosis of Altered Thought Processes with Personal Hygiene Needs?
    a. "What would you like to do first, brush your teeth?"
    b. "Where is your toothbrush?"
    c. "When would you like to have your bath?"
    d. "Would you like to brush your teeth, or do you want me to do it for you? It's good to do things for yourself."

13. Which of the following positions would be most appropriate for a patient with right-sided paralysis following a stroke?
    a. on the side with support to the back, with pillows to keep the body in alignment, hips slightly flexed, and hands tightly holding a rolled washcloth
    b. on the side with support to the back, pillows to keep the body in alignment, hips slightly flexed, and a washcloth placed so that fingers are slightly curled
    c. on the back with two large pillows under the head, a pillow under the knees, and a footboard
    d. on the back with no pillows used, with trochanter rolls and a footboard

14. To prevent infection in a patient with a subdural intracranial pressure monitoring system in place, the nurse should
    a. Use aseptic technique when cleaning the insertion site and connections.
    b. Use clean technique for cleansing connections and aseptic technique for the insertion site.
    c. Use sterile technique when cleansing the insertion site.
    d. Close any leaks in the tubing with tape.

15. Ms. Seymour, aged 27, recently has been diagnosed with multiple sclerosis. In assisting Ms. Seymour to adapt to her altered lifestyle, which of the following information would be important to include in patient teaching?
    a. the effects that stress and tiredness have on symptoms
    b. the need for small, frequent meals
    c. the need for vigorous exercise
    d. the positive effects of a high-protein diet

ANSWER KEY

1. **Correct response: *b***
   The first sign of downward pressure on the reticular activating system in the brain stem decreases responsiveness.
   a. Pupillary changes occur later.
   c. Systolic blood pressure increases.
   d. Temperature changes vary and may not be present even with severe decreases in responsiveness.
   Comprehension/Physiologic/Assessment

2. **Correct response: *c***
   Protecting the patient by moving objects so that the arms and legs do not hit them and placing a soft object under the head are the most important immediate interventions.
   a. Trying to force a tongue blade or other object into the mouth may damage teeth.
   b. Nothing is gained by elevating the patient's head since breathing will return to normal after the activity stops.
   d. Restraining movement may result in injury or stiffness following the seizure.
   Application/Safe care/Evaluation

3. **Correct response: *a***
   Pain, particularly on movement of the neck, results from blood leakage into the CSF; time will be required for it to be absorbed.
   b and c. Lack of oxygen and increased CSF production usually do not occur.
   d. Neurotransmitters are not involved in the process.
   Knowledge/Physiologic/Analysis (Dx)

4. **Correct response: *d***
   Bladder infections result from a variety of causes in many patients with neurologic problems. Elevated temperature occurs in urinary and respiratory infections. A negative urine culture would be another indicator of the absence of infection.
   a. Cystography is done to evaluate

   bladder function, not detect infection.
   b and c. Pain on urination or oliguria are indicators of infection.
   Comprehension/Physiologic/Evaluation

5. **Correct response: *b***
   Patients with decreased arousal frequently have airway problems caused by immobility or by pathology in the brain stem. Attention to respirations and frequent assessment of airway for suctioning are indicated.
   a. Decreased cardiac output would not cause moist sound.
   c. The breathing pattern may be altered, but moist sounds do not indicate a change in pattern.
   d. Anxiety may result from difficulties in breathing, but this patient probably is not alert enough to experience anxiety.
   Application/Physiologic/Analysis (Dx)

6. **Correct response: *c***
   A number of areas of the brain are involved in cognition and thinking, but damage to the prefrontal area frequently results in impaired judgment and insight.
   a. Vision problems may occur with pathology in the occipital lobe or in the pituitary area (optic chiasm).
   b. Swallowing problems result from damage to cranial nerves IX in the brain stem.
   d. Hearing impairment commonly occurs with damage to the CN VIII.
   Comprehension/Safe care/Assessment

7. **Correct response: *d***
   This patient needs to learn to scan her entire visual field.
   a, b, and c. These interventions are not as appropriate as d.
   Analysis/Health promotion/Implementation

8. **Correct response: *c***
   Providing a patient with information about expected sensations often helps decrease anxiety. The contrast media fre-

quently causes a burning sensation as it passes through the cerebral arteries.

a. Patients rarely receive general anesthesia for an angiogram.

b. The test usually takes less than an hour.

d. Various complications—such as airway obstruction and vasospasm with sensory and motor deficits—may occur after an angiogram.

Application/Health promotion/ Implementation

9. **Correct response: d**

Most aphasias involve both expressive and receptive components although one may dominate. The speech center is most often found on the nondominant side; the left side of the brain controls the right side of the body.

a, b, and c. These deficits would not be expected in this patient.

Analysis/Physiologic/Assessment

10. **Correct response: d**

Immobilization in alignment will prevent possible fractures or dislocated bone from damaging the spinal cord.

a. Monitoring the patient is important but secondary to immobilization.

b. Flexing the neck can cause spinal cord damage.

c. Patients with suspected back injuries should avoid movement until evaluation rules out cord damage.

Application/Safe care/Implementation

11. **Correct response: a**

It often takes time for an aphasic person to select a proper word; the nurse should let the person try to express himself or herself without letting the person become too frustrated.

b, c, and d. These interventions would not be appropriate in this situation.

Analysis/Psychosocial/Implementation

12. **Correct response: b**

Simple directions are most appropriate; this patient probably is not capable of making decisions at this time.

a, c, and d. Because all of these statements ask the patient to make a decision, they would be inappropriate in this situation.

Analysis/Psychosocial/Planning

13. **Correct response: b**

The optimum position is one that approximates normal body functioning.

a. Curling the fingers tightly can lead to contractures.

c and d. Placing too many pillows under the head may interfere with breathing and pull the rest of the body out of alignment.

Analysis/Health promotion/Evaluation

14. **Correct response: c**

Utmost care is needed to prevent introducing organisms into the subdural space; therefore, sterile technique is required.

a and b. Sterile technique is required.

d. Leaking tubing should be replaced.

Application/Safe care/Planning

15. **Correct response: a**

Studies have shown that stress and fatigue adversely affect the course of the disease. Teaching stress management techniques and helping the patient adjust her schedule to ensure adequate rest will be beneficial.

b. Small, frequent feedings are not a priority in a patient with MS.

c. Vigorous exercise can lead to fatigue.

d. Increased protein intake is not associated with MS treatment.

Application/Health promotion/Planning

Eye, Ear, Nose, Sinus, and Throat Disorders

I. Anatomy and physiology: eyes

A. Structure

1. Anatomically, the eye can be divided into three layers, or coats (outer, middle, and inner) and the refractive media.

2. The outer, protective layer consists of the:

   a. Sclera: white, opaque, fibrous connective tissue

   b. Cornea: the anterior continuation of the sclera, transparent and avascular

3. The middle, vascular layer (also known as the uveal tract) includes the:

   a. Choroid: a thin, pigmented membrane containing blood vessels that supply eye tissues

   b. Ciliary body: the anterior continuation of the choroid containing muscles that change the shape of the lens to focus vision

   c. Iris: the central extension of the ciliary body consisting of two muscles and a central opening, the pupil, which constricts and dilates to regulate the amount of light entering the eye's interior (constricts with strong light and near vision, dilates with dim light and far vision)

4. The inner, neural layer—the retina—contains layers of nerve cells, including rods and cones, that translate lightwaves into neural impulses for transmission to the brain.

5. Refractive media include the:

   a. Cornea

   b. Aqueous humor, watery fluid filling the eye's anterior chamber that serves as a refracting medium and maintains the hydrostatic intraocular pressure (IOP)

   c. Lens, a biconvex crystalline body located behind the pupil that changes shape for accommodation (focusing)

   d. Vitreous humor, a jellylike substance filling the posterior cavity behind the lens, acting as a refractive medium and maintaining the shape of the eye

B. Function

1. Vision depends on a complex coordination of ocular structures that mediate passage of light rays reflected from an external object to the retina and transmit visual images to the brain for interpretation.

2. Normally, light passes through the refractive media to the retina, where an inverted and reversed image forms.

3. In the retina, rods and cones convert the projected image into nerve impulses and transmit them to the optic nerve.

4. Impulses travel along the optic nerve to the brain's optic chiasm and then to the cerebral cortex, where they are interpreted as sight.

II. Overview of eye disorders

A. Assessment

1. The visual fields confrontation test evaluates the peripheral extent of visual fields (other than central reading vision); normal findings include 60 degrees nasally, 50 degrees upward, 90 degrees temporally, 70 degrees downward.

2. IOP measurement requires a tonometer applied to the cornea. Normal IOP ranges from 12 to 21 mmHg; pressure is increased in glaucoma.

3. Visual acuity testing uses a Snellen chart to evaluate for visual acuity and newsprint to assess near vision. Normal visual acuity is considered to be $20/20$, in which the numerator represents the distance from the person to chart and the denominator the distance at which a normal eye can read the line; the larger the denominator, the poorer the vision.

4. Used to prescribe corrective lenses, the refraction test has the person read a Snellen chart through various corrective lenses to measure errors of focus: myopia (nearsightedness), hyperopia (farsightedness), astigmatism (inability to focus horizontal and vertical rays on retina).

5. Ophthalmoscopic examination evaluates blood vessels and structures of the posterior eye (fundus), detecting retinal changes due to neurologic or vascular conditions.

B. Psychosocial implications

1. A patient with a visual problem may experience coping difficulties related to:
   a. Unknown prognosis
   b. Chronicity or long-term nature of the condition

2. The patient also may experience self-concept changes associated with:
   a. Altered body image due to blindness or the need to wear eyeglasses
   b. Potential for loss of independence

3. The patient may have to adjust to lifestyle changes related to potential changes in:
   a. Role performance
   b. Occupational performance, with possibility of job loss
   c. Self-care ability

4. Changes in social interaction patterns related to vision problems may lead to:
   a. Depression
   b. Isolation

C. Medications used to treat eye problems

1. *Miotics* are used to lower IOP in glaucoma by constricting pupils and promoting outflow of aqueous humor; agents include:
   a. Parasympathomimetic (cholinergic) drugs: pilocarpine hydrochloride (e.g., Pilocar), carbachol (e.g., Carbacel)
   b. Cholinesterase inhibitors: echothiophate iodide (e.g., Echodide), physostigmine salicylate (e.g., Eserine Salicylate)

2. *Mydriatics* are used to dilate the pupil for intraocular assessment and to accommodate refraction; *cycloplegics*, to paralyze ciliary accommodative muscles before refraction. Drugs used include:
   a. Parasympatholytic (anticholinergic) drugs, with combined mydriatic and cycloplegic effects: atropine sulfate (e.g., Atropisol), scopolamine hydrobromide (e.g., Isopto Hyoscine)

      b.   Sympathomimetic (adrenergic) drugs, used for mydriasis and vasoconstriction and in open-angle glaucoma to reduce IOP, but not to induce cycloplegia: adrenaline, phenylephrine hydrochloride (e.g., Neo-Synephrine)

   3.   *Corticosteroids* are administered to treat nonpyrogenic inflammation (due to allergy or injury); agents include:
      a.   Dexamethasone (e.g., Maxidex Ophthalmic Solution)
      b.   Prednisolone acetate (e.g., Econopred) and prednisolone sodium phosphate (e.g., Metreton Ophthalmic)
      c.   Fluorometholone (e.g., Fluor-Op)

   4.   *Carbonic anhydrase inhibitors*, such as acetazolamide (e.g., Diamox), are used to control IOP in glaucoma by reducing aqueous humor formation.

   5.   Used to treat glaucoma, *beta-adrenergic blockers* decrease formation of aqueous humor and prevent the sympathetic response of pupil dilation; agents include:
      a.   Timolol maleate (e.g., Timoptic)
      b.   Betaxolol hydrochloride (Betoptic)

   6.   *Hyperosmotic agents* reduce IOP by increasing blood osmolality and are administered for acute IOP increase and preoperatively; agents include:
      a.   Mannitol (Osmitrol)
      b.   Glycerol (e.g., Osmoglyn)

III. General nursing interventions in eye care
A. Ophthalmic medication administration
   1.   Ensure that all eye medications are sterile.
   2.   Do not use unlabeled, cloudy, or discolored solutions.
   3.   Avoid contact with the eye to prevent contaminating the medication bottle or tube tip.
   4.   Treat each eye separately (i.e., separate medication and equipment); treat the uninfected eye first to avoid cross contamination.
   5.   To instill eye drops:
      a.   Tilt the patient's head back slightly; expose the lower conjunctival sac by pulling down gently on the cheekbone.
      b.   Have the patient look up.
      c.   Resting your hand on the patient's forehead for support, to prevent eye injury during administration, instill the prescribed amount of medication onto the lower conjunctiva.
      d.   Close the lid gently and press on the nasal–lacrimal canal (inner canthus) to prevent systemic drug absorption and resulting side effects.

   e.   Wipe excess secretions with a sterile cotton ball, wiping from the inner to the outer canthus.
6. To instill eye ointment:
   a.   Follow the same basic procedure as for instilling eye drops.
   b.   Have the patient close the lid and roll the eye after instillation.

B.   Eye patch application
1.   Have the patient close both eyes during patch application.
2.   Apply the patch and secure it with two strips of tape extending from the midforehead to the lateral cheekbone.
3.   Never apply pressure unless prescribed; if pressure is indicated, use two or three pads and more tape.
4.   Never change an eye patch without a physician's order.

C.   Eye shield application
1.   Apply an eye shield, alone or over an eye patch, to protect the eye from pressure or irritation.
2.   Rest the shield on the bony prominences of the brow, cheek, and nose, and secure it in place with strips of transparent tape in the same manner as for an eye patch (medial top to lateral bottom).

IV.   General nursing interventions in eye surgery

A.   Preoperative care
1.   Explain expected preoperative procedures (e.g., sedation, local or general anesthetic) to reduce anxiety associated with the unfamiliar and unexpected.
2.   For the same reason, explain what to expect postoperatively (e.g., eye patch application, prescribed positioning, activity restrictions, ophthalmic medication use, measures to prevent increased IOP, a small amount of serous drainage and subjunctival hemorrhage postoperatively, and eyelid edema for several days).

B.   Postoperative care
1.   Take precautions to prevent increased IOP, such as:
   a.   Instructing the patient to lie on the unoperated side
   b.   Avoiding constipation (e.g., by administering stool softeners)
   c.   Encouraging the patient to avoid sneezing or coughing (or to cough with the mouth open, if necessary)
   d.   Administering an antiemetic to a nauseous patient to prevent vomiting
   e.   Washing the patient's hair, when allowed, with the neck hyperextended rather than flexed
   f.   Instructing the patient to avoid excessive exertion, such as lifting and pushing objects

2. Take precautions to prevent injury, such as:
   a. Orienting the patient to the hospital environment
   b. Keeping a call bell and other needed items within the patient's reach and in a consistent place
   c. Keeping the bed in a low position with the side rails up
   d. Providing adequate room light, or dimming lights if the patient experiences photophobia
   e. Assisting the patient with ambulation, if indicated
   f. Advising the patient not to rub the eyes or touch an eye patch
3. Relieve postoperative discomfort with proper positioning and analgesics as prescribed; avoid opiates, which may cause vomiting or constipation.
4. Instruct the patient to report any sharp pain or feelings of pressure in the eye, which may indicate hemorrhage, increased IOP, or infection.
5. Promote mobility within postoperative restrictions; post any prescribed activity restrictions on the patient's bed.
6. Prevent sensory deprivation by:
   a. Rooming the patient with another well-oriented, active person if possible
   b. Providing sensory stimulation (e.g., talk to the patient often, provide a radio or TV, encourage frequent visitation by family and friends)
   c. Frequently reorienting the patient to the environment and the date and time of day
7. Promote adequate nutrition; assist the patient with eating and drinking, as necessary, to ensure adequate intake and prevent choking and aspiration.
8. Teach the patient to report signs and symptoms of potential complications, such as coughing, marked restlessness, sharp eye pain, or any eye pain unrelieved by analgesics.
9. Teach appropriate self-care measures, which may include:
   a. Not removing an eye patch unless specifically ordered
   b. Wearing an eye shield at night or when lying down
   c. Taking sponge baths or showers without getting water on the face
   d. Wearing dark glasses and dimming room lights if experiencing photophobia or using dilating drops
   e. Using medications as prescribed

V. Retinal detachment

A. Description: separation of the retina from the choroid in the posterior eye

B. Etiology and incidence

1. Retinal detachment may result from trauma, age-related degenerative changes, or cataract removal.

2. It most commonly affects persons older than age 40.

C. Pathophysiology

1. Retinal layers separate from the choroid, creating a subretinal space.
2. Vitreous fluid seeps between these layers, disrupting choroidal blood supply.
3. Detachment may be partial, causing varying degrees of visual deficits, or total, causing blindness in the affected eye.
4. In most cases, surgery is indicated to reattach the retina.

D. Assessment findings

1. Clinical manifestations typically include:
   a. Recurrent flashes of light and floating spots initially
   b. Progressive blurring of vision in the affected eye, followed by visual field deficits, with the area of visual loss depending on the area of detachment
2. The patient is commonly anxious, confused, and fearful of blindness.
3. Ophthalmoscopic examination may reveal an area of gray, opaque retina, possibly with fold, holes, or tears.

E. Nursing diagnoses

1. Anxiety
2. High Risk for Injury
3. Knowledge Deficit
4. Impaired Physical Mobility
5. Pain
6. Sensory and Perceptual Alteration: Visual

F. Planning and implementation

1. Provide information regarding surgical options, which may include:
   a. Creating localized chorioretinal adhesions to reapproximate the retina and choroid through cryotherapy, photocoagulation, laser surgery
   b. Sealing the retina to the choroid with scleral buckling surgery
   c. Injecting an intraocular gas bubble to promote adhesion
2. Limit mobility by:
   a. Positioning the patient in bed preoperatively, as prescribed (usually with the detached area dependent), and instructing the patient to avoid lying face down, stooping, or bending
   b. Enforcing bedrest for 1 day postoperatively, positioned supine or on the unoperated side unless directed otherwise

3. Promote adaptation to perceptual impairment:
   a. Preoperatively, patch both eyes if detachment threatens the macula; administer mydriatics or cycloplegics for wide dilation, as prescribed.
   b. Postoperatively, patch the surgical eye for 1 to 4 hours; administer dilating drops or combination antibiotic–steroid drops, as prescribed; encourage visitors, socialization, sensory stimulation, and diversional activities.
4. Relieve discomfort
   a. Preoperatively, administer sedation as prescribed, promote comfort and relaxation, and minimize eye strain.
   b. Postoperatively, administer mild analgesics for discomfort, and apply cool or warm compresses to swollen eyelids.
5. Provide postoperative instructions, covering:
   a. Activities allowed and restricted
   b. Position prescribed
   c. Resumption of activity: resuming ADLs gradually and as tolerated, commonly resuming light work in 3 weeks and normal activity in 6 weeks; avoiding heavy lifting, deep bending, or stooping (possibly for life); avoiding bumping or otherwise injuring the head

G. Evaluation
1. The patient adheres to activity and positioning requirements.
2. The patient displays low anxiety during the period of visual impairment.
3. The patient reports adequate comfort level following surgery.
4. The patient follows recommendations for activity resumption.
5. The patient remains free of eye and other injuries.

VI. Glaucoma

A. Description
1. Glaucoma refers to a group of disorders characterized by abnormally elevated IOP, which can damage the optic nerve.
2. Types include:
   a. Chronic open-angle glaucoma
   b. Acute closed-angle (or narrow-angle) glaucoma

B. Etiology and incidence
1. Glaucoma may be congenital and usually is acquired (hereditary tendency).
2. The second most common cause of blindness in the United States, glaucoma affects about 2% of the population older than age 40.

C. Pathophysiology

1. In chronic open-angle glaucoma, obstruction to outflow of aqueous humor through the trabecular meshwork to canal of Schlemm leads to increased IOP. It usually is bilateral.

2. Increased IOP eventually destroys optic nerve function, causing blindness.

3. Acute closed-angle glaucoma typically involves sudden, complete unilateral closure with pupil dilation stimulated by dark environment, emotional stress, or mydriatic drugs. It is considered a medical emergency; delay in treatment leads to blindness within several days of onset.

D. Assessment findings

1. Clinical manifestations of chronic open-angle glaucoma typically include:
   a. No early symptoms
   b. Insidious visual impairment, blurring
   c. Diminished accommodation
   d. Gradual loss of peripheral vision (tunnel vision)
   e. Mild aching of eyes
   f. Halos around lights later with elevated IOP

2. Acute narrow-angle glaucoma is commonly marked by:
   a. Transitory attacks of diminished visual acuity
   b. Colored halos around lights
   c. Reddened eye with excruciating pain
   d. Headache
   e. Nausea and vomiting

3. Important diagnostic tests for glaucoma include:
   a. Tonometry, which detects elevated IOP
   b. Slit-lamp examination
   c. Gonioscopy to differentiate between chronic open-angle and acute closed-angle glaucoma

E. Nursing diagnoses

1. Anxiety
2. High Risk for Injury
3. Knowledge Deficit
4. Sensory and Perceptual Alterations: Visual

F. Planning and implementation

1. Manage chronic open-angle glaucoma with prescribed pharmacologic agents to reduce IOP, which may include:
   a. Miotics
   b. Beta-adrenergic blockers
   c. Carbonic anhydrase inhibitors

2. Provide information about laser trabeculoplasty if medication therapy proves ineffective.

3. Provide information regarding management of acute narrow-angle glaucoma, including:

        a.   Immediate surgical opening of the eye chamber

        b.   Carbonic anhydrase inhibitors intravenously (IV) or intramuscularly (IM) to restrict production of aqueous humor

        c.   Osmotic agents (mannitol, glycerol)

        d.   Surgical or laser peripheral iridectomy after acute episode is relieved

        e.   Prophylactic peripheral iridectomy of the unaffected eye before discharge

   4. Provide general preoperative and postoperative care and teaching (see Section IV).

   5. Teach the patient about specific safety precautions, including:

        a.   Avoiding mydriatics like atropine, which may precipitate acute glaucoma in a patient with narrow angle glaucoma

        b.   Carrying prescribed medications at all times

        c.   Carrying a Med-alert card or wearing a bracelet stating the type of glaucoma and need for medication

        d.   Taking extra precautions at night (e.g., use handrails, provide extra lighting to compensate for impaired pupil dilation from miotic use)

G. **Evaluation**

   1. The patient verbalizes understanding of prescribed medications and demonstrates appropriate administration technique.

   2. The patient verbalizes the importance of carrying a Med-alert card specifying his or her glaucoma.

   3. The patient verbalizes understanding of the need to avoid activities that can increase IOP.

   4. The patient demonstrates compliance with the postoperative regimen.

VII. **Cataracts**

A. **Description: gradually progressive opacity of the lens or lens capsule that leads to visual loss**

B. **Etiology and incidence**

   1. The most common cause of cataracts is aging; about 85% of persons older than age 80 experience this problem to some degree.

   2. Other possible causes include trauma, drug or chemical toxicity, genetic defects, and secondary effects of other diseases.

C. **Pathophysiology**

   1. Altered nutrient metabolism within the lens triggers cataract formation.

   2. The lens becomes cloudy and has reduced accommodative power.

3. Light rays cannot pass through the opaque lens to the retina, causing vision loss.

4. Cataracts develop bilaterally, but progression varies in each eye.

D. Assessment findings

1. Clinical manifestations include:

   a. Progressively worsening blurred vision

   b. Cloudy appearing lens

   c. No pain or eye redness

2. Ophthalmoscopic or slit-lamp examination confirms diagnosis.

E. Nursing diagnoses

1. Anxiety

2. Knowledge Deficit

3. Pain

4. Sensory and Perceptual Alteration: Visual

F. Planning and implementation

1. Provide information regarding lens extraction surgery, covering:

   a. Preoperative medications: sympathomimetic medication instilled in eye to dilate and vasoconstrict; mannitol IV or glycerol PO administered (after antiemetic) to reduce IOP

   b. What to expect after lens removal: patient becomes aphakic (without lens); patient may experience hyperopia (farsightedness); with one eye aphakic and the other with lens, patient will experience diplopia (double vision)

   c. What to expect after lens removed with intraocular lens (IOL) insertion: patient becomes pseudophakic (has false lens); IOL enables immediate binocular vision if vision good in other eye; vision will be fine-tuned with glasses

2. Relieve postoperative discomfort with analgesics and atropine eye drops as prescribed. Instruct the patient to report severe eye pain immediately; this may indicate increasing IOP or hemorrhage.

3. Provide postoperative teaching, covering:

   a. Discharge, which usually occurs a few hours after surgery

   b. The need for a patch and shield over the operative eye

   c. Patch change by the surgeon the second postoperative day

   d. The need for eye protection: wearing glasses during day (sunglasses at first), using an eye shield at night to prevent rubbing the eye, avoiding straining, lying on back or unoperated side when in bed, reading only in moderation, maintaining sedentary lifestyle for 2 weeks

4. Assist the patient with adaptation to altered vision and rehabilitative requirements; explain the need to:

   a. Wear temporary thick convex cataract glasses if one eye is aphakic and the other has poor visual acuity.

   b. Wear an eye patch over a glass or phakic eye for binocular vision, if one eye is aphakic and the other phakic (with lens).

   c. Turn the head to the side to scan the entire visual field to compensate for impaired peripheral vision.

   d. Compensate for altered spatial relationships.

   e. Wear permanent glasses prescribed after healing is complete in 2 to 12 months.

   f. Use steroid–antibiotic drops postoperatively, if an IOL was inserted.

   g. Use cycloplegic drops for 1 to 2 months postoperatively, if no IOL was inserted.

G. Evaluation

1. The patient verbalizes the need to take precautions and avoid complications.

2. The patient exhibits positive adjustment to altered vision and rehabilitative requirements.

VIII. Anatomy and physiology: ears

A. Structure

1. External ear

   a. Structures of the external ear include the auricle, external auditory canal, and tympanic membrane (eardrum).

   b. The auricle and external auditory canal receive and direct sound waves to the tympanic membrane.

2. Middle ear

   a. Ossicles (consisting of the malleus, incus, and stapes) move and conduct sound waves from the external ear to inner ear.

   b. The eustachian tube equalizes pressure on both sides of the tympanic membrane.

   c. The middle ear communicates with mastoid air cells of the temporal bone.

3. Inner ear (labyrinth)

   a. The vestibule contains receptors that respond to the position of the head as it relates to gravity.

   b. The cochlea contains the organ of Corti (receptor end organ of hearing).

      c.   Semicircular canals contain sensory organs of equilibrium.

    4.   The acoustic nerve (CN VIII) connects the cochlea, semicircular canals, and vestibular receptors with the brain.

B.   **Function**

    1.   The ears are involved in both the hearing and position sense (balance and equilibrium).

    2.   In hearing, sound waves are directed by the external ear through the external auditory meatus where they strike the tympanic membrane, causing it to vibrate.

    3.   These vibrations trigger movement of the ossicles in the middle ear, whose stapes transmit the vibrations through the fluid in the inner ear to the cochlea and the organ of Corti.

    4.   Movement in the organ of Corti stimulates the sensory ends of the cochlear branch of the acoustic nerve (CN VIII), which sends impulses to the temporal lobe for interpretation as sound.

    5.   For position sense, fluid in the semicircular canals of the inner ear responds to body movement by stimulating nerve cells that line the canals. These cells transmit impulses through the vestibular branch of the acoustic nerve to the brain for maintenance of balance and equilibrium.

IX.   **Overview of ear disorders**

    A.   **Assessment**

        1.   Tympanic membrane inspection involves straightening the external auditory canal of an adult by pulling the auricle up and back while tilting the patient's head slightly; normal findings include an intact, shiny, pearly gray, concave membrane that moves with swallowing.

        2.   Hearing acuity can be screened by having the patient identify at what point near the ear that he or she can hear a whispered voice or ticking watch; normally, the patient should hear the sound at a distance of 2 feet or so.

        3.   The Weber test evaluates bone conduction with a tuning fork placed on the midline of the head; normally, the tone is heard equally in both ears by bone conduction.

        4.   The Rinne test uses a tuning fork to evaluate air conduction and bone conduction; normally, air conduction is greater than bone conduction (positive Rinne).

        5.   Audiometry should be performed by an audiologist certified by the American Speech and Hearing Association.

        6.   Assessment of nose and throat should accompany ear assessment because infection in these areas may lead to ear problems.

    B.   **Psychosocial implications**

        1.   A patient with a hearing problem may experience coping difficulties related to:

a. Unknown prognosis

b. Chronicity or long-term nature of the condition

2. The patient also may experience self-concept changes associated with:

a. Altered body image due to deafness or the need for a hearing aid

b. Potential for loss of independence

3. The patient may have to adjust to lifestyle changes related to potential changes in:

a. Role performance

b. Occupational performance, with possibility of job loss

c. Self-care ability

4. Changes in social interaction patterns related to hearing problems may lead to:

a. Depression

b. Isolation

C. **Medications used to treat ear problems**

1. *Anticerumen agents* such as carbamide peroxide (e.g., Debrox drops) are administered to soften impacted cerumen and enable its removal.

2. *Antivertigo agents*, used in Menière's disease to control vertigo, include:

a. Atropine sulfate

b. Diazepam (Valium)

c. Dimenhydrinate (Dramamine)

d. Meclizine hydrochloride (e.g., Antivert)

3. Other drugs used to treat Menière's disease include *diuretics* such as acetazolamide (e.g., Diamox) and chlorothiazide (e.g., Diuril) and *vasodilators* such as nicotinic acid, tolazoline hydrochloride (Priscoline), and methantheline bromide (Banthine).

X. **Conductive hearing loss**

A. **Description**

1. Conductive hearing loss refers to various problems involving impaired passage of sound from the external ear to the inner ear.

2. Specific conditions include:

a. Cerumen impaction

b. External otitis

c. Serous otitis media

d. Suppurative otitis media

e. Otosclerosis

B. **Etiology and incidence**

1. Cerumen impaction usually occurs in persons who naturally produce large amounts of cerumen.

2. Causes of external otitis media include infection (bacterial or

fungal), excessive moisture in the suditory canal (swimmer's ear), and trauma.

    3.   Serous otitis media may result from eustachian tube obstruction, sudden changes in atmospheric pressure, allergy, and viral disease.

    4.   Suppurative otitis media may follow viral disease, tympanic membrane perforation, or prolonged forceful nose blowing. It is most common in infants and young children because of their immature and relatively poorly draining eustachian tubes.

    5.   Otosclerosis appears to be a hereditary condition; it affects women twice as often as men and typically develops between ages 15 and 30.

C. Pathophysiology

    1.   Impacted cerumen in external ear can block sound from reaching the tympanic membrane.

    2.   External otitis media involves inflammation of the external ear, with crust formation and edema in the auditory canal.

    3.   Serous otitis media involves sterile fluid accumulation in the middle ear. It may be acute or chronic; frequent recurrences can threaten hearing.

    4.   Suppurative otitis media involves pus accumulation in the middle ear and possibly extending into adjacent structures. Chronic recurrence may lead to tympanic membrane perforation.

    5.   In otosclerosis, spongy bone grows over the normal bony labyrinth, causing the footplate of the stapes to become fixed in the oval window of the otic capsule.

D. Assessment findings

    1.   Cerumen impaction is often visible; the patient demonstrates some degree of hearing loss.

    2.   External otitis media is commonly marked by:

        a.   Itching and pain

        b.   Watery or purulent discharge

    3.   Manifestations of serous otitis media include:

        a.   Plugged feeling in ear

        b.   Reverberation of the patient's own voice

        c.   Hearing loss

    4.   Suppurative otitis media typically produces:

        a.   Throbbing ear pain

        b.   Fever, hearing loss, nausea, and vomiting

        c.   Feeling of increased pressure in the ear

        d.   Bright red, bulging or retracted tympanic membrane

        e.   Possible tympanic membrane rupture with discharge (otorrhea)

    5. Otosclerosis may be marked by:
        a. Reduced air conduction compared to bone conduction on Rinne test
        b. Mixed hearing loss or sensorineural hearing loss
        c. Tinnitus

E. Nursing diagnoses
    1. Knowledge Deficit
    2. High Risk for Injury
    3. Impaired Physical Mobility
    4. Pain
    5. Sensory and Perceptual Alteration: Auditory
    6. Social Isolation

F. Planning and implementation
    1. Instruct the patient in general ear care and hearing protection measures, including:
        a. Protecting the ears from loud noises with plugs, muffs, and so forth
        b. Chewing gum or sucking hard candy when flying to open the eustachian tube and allow air into middle ear
        c. Never inserting any object into the auditory canal beyond the extent of vision
        d. Inserting no object smaller than the finger into the ear
        e. Blowing the nose with the mouth open and both nostrils open to prevent forcing contaminated material into the middle ear
    2. If appropriate, remove impacted cerumen by first softening it with peroxide or glycerol instillation, then irrigating out softened wax after 2 or 3 days.
    3. Provide care to a patient with tympanic membrane perforation as follows:
        a. Maintain strict asepsis.
        b. Do not irrigate the ear.
        c. Protect from water contamination by having the patient wear ear plugs and a bathing cap.
        d. Recognize a patient at risk for labyrinthitis or meningitis.
    4. For a patient with hearing impairment, enhance communication:
        a. Do not rely on the hospital's intercom system.
        b. Do not exclude the patient from conversations in the room.
        c. Avoid startling the patient; get the patient's attention before speaking to him or her.
        d. Ensure adequate lighting; face the person, speak

slowly and distinctly with voice slightly raised (but without shouting), use nonverbal cues.

    e.   Use a message board if necessary.

    f.   Insert a hearing aid if indicated.

5.   Treat external otitis media with topical antibiotics and steroids, gentle debridement, and acid–alcohol solutions to sterilize the auditory canal as prescribed.

6.   Prepare a patient with serous otitis media for treatment, which may include:

    a.   Needle aspiration

    b.   Myringotomy (incision into the tympanic membrane to relieve pressure and remove pus)

7.   Provide prescribed treatments for a patient with suppurative otitis media, which may include:

    a.   Systemic antibiotics (for at least 7 days)

    b.   Nasal decongestants

    c.   Analgesics

    d.   Heat and cold applications

8.   If indicated, prepare a patient with suppurative otitis media for surgery, which may involve:

    a.   Mastoidectomy (if the mastoid is involved)

    b.   Myringoplasty (repair of perforated tympanic membrane)

    c.   Tympanoplasty (replacement or rebuilding of middle ear structures)

9.   Prepare a patient with otosclerosis for surgery, as indicated, which may include:

    a.   Stapedectomy (replacement of diseased ossicles with prostheses)

    b.   Fenestration (creation of a new window into the labyrinth to provide a new pathway for sound)

10.   Prepare a patient undergoing ear surgery for postoperative expectations and requirements:

    a.   Inform the patient that hearing may not improve noticeably until swelling leaves the operative area and packs are removed.

    b.   Explain expected postoperative restrictions on positioning and movement.

    c.   Instruct the patient not to sneeze, cough, blow his or her nose, or touch the ear or dressing until allowed.

11.   Take steps to prevent postoperative injury due to postoperative complications:

    a.   Monitor for signs and symptoms of infection (e.g., temperature elevation, headache, drainage).

    b.   Do not disturb the inner dressing.

    c.   Avoid applying pressure to the ear or ear dressing, which could dislodge a graft or prosthesis.

        d. If the patient experiences vertigo, note nystagmus and record the direction of eye movement and effects of position changes.

        e. Observe for signs of facial nerve injury (e.g., inability to frown, wrinkle forehead, close eyes, bare teeth, or pucker lips). (*Note:* Injury may be temporary, due to swelling, or it may be permanent.)

        f. Protect the eye if facial nerve injury occurs.

        g. Instruct the patient to report tinnitus, fluctuating hearing, or vertigo.

12. Promote mobility within postoperative restrictions:

        a. Maintain bedrest for up to 48 hours.

        b. Position the patient on his or her side with the operative ear up, to prevent displacement of graft; with operative ear down, to enhance drainage; or on the unoperative side, to minimize nausea and vomiting.

13. Relieve postoperative discomfort and guard against injury by:

        a. Maintaining the prescribed position

        b. Keeping the bed rails up and assisting the patient with ambulation

        c. Teaching the patient to use hand rails (vertigo may threaten safety) and avoid contraindicated or sudden movements

        d. Avoiding jarring the patient or the bed

        e. Instructing the patient to breathe deeply through an open mouth

        f. Medicating for pain or nausea as indicated

        g. Providing a light or liquid diet to control nausea as necessary

14. Provide the patient with self-care instructions, including:

        a. Avoiding getting the ear wet to prevent infection

        b. Avoiding persons with upper respiratory infection

        c. Avoiding bending, straining, and flying until allowed in the postoperative stapedectomy period

        d. Taking the full course of prescribed medications, even after symptoms are relieved

        e. Taking care to prevent burns with a hair dryer if the auricle is numb

G. Evaluation

1. The patient demonstrates understanding of effective ear care and hearing protection measures.

2. The patient is free of discomfort and complications postoperatively.

3. The patient verbalizes understanding of self-care and follow-up instructions.

XI. Menière's disease

    A. Description: a chronic disorder of the inner ear involving sensorineural hearing loss, severe vertigo, and tinnitus

    B. Etiology and incidence

        1. The cause of Menière's disease is unknown; it is associated with aging and may follow middle ear infection or head trauma.

        2. It affects men slightly more often than women and most commonly occurs between ages 40 and 50.

    C. Pathophysiology

        1. Menière's disease appears to involve overproduction or decreased absorption of endolymph, with resultant degeneration of vestibular and cochlear hair cells.

        2. Recurrent attacks result in progressive sensorineural hearing loss (especially low tones), usually unilateral in nature.

    D. Assessment findings

        1. Menière's disease may produce:

            a. Sudden episodes of severe whirling vertigo, with the inability to stand or walk; an episode may last up to several hours

            b. Buzzing tinnitus that worsens before and during an episode

            c. Nausea, vomiting, and diaphoresis

            d. Possibly brief loss of consciousness with nystagmus

        2. Audiometric testing reveals sensorineural hearing loss.

    E. Nursing diagnoses

        1. Anxiety

        2. High Risk for Injury

        3. Knowledge Deficit

        4. Pain

        5. Sensory and Perceptual Alteration: Auditory

        6. Social Isolation

    F. Planning and implementation

        1. Provide a safe, quiet, dimly lit environment, and enforce bedrest during acute episodes.

        2. Provide emotional support and reassurance to alleviate anxiety.

        3. Relieve discomfort with:

            a. Atropine sulfate or diazepam for vertigo as prescribed

            b. Proper positioning for comfort: affected ear uppermost

        4. Provide self-care instructions, covering:

            a. The nature of the disorder

            b. Self-administration of atropine sulfate for episodes

       c.   Other medications as prescribed (e.g., antihistamines, vasodilators, diuretics, mild sedatives)

       d.   The need for a low-salt diet

       e.   The importance of avoiding stimulants and vasoconstrictors (e.g., coffee, decongestants, alcohol)

  5.   Discuss potential treatment options:

       a.   Conservative management: psychotherapy, allergic hyposensitization, low sodium diet, antihistamines, vasodilators, steroids, antiemetics

       b.   Surgery: sac decompression, shunts, ultrasound, labyrinthectomy

G. Evaluation

  1.   The patient reports relief of symptoms due to exacerbation of Menière's disease.

  2.   The patient remains free from injury during episode.

  3.   The patient verbalizes understanding of the prescribed self-care regimen and the importance of compliance.

XII. Anatomy and physiology: nose and sinuses

A. Nose

  1.   The nasal passages, or turbinates, are three bony structures (superior, middle, and inferior) located between the roof of the mouth and the frontal, ethmoid, and sphenoid bones of the skull.

  2.   The lining of the nasal turbinates is highly vascular; the nasal vestibule just inside the nares contains cilia—tiny hairs that filter inspired air.

  3.   Nasal passages filter, warm, and humidify inspired air.

  4.   Enervated by the olfactory nerve (CN I), the nose provides the function of olfaction (smell); the senses of taste and smell are closely related.

B. Sinuses

  1.   The four paranasal sinuses (frontal, maxillary, ethmoidal, and sphenoidal) are air cavities located around and draining into the nasal turbinates.

  2.   The sinuses produce mucus for the nasal cavity and give timbre and resonance to the voice.

XIII. Overview of nose and sinus disorders

A. Nose and olfactory function assessment

  1.   Assess olfaction by having person identify various odors.

  2.   Insert speculum blades ½ inch into nares, resting index finger on side of patient's nose.

  3.   Inspect for pallor, edema, masses, polyps, redness.

B. Sinus assessment

  1.   Inspect the nasal mucosa for redness and discharge.

  2.   Palpate the frontal and maxillary sinuses for tenderness.

XIV. **Epistaxis**

    A. Description: severe nosebleed

    B. Etiology

        1. Epistaxis may be spontaneous or may result from trauma (usually nose picking).

        2. It also may be associated with chemical irritation, acute or chronic infection (such as rhinitis or sinusitis), purpura, leukemia and other blood dyscrasias, hypertension, anticoagulant therapy, or deviated septum.

    C. Pathophysiology

        1. In children, epistaxis usually originates in the anterior nose and tends to be mild; in adults, it tends to originate in the posterior nose and be more severe.

        2. Slight to moderate epistaxis usually causes no complications; however, severe bleeding (persisting longer than 10 minutes after pressure is applied) may cause blood loss up to 1 L/ hour.

    D. Assessment findings

        1. Clinical manifestations may include:

            a. Bleeding through the nares, blood trickling into the oropharynx

            b. Blood in the corners of eyes (through the lacrimal ducts)

            c. Blood in the auditory canal if the tympanic membrane is perforated

        2. Nasal inspection with a bright light and speculum may locate the source of bleeding.

    E. Nursing diagnoses

        1. Ineffective Airway Clearance

        2. High Risk for Injury

        3. Pain

    F. Planning and implementation

        1. Intervene to control bleeding, as follows:

            a. Have the patient sit upright, breathe through the mouth, and refrain from talking.

            b. Compress the soft outer portion of the nares against the septum for 5 to 10 minutes.

            c. Instruct the patient to avoid nose blowing during or after the episode.

        2. If pressure does not control bleeding, insert anterior packing or posterior packing as appropriate. Keep scissors and a hemostat on hand to cut the strings and remove the packing in the event of airway obstruction.

        3. Monitor bleeding: Inspect for blood trickling into the poste-

rior pharynx; observe for hemoptysis, hematemesis, frequent swallowing or belching; instruct the patient not to swallow but to spit out any blood.

4. If indicated, provide information regarding electrocautery.

G. Evaluation

1. The patient remains calm and exhibits no or only minor breathing difficulty.
2. Bleeding is controlled.
3. The patient reports adequate pain relief.

XV. Anatomy and physiology: throat

A. Larynx

1. Transition between upper and lower airways
2. Permits vocalization

B. Epiglottis

1. Part of larynx that protects lower airway
2. Covers larynx during swallowing

XVI. Overview of throat disorders

A. Assessment

1. Examine the posterior pharynx with a warmed mirror (to prevent fogging) and tongue depressor, instructing the patient to open the mouth wide and take a deep breath to flatten the posterior tongue.
2. Observe color and symmetry; note any exudate, ulcerations, or swelling.
3. Palpate the neck for enlarged lymph nodes.
4. Palpate the neck to assess position and mobility of the trachea; lateral deviation may indicate a mass in the neck or mediastinum.

B. Psychosocial implications

1. The patient with laryngeal cancer may experience coping difficulties related to:
   a. Unknown progression of symptoms
   b. Chronicity or long-term nature of the disease
   c. Fear of death
   d. Altered communication
2. The patient also may experience self-concept changes due to:
   a. Body image change after laryngectomy
   b. Potential loss of independence
   c. Altered role performance
3. Disease-related changes in social interaction patterns may result in:
   a. Depression
   b. Isolation

XVII. Foreign body aspiration

A. Description: partial or total occlusion of the larynx or lower airway by an aspirated object

B. Etiology
  1. Children may aspirate a variety of objects.
  2. Food is the most common cause of airway obstruction in adults.

C. Pathophysiology
  1. Objects may be aspirated into the upper airway or lower airway (below the larynx).
  2. Aspirated objects can enter the right main bronchus.
  3. Complete airway obstruction may rapidly lead to cardiopulmonary arrest.

D. Assessment findings
  1. Clinical manifestations of airway obstruction commonly include:
     a. Signs of respiratory distress
     b. Weak, ineffective cough
     c. High-pitched noises on inspiration
     d. Clutching of neck with hands
     e. Inability to speak with complete obstruction
  2. Cyanosis and loss of consciousness may occur with complete obstruction.

E. Nursing diagnoses
  1. Anxiety
  2. Ineffective Breathing Pattern

F. Planning and implementation
  1. If the patient is able to speak, indicating partial airway obstruction:
     a. Position for optimal ventilation.
     b. Encourage coughing.
  2. If the patient is unable to speak, indicating complete obstruction:
     a. Call for help immediately.
     b. Perform abdominal thrust (Heimlich maneuver); use lower sternal thrust for an obese or pregnant victim.
     c. Remove an object in the larynx with a finger or forceps via laryngoscopy.
     d. Remove an object in the lower airway through bronchoscopy.
     e. Prepare to assist with emergency cricothyroidotomy if necessary.
  3. Help relieve anxiety:
     a. Do not leave the patient unattended.
     b. Encourage the patient to resume a normal breathing

pattern and to talk about the episode after obstruction is relieved.

G. **Evaluation**
1. The patient breathes without difficulty.
2. The patient demonstrates anxiety relief after airway clearance and discussion of the episode.

XVIII. Laryngeal cancer
A. **Description: neoplasm of the larynx; types include:**
   1. Intrinsic: involving the vocal cords
   2. Extrinsic: involving another part of the larynx
B. **Etiology and incidence**
   1. Predisposing factors to laryngeal cancer include:
      a. Familial tendency
      b. Cigarette smoking
      c. Chronic vocal straining
      d. Prolonged alcohol ingestion
   2. Laryngeal cancer is the most common cancer of the head and neck; incidence is highest in men between age 50 and 65.
C. **Pathophysiology**
   1. Most laryngeal tumors are slow-growing squamous cell carcinomas.
   2. Intrinsic tumors are typically slow growing with little tendency to spread.
   3. More rapid-growing extrinsic tumors may spread to the lymph nodes of the neck or to the thyroid gland.
   4. Prognosis generally is favorable with early detection and treatment.
D. **Assessment findings**
   1. The earliest and predominant sign of intrinsic laryngeal cancer is persistent hoarseness.
   2. Extrinsic laryngeal cancer commonly is marked by:
      a. No early hoarseness
      b. Throat pain and burning when drinking hot or acidic liquids (e.g., orange juice)
      c. Pain possibly radiating to the ear
      d. Possibly enlarged lymph nodes or lump in the neck with metastasis
   3. Late symptoms of both types include:
      a. Dysphagia and hoarseness
      b. Dyspnea, cough, hemoptysis, foul-smelling breath
      c. Weight loss
   4. Studies that aid diagnosis include laryngoscopy, CT scan, laryngography, tissue biopsy, and chest radiograph (to detect metastases).

E. **Nursing diagnoses**
1. Ineffective Airway Clearance
2. Anxiety
3. Ineffective Breathing Pattern
4. Impaired Verbal Communication
5. High Risk for Injury
6. Knowledge Deficit
7. Altered Nutrition: Less Than Body Requirements

F. **Planning and implementation**
1. Provide information regarding treatments, which may include:
   a. Radiation therapy
   b. Combination therapy, including chemotherapy
   c. Partial laryngectomy for intrinsic type; retains normal airway and phonation
   d. Radical neck dissection or modified radical neck on involved side
   e. Total laryngectomy: pharyngeal opening closed; speech and breathing altered; all airflow is through permanent tracheostomy
   f. Total laryngectomy with laryngoplasty: dermal tube allows exhalation of air into pharyngeal cavity; patient closes permanent tracheostomy opening with finger to speak; speech production is similar to normal
2. Determine the patient's understanding of the treatment plan; answer questions, address concerns, and clarify any misconceptions.
3. Encourage the patient and family members to ventilate feelings and concerns related to diagnosis, prognosis, treatment, recovery, and altered function.
4. Prepare the patient and family for expected postoperative alterations in breathing, speech, and appearance as appropriate.
5. Plan for an alternative means of communication before surgery (e.g., message board, magic slate, use of call bell, hand signals).
6. Initiate a preoperative evaluation by a speech pathologist if indicated.
7. Refer the patient and family to support groups, such as the American Cancer Society and laryngectomy groups (e.g., Lost Chord Club, New Voice Club).
8. Promote adequate ventilation postoperatively:
   a. Place the patient in Fowler's position after recovery from anesthesia.
   b. Turn the patient frequently to promote ventilation and drainage.
   c. Provide laryngectomy care; suction as needed.

     d.   Assess diaphragmatic movement on the affected side; nerve damage may occur during surgery.

     e.   Observe for signs of impaired gas exchange: restlessness, labored breathing, apprehension, increased pulse rate.

     f.   Administer pain medications as needed; avoid medications that can depress respiration.

     g.   Encourage early ambulation.

9. Prevent postoperative infection and hemorrhage at the laryngectomy site:

     a.   Clean the stoma daily with saline or prescribed solution.

     b.   Monitor wound drainage.

10. Provide an alternative means of communication postoperatively:

     a.   Keep the call bell readily available at all times.

     b.   Provide a magic slate or flash cards.

     c.   Instruct the patient in rudiments of lip reading or sign language.

     d.   Have electronic devices accessible as appropriate.

11. Encourage the patient to work with the speech pathologist; esophageal speech training for total laryngectomy typically begins 1 week after surgery.

12. If indicated, prepare the patient for tracheoesophageal puncture and prosthesis fitting after laryngectomy healing is complete.

13. Promote adequate nutrition:

     a.   Provide enteral feeding using nasogastric tube, total parenteral nutrition if nutritionally debilitated, or enteral feeding via cervical pharyngectomy (initial tube placement by surgeon; subsequent placements by nurse) as indicated.

     b.   Discuss the decreased sense of taste and smell that commonly occurs postoperatively; reassure the patient that these senses should improve over time.

     c.   Provide frequent oral hygiene.

     d.   Assess for swallowing difficulty due to swelling, alteration of structure, or nerve damage from surgery; assure the patient that swallowing will be easier once the laryngectomy tube is removed (3 to 6 weeks postoperatively).

     e.   After tube removal, begin oral feeding with thick liquids (which are easier to swallow), introducing solid foods as tolerated.

14. Assist the patient in adapting to home maintenance management:

     a.   Encourage gradual assumption of self-care.

       b.   Teach tracheal and stomal care: expect frequent coughing initially with tracheal breathing; maintain clear airway; support neck when changing positions at first; wipe stoma after coughing; cleanse around stoma twice daily (lubricate skin with non–oil-based ointment); provide adequate hydration and humidification of environment; avoid air conditioning.

       c.   Teach laryngectomy protection: prevent water from entering the stoma; take tub baths or use a hand-held shower (swimming not recommended); protect stoma from hair sprays, loose hair, and powders; carry an identification card or wear a bracelet informing first-aid providers of special resuscitation requirements.

  15. Teach airway care for a patient discharged with a laryngectomy tube in place.

G. **Evaluation**

  1. The patient demonstrates effective communication method(s).

  2. The patient expresses a hopeful attitude about recovery.

  3. The patient exhibits effective ventilation without difficulty or signs of hypoxia or hypercapnia postoperatively.

  4. The patient exhibits no signs of hemorrhage or infection.

  5. The patient maintains adequate nutritional status.

  6. The patient verbalizes understanding of appropriate self-care techniques for airway management and laryngectomy protection.

Bibliography

Brunner, L. S., & Suddarth, D. S. (1986). *The Lippincott manual of nursing practice* (4th ed.). Philadelphia: J. B. Lippincott.

Brunner, L. S., & Suddarth, D. S. (1988). *Textbook of medical-surgical nursing* (6th ed.). Philadelphia: J. B. Lippincott.

Luckmann, J., & Sorensen, K. C. (1987). *Medical-surgical nursing: A psychophysiologic approach* (3rd ed.). Philadelphia: W. B. Saunders.

Sorensen, K. C., & Luckmann, J. (1986). *Basic nursing: A psychophysiologic approach* (2nd ed.). Philadelphia: W. B. Saunders.

STUDY QUESTIONS

1. In order to prevent systemic side effects from drug absorption during eye drop instillation, the nurse should
   a. Press on the outer canthus of the eye.
   b. Press on the inner canthus of the eye.
   c. Have the patient close his or her eyes tightly.
   d. Have the patient lie supine a few minutes.

2. Mr. Close, aged 35, has been admitted to the hospital with retinal detachment at the inner aspect of his right eye. Correct preoperative positioning of Mr. Close would be
   a. Fowler's position
   b. supine with a small pillow
   c. right side-lying
   d. left side-lying

3. Following surgical repair of his detached retina, Mr. Close complains of periocular aching. Which drug would be the *most* appropriate analgesic at this time?
   a. Tylenol
   b. Codeine
   c. Demerol
   d. Morphine

4. Postoperatively, Mr. Close has both eyes patched. The nurse hears him calling for his dog, Joey, and he says he wants to check the gate to make certain it's locked. An appropriate nursing diagnosis for this behavior would be
   a. Ineffective Coping related to knowledge deficit
   b. Anxiety and Fear related to loss of vision
   c. Visual Sensory and Perceptual Alterations related to loss of vision
   d. High Risk for Social Isolation related to vision loss

5. Mr. Lee, aged 73, has been admitted to the hospital for surgical correction of glaucoma. During the nursing history, he tells the nurse that he has
   a. been seeing flashes of light and floaters
   b. recently had a driving accident while changing lanes
   c. been having headaches, nausea, and redness of his eyes
   d. been having more frequent episodes of double vision

6. The *most* relevant nursing diagnosis for the patient admitted for surgical correction of glaucoma would be
   a. Anxiety and Fear related to loss of vision
   b. Altered Comfort: Acute Pain
   c. Self-Care Deficit related to impaired vision
   d. High Risk for Injury due to increased intraocular pressure

7. The evaluation of management of the patient with acute closed angle glaucoma is that the patient
   a. has miosis established
   b. has mydriasis established
   c. reports relief of eye pain
   d. reports relief of nausea and vomiting

8. A nursing history of a patient with cataract would most likely include patient complaints of
   a. eye pain
   b. floaters
   c. eye redness
   d. blurred vision

9. The *priority* nursing diagnosis for a patient admitted to the hospital with an acute episode of Menière's disease should be
   a. Altered Comfort due to vertigo
   b. Altered Comfort due to nausea and vomiting
   c. High Risk for Fluid Volume Deficit due to vomiting
   d. High Risk for Injury due to vertigo

10. Ms. May, aged 46, has been admitted to the hospital with a history of worsening Menière's disease. During an acute episode, her chief complaint would be
    a. vertigo
    b. dizziness
    c. severe ear pain

d. sudden deafness

11. Ms. May receives self-care instructions before being discharged from the hospital. The nurse evaluates that the patient understands her diet prescription, which is
    a. high in protein
    b. high in salt
    c. low in protein
    d. low in salt

12. Appropriate hygienic teaching for nose blowing includes having the individual blow with
    a. both nostrils open and mouth open
    b. both nostrils open and mouth closed
    c. alternate nostrils open and mouth closed
    d. alternate nostrils open and mouth open

13. Mr. Lewis, aged 27, has just returned from having nasal surgery with posterior packing in place. The nurse plans intervention toward control of bleeding by observing that Mr. Lewis
    a. appears to be anxious
    b. has discoloration about his eyes
    c. is frequently swallowing
    d. has a tarry stool

14. The nurse who is admitting a patient scheduled for a total laryngectomy determines that the patient understands the consequences of the planned surgery when he states

a. "I'll be breathing and talking as usual after surgery."
b. "I'll be breathing as usual but talking differently after surgery."
c. "I'll be breathing through my neck, but my talking will be the same after surgery."
d. "I'll be breathing through my neck and will have to talk in a new way after surgery."

15. Mr. Cole, aged 61, has been admitted with squamous cell carcinoma of the larynx and is scheduled to have a total laryngectomy. During the preoperative period, it is most important that the nurse:
    a. explain the surgery and obtain informed consent for it
    b. prearrange an alternative communication system with Mr. Cole
    c. have someone with this type of surgery visit Mr. Cole
    d. teach Mr. Cole how to suction himself effectively and confidently

16. Postoperatively, Mr. Cole returns with a cervical pharyngotomy tube in place. The nurse understands that this tube
    a. will need to be irrigated frequently at first
    b. will need to be suctioned frequently at first
    c. is inserted for feeding with no danger of entering the airway
    d. will be used to decompress the stomach postoperatively

ANSWER KEY

1. *Correct response: b*
    Pressing the inner canthus occludes the nasal–lacrimal canal, where absorption takes place.
    a. The outer canthus does not communicate with a duct.
    c. Squeezing the eyes shut might express the medication.
    d. Position would not affect flow into the canal.
    Comprehension/Physiologic/Implementation

2. *Correct response: d*
    The patient generally is positioned so that the detached area is dependent.
    a, b, and c. The other positions would not accomplish this goal of management.
    Analysis/Safe care/Planning

3. *Correct response: a*
    Discomfort is usually mild.
    b. Codeine is constipating and may lead to straining and increased IOP.
    c. Demerol often causes nausea and vomiting.
    d. Morphine causes both nausea and vomiting and constipation, which should be avoided after eye surgery.
    Comprehension/Physiologic/Implementation

4. *Correct response: c*
    Sensory deprivation with both eyes patched can lead to perceptual impairment with confusion and memory dysfunction.
    a, b, and d. Although the other diagnoses are also appropriate for the patient with eye surgery and loss of vision, the nurse should recognize Mr. Close's behavior as Disorientation and Thought Disturbance due to sensory deprivation.
    Analysis/Psychosocial/Analysis (Dx)

5. *Correct response: b*
    a. Gradual loss of peripheral vision is characteristic of glaucoma, whereas flashes of light and floaters are characteristic of retinal detachment.
    c. Nausea, headache, and eye redness are seen with an episode of acute (sudden) narrow-angle closure.
    d. Double vision occurs when one eye has a lens and the other is aphakic.
    Knowledge/Physiologic/Assessment

6. *Correct response: d*
    The nursing diagnosis reflects the nurse's understanding of the primary pathophysiology of glaucoma (increased IOP).
    a, b, and c. The other diagnoses also should be incorporated into the plan of care.
    Knowledge/Health promotion/Analysis (Dx)

7. *Correct response: a*
    Acute closed-angle glaucoma is a medical emergency; the immediate goal is to open the angle with miotics to prevent blindness.
    b, c, and d. Eye dilation would aggravate the emergency and cause discomfort, nausea, and vomiting.
    Analysis/Physiologic/Evaluation

8. *Correct response: d*
    a and c. Cataracts lead to progressive worsening and blurring of vision and are not associated with eye pain or redness (seen in glaucoma).
    b. Floaters are characteristic of retinal detachment.
    Application/Physiologic/Assessment

9. *Correct response: d*
    Vertigo is the outstanding symptom of Menière's.
    a. The severe rotational whirling sensation makes the patient unable to stand or walk without falling.
    b. Discomfort is usually associated with a feeling of pressure.
    c. Nausea is often present and may lead to fluid loss, but the chance of

a patient fall is more of a priority nursing concern for patient safety.
Analysis/Safe care/Analysis (Dx)

10. **Correct response: a**
    Menière's is characterized by sudden severe episodes of vertigo during which the patient has a sensation of spinning.
    b. Dizziness should be distinguished from true rotational vertigo.
    c and d. A feeling of pressure but not pain is also characteristic, and hearing loss is progressive, not sudden.
    Application/Physiologic/Assessment

11. **Correct response: c**
    It is thought that Menière's is due to edema of the semicircular canals; a low-salt diet is often prescribed as well as diuretic drugs.
    a, b, and d. High-salt foods should be avoided, but protein intake should have no relation to Menière's (hypoproteinemia might aggravate edema).
    Application/Health promotion/Evaluation

12. **Correct response: a**
    Keeping both nostrils and mouth open prevents forcing contaminated material into the middle ear (otitis media).
    b, c, and d. All other responses would increase risk of middle ear infection.
    Application/Health promotion/ Implementation

13. **Correct response: c**
    Trickling down the posterior pharynx (noted with flashlight) and swallowing, belching, or hematemesis indicate continued bleeding.
    a. Anxiety is common due to the necessity to mouth-breathe.
    b. Black eyes occur with surgical trauma and are expected.

    d. Tarry stools indicate previous, but not current, bleeding.
    Analysis/Safe care/Planning

14. **Correct response: d**
    All airflow is through a permanent tracheostomy with a total laryngectomy, necessitating esophageal speech or use of an electronic device.
    a. Breathing and talking are unchanged with partial laryngectomy.
    b. All airflow will be through the neck.
    c. Even with laryngoplasty, the tracheostomy is occluded during speech.
    Application/Safe care/Analysis (Dx)

15. **Correct response: b**
    Since all airflow will be through the neck and the larynx will be removed, some form of communication must be assured before surgery (e.g., magic slate, signals).
    a. It is the surgeon's responsibility to explain surgery.
    c. If possible, psychologic preparation is enhanced with a visit from another laryngectomy patient.
    d. Suctioning is easier to teach postoperatively with a tracheostomy present.
    Application/Health promotion/Planning

16. **Correct response: c**
    The pharyngotomy tube is inserted without danger of entering the trachea and is used for nutrition postoperatively.
    a. This type of tube is inserted initially by the surgeon, then inserted by the nurse for subsequent feedings.
    b. Insertion of an nasogastric tube may be preferred by some surgeons.
    d. The tube is neither irrigated nor suctioned but is used for intermittent feeding.
    Analysis/Safe care/Implementation

Musculoskeletal Disorders

16

I. Anatomy and physiology

A. Structure

1. The body contains 206 different bones; types include:
   a. Long bones (e.g., femur, humerus, radius)
   b. Short bones (e.g., tarsals, carpals)
   c. Flat bones (e.g., skull, sternum, ribs, ilium)
   d. Irregular bones (e.g., mandible, vertebrae, ear ossicles)
   e. Sesamoid bones (e.g., patella)
2. Articulations (joints) are of various types:
   a. Synarthroses (fixed) (e.g., skull sutures)
   b. Amphiarthroses (slightly movable; e.g., vertebral joints)
   c. Diarthroses (freely movable; e.g., hip, knee, wrist)
3. The skeletal muscle system includes:
   a. Fasciculi: bundles of muscle fibers covered with connective tissue
   b. Muscle sheaths: connective tissue covering groups of muscle bundles
4. Ligaments are strong fibrous connective tissue binding bones.
5. Tendons are strong, fibrous, nonelastic connective tissue extending from muscle sheath.

6. Cartilage types include:
   a. Hyaline: pearly, blue cartilage covering articular bone surfaces
   b. Fibrocartilage: white, tough, fibrous tissue found in knee
   c. Yellow: elastic, fibrous cartilage found in larynx, external ear

B. Function
   1. Bone functions include:
      a. Protection of vital organs
      b. Support for body tissue
      c. Assistance in movement through leverage and attachment for muscles
      d. Hematopoiesis (red blood cell production)
      e. Storage of mineral salts
   2. Functions of freely movable joints include:
      a. Abduction: away from midline
      b. Adduction: toward midline
      c. Circumduction: circle movement
      d. Extension: straightening
      e. Flexion: bending
      f. External rotation: laterally turning on axis
      g. Internal rotation: medially turning on axis
      h. Supination: facing upward
      i. Pronation: facing downward
   3. Skeletal muscle functions include:
      a. Facilitation of voluntary body movement through contraction
      b. Maintenance of body posture
      c. Production of body heat
   4. Ligaments provide joint stability and allow restricted joint movement.
   5. Tendons bind muscles to bones.
   6. Cartilage functions include:
      a. Absorption of weight, shock, stress, and strain
      b. Protection of bones, joints, and joint tissue

II. Overview of musculoskeletal disorders
   A. Assessment
      1. Health history should cover:
         a. Biographic data (age and sex; socioeconomic status and living conditions, including layout of home, conditions that may affect condition or rehabilitation; occupation, including the amount and type of physical activity required)
         b. Exercise patterns: type, frequency, amount of energy expenditure

      c. Hobbies: type, amount of energy expenditure involved

      d. Diet: type, frequency, and amount of food consumption, including proteins, carbohydrates, calcium, other nutrients

      e. Drug, tobacco, and alcohol intake (include both prescribed and over-the-counter drugs)

      f. Family history of musculoskeletal problems

      g. Past history of illnesses, conditions, medication use

2. The nurse also should elicit information on the patient's present problem, including:

      a. Onset and course

      b. Symptoms (e.g., pain, swelling, altered movement, color changes, stiffness, deformity, sensory changes)

      c. Treatment received

      d. Perception of problem and expectations of outcome

      e. Lifestyle impacts

      f. Any other concurrent health problems

3. Physical examination involves:

      a. Upright body alignment: posture

      b. Bone discrepancies: contour, length, alignment, symmetry

      c. Bone motion: smoothness

      d. Gait: coordination, rhythm, stride, balance

      e. Joint alignment, symmetry, size, shape, contour, stability, tenderness, heat, swelling

      f. Joint movement: range, smoothness, pain, crepitus, clicks

      g. Muscle mass: shape, size, contour, symmetry, firmness

      h. Muscle strength: symmetry, resistance, contractility

      i. Muscle discrepancies: hypertrophy, atrophy, fasciculation, spasms

B. Laboratory studies and diagnostic tests

1. Roentgenography (radiography, radiograph, photographic images) detects musculoskeletal structure, integrity, texture, or density problems; allows evaluation of disease progression, treatment efficacy.

2. Bone scans detect skeletal trauma and disease.

3. Arthrography studies soft tissue structure and contours of joint cavities.

4. Arthrocentesis allows analysis of synovial fluid, blood, or pus aspirated from a joint cavity.

5. Myelography can detect herniation, tumor, and congenital or degenerative conditions of the spinal canal.

6. Electromyography (EMG) measures muscle electrical impulses for diagnosis of muscle or nerve disease.

7. Biopsy (aspiration, punch, needle, or incision) studies bone, synovium, or muscle tissue.

8. Computed tomography (CT) scans study soft tissue, bone, and the spinal cord; provide a three-dimensional, cross-sectional image.

9. Magnetic resonance imaging allows study of soft tissue in multiple planes of the body.

10. Relevant laboratory studies include:
    a. Complete blood count: indicates anemias, hemorrhage, infections, neoplastic conditions, lupus erythematosus, blood dyscrasias, allergies, stress, and so forth
    b. Alkaline phosphatase: increased in osteoblastic activity, inflammatory conditions
    c. Creatinine phosphokinase: elevation may indicate skeletal muscle necrosis, atrophy, or trauma
    d. Lactic dehydrogenase: elevation may indicate skeletal muscle damage
    e. Serum calcium: increased during immobility, bone demineralization; decreased in hypomalabsorption and malnutrition
    f. C-reactive protein: may be positive in lupus erythematosus, strep infections, cancer, and so forth
    g. Rheumatoid factor: may be positive in rheumatoid arthritis, lupus erythematosus, sarcoidosis, and so forth

C. **Psychosocial implications**
   1. A patient with a serious musculoskeletal problem may experience coping difficulties related to:
      a. Progressive nature of the disorder
      b. Long-term nature of healing or chronicity of condition
   2. The patient also may have self-concept concerns related to fear of:
      a. Role changes toward increased dependence
      b. Body image changes related to loss of structural integrity
   3. The patient also expresses concern over possible lifestyle changes related to:
      a. Impaired physical ability or mobility
      b. Changes in occupational ability, with possibility of job loss
   4. Social interaction changes related to pain and limited mobility can result in:
      a. Isolation
      b. Depression

III. Cast application

A. Overview

1. Casts are solid dressings applied to a limb or other body part; types include:
   a. Short arm: extends from below elbow to proximal palmer crease

  b. Long arm: extends from axillary fold to proximal palmer crease

  c. Short leg: extends from below knee to base of toes

  d. Long leg: extends from upper third of thigh to base of toes

  e. Spica: extends from midtrunk covering one or both extremities

  f. Body: encases trunk of body

  g. Splint: bivalved cast providing immobilization, allowing for swelling

 2. Casts are applied to:

  a. Immobilize a body part in a specific position

  b. Exert uniform compression to soft tissue

  c. Provide for early mobilization of unaffected body parts

  d. Correct or prevent deformities

  e. Stabilize and support unstable joints

B. **Assessment**

 1. Evaluate the patient's pain, noting severity, nature, exact location, source, and alleviating and exacerbating factors.

 2. Assess movement of distal parts, and evaluate the patient's capability for physical mobility.

 3. Evaluate the patient's ability to learn essential procedures.

 4. Perform regular neurovascular checks of the affected limb; look for:

  a. Signs of circulatory compromise (pallor, bluish discoloration, diminished peripheral pulses)

  b. Excessive redness, warmth, and swelling

  c. Altered capillary refill time

C. **Nursing diagnoses**

 1. Pain

 2. Altered Tissue Perfusion: Peripheral

 3. High Risk for Impaired Skin Integrity

 4. Altered Role Performance

 5. Self-Care Deficit

D. **Planning and implementation**

 1. Prepare for cast application:

  a. Explain the procedure and what to expect to the patient.

  b. Obtain informed consent if an operative procedure is required.

  c. Clean the skin of the affected part thoroughly.

  d. Inspect for and document any skin lesions, discolorations, or nonremovable foreign material.

 2. Assist with cast application:

  a. Prepare the room and a container of cool water.

  b. Apply a stockinette or padding as ordered.

     c.   Assist the physician during application as needed.

3.   After cast application, provide cast care:
- a.   Support an exposed cast with the palms of your hands to prevent indentations.
- b.   Ensure that the stockinette is pulled over rough edges of the cast.
- c.   Elevate the casted extremity above the level of the heart.
- d.   Provide adequate covering and warmth to uncasted areas.
- e.   Expose a fresh plaster cast to circulating air, uncovered, until dry (24 to 72 hours); expose a fresh synthetic cast until it's completely set (about 20 minutes).
- f.   Assess for plaster cast dryness: wet (musty odor, cool, damp, gray, dull color); dry (no odor, white, shiny, resonant sound when percussed).
- g.   Instruct the patient not to allow the cast to become wet. Tell him or her to dry a synthetic cast with a hair dryer on cool setting if it gets wet.

4.   Initiate pain relief measures if indicated, which may include:
- a.   Position changes
- b.   Elevation of body part
- c.   Analgesics as prescribed
- d.   Nonpharmacologic pain relief measures (e.g., guided imagery, relaxation, distraction)

5.   Observe for signs of cast syndrome—development of gastric and intestinal ileus due to compression of the mesenteric artery—in a patient with a body or hip spica cast; note abdominal pain and distention, nausea and vomiting, elevated blood pressure, tachycardia, tachypnea, and acute anxiety. Notify the doctor immediately if you suspect cast syndrome—if untreated, it may rapidly be fatal.

6.   Notify the physician immediately if signs of other complications develop.

7.   Apply cold packs as prescribed to reduce swelling.

8.   Instruct the patient to keep a casted extremity elevated while sitting or reclining and to change position slowly and carefully while supporting the casted extremity.

9.   Provide patient teaching, covering:
- a.   Isometric exercises to strengthen muscles covered by the cast
- b.   Muscle-strengthening exercises for the upper body if crutches are to be used
- c.   The need to promptly report cast breaks and signs and symptoms of complications
- d.   The importance of never inserting sharp objects (e.g., coat hanger to scratch itchy skin) under the cast
- e.   Appropriate cast care measures, depending on type

      f.   Safety precautions (e.g., avoid walking on wet floors)

      g.   Skin care and muscle-strengthening exercises for the affected body part after cast removal

  10.   Reinforce physician instructions on the amount of weight-bearing allowed.

  11.   Encourage mobility and active participation in self-care.

  12.   Ensure proper technique and procedure in cast removal.

E. Evaluation

  1.   The patient reports reduced pain and discomfort.

  2.   The patient exhibits adequate tissue perfusion.

  3.   The patient maintains independence in self-care activities within limitations.

  4.   The patient maintains mobility in unaffected body parts.

  5.   The patient exhibits minimal muscle atrophy in the affected body part.

  6.   The patient remains free of complications of immobility.

  7.   The patient verbalizes or demonstrates knowledge of treatments, cast care, safety measures, and signs and symptoms of complications.

IV. Traction application

A. Overview

  1.   Traction is an orthopedic treatment that involves placing tension on a limb, bone, or muscle group using various weight and pulley systems.

  2.   Types of traction include:

      a.   Continuous: uninterrupted, used to treat fractures, dislocations

      b.   Intermittent: applied for specified periods to reduce muscle spasms

      c.   Running: straight pulling force in one plane

      d.   Balanced suspension: exertion of pull while supported by hammock or splint held by balanced weights

      e.   Skin traction: weight applied and held to skin with tape or foam or Velcro splint

      f.   Skeletal traction: weight applied and attached to metal inserted into bone (pins, wires, tongs)

  3.   Traction is applied to:

      a.   Decrease muscle spasms

      b.   Reduce, align, and immobilize fractures

      c.   Correct or prevent deformity

      d.   Increase space between joint surfaces

B. Assessment

  1.   Monitor skin integrity of the affected part before and after traction placement; also assess bony prominences and pin insertion sites.

2. Assess cardiovascular status, noting color, temperature, capillary refill time, and pulses in the affected extremity or area; evaluate for edema.
3. Monitor respiratory status, including rate and pattern, breath and lung sounds, and ability to cough and deep breathe.
4. Assess for pain, paresthesias, or other sensations in affected areas.
5. Evaluate muscle strength and tone and mobility in affected and unaffected areas.
6. Assess mental status, noting level of orientation, effectiveness of coping, and behavior.
7. Regularly check the condition of the traction equipment: ropes, pulleys, weights.
8. Evaluate the patient's knowledge of the treatment regimen and its purpose.

C. Nursing diagnoses
1. High Risk for Infection
2. Impaired Physical Mobility
3. Pain
4. Altered Role Performance
5. Self-Care Deficit
6. High Risk for Impaired Skin Integrity
7. Altered Tissue Perfusion: Peripheral

D. Planning and implementation
1. Place a bedboard under the patient's mattress to ensure extra firm support.
2. Use a special mattress to preserve skin integrity.
3. Turn and reposition the patient regularly within the limitations of traction.
4. Keep bed linen free of wrinkles to protect skin.
5. Provide frequent skin care to areas of potential pressure.
6. Provide patient teaching, covering:
   a. Active exercises for unaffected body parts
   b. Use of a trapeze, if indicated
   c. Deep breathing exercises to be done hourly
7. Promote self-care within traction limitations.
8. Increase the patient's fluid intake to 2000 to 2500 mL/day.
9. Provide a balanced diet high in fiber and protein.
10. Assess nerve and circulatory function every 2 hours.
11. Assess areas over traction tape for tenderness, skin irritation.
12. Inspect skeletal traction sites for signs of irritation or infection.
13. Assess pin entrance and exit sites and areas surrounding pin sites at least twice a day.
14. Cleanse pin sites as prescribed.
15. Never remove weights unless prescribed or in an emergency.

E. Evaluation
1. The patient reports reduced pain and discomfort.
2. The patient exhibits adequate tissue perfusion.
3. The patient maintains independence in self-care activities within limitations.
4. The patient maintains mobility in unaffected body parts.
5. The patient exhibits minimal muscle atrophy in the affected body part.
6. The patient remains free of complications of immobility and problems related to pressure and open skin areas.

V. Orthopedic surgery

A. Overview
1. Orthopedic surgery refers to various surgical procedures involving the skeletal system and its joints, muscles, and associated structures.
2. Specific procedures include:
    a. Open reduction: reduction and alignment of fracture through surgical opening
    b. Internal fixation: stabilization of reduced fracture with screws, plates, nails, or pins
    c. Bone graft: placement of bone tissue for healing, stabilization, or replacement
    d. Arthroplasty: joint repair through small arthroscope to avoid large incision
    e. Arthrodesis: immobilization of joint through fusion
    f. Joint replacement: replacement of joint surface with metal or plastic materials
    g. Tendon transfer: movement of tendon insertion to improve function
    h. Tenotomy: cutting tendon
    i. Fasciotomy: removal of muscle fascia relieving constriction
    j. Osteotomy: alignment of bone by removal of wedge
3. Orthopedic surgery is performed to:
    a. Reconstruct diseased or injured musculoskeletal structures
    b. Replace a diseased or damaged bone or joint
    c. Remove a diseased or damaged bone or joint
    d. Repair an injured bone or joint

B. Assessment
1. Preoperative assessment should cover:
    a. Past medical history (e.g., responses to surgery, medications, treatments)
    b. Current medications and conditions (e.g., colds, infections, steroids)

    c.   Nutritional and hydration status: protein, calorie, and fluid intake

    d.   The patient's knowledge of the surgical procedure and treatment regimen

    e.   Skin integrity

    f.   Routine preoperative assessments

  2. Postoperative assessment should include:

    a.   Cardiovascular status: blood pressure, pulse, temperature, blood loss, skin color, capillary refill, pulses and skin temperature of affected extremity

    b.   Respiratory status: rate and pattern, effectiveness of gas exchange, coughing, and deep breathing

    c.   Neurologic status (e.g., nature and degree of pain, nerve function of affected extremity, paresthesia distal to treatment modality)

    d.   Urinary elimination (e.g., voiding frequency, amount, color)

    e.   Integumentary (e.g. condition of skin at pressure areas and the treatment site)

    f.   Nutritional and hydration status: amount and type of intake

    g.   Safety and effectiveness of orthopedic apparatus

    h.   Other routine postoperative assessments

C. **Nursing diagnoses**

  1. Preoperative:

    a.   High Risk for Infection

    b.   Pain

  2. Postoperative:

    a.   Body Image Disturbance

    b.   Impaired Physical Mobility

    c.   Pain

    d.   Altered Role Performance

    e.   Self-Care Deficit

    f.   Self-Esteem Disturbance

    g.   Impaired Skin Integrity

D. **Planning and implementation**

  1. Preoperative

    a.   Reinforce the physician's explanations of the surgery and related procedures.

    b.   Relieve pain and discomfort with therapeutic techniques or analgesics as prescribed.

    c.   Provide meticulous skin preparation using aseptic technique as prescribed.

    d.   Acquaint the patient with postoperative treatment devices, procedures, exercises, and other expected measures.

      e. Provide routine preoperative nursing care (see Chapter 24, Perioperative Nursing).

2. Postoperative

    a. Monitor blood loss at the operative site; suction drainage as necessary.

    b. Administer analgesics and perform therapeutic measures to relieve pain and discomfort as necessary.

    c. Turn and reposition the patient and exercise unaffected body parts every 2 hours or as prescribed.

    d. Elevate the operative extremity to minimize swelling.

    e. Promote early ambulation as prescribed.

    f. Administer prophylactic antibiotics as prescribed.

    g. Develop an individualized exercise program within the patient's limitations.

    h. Instruct the patient in proper use of assistive devices, if indicated.

    i. Encourage a well-balanced diet with increased protein and vitamin intake.

    j. Provide other routine postoperative nursing measures (see Chapter 24, Perioperative Nursing).

E. Evaluation

1. Preoperative

    a. The patient reports control of pain and discomfort.

    b. The patient verbalizes knowledge of the purpose and expectations of the prescribed treatment regimen.

    c. The patient remains free of infection before surgery.

    d. The patient maintains good nutritional status.

2. Postoperative

    a. The patient reports progressive relief of pain and discomfort.

    b. The patient demonstrates independence in self-care activities within limitations.

    c. The patient remains free of complications related to immobility.

    d. The patient verbalizes understanding of the prescribed treatment regimen and demonstrates proper use of any assistive devices.

    e. Wound healing occurs without complications.

VI. Arthroplasty

  A. Overview

1. Arthroplasty refers to reconstruction or replacement of a diseased or damaged joint.

2. Arthroplasty is performed to:

    a. Reduce or eliminate pain

    b. Restore function

    c. Provide joint stability

    d. Prevent complications

  3. Common types include:

    a. Total hip replacement: replacement of a severely damaged hip joint with metal or synthetic ball and socket

    b. Total knee replacement: replacement of tibial, femoral, and patellar joint surfaces for a severely damaged knee joint

B. Assessment

  1. Preoperative and postoperative assessment is similar to that for any patient undergoing orthopedic surgery (see Section V.C).

  2. Also assess for signs and symptoms of:

    a. Joint dislocation (e.g., shortened extremity, increasing discomfort, impaired movement)

    b. Infection; pain, fever, redness, swelling, dislocation

    c. Thromboembolism (a major, life-threatening complication that may follow total hip replacement): see Chapter 8, Peripheral Vascular Disorders, Section IV

C. Nursing diagnoses

  1. Body Image Disturbance

  2. High Risk for Infection

  3. Impaired Physical Mobility

  4. Pain

  5. Altered Role Performance

  6. Self-Care Deficit

  7. Self-Esteem Disturbance

  8. Impaired Skin Integrity

D. Planning and implementation

  1. For total hip replacement:

    a. See Orthopedic surgery, Section V.E.

    b. Position the patient supine and on the unoperated side, supporting the entire operative leg in abducted position with wedges, sandbags, or pillows; may turn the patient to the operative side if prescribed.

    c. Keep the head of the bed flat, elevated only 45 to 50 degrees for short periods during the first 24 hours post-surgery.

    d. Avoid hip flexion beyond 90 degrees.

    e. Prevent external rotation of the leg with a pillow splint.

    f. Administer anticoagulants as prescribed; monitor for side effects.

    g. Apply antiembolic hose as prescribed.

    h. Encourage early ambulation and progressive weight bearing as prescribed.

    i. Instruct the patient to pivot on the operated leg when turning.

j.   Teach proper use of a walker or crutches; consult with a physical therapist as needed.

k.   Encourage the patient to obtain a raised toilet seat for use after discharge, to prevent inappropriate hip flexion.

l.   Instruct the patient to avoid activities causing hip flexion beyond 90 degrees (e.g., sitting in low chairs, riding in small cars) for 6 to 12 weeks after surgery.

m.   Instruct the patient to sit with the knees apart and to avoid crossing the legs.

n.   Assist in patient teaching for stretching, exercise, and rest.

o.   Teach the patient signs and symptoms of joint complications (e.g., displacement, infection, bleeding) to watch for and promptly report.

2.   For total knee replacement:

    a.   See Orthopedic surgery, Section V.E.

    b.   Allow transfer out of the bed to a chair; use an extension splint as prescribed.

    c.   Promote progressive weight bearing as prescribed.

    d.   Instruct the patient in flexion exercises when prescribed.

    e.   Monitor response to continuous passive motion machine on the operative leg.

    f.   Teach the patient the importance of avoiding hyperflexion of the knee, jogging, jumping, heavy lifting, and obesity.

E. Evaluation

1.   The patient reports relief of pain and discomfort.

2.   The patient remains free of complications such as infection, thromboembolism, and dislocation.

3.   The patient verbalizes or demonstrates adequate knowledge of treatments, medications, and assistive devices.

4.   The patient demonstrates the prescribed exercise regimen effectively and appropriately.

VII. Sprains and strains

A. Description

1.   A *sprain* is a complete or incomplete tear in the supporting ligaments surrounding a joint.

2.   A *strain* is an overstretching injury to a muscle or tendon.

B. Etiology

1.   Sprains commonly result from a wrenching or twisting motion that disrupts the stabilizing action of ligaments; common locations include the ankle, knee, wrist, thumb, shoulder, neck, and lower back.

2.   Strains typically result from excessively vigorous movement in understretched or overstretched muscles and tendons; com-

monly affected areas include the groin, hamstring, calf, shoulder, and back muscles, and the Achilles tendon.

C. **Assessment findings**
      a. Pain and discomfort, especially on joint movement
      b. Swelling, possibly ecchymoses
      c. Decreased joint motion and function
      d. Feeling of joint looseness with severe sprain
  2. Manifestations of strains include:
      a. Pain: sudden, severe, incapacitating with acute strain; gradual onset of soreness and tenderness with chronic strain
      b. Swelling
      c. Ecchymoses developing several days following injury
  3. Radiographs are commonly done to rule out fracture or dislocation.

D. **Nursing diagnoses**
  1. High Risk for Injury
  2. Impaired Physical Mobility
  3. Pain
  4. Altered Tissue Perfusion: Peripheral

E. **Planning and implementation**
  1. For a patient who sustains a sprain:
      a. Elevate or immobilize the affected joint, and apply ice packs immediately.
      b. Assist with tape, splint, or cast application as necessary.
      c. Instruct the patient in use of assistive device (e.g., crutches), if indicated.
      d. Prepare the patient with a severe sprain for surgical repair or reattachment, if indicated.
      e. Instruct the patient in prescribed weight-bearing activities and activity restrictions.
      f. Provide pain relief with prescribed medications and other comfort measures.
  2. For a patient suffering muscle or tendon strain:
      a. Instruct the patient to allow the muscle or tendon to rest and repair itself by avoiding use for approximately 1 week, then progressing activity gradually until healing is complete.
      b. Teach appropriate stretching exercises to be performed after healing to help prevent reinjury.
      c. Prepare the patient for surgical repair in severe injury.

F. **Evaluation**
  1. For sprains:
      a. The patient reports reduced pain.
      b. The patient states appropriate measures to enhance comfort and promote healing.

       c.   The patient exhibits adequate tissue perfusion in the affected area.

       d.   The patient demonstrates proper care of cast or use of assistive device.

       e.   The patient demonstrates proper performance of prescribed rehabilitative exercises.

  2. For strains:

       a.   The patient reports decreased pain and weakness within 3 to 5 days after injury.

       b.   The patient resumes normal activity without further injury following healing.

VIII. Dislocations

A. **Description: displacement of a bone from its normal articulation with a joint**

B. **Etiology**

  1. A dislocation may be congenital (e.g., congenital hip displacement) or may result from trauma (e.g., abnormal twisting) or disease of surrounding joint tissue (e.g., Paget's disease).

  2. Common locations of dislocation include the shoulder, elbow, wrist, digits, hip, knee, ankle, and vertebrae.

C. **Pathophysiology**

  1. Traumatic dislocation may cause severe stress to associated joint structures, interrupting blood supply and causing nerve damage.

  2. If untreated, this may lead to avascular necrosis or nerve palsy in the affected area.

D. **Assessment findings**

  1. Common signs and symptoms of dislocation include:

       a.   Pain

       b.   Visible disruption of joint contour

       c.   Swelling

       d.   Ecchymoses

       e.   Impaired joint mobility

       f.   Change in extremity length

       g.   Change in axis of dislocated bones (rotation)

  2. Severe dislocation may produce circulatory or sensory changes in the affected joint and limb.

  3. Radiograph findings may confirm dislocation.

E. **Nursing diagnoses**

  1. High Risk for Injury

  2. Impaired Physical Mobility

  3. Pain

  4. Altered Tissue Perfusion: Peripheral

F. **Planning and implementation**

  1. Immobilize the affected joint during transport to medical care.

2. Assist the physician in reducing displaced parts as necessary.
3. Keep the joint immobilized as prescribed, using bandages, splints, a cast, or traction.
4. Assess for signs of circulatory or neurologic impairment.
5. After removal of the immobilizing device, instruct the patient to exercise the joint as prescribed to promote return to normal function.
6. Instruct the patient in the use of assistive devices (e.g., crutches) as indicated.

G. Evaluation

1. The patient reports reduced pain.
2. The patient states appropriate measures to enhance comfort and promote healing.
3. The patient exhibits adequate tissue perfusion and sensory function in the affected area.
4. The patient demonstrates proper care of cast or use of assistive device.
5. The patient demonstrates proper performance of prescribed rehabilitative exercises and safety precautions to prevent reinjury.

IX. Fractures

A. Description

1. A fracture is a traumatic injury interrupting bone continuity.
2. Fractures are classified according to type and extent as:
    a. Closed simple, uncomplicated: not causing a break in the skin
    b. Open compound, complicated: involving trauma to surrounding tissue and a break in the skin
    c. Incomplete: partial cross-section break with incomplete bone disruption
    d. Complete: complete cross-section break severing the periosteum
    e. Impact: fracture ends forcibly wedged together
    f. Comminuted: several breaks of bone with splinters, fragments
    g. Displaced: separation of fragments at fracture site
    h. Complicated: involving injury to surrounding tissue
    i. Articular: involving a joint surface
    j. Extracapsular: a break near but not in a joint capsule
    k. Intracapsular: involving a joint capsule
    l. Epiphyseal: break in long bones involving ossification center

B. Etiology

1. Fractures can result from crushing force or direct blow.
2. Torsion fractures can occur from sudden twisting motion; persons with osteoporosis are at particular risk.

3. Extremely forceful muscle contraction also can cause fractures.

C. Pathophysiology

1. Fracture occurs when stress placed on a bone exceeds the bone's ability to absorb it.
2. Stages of normal fracture healing include:
   a. Inflammation
   b. Cellular proliferation
   c. Callus formation
   d. Callus ossification
   e. Mature bone remodeling
3. Potential complications of fracture include:
   a. Life-threatening systemic fat embolus, most commonly developing within 24 to 72 hours after fracture
   b. Nonunion of the fracture site
   c. Arterial damage during treatment
   d. Compartment syndrome
   e. Infection, possibly sepsis
   f. Hemorrhage, possibly leading to shock

D. Assessment findings

1. Clinical manifestations of fracture may include:
   a. Pain
   b. Swelling
   c. Tenderness
   d. Abnormal movement and crepitus
   e. Loss of function
   f. Ecchymoses
   g. Visible deformity
   h. Paresthesias and other sensory abnormalities
2. Radiograph and other imaging studies may identify the site and type of fracture.

E. Nursing diagnoses

1. Body Image Disturbance
2. High Risk for Infection
3. High Risk for Injury
4. Impaired Physical Mobility
5. Pain
6. Altered Role Performance
7. Self-Care Deficit
8. Self-Concept Disturbance
9. Altered Tissue Perfusion: Peripheral

F. Planning and implementation

1. Immobilize a fractured extremity with splints before moving the patient.
2. Avoid straightening the injured body part if a joint is involved.
3. Cover any breaks in the skin with clean or sterile dressings.

4. Support the affected body part above and below the fracture site when moving the patient.
5. Explain all procedures and treatments, emphasizing the importance of the patient's participation in the treatment regimen.
6. Provide nonpharmacologic interventions (e.g., relaxation, massage, guided imagery) to help relieve pain.
7. Administer analgesics as ordered.
8. Elevate the injured extremity above the level of the patient's heart for the first 24 hours or as directed.
9. Apply cold packs as ordered for the first 24 hours.
10. Assist the patient with active range-of-motion exercises to unaffected body parts, to help maintain function.
11. Promote the patient's participation in self-care activities within limitations of the injury and treatment regimen.
12. Explain prescribed activity restrictions and necessary lifestyle modifications due to impaired mobility.
13. Teach the proper use of assistive devices as indicated.
14. Provide appropriate nursing interventions associated with prescribed treatment modalities (see Sections III, IV, and V as appropriate).
15. Monitor closely for signs and symptoms of complications.

G. **Evaluation**
1. The patient participates actively in pain management.
2. The patient reports relief of pain and discomfort.
3. The patient exhibits adequate tissue perfusion.
4. The patient demonstrates normal movement in unaffected body parts.
5. The patient participates in muscle-strengthening exercises of affected body parts, if indicated.
6. The patient maintains independence in self-care within limits of the injury and treatment plan.
7. The patient actively participates in the prescribed medical regimen.
8. The patient remains free of potential systemic complications.
9. The patient regains maximum use of the affected body part.

X. **Compartment syndrome**
A. **Description: a condition involving increased pressure and constriction of nerves and vessels within an anatomic compartment (e.g., the volar compartment of the forearm and the anterior and deep posterior compartments of the leg)**
B. **Etiology**
1. Compartment syndrome can result from one of two mechanisms:
   a. Decrease in compartment size
   b. Increase in compartment contents

2. Decrease in compartment size may result from closure of fascial defects or excessively tight bandages, casts, or splints.

3. Increase in compartment contents can result from swelling, bleeding, or muscle hypertrophy.

C. Pathophysiology

1. The primary problem in compartment syndrome is decreased tissue perfusion due to vessel constriction.

2. Compromised tissue and cellular perfusion persisting longer than 4 to 6 hours can cause nerve and muscle ischemia, resulting in permanent damage (e.g., Volkmann's ischemic contracture).

D. Assessment findings

1. Early detection of compartment syndrome is essential to enable prompt intervention aimed at relieving pressure and preventing tissue and nerve damage.

2. Clinical manifestations of compartment syndrome may include:

    a. Cardiovascular effects: diminished capillary refill, cyanotic nailbeds, pulselessness distal to the involved area

    b. Neurologic effects: deep, throbbing, unrelenting pain in the affected area; paresthesias; paralysis distal to the involved area

    c. Musculoskeletal effects: hard, swollen muscle, weakness with muscle stretch deterioration

E. Nursing diagnoses

1. High Risk for Injury

2. Pain

3. Altered Tissue Perfusion: Peripheral

F. Planning and implementation

1. Recognize that this condition represents a medical emergency requiring prompt intervention.

2. Elevate the affected extremity to the heart level and apply cold packs to control edema.

3. Release constrictive dressings immediately.

4. If indicated, bivalve a constrictive cast by splitting it along both sides to release pressure; leave the cast in place for support, however.

5. If pressure is not relieved in 1 to 2 hours, prepare the patient for fasciotomy, and assist with the procedure as necessary.

6. Promote correction of deformities with physical therapy and exercise as prescribed.

G. Evaluation

1. The patient exhibits increased tissue perfusion.

2. The patient reports decreased pain.

3. The patient demonstrates adequate functioning in the affected limb.

4. The patient displays no resulting injury after compartment release.

XI. Osteoarthritis

(*Note:* See Chapter 12, Immunologic Disorders, for a discussion of rheumatoid arthritis.)

A. **Description: a slowly progressive degenerative joint disease characterized by variable changes in weight-bearing joints**

B. **Etiology and incidence**

1. Of unknown cause, osteoarthritis is associated with obesity, aging, trauma, genetic predisposition, and congenital abnormalities.
2. The most common form of arthritis, osteoarthritis affects both sexes about equally, with onset generally after age 40.

C. **Pathophysiology**

1. Osteoarthritis causes deterioration of the joint cartilage and formation of reactive new bone at joint margins and in subchondral areas.
2. Disability varies from limitation of finger movement to severe hip and knee degeneration.
3. Progression is also variable; joints with minor deterioration may remain stable for years.

D. **Assessment findings**

1. Clinical manifestations of osteoarthritis include:
   a. Pain and muscle spasm, more pronounced after exercise, at night, and in the early morning
   b. Limited motion in affected joints
   c. Joint "grating" on movement
   d. Flexion contractures, primarily in the hip and knee
   e. Joint tenderness, Heberden's nodes in interphalangeal joints
2. Radiographs may confirm diagnosis.

E. **Nursing diagnoses**

1. Body Image Disturbance
2. Impaired Physical Mobility
3. Pain
4. Altered Role Performance
5. Self-Care Deficit

F. **Planning and implementation**

1. Apply warm compresses or diathermy to sore joints.
2. Massage surrounding muscles, not overinflamed joints.
3. Promote adequate rest and reduction of stress.
4. Position the patient to prevent flexion deformity using foot board, splints, sandbags, wedges, or pillows as needed.
5. Remove splints routinely, if used, to exercise joints.

6. Plan activities that promote optimal function and independence.
7. Consult with a physical therapist for an exercise plan.
8. Teach the patient about:
   a. Prescribed medication use (e.g., analgesics, nonsteroidal antiinflammatory drugs)
   b. Prescribed exercises (only within tolerance level and with modified weight bearing using assistive devices as indicated)
   c. Use of assistive devices, if needed, for activities of daily living (ADLs)
   d. Correct posture techniques while standing and sitting
9. Prepare the patient for surgical treatment as indicated (e.g., osteotomy, arthroplasty, total joint replacement).
10. Caution against resorting to nontraditional treatments by nonmedical groups, but respect the patient's right to choose such a treatment if he or she obtains relief.

G. Evaluation
1. The patient reports reduced pain.
2. The patient maintains or increases joint movement and muscle strength.
3. The patient verbalizes understanding of prescribed medications, exercise, and other aspects of treatment.
4. The patient participates in ADLs to the greatest level possible within disease limitations.

XII. Gouty arthritis
A. Description: a metabolic disease marked by urate crystal deposits in joints throughout the body, causing local irritation and inflammatory responses
B. Etiology and incidence
1. Gouty arthritis apparently is linked to a genetic deficit in purine metabolism.
2. It affects men older than age 30 almost exclusively.

C. Pathophysiology
1. Gout is characterized by formation of tophus deposits in soft tissues and urate crystals in joint synovia.
2. It primarily affects joints in the feet (especially the great toe) and legs, but may strike in any joint.
3. The disorder follows a variable course of periodic attacks, often with years-long symptom-free periods between attacks.
4. Eventually, it can lead to chronic disability and, in some cases, severe hypertension and progressive renal failure.

D. Assessment findings
1. The patient commonly reports sudden attacks, usually at night, with periodic remissions and exacerbations.

    2. Typical manifestations include:
- a. Pain, usually monarticular, acute, crushing, and pulsating
- b. Joint swelling and inflammation
- c. Intolerance to the weight of bed linens over the affected joint
- d. Pruritus or skin ulceration over the affected joint

    3. Severe disease may produce signs of renal involvement (e.g., oliguria, low back pain, hypertension).

    4. Laboratory findings may include:
- a. Urate crystals in synovial fluid
- b. Hyperuricemia
- c. Elevated serum uric acid level

    5. In advanced disease, radiograph may show joint damage.

E. Nursing diagnoses
1. Body Image Disturbance
2. Altered Nutrition: Less Than Body Requirements
3. Pain
4. Altered Role Performance
5. Self-Care Deficit
6. Impaired Skin Integrity

F. Planning and implementation
1. Administer prescribed medications to control acute attacks, which may include:
   - a. Antiuric acid agents (administered until the patient experiences nausea, vomiting, and diarrhea—indicating therapeutic blood level—then discontinued)
   - b. Probenecid or allopurinol
   - c. Nonsteroidal antiinflammatory drugs
   - d. Analgesics
2. Apply ice to affected joints.
3. Maintain strict bedrest for 24 hours after an attack.
4. Elevate affected limbs.
5. Provide a bed cradle to keep bed linen off affected joints.
6. Teach the patient about:
   - a. The prescribed medication regimen
   - b. The need to increase fluid intake to 3 L/day
   - c. Diet modifications to limit foods high in purine (e.g., organ meats, anchovies, sardines, shellfish, chocolate, meat extracts)

G. Evaluation
1. The patient reports reduced pain.
2. The patient experiences minimal skin irritation over affected joints.
3. The patient demonstrates minimal side effects to the medication regimen.

4. The patient verbalizes knowledge of prescribed medications, dietary modifications, and other treatments.
5. The patient demonstrates reduced frequency and severity of acute attacks.
6. The patient participates in self-care activities and ADLs to the limit of his ability.

XIII. Bone tumors

A. Description

1. Bone tumors can be either benign or malignant.
2. Types include:
   a. Osteochondroma: benign tumor usually at the ends of long bones
   b. Ecchondroma: painful, benign tumor of hyaline cartilage
   c. Osteogenic sarcoma: highly metastasizing, malignant bone tumor
   d. Chondrosarcoma: malignant tumor of hyaline cartilage
   e. Multiple myeloma: malignant tumor arising from bone marrow

B. Etiology and incidence

1. The etiology of bone cancer is unclear.
2. Bone cancer is relatively rare; only an estimated 6000 new bone and soft tissue sarcomas occur each year in the United States.
3. Various types predominate in certain age groups:
   a. Osteochondroma: childhood and adolescence
   b. Ecchondroma: childhood and adolescence
   c. Osteogenic sarcoma: younger than age 25
   d. Chondrosarcoma: adult males
   e. Multiple myeloma: between age 50 and 70

C. Pathophysiology

1. Benign bone tumors usually are slow growing and well circumscribed.
2. Primary malignant bone tumors arise from bone tissue cells or bone marrow components. Cellular characteristics and disease progression vary with type and location.
3. Primary tumors tend to readily involve contiguous tissues and metastasize to the lungs early.

D. Assessment findings

1. Clinical manifestations are highly variable but may include:
   a. Bone pain, possibly severe and persistent or only mild
   b. Varying degrees of movement limitation
   c. Palpable, fixed mass on bone
   d. Sensory disturbance in affected areas secondary to nerve compression

         e.   Pathologic fracture in affected bone

         f.   Systemic effects (e.g., weight loss, mild fever, malaise)

   2. Important laboratory studies and diagnostic tests include:

         a.   Chest radiograph to detect lung metastases

         b.   Bone scan to detect extension of bone lesions

         c.   Biopsy for tumor identification

         d.   Arteriography

         e.   Urinalysis and blood chemistries (Elevated alkaline phosphatase is a common finding.)

E. **Nursing diagnoses**

   1. Ineffective Family Coping

   2. Ineffective Individual Coping

   3. High Risk for Injury

   4. Pain

   5. Altered Role Performance

   6. Self-Care Deficit

F. **Planning and implementation**

   1. Provide pain relief through analgesic administration or therapeutic techniques as prescribed.

   2. Assist with position change and ambulation to prevent stress on affected, weakened bones.

   3. Provide patient or family teaching, covering:

         a.   Use of assistive devices as ordered

         b.   Action and possible side effects of chemotherapeutic drugs

         c.   Medication and treatment regimens for home care

   4. Encourage the patient and family members to express feelings and concerns; convey an accepting, reassuring demeanor.

   5. Prepare the patient for surgery and possible limb salvage or amputation as indicated. (Malignant tumors are thoroughly removed with wide excision, resection of the affected part, or amputation of the entire limb to prevent metastasis.)

   6. Refer the patient and family to appropriate support groups.

   7. Encourage the patient's maximum independence within limitations of the condition.

G. **Evaluation**

   1. The patient reports adequate pain relief.

   2. The patient experiences no injuries, including pathologic fractures.

   3. The patient (and family members as appropriate) verbalize understanding of the prescribed treatment regimen.

   4. The patient and family members demonstrate appropriate coping skills in dealing with the disease and its prognosis.

   5. The patient maintains independence in ADLs living within limitations imposed by the disease.

XIV. Osteomyelitis

A. Description: severe pyogenic bone infection

B. Etiology and incidence

    1. Osteomyelitis can result from trauma or secondary infection (most commonly with *Staphylococcus aureus*).

    2. It tends to affect persons with low resistance or with decreased blood flow to a trauma site.

    3. Blood-borne osteomyelitis (hematogenic) is more common in children secondary to throat infection.

    4. Osteomyelitis secondary to trauma or orthopedic surgical procedures is more common in older persons.

C. Pathophysiology

    1. Blood stream circulation of infectious microbes to susceptible bone leads to:

        a. Inflammation

        b. Increased vascularity

        c. Edema

    2. The organisms grow and form pus within the bone, and abscess formation may occur.

    3. This deprives the bone of its blood supply, eventually leading to necrosis.

    4. Necrosis stimulates new bone formation (involucrum) by the periosteum; this pushes old bone (sequestrum) out of the abscess or a sinus.

D. Assessment findings

    1. Osteomyelitis is commonly marked by:

        a. Localized bone pain

        b. Tenderness, heat, and swelling in the affected area

        c. Guarding of the affected area

        d. Restricted movement in affected area

        e. Systemic symptoms (e.g., high fever and chills [acute osteomyelitis], low-grade fever and generalized weakness [chronic osteomyelitis])

        f. Purulent drainage from a skin abscess

    2. Laboratory studies may reveal:

        a. Leukocytosis on WBC count

        b. Elevated erythrocyte sedimentation rate

        c. The causative organism identified on blood culture

        d. Bone involvement in advanced disease demonstrated by radiograph and bone scan

E. Nursing diagnoses

    1. High Risk for Injury

    2. Impaired Physical Mobility

    3. Pain

    4. Impaired Skin Integrity

F. **Planning and implementation**
1. Control pain by administering prescribed analgesics and providing comfort measures.
2. Support an affected limb above and below the affected area.
3. Elevate the affected limb to reduce swelling.
4. Administer antibiotics as prescribed to treat infection.
5. Provide local treatments as prescribed (e.g., warm saline soaks).
6. Provide a diet high in protein and vitamins C and D to promote healing.
7. Teach the patient about:
    a. Activity restrictions
    b. Self-care techniques
    c. Home wound care and IV therapy, if ordered
8. Prepare the patient for surgical debridement, bone grafting, or amputation as appropriate.

G. **Evaluation**
1. The patient reports adequate pain control.
2. The patient performs ADLs within activity restrictions.
3. The patient demonstrates self wound care and IV therapy, if prescribed.
4. The patient states signs and symptoms of further complications to watch for and report.

Bibliography

Brunner L. S, & Suddarth, D. S. (1986). *The Lippincott manual of nursing practice* (4th ed.). Philadelphia: J. B. Lippincott.

Brunner L. S., & Suddarth, D. S. (1988). *Textbook of medical-surgical nursing* (6th ed.). Philadelphia: J. B. Lippincott.

Doenges, M. E., Moorhouse, M. F., & Geissler, A. C. (1989). *Nursing care plans: Guidelines for planning patient care* (2nd ed.). Philadelphia: F. A. Davis.

Jaffe, M. S., & Melson, K. A. (1988). *Laboratory and diagnostic cards: Clinical implications and teaching.* St. Louis: C. V. Mosby.

Luckman, J., & Sorenson K. C. (1987). *Medical-surgical nursing: A psychophysiologic approach* (3rd ed.). Philadelphia: W. B. Saunders.

Mourad, L. A., & Droste, M. M. (1988). *The nursing process in the care of adults with orthopedic conditions* (2nd ed.). New York: John Wiley & Sons.

STUDY QUESTIONS

1. On her way to work one morning, a nurse comes across an automobile accident. One victim's arm is grossly deformed with ends of the humerus protruding through the skin. Emergency care for this type of injury should include
   a. applying gentle traction to align the fractured bone ends, then splinting the entire extremity in corrected position
   b. covering the broken skin and bone ends with a clean material, then splinting in the position of the deformity
   c. wrapping a tight, clean covering around the broken skin and bone ends, then applying gentle traction to the fracture
   d. leaving the broken skin and bone fragments uncovered and splinting the deformed arm above the elbow at the fracture site

2. Ms. Boyd, aged 33, is being treated for fractures of the femur and pelvis following an accident. While caring for Ms. Boyd, the nurse observes a sudden change in her condition and determines that she displays symptoms of a systemic fat embolism. Based on this information, all the following nursing diagnoses likely would be appropriate *except*
   a. Ineffective Thermoregulation
   b. Altered Thought Processes
   c. Altered Tissue Perfusion: Cardiopulmonary
   d. Impaired Gas Exchange

3. Mrs. Hunt, aged 76, is receiving treatment for osteoarthritis. The nurse would evaluate the effectiveness of her analgesic medications by noting which of the following?
   a. The patient increases motion in joints that have contractures.
   b. The patient demonstrates disappearance of Heberden's nodes.
   c. The patient reports decreased pain after exercise and at night.

   d. The patient demonstrates the ability to perform ADLs.

4. Which patient statement would alert the nurse for the potential complication of cast syndrome in a patient with a hip spica cast?
   a. "I have sensitive skin to warm, dry environments."
   b. "I become highly emotional when I feel confined in small spaces."
   c. "I had a postoperative infection when I had my appendix removed."
   d. "I felt more pain in my hip yesterday than I do today."

5. Mr. Bell, aged 50, is diagnosed with gouty arthritis and is started on a low purine diet. The nurse's teaching plan should include instructing Mr. Bell to avoid which of the following foods?
   a. citrus fruits
   b. green vegetables
   c. organ meats
   d. fresh fish

6. Mr. Steiner, aged 24, has been diagnosed with osteogenic sarcoma of the femur and is receiving chemotherapy. Which of the following nursing diagnoses would be of most importance when planning activities for Mr. Steiner?
   a. Altered Role Performance related to discomfort, pain, and impaired mobility
   b. Impaired Skin Integrity related to inflammatory response to chemotherapy
   c. High Risk for Injury: pathologic fracture related to effects of tumor and chemotherapy
   d. Ineffective Individual Coping related to diagnosis and treatment regimen

7. Mrs. Moore, aged 45, is awaiting surgical fixation of a fractured hip. If the physician orders Buck's traction until surgery is performed, the nurse should plan for which of the following traction applications?

a. continuous, balanced suspension skeletal traction
b. intermittent, running skeletal traction
c. continuous, running skin traction
d. intermittent, balanced suspension skin traction

8. Which priority nursing intervention should be included in the plan of care following application of Buck's traction to Mrs. Moore's leg?
   a. turning and repositioning with pillows every hour to prevent deformity
   b. cleaning the traction application site every 8 hours to improve circulation
   c. checking the traction ropes and pulleys every hour for proper alignment
   d. checking nerve and circulatory function every 2 hours in the affected leg

9. Mrs. Taylor, aged 74, suffers from degenerative joint disease due to osteoarthritis and is admitted for a total joint replacement of the right hip. During the preoperative period, the nurse should focus assessment primarily on
   a. local and systemic infections
   b. self-care ability
   c. response to pain medications
   d. range of motion in the affected joint

10. Following arthroplasty, the nurse should maintain correct position of Mrs. Taylor's operative leg by
    a. placing an abductor wedge or pillows between the legs
    b. placing sandbags or pillows to keep leg adducted
    c. elevating the affected leg on two pillows or supports
    d. positioning her supine and on the operative side

11. When discussing physical activities with Mrs. Taylor, the nurse should instruct her to
    a. Avoid weight bearing until the hip is completely healed.
    b. Intermittently cross and uncross legs several times daily.

c. Maintain hip flexion at 90 degrees when sitting.
d. Limit hip flexion to only 45 to 60 degrees.

12. Before discharge, the nurse reviews the signs and symptoms of joint dislocation with Mrs. Taylor. The nurse would determine that Mrs. Taylor understands the instructions by her identification of which of the following symptoms?
    a. positive Homans' sign and inability to bear weight
    b. painless, sudden deformity of the affected hip joint
    c. severe hip pain with shortening of the extremity
    d. severe pain and swelling of the affected hip joint

13. As part of treatment of gouty arthritis for Mrs. Martin, aged 66, the physician orders antiuric acid medication to be given in large doses until the maximum safe dosage can be determined. The nurse would determine the maximum dosage and the need for dosage reduction by asking Mrs. Martin to report which of the following symptoms?
    a. bleeding gums and bruising
    b. nausea, vomiting, and diarrhea
    c. gastric irritation and heartburn
    d. blurred vision and nausea

14. Mr. Peterson, aged 38, underwent a below-knee right leg amputation. Several days after surgery, he reports to the nurse that he feels a crushing pain in his right foot and lower leg. Which of the following nursing diagnoses would the nurse most likely add to Mr. Peterson's care plan to address his pain?
    a. Pain related to excessive pressure on bony prominence
    b. Dysfunctional Grieving related to loss of body part
    c. Ineffective Coping related to denial of loss of body part
    d. Pain related to phantom sensations

ANSWER KEY

1. **Correct response: b**
   The fracture described is an open, compound fracture. Emergency care for this type of fracture is to prevent movement until the limb is immobilized. The wound should first be covered with a clean (or sterile if available) dressing to prevent further contamination, then splinted with as little movement as possible.

   a, c, and d. No attempts to align or reduce the fracture should be made, and the bone fragments should not be touched or pushed back into place.

   Application/Safe care/Implementation

2. **Correct response: a**
   This diagnosis is not specifically associated with fat embolism.

   b, c, and d. Systemic fat embolism most commonly occurs in patients with fractures of the pelvis or long bones, crush injuries, or multiple fractures. Numerous fat globules mobilize from the fracture site, enter the blood stream, and travel to distal areas where they lodge and obstruct blood flow. Signs and symptoms of fat embolism include mental signs such as agitation, confusion, delirium, or coma; respiratory signs such as tachypnea, dyspnea, crackles, and wheezes; and pallor or cyanosis. These manifestations indicate an emergency condition warranting immediate intervention.

   Analysis/Physiologic/Analysis (Dx)

3. **Correct response: c**
   Patients with osteoarthritis experience increased joint pain after exercise, at night, and early morning. Pain medication should relieve the pain during these times.

   a, b, and d. These observations would not specifically reflect analgesic effectiveness.

   Knowledge/Health promotion/Evaluation

4. **Correct response: b**
   A patient immobilized in large casts may experience either psychologic or physiologic complications. The psychologic complication is a claustrophobic reaction involving acute anxiety and possible irrational behavior. Physiologic effects may include tachypnea, diaphoresis, dilated pupils, tachycardia, and elevated blood pressure related to the acute anxiety. Patients who report problems with claustrophobia are at risk for this complication.

   a and c. These findings would alert the nurse to possible infection.

   d. This finding is related to progress, not cast syndrome.

   Analysis/Psychosocial/Assessment

5. **Correct response: c**
   Patients with gouty arthritis have a disorder in purine metabolism with abnormal amounts of urates in the body. Urate crystals become deposited in parts of the body causing local irritation and an inflammatory response. Treatment usually consists of lowering the serum urate level to dissolve crystalline deposits through dietary restrictions. Foods high in purine that should be avoided are organ meats, anchovies, sardines, shell fish, chocolate, and meat extracts.

   a, b, and d. The other foods listed are all important to a well-balanced diet.

   Comprehension/Health promotion/Planning

6. **Correct response: c**
   Osteogenic sarcoma is a primary malig-

nant bone tumor affecting bone cells. The tumor and chemotherapy leaves the bone weakened and makes the patient more vulnerable to pathologic fractures. The nurse should prevent stress on the weakened bone by assisting the patient with position changes and ambulation.

a, b, and d. Although these diagnoses may be relevant and important to care, they are not the most important.

Comprehension/Safe care/Analysis (Dx)

7. *Correct response: c*
Continuous traction is used to treat fractures, whereas intermittent traction is used to treat muscle spasms or to reduce pain. In this situation, the patient has a fractured femur and therefore needs the continuous pull to immobilize the fracture until surgery is performed. The nurse should always assume traction is continuous unless otherwise ordered by the physician. Buck's traction is an extension traction that exerts a straight pull on the leg. The traction is applied to the skin of the lower leg using tape, sponge rubber, or plastic materials.

a, b, and d. These other forms of traction would be inappropriate for this type of injury.

Knowledge/Physiologic/Planning

8. *Correct response: d*
Neurologic and circulatory checks should be done every 2 hours for a patient in traction to detect complications early.

a. A patient receiving traction should be turned and positioned correctly about every 2 hours unless he or she is placed on a special mattress to prevent pressure ulcers.

b. The traction tape should remain in place, but the area should be palpated to determine tenderness caused from pressure, decreased circulation, or nerve pressure.

c. The nurse should check the ropes, pulleys, and weights for proper alignment and traction pull every 8 hours.

Application/Physiologic/Implementation

9. *Correct response: a*
Infection is a major concern for any patient undergoing orthopedic surgery. It can be especially harmful for patients with joint replacements because infection may prevent achieving a functional joint postoperatively and necessitate another surgical procedure.

b, c, and d. Although these all may be important factors to assess, infection represents the primary concern.

Application/Safe care/Assessment

10. *Correct response: a*
Following total hip replacement, the patient should be kept flat while in a recumbent position with the affected extremity in an abducted position. This is accomplished by placing an abduction wedge or pillows between the patient's legs.

b. Adduction of the affected leg could cause dislocation of the hip replacement.

c. Hip flexion should never be beyond 45 to 60 degrees when elevating the leg or while sitting.

d. The patient should be turned only 45 degrees on the unoperated side with full support to the operative leg to keep it in the abduction position.

Application/Physiologic/Implementation

11. *Correct response: d*
Following a total hip replacement, the patient should be instructed to avoid any activities that cause hip adduction (crossing legs), flexion beyond 90 degrees (sitting in low chairs or on low toilet seats), and rotation (pivoting on affected leg).

a. Progressive weight-bearing exercises are encouraged early depending on physician's orders.

b. Crossing the legs causes hip adduction, which is contraindicated following hip replacement surgery.

c. The patient should be taught to limit hip flexion to only 45 to 60 degrees.

Application/Safe care/Implementation

12. **Correct response: c**

Dislocation of the hip prosthesis is a complication from extreme positions of hip adduction or flexion or from infection of the operative area. Signs and symptoms of hip dislocation include severe hip pain, shortening of the extremity, internal or external rotation of the extremity, and inability to move the hip.

a. A positive Homans' sign indicates thrombophlebitis, an unrelated complication.

b. Hip dislocation invariably produces pain.

d. Swelling may or may not occur with dislocation.

Analysis/Health promotion/Evaluation

13. **Correct response: b**

Antiuric acid medications are commonly prescribed to control acute attacks. Larger doses and high blood levels are needed. Doses are usually prescribed to the maximum level tolerated, determined by the appearance of symptoms such as nausea, vomiting, and diarrhea.

a, c, and d. These signs and symptoms represent side effects of aspirin and must be addressed separately (e.g., giving enteric-coated tablets to reduce gastric irritation).

Analysis/Physiologic/Evaluation

14. **Correct response: d**

Patients often experience phantom pain or sensations following a limb amputation. This pain is felt in the part that has been amputated, and patients experience feelings that the part still remains. They may feel a crushing, cramping, or twisting of the amputated part. The nurse must acknowledge that these sensations are real to the patient and help the patient deal with them.

a. Severe pain at the operative site may indicate excessive pressure on the bony prominence or hematoma formation.

b and c. Physiologic pain is not usually associated with the grieving process or with ineffective coping.

Application/Physiologic/Analysis (Dx)

Liver, Biliary, and Pancreatic Disorders

I. Anatomy and physiology
 - A. Structure
 - B. Function

II. Overview of liver, biliary system, and pancreatic disorders
 - A. Assessment
 - B. Laboratory studies and diagnostic tests: liver
 - C. Laboratory studies and diagnostic tests: biliary system
 - D. Laboratory studies and diagnostic tests: pancreas
 - E. Psychosocial implications

III. Jaundice
 - A. Description
 - B. Etiology and incidence
 - C. Pathophysiology
 - D. Assessment findings
 - E. Nursing diagnoses
 - F. Planning and implementation
 - G. Evaluation

IV. Portal hypertension
 - A. Description
 - B. Etiology and incidence
 - C. Pathophysiology
 - D. Assessment findings
 - E. Nursing diagnoses
 - F. Planning and implementation
 - G. Evaluation

V. Hepatic encephalopathy
 - A. Description
 - B. Etiology and incidence
 - C. Pathophysiology
 - D. Assessment findings
 - E. Nursing diagnoses

 - F. Planning and implementation
 - G. Evaluation

VI. Hepatitis
 - A. Description
 - B. Etiology and incidence
 - C. Pathophysiology
 - D. Assessment findings
 - E. Nursing diagnoses
 - F. Planning and implementation
 - G. Evaluation

VII. Cirrhosis
 - A. Description
 - B. Etiology and incidence
 - C. Pathophysiology
 - D. Assessment findings
 - E. Nursing diagnoses
 - F. Planning and implementation
 - G. Evaluation

VIII. Bleeding esophageal varices
 - A. Description
 - B. Etiology and incidence
 - C. Pathophysiology
 - D. Assessment findings
 - E. Nursing diagnoses
 - F. Planning and implementation
 - G. Evaluation

IX. Liver cancer
 - A. Description
 - B. Etiology and incidence
 - C. Pathophysiology
 - D. Assessment findings
 - E. Nursing diagnoses
 - F. Planning and implementation

I. Anatomy and physiology

  A. **Structure**

    1. Liver

      a. Located in the right upper abdominal quadrant, the liver is divided into four lobes: the left, right, caudate, and quadrate lobes.

      b. The lobes are further subdivided into smaller units known as lobules.

      c. Blood supply to the liver is supplied from the portal vein (75%), which drains the gastrointestinal (GI) tract, and from the hepatic artery (25%).

      d. The liver contains various cell types, including hepatocytes (liver cells) and Kupffer cells (phagocytic cells that engulf bacteria).

    2. Biliary system

      a. Canaliculi, the smallest bile ducts located between liver lobules, receive bile from hepatocytes.

      b. The canaliculi form larger bile ducts, which lead to the hepatic duct.

      c. The hepatic duct from the liver joins the cystic duct

from the gallbladder to form the common bile duct, which empties into the duodenum.

    d.   Flow of bile into the intestine is controlled by the sphincter of Oddi.

    e.   The gallbladder is a hollow, pear-shaped organ, 3 to 4 in long, attached to the liver under the right lobe.

    f.   The gallbladder normally holds 30 to 50 mL of bile and can hold up to 70 mL when fully distended.

  3. Pancreas

    a.   A slender, fish-shaped organ, the pancreas lies horizontally in the abdomen behind the stomach and extends roughly from the duodenum to the spleen.

    b.   The functional pancreatic exocrine unit is the secreting acinus.

    c.   Pancreatic acini are arranged in lobules with channels that extend to the main lobular duct.

    d.   The acini normally produce between 1200 and 3000 mL of pancreatic juice daily.

B. **Function**

  1. Liver functions include:

    a.   Regulating blood glucose level; makes glycogen, which is stored in hepatocytes

    b.   Synthesizing glucose from amino acids of lactate through gluconeogenesis

    c.   Converting ammonia produced from gluconeogenetic by-products and bacteria to urea

    d.   Synthesizing plasma proteins such as albumin, globulins, clotting factors, and lipoproteins

    e.   Breaking down fatty acids into ketone bodies

    f.   Storing vitamins and trace metals

    g.   Affecting drug metabolism

    h.   Secreting bile

  2. Continuously formed by hepatocytes (about 1 L/day), bile comprises:

    a.   Water, electrolytes, lecithin, fatty acids, cholesterol

    b.   Bilirubin: pigment derived from breakdown of hemoglobin; conjugated with glucuronic acid by hepatocytes, producing direct or conjugated bilirubin that is secreted into bile

    c.   Bile salts: (made from cholesterol) emulsify fat, reabsorbed in distal ileum and returned to the liver via the portal vein

  3. Metabolic functions of the biliary system include:

    a.   Draining bile from hepatocytes to the gallbladder by way of the biliary tree

    b.   Storing bile in the gallbladder and releasing it to the duodenum, mediated by the hormone cholecystokinin

4. The pancreas has both endocrine and exocrine functions. (Endocrine functions are discussed in Chapter 10, Endocrine and Metabolic Disorders.) Exocrine functions include:
   a. Producing pancreatic juice, which contains three types of digestive enzymes: amylase (hydrolyzes carbohydrate to disaccharides), lipase (hydrolyzes fat to fatty acids and glycerol), trypsin (proteolytic enzymes that split proteins); controlled by the vagus and two hormones, pancreozymin and secretin
   b. Secreting water and bicarbonate to neutralize gastric juice

II. Overview of liver, biliary system, and pancreatic disorders
A. Assessment
1. Assess liver size by percussing the upper and lower liver borders.
2. Record the level at which the lower border descends below the right costal margin.
3. Palpate the liver, if possible, to assess:
   a. Consistency
   b. Pain
   c. Shape
   d. Presence of firmness or nodules

B. Laboratory studies and diagnostic tests: liver
1. Liver function tests include:
   a. Alkaline phosphatase
   b. Serum glutamic-pyruvic transaminase (SGPT)—now more commonly known as ALT—and serum glutamic-oxaloacetic transaminase (SGOT)—now known as AST
   c. Lactic dehydrogenase (LDH)
   d. Serum proteins
   e. Direct and indirect bilirubin
   f. Serum ammonia
   g. Clotting factors
   h. Serum lipids
2. Liver biopsy, sampling of liver tissue by needle aspiration for histology, is done to establish diagnosis of specific liver disease.
3. Other important liver studies include:
   a. Computed tomography (CT) scan to detect neoplasms, cysts, abscesses, and hematomas
   b. Angiography to visualize hepatic circulation or masses
   c. Splenoportography to determine adequacy of portal blood flow
   d. Liver scan to demonstrate liver size and shape

C. Laboratory studies and diagnostic tests: biliary system
1. Ultrasonography can detect calculi (gallstones) or a dilated common bile duct.

2.   Radionuclide imaging of the biliary tree and gallbladder can aid diagnosis of acute cholecystitis.
3.   Cholecystography detects gallstones and assesses the gallbladder's ability to fill, concentrate, and contract.
4.   Endoscopic retrograde cholangiopancreatography (ERCP) allows direct visualization of the common bile ducts and pancreatic duct.
5.   Percutaneous transhepatic cholangiography is useful in distinguishing jaundice caused by liver disease.

D.   Laboratory studies and diagnostic tests: pancreas
1.   Blood studies include:
     a.   Serum amylase and lipase: important aids in diagnosing pancreatitis
     b.   White blood cell count: usually elevated in pancreatitis
     c.   Serum bilirubin levels: possibly elevated in pancreatic dysfunction
2.   Radiographic studies of the abdomen and chest may differentiate pancreatitis from other disorders.
3.   Ultrasonography and CT scanning are used to identify increased pancreas size and to detect pancreatic cysts, pseudocysts, or tumors.
4.   Stool analysis evaluates fat content: normally around 20%, may range from 50% to 90% in pancreatic disease.
5.   ERCP is the most helpful study in the diagnosis of pancreatitis; it also enables tissue biopsy for analysis and differentiating pancreatitis from carcinoma.

E.   Psychosocial implications
1.   The patient with a liver, biliary, or pancreatic disorder may experience coping difficulty related to:
     a.   Progressive nature of the disorder
     b.   Chronicity of the disorder
     c.   Fear of death
     d.   Limitations in function
     e.   Pain
     f.   Guilt associated with the disorder's cause
2.   The patient also may express self-concept concerns related to fear of:
     a.   Role changes toward increased dependence
     b.   Loss of sexuality and sexual function
     c.   Body image changes
3.   Common lifestyle concerns may be related to potential changes in:
     a.   Physical and functional ability
     b.   Work performance, with possible job loss
     c.   Self-care ability

4.   Disease-related changes in social interactions may result in:
  a.   Depression
  b.   Isolation
  c.   Rejection
  d.   Hopelessness

III. Jaundice

A.   Description: a symptom or syndrome characterized by increased bilirubin concentration in blood; classified as hemolytic, hepatocellular, or obstructive

B.   Etiology and incidence

1.   Hemolytic jaundice can result from:
  a.   Transfusion reaction
  b.   Hemolytic anemia
  c.   Severe burns
  d.   Autoimmune hemolytic anemia

2.   Causes of hepatocellular jaundice include:
  a.   Hepatitis
  b.   Yellow fever
  c.   Alcoholism

3.   Obstructive jaundice may be:
  a.   Extrahepatic, caused by bile duct plugging from gallstones, an inflammatory process, tumor, or pressure from enlarged gland
  b.   Intrahepatic, resulting from pressure on channels from inflamed liver tissue or exudate

4.   Jaundice also may be hereditary.

C.   Pathophysiology

1.   Hemolytic jaundice, caused by increased destruction of red blood cells, results in the inability to excrete bilirubin as quickly as it forms.

2.   Hepatocellular jaundice results from the inability of diseased liver cells to clear normal amounts of bilirubin, due to defective uptake, consumption, or transport mechanisms.

3.   Bile deposition in the skin, mucous membranes, and sclera results in characteristic yellow tinging of these structures.

D.   Assessment findings

1.   Clinical manifestations of jaundice include:
  a.   Dark, foamy urine due to increased bile in urine
  b.   Light or clay-colored stools due to lack of bile in the small bowel
  c.   Pruritus due to increased bile acids in skin
  d.   Inability to tolerate fatty foods due to absence of bile in the small intestine

2.   The patient may be mildly or severely ill with other symptoms

such as anorexia, fatigue, nausea, weakness, and possible weight loss.

   3. Laboratory study findings in jaundice may include:
      a. Conjugated bilirubin (direct): normal or elevated
      b. Unconjugated bilirubin (indirect): normal or elevated
      c. Total bilirubin: elevated
      d. Urine bilirubin: absent or elevated
      e. Urine urobilinogen: decreased or increased
      f. Fecal urobilinogen: elevated, decreased, or absent
      g. AST (or SGOT): normal or elevated
      h. ALT (or SGPT): normal or elevated
      i. Partial thromboplastin time: normal or prolonged

E. **Nursing diagnoses**
   1. Activity Intolerance
   2. Anxiety
   3. Altered Nutrition: Less Than Body Requirements
   4. High Risk for Impaired Skin Integrity

F. **Planning and implementation**
   1. Assess the patient's level of activity.
   2. Intervene to reduce anxiety; reinforce the physician's explanations of the cause and expected outcome of jaundice, and encourage the patient to express feelings and concerns.
   3. Assess dietary intake and nutritional status; promote a high carbohydrate intake, with protein intake consistent with that recommended for hepatic encephalopathy.
   4. Assess for pruritus, and provide frequent skin care.

G. **Evaluation**
   1. The patient verbalizes understanding of appropriate carbohydrate and protein intake.
   2. The patient exhibits decreased anxiety.
   3. The patient exhibits decreased jaundice and pruritus.

IV. Portal hypertension

A. **Description: elevated pressure in the portal vein associated with increased resistance to blood flow through the porta hepatis**

B. **Etiology and incidence**
   1. Major causes of portal hypertension include:
      a. Cirrhosis
      b. Mechanical obstruction (e.g., thrombosis, tumor)
   2. Incidence information is similar to that for cirrhosis.

C. **Pathophysiology**
   1. Obstruction of portal venous flow through the liver leads to:
      a. Formation of esophageal, gastric, and hemorrhoidal varicosities due to increased venous pressure
      b. Accumulation of fluid in the abdominal cavity (ascites)

2. The spleen and other organs that empty into the portal system also undergo the effects of congestion.

D. Assessment findings

1. Signs and symptoms of portal encephalopathy include:
   a. Shifting dullness or fluid wave on abdominal percussion
   b. Dilated abdominal vessels radiating from the umbilicus (caput medusae)
   c. Enlarged, palpable spleen
   d. Bruits detected over the upper abdominal area due to esophageal and gastric varicosities
2. Important diagnostic tests include portal pressure measurement, liver scans, splenoportography, abdominal angiography, and liver biopsy.

E. Nursing diagnoses

1. Activity Intolerance
2. Body Image Disturbance
3. Decreased Cardiac Output
4. Fear
5. Fluid Volume Excess
6. High Risk for Injury
7. Pain
8. High Risk for Impaired Skin Integrity
9. Altered Tissue Perfusion: Cardiopulmonary and Renal

F. Planning and implementation

1. Measure and record abdominal girth and body weight daily.
2. Administer diuretics and Aldactone (aldosterone blocking agent), as ordered, to reduce fluid retention.
3. Assess fluid balance, monitoring intake and output carefully.
4. Monitor for adverse effects of diuretic therapy (e.g., fluid and electrolyte disturbances such as hypovolemia, hypokalemia, and hyponatremia). Keep in mind that diuretic therapy also can precipitate encephalopathy.
5. Encourage the patient to verbalize feelings about any body image and self-concept changes.
6. Observe the patient closely for signs and symptoms of vascular collapse following paracentesis (removal of fluid from the peritoneal cavity).
7. If indicated, prepare the patient for peritoneojugular (LeVeen) shunting to shunt ascitic fluid to the venous system.

G. Evaluation

1. The patient exhibits reduced abdominal girth and body weight.
2. The patient maintains adequate electrolyte balance.
3. The patient verbalizes feelings about body image and self-concept.

4. The patient exhibits no evidence of vascular collapse.

V. Hepatic encephalopathy

A. Description: a neurologic syndrome developing as a complication of liver disease; may be acute and self-limiting or chronic and progressive

B. Etiology and incidence

1. Possible causes of hepatic encephalopathy include:
   a. Severe liver injury
   b. Hepatocellular failure
   c. Portal shunting directly from the portal system to systemic venous circulation
   d. Increased serum ammonia levels secondary to GI bleeding, high-protein diet, or bacterial growth in the intestine and uremia
2. Incidence information is similar to that for cirrhosis.

C. Pathophysiology

1. Hepatic encephalopathy results from accumulation of ammonia and other identified toxic metabolites in blood due to the liver cells' inability to convert ammonia to urea.
2. Increased blood ammonia concentration leads to neurologic dysfunction and possible brain damage.

D. Assessment findings

1. Clinical manifestations include:
   a. Neurologic dysfunction progressing from minor mental aberrations and motor disturbances to coma
   b. Asterixis or flapping tremor of hands (also called liver flap)
2. Laboratory tests may reveal:
   a. Elevated serum ammonia level
   b. Elevated serum bilirubin level
   c. Prolonged prothrombin time

E. Nursing diagnoses

1. Ineffective Airway Clearance
2. High Risk for Injury
3. Sensory and Perceptual Alterations
4. Impaired Skin Integrity

F. Planning and implementation

1. Closely monitor neurologic status for any changes.
2. Measure and record daily fluid intake and output and body weight.
3. Take vital signs every 4 hours, assessing for changes from baseline.
4. Assess for signs and symptoms of infection.
5. Evaluate serum ammonia values daily.

6. Reduce or eliminate the patient's dietary protein intake if you detect evidence of impending coma.
7. Administer a high cleansing enema to reduce ammonia absorption.
8. Administer an antibiotic, such as neomycin, to act as an intestinal antiseptic agent as ordered.
9. Monitor electrolyte status and intervene as indicated to correct any imbalances.
10. Administer conservative doses of sedative or analgesic drugs, as prescribed, and monitor closely following administration.
11. Administer lactulose, as ordered, to keep ammonia in its ionized state and to trigger catharsis.

G. **Evaluation**
1. The patient exhibits increased level of consciousness.
2. The patient maintains adequate intake and output.
3. The patient maintains vital signs within normal ranges.
4. The patient exhibits normal serum ammonia level.
5. The patient displays no evidence of infection or injury.

VI. Hepatitis

A. **Description: an inflammatory disorder of the liver parenchyma occurring in four types: hepatitis A, hepatitis B, non-A and non-B hepatitis, and toxic or drug-induced hepatitis**

B. **Etiology and incidence**
1. Hepatitis usually results from viral infection; however, it also can result from toxicity or certain drugs.
2. The hepatitis A virus (an RNA virus) may be transmitted via the fecal–oral route or from contaminated food or water. This virus is endemic in some parts of the world; children younger than 15 years are at greatest risk.
3. The hepatitis B virus (a DNA virus) may be transmitted parenterally or by intimate contact with carriers; persons with acute disease; or contaminated instruments, syringes, or needles. Incidence is greatest in areas with high population densities and poor hygienic conditions.
4. Non-A, non-B hepatitis (linked to an unidentifiable virus) can result from transfusion of contaminated blood products, exposure to infected persons in renal transplant and dialysis units, or parenteral drug abuse.
5. Toxic or drug-induced hepatitis results from chemicals or medications that damage the parenchyma (e.g., carbon tetrachloride, halothane, acetaminophen).

C. **Pathophysiology**
1. After exposure to a hepatitis virus, incubation period varies: typically about 30 days for hepatitis A, 90 days for hepatitis B, and 50 days for non-A, non-B hepatitis.

2. Hepatocellular damage results from the body's immune response to the virus or toxin and is characterized by diffuse inflammatory infiltration with local necrosis.

3. Bile flow is interrupted, anitigen–antibody complexes activate the complement system, bilirubin diffuses into tissues, bile salts accumulate, and hepatomegaly and splenomegaly occur.

4. In uncomplicated cases, hepatocellular repair usually is completed within 3 to 4 months of onset.

5. Possible complications include fulminating hepatitis (a rare but life-threatening condition), chronic hepatitis, a chronic carrier state for hepatitis B surface antigen, cholestatic hepatitis, aplastic anemia, and pancreatitis.

D. Assessment findings

1. Hepatitis A is commonly marked by:
   a. Initially, headache, malaise, fatigue, anorexia, lethargy, fever, flulike respiratory symptoms
   b. In the icteric phase, dark urine, scleral icterus, jaundice, liver tenderness and perhaps enlargement
   c. Elevated serum transaminase levels, presence of hepatitis virus antibodies

2. Hepatitis B resembles hepatitis A clinically but usually with more severe manifestations. Fever and respiratory symptoms are rare; arthralgias and rash may occur.

3. Non-A, non-B, and toxic or drug-induced hepatitis typically resemble viral hepatitis in onset and symptoms; may progress to hepatic failure.

E. Nursing diagnoses

1. Activity Intolerance
2. Fatigue
3. Knowledge Deficit
4. Altered Nutrition: Less Than Body Requirements
5. Altered Sexuality Patterns
6. Social Isolation

F. Planning and implementation

1. Ensure the patient receives adequate fluid intake, sufficient rest, and proper nutrition.
2. Intervene to provide symptomatic relief as appropriate.
3. Administer blood transfusions or electrolyte supplements as ordered.
4. Teach the patient health maintenance measures related to the type of hepatitis, which may include:
   a. Hepatitis A: good sanitation and personal hygiene practices, effective sterilization procedures, administration of immune globulin
   b. Hepatitis B: administration of specific hepatitis B im-

mune globulin, hepatitis B vaccine for preexposure, immunization of high-risk persons

    c.   Non-A, non-B hepatitis: mandatory screening of blood donors, avoidance of certain medications and alcohol

    d.   Toxic or drug-induced hepatitis: avoidance of the causative agent

G. Evaluation

    1.   The patient maintains adequate fluid and nutrient intake.

    2.   The patient reports decreased fatigue.

    3.   The patient verbalizes understanding of preventive measures and self-care to maintain health status.

VII. Cirrhosis

  A. Description: a chronic degenerative liver disease marked by diffuse destruction and fibrotic regeneration of hepatic cells; classified as Laennec's, posthepatic, and biliary cirrhosis

  B. Etiology and incidence

    1.   Major causes of cirrhosis include:

        a.   Alcoholism and chronic nutritional deficiencies (Laennec's cirrhosis)

        b.   Bile duct disorders that suppress bile flow (biliary cirrhosis)

        c.   Various types of hepatitis (posthepatic cirrhosis)

    2.   Incidence is twice as high in men than in women; peak incidence occurs between ages 40 and 60.

  C. Pathophysiology

    1.   In cirrhosis, liver cells are injured or destroyed and replaced with scar tissue. Regeneration of liver tissue is patchy, resulting in a characteristic "hobnail" appearance.

    2.   Fibrosis and other changes in hepatocytes and reticular cells, as well as vascular and bile duct changes, lead to decreased blood and bile flow. Obstructed blood flow results in portal hypertension and esophageal varices.

    3.   Impaired hepatic functions include gluconeogenesis, detoxification of drugs and alcohol, bilirubin metabolism, vitamin absorption, and hormonal metabolism.

  D. Assessment findings

    1.   Clinical manifestations include:

        a.   Enlarged, firm liver

        b.   Chronic dyspepsia

        c.   Constipation or diarrhea

        d.   Gradual weight loss

        e.   Ascites

        f.   Splenomegaly

        g.   Spider telangiectases

        h.   Dilated abdominal blood vessels

   i. Signs and symptoms of portal hypertension (late)
  2. Laboratory study results may include:
   a. Destruction and fibrosis of liver tissue seen on biopsy
   b. Abnormal thickening and masses revealed on liver scan
   c. Elevated ALT, AST, and LDH levels
   d. Hypoalbuminemia
   e. Elevated prothrombin time
   f. Reduced bromsulphalein dye excretion

E. Nursing diagnoses
  1. Activity Intolerance
  2. High Risk for Injury
  3. Altered Nutrition: Less Than Body Requirements
  4. High Risk for Impaired Skin Integrity
  5. Altered Thought Processes

F. Planning and implementation
  1. Promote adequate rest and relaxation.
  2. Ensure good nutritional intake.
  3. Prevent threats to skin integrity.
  4. Minimize the risk of bleeding.
  5. Minimize metabolic derangements that can cause further deterioration of mental status.

G. Evaluation
  1. The patient demonstrates independence in activities.
  2. The patient exhibits improved nutritional status.
  3. The patient exhibits improved skin integrity.
  4. The patient demonstrates reduced risk of bleeding.
  5. The patient demonstrates improved mental status.

VIII. Bleeding esophageal varices

A. Description: a hemorrhagic process involving dilated, tortuous veins in the submucosa of the lower esophagus

B. Etiology and incidence
  1. The most common cause is portal hypertension resulting from obstructed portal venous circulation.
  2. Incidence information is similar to that for cirrhosis.

C. Pathophysiology
  1. Portal hypertension results in the development of collateral circulation in the lower esophagus as venous blood diverted from the GI tract and spleen due to portal obstruction seeks an outlet.
  2. These collateral veins become tortuous, dilated, and fragile due to excessive intraluminal pressure and are particularly prone to ulceration and hemorrhage.
  3. Ruptured esophageal varices are the most common cause of death in patients with hepatic cirrhosis.

D. **Assessment findings**
1. Present with hematemesis and melena, if ulcerated massive hemorrhage occurs
2. Signs of hepatic encephalopathy
3. Dilated abdominal veins
4. Ascites
5. Endoscopy confirms diagnosis

E. **Nursing diagnoses**
1. Activity Intolerance
2. Decreased Cardiac Output
3. Fear
4. High Risk for Injury
5. Pain
6. High Risk for Impaired Skin Integrity
7. Altered Thought Processes

F. **Planning and implementation**
1. Monitor vital signs and urinary output to evaluate fluid balance.
2. Assess level of consciousness.
3. Administer Pitressin therapy, as prescribed, monitoring for angina due to the drug's severe vasoconstrictive effects.
4. If the physician performs balloon tamponade to control bleeding, explain the procedure to the patient to reduce fear and enhance his or her cooperation with insertion and maintenance of the esophageal tamponade tube, and monitor closely to prevent accidental removal or displacement of the tube with resultant airway obstruction.
5. If the physician orders iced saline lavage, focus nursing interventions on:
   a. Ensuring nasogastric tube patency to prevent aspiration
   b. Observing gastric aspirate for evidence of bleeding
   c. Protecting the patient from chilling
6. After injection sclerotherapy, if performed, assess for:
   a. Aspiration
   b. Esophageal perforation
   c. Rebleeding
7. After portal-systemic surgical intervention, if done, monitor for such complications as:
   a. Development of systemic encephalopathy
   b. Liver failure
   c. Rebleeding

G. **Evaluation**
1. The patient verbalizes understanding of the disorder and procedures used.
2. The patient communicates needs and fears.

3.   The patient reports reduced fear related to potential hemor-
     rhage.
4.   The patient maintains a patent airway with no aspiration.
5.   The patient maintains good skin integrity.
6.   The patient remains free of massive hemorrhage.
7.   The patient reports increased comfort resulting from treat-
     ment.

IX. Liver cancer

A. Description: a rare form of cancer with a high mortality rate; may be primary (benign or malignant) or metastatic

B. Etiology and incidence

1.   Adenoma, a benign primary tumor, is associated with use of oral contraceptives or androgens; incidence is increasing, primarily in women.
2.   Occurring most frequently in men, hepatoma (or hepatocellular carcinoma)—the most common malignant primary tumor—has been linked to various factors, including hepatitis B, chronic liver disease, anabolic steroid use, and long-term androgen therapy.
3.   Metastatic liver cancer is associated with approximately one half of all late cancer cases. In the United States, it is up to 20 times more prevalent than primary liver tumors.

C. Pathophysiology

1.   Primary liver tumors originate in hepatocytes, connective tissue, or blood vessels (hepatomas) or in intrahepatic bile ducts (cholangiomas).
2.   Metastatic cancer can spread from virtually any body area but is most commonly associated with breast, lung, and colon cancer.
3.   Processes of liver metastasis include:
     a.   Extension from adjacent organs
     b.   Migration by way of the hepatic arterial system or the portal venous system
     c.   Seeding from peritoneal migration
4.   Although benign, adenomas carry a high risk of rupture due to their high vascularity.
5.   Malignant liver cancer is almost always fatal, with death occurring an average of 6 months after diagnosis.

D. Assessment findings

1.   Possible clinical manifestations of hepatoma include:
     a.   Recent weight loss
     b.   Weakness, fatigue
     c.   Hepatomegaly
     d.   Jaundice
     e.   Ascites

    f. Liver mass detected on palpation
   2. Pertinent laboratory studies may reveal:
     a. Anemia
     b. Elevated alkaline phosphatase
     c. Hypoproteinemia
     d. Decreased activity on liver function studies
     e. Fillings defects revealed on liver scans
   3. Positive tissue biopsy confirms diagnosis.

E. Nursing diagnoses
   1. Ineffective Breathing Pattern
   2. Fear
   3. High Risk for Infection
   4. Altered Nutrition: Less Than Body Requirements
   5. Pain
   6. Altered Role Performance
   7. High Risk for Impaired Skin Integrity

F. Planning and implementation
   1. Provide emotional support for the patient and family, and help them cope with the diagnosis of cancer and its typically poor prognosis.
   2. Teach the patient and family about the prescribed treatment plan, which may include radiation therapy, chemotherapy, or surgery (resection or liver transplantation).
   3. If the physician institutes percutaneous biliary drainage to by-pass obstructed biliary ducts, teach the patient catheter care and signs of infection to watch for and report.
   4. If liver transplantation was performed, provide postoperative care, including:
     a. Administering prescribed immunosuppressive drugs to prevent tissue rejection
     b. Monitoring for and reporting signs of transplant rejection
   5. Arrange for home health care follow-up after discharge.

G. Evaluation
   1. The patient reports minimal discomfort and adequate pain control.
   2. The patient displays minimal respiratory compromise.
   3. The patient maintains adequate nutritional status.
   4. The patient exhibits improved skin and tissue integrity.
   5. The patient remains free of infection.
   6. The patient and family members communicate fears and receive adequate emotional support.

X. Cholelithiasis and cholecystitis
  A. Description
   1. Cholelithiasis refers to calculi formation in the gallbladder.

2. Cholecystitis is acute or chronic inflammation of the gall-bladder.

B. Etiology and incidence
1. Gallstone formation results from changes in bile components or bile stasis, which may be associated with such factors as:
   a. Infection
   b. Cirrhosis
   c. Pancreatitis
   d. Celiac disease
   e. Diabetes mellitus
   f. Pregnancy
   g. Oral contraceptive use
2. Cholelithiasis is extremely common, affecting approximately 20% of the population in the United States. It is the fifth leading cause of hospitalization in adults and is associated with about 90% of all gallbladder disease in the United States.
3. Incidence is greater in women than in men before age 50 and approximately equal in both sexes after age 50.
4. Acute cholecystitis may be calculous (with gallstones) or acalculous (without gallstones) and can result from:
   a. Obstruction of the cystic duct with an impacted gall-stone (90% to 95% of cases)
   b. Tissue damage due to trauma, massive burns, or surgery
   c. Gram-negative septicemia
   d. Multiple blood transfusions
   e. Prolonged fasting
   f. Hypertension
   g. Overuse of narcotic analgesics
5. Although chronic cholecystitis may follow acute cholecystitis, it often occurs independently; it is almost always associated with gallstone formation.
6. Acute cholecystitis is most common in middle-aged persons; the chronic form most often affects the elderly. Incidence of either type is greater in women than in men (ratio of about 3:1).

C. Pathophysiology
1. Calculi usually form from solid constituents of bile; the three major types are:
   a. Cholesterol gallstones, the most common type, thought to form in supersaturated bile
   b. Pigment gallstones, formed mainly of unconjugated pigments in bile precipitate
   c. Mixed types, with characteristics of pigment and cholesterol stones
2. Up to one half of persons with gallstones are asymptomatic and require no intervention.

3. In some cases, however, gallstones can obstruct the cystic duct, causing cholecystitis, or the common bile duct, where they are termed choledocholithiasis.

4. In cholecystitis, inflammation causes the gallbladder wall to become thickened and edematous and the cystic lumen to increase in diameter.

5. Submucosal hemorrhage, mucosal ulceration, and polymorphonuclear infiltration follow.

6. If inflammation spreads to the common bile duct, obstruction of bile drainage can lead to jaundice.

7. Other possible complications include:
   a. Empyema (pus-filled gallbladder)
   b. Perforation
   c. Emphysematous cholecystitis

8. Treatment for cholelithiasis and cholecystitis may involve:
   a. Chenodeoxycholic acid to dissolve gallstones (effective in dissolving about 60% of radiolucent gallstones)
   b. Nonsurgical removal (e.g., lithotripsy or extracorporeal shock wave therapy)
   c. Surgical treatment (e.g., cholecystectomy [gallbladder removed after ligation of cystic duct and artery], choledochostomy [incision into the common bile duct for calculi removal], cholecystomy [gallbladder opened; stones, bile, or pus removed; drainage tube placed])

9. Pigment gallstones cannot be dissolved and must be surgically removed.

D. Assessment findings

1. Many patients with cholelithiasis are asymptomatic.

2. Possible clinical manifestations include:
   a. Episodic (commonly following a high-fat meal), cramping pain in the right upper abdominal quadrant or the epigastrium, possibly radiating to the back near the right scapular tip (biliary colic)
   b. Nausea and vomiting
   c. Fat intolerance
   d. Fever and leukocytosis
   e. Signs and symptoms of jaundice

3. Biliary ultrasonography (cholecystosonography) can detect gallstones in most cases.

4. Acute cholecystitis is commonly marked by:
   a. Biliary colic
   b. Tenderness and rigidity in the right upper quadrant elicited on palpation (Murphy's sign)
   c. Fever
   d. Nausea and vomiting
   e. Fat intolerance

       f.   Signs and symptoms of jaundice

  5. Manifestations of chronic cholecystitis commonly include:

       a.   Pain, less severe than in the acute form

       b.   Fever, also less severe than in the acute form

       c.   Fat intolerance

       d.   Heartburn

       e.   Flatulence

  6. Laboratory and diagnostic study findings in acute or chronic cholecystitis may include:

       a.   Leukocytosis

       b.   Elevated alkaline phosphatase

       c.   Detection of gallstones on ultrasonography

       d.   Inability to visualize the gallbladder on HIDA scanning or oral cholecystography

E. **Nursing diagnoses**

  1. High Risk for Fluid Volume Deficit

  2. High Risk for Infection

  3. Altered Nutrition: Less Than Body Requirements

  4. Pain

  5. High Risk for Impaired Skin Integrity

F. **Planning and implementation**

  1. Intervene as necessary to relieve pain; administer prescribed analgesics.

  2. Promote adequate rest.

  3. Administer antibiotics and antacids as prescribed.

  4. Assess nutritional status, and promote a high-protein, high-carbohydrate, low-fat diet.

  5. Monitor fluid balance, and administer IV fluids as prescribed.

  6. Monitor for signs and symptoms of possible complications.

  7. Teach the patient about planned treatments; prepare him or her for scheduled procedures as appropriate.

G. **Evaluation**

  1. The patient reports only minimal discomfort.

  2. The patient remains free of infection.

  3. The patient maintains adequate fluid volume.

  4. The patient exhibits intact, uncompromised skin integrity with no evidence of jaundice.

  5. The patient maintains adequate nutritional status and verbalizes understanding of dietary recommendations to help control symptoms.

XI. **Acute pancreatitis**

  A. **Description: inflammation of the pancreas ranging from a relatively mild, self-limiting disorder to rapidly fatal acute hemorrhagic pancreatitis**

  B. **Etiology and incidence**

    1. The major causes of acute pancreatitis are:

        a. Alcoholism
        b. Cholecystitis
        c. Surgery involving or near the pancreas

    2. Other possible predisposing factors include:
        a. Viral hepatitis
        b. Mumps
        c. Peptic ulcer disease
        d. Periarteritis
        e. Hyperlipidemia
        f. Hypercalcemia
        g. Anorexia nervosa
        h. Shock with ischemia
        i. Trauma to the pancreas
        j. ERCP
        k. Use of medications such as thiazide diuretics, furosemide, valproic acid, estrogens, tetracycline, azathioprine, mercaptopurine, sulfonamides, and glucocorticoids

    3. Men most commonly develop pancreatitis related to alcoholism, trauma, or peptic ulcer; in women, pancreatitis is most commonly associated with cholecystitis.

C. Pathophysiology

    1. Acute pancreatitis involves various pathologic changes, ranging from edema and inflammation to necrosis and hemorrhage.

    2. Abnormal pancreatic enzyme activation in the pancreas (instead of in the GI tract) causes the pancreas to begin to digest itself.

    3. Kinin activation alters cell membrane permeability, causing a loss of protein-rich fluid into the tissues and peritoneal cavity and producing hypovolemia.

D. Assessment findings

    1. Clinical manifestations of acute pancreatitis include:
        a. Abdominal tenderness with back pain
        b. GI problems: nausea, vomiting, diarrhea, steatorrhea
        c. Fever
        d. Jaundice
        e. Mental confusion
        f. Flank or umbilical bruising
        g. Hypotension
        h. Signs of hypovolemia
        i. Respiratory distress may occur

    2. Laboratory studies may reveal elevated amylase, lipase, and WBC levels.

E. Nursing diagnoses

    1. Ineffective Breathing Patterns
    2. Fluid Volume Deficit

      3. Altered Nutrition: Less Than Body Requirements

      4. Pain

  F. **Planning and implementation**

      1. Administer prescribed pain medications. (Demerol is the drug of choice to prevent spasms at the sphincter of Oddi.)

      2. Perform nasogastric suction as needed.

      3. Assess fluid and electrolyte status, and provide replacement therapy as indicated.

      4. Administer blood transfusions and parenteral nutrition as prescribed.

      5. Maintain optimal respiratory status; place the patient in semi-Fowler's position to decrease pressure on the diaphragm, and teach the patient coughing and deep breathing techniques.

      6. Administer cimetidine as prescribed, to reduce gastric acidity.

  G. **Evaluation**

      1. The patient reports decreased pain.

      2. The patient exhibits improved fluid and nutritional status.

      3. The patient demonstrates adequate respiratory function.

XII. **Chronic pancreatitis**

  A. **Description: progressive pancreatic inflammation resulting in permanent structural damage to pancreatic tissue**

  B. **Etiology**

      1. Chronic pancreatitis typically results from repeated episodes of acute pancreatitis and incidence.

      2. More than half of all cases of chronic pancreatitis are associated with alcoholism.

  C. **Pathophysiology**

      1. With repeated attacks of pancreatitis, pancreatic cells are progressively replaced with fibrous tissue, causing increased pressure within the pancreas.

      2. Eventually, this results in mechanical obstruction of the pancreatic duct, common bile duct, and duodenum.

      3. Other effects include atrophy of the ductal epithelium, inflammation, and destruction of pancreatic cells.

  D. **Assessment findings**

      1. Chronic pancreatitis is commonly marked by:

         a. Pain

         b. Weight loss

         c. Steatorrhea

         d. Anorexia

      2. Laboratory study findings typically reveal:

         a. Pancreatic calcification detected on ERCP

         b. Abnormal glucose tolerance test

  E. **Nursing diagnoses**

      1. Diarrhea

2. Altered Nutrition: Less Than Body Requirements
3. Pain

F. Planning and implementation

1. Provide symptomatic treatment, focusing on relieving pain, promoting comfort, and treating new attacks.
2. Manage any endocrine or exocrine insufficiency as appropriate:
   a. Diabetes mellitus: Initiate dietary and insulin therapy as prescribed.
   b. Fat malabsorption: Administer pancreatic enzymes and fat-soluble vitamins as prescribed.
3. Help the patient reduce pancreatic secretions by:
   a. Promoting a low-fat diet
   b. Encouraging avoidance of caffeine and alcohol
   c. Instructing in the use of antacids or cimetidine as prescribed
4. Prepare the patient for surgery to relieve pain and drain cysts, if indicated.

G. Evaluation

1. The patient reports only minimal discomfort.
2. The patient maintains adequate nutritional status.
3. The patient reports reduced frequency of diarrhea and steatorrhea.

XIII. Pancreatic cancer

A. Description: tumors, most commonly adenocarcinomas, of the pancreas

B. Etiology and incidence

1. Pancreatic cancer is linked to such factors as:
   a. Exposure to chemicals
   b. High-fat diet
   c. Cigarette smoking
   d. Chronic pancreatitis
2. Pancreatic cancer is second only to colon cancer as a cause of GI cancer-related death. Incidence is greater in men than in women; peak incidence occurs between age 55 to 65.

C. Pathophysiology

1. Carcinoma may arise in any portion of the pancreas (head, body, or tail), producing clinical manifestations that vary, depending on the location.
2. The overall 5-year survival rate for all patients with pancreatic cancer is less than 5%.
3. Treatment may involve:
   a. Surgery, aimed at either cure or symptom palliation
   b. Chemotherapy
   c. Radiation therapy for palliation

D. Assessment findings
1. The following may be initial manifestations or may develop only when cancer is in an advanced stage:
    a. Anorexia
    b. Weight loss
    c. Abdominal pain
    d. Jaundice
    e. Diarrhea or steatorrhea
    f. Palpable epigastric mass
2. Laboratory and diagnostic studies may reveal:
    a. Elevated serum alkaline phosphatase level (in 80% of patients)
    b. Elevated carcinoembryonic antigen (CEA), LDH, AST, and serum amylase levels
    c. Hyperglycemia
    d. Pancreatic structural abnormalities demonstrated on upper GI series
    e. Mass demonstrated by ultrasonography or CT scan of the pancreas
    f. Pancreatic duct stricture seen on ERCP
    g. Tissue biopsy positive for malignancy

E. Nursing diagnoses
1. Ineffective Breathing Patterns
2. Altered Nutrition: Less Than Body Requirements
3. Pain
4. Impaired Tissue Integrity

F. Planning and implementation
1. Assess the patient's level of pain frequently. Intervene as necessary to relieve pain: administer pain medication as prescribed, and assist the patient in assuming positions of comfort.
2. Assess for and report any changes affecting nutritional needs. Administer parenteral nutrition as prescribed.
3. Monitor serum glucose level, and observe for signs of hyperglycemia.
4. Administer pancreatic enzymes, if ordered, when enteral diet is resumed.
5. Prepare the patient for pancreatoduodenectomy (removal of most of the pancreas to excise a resectable tumor), if indicated.
6. After surgery, provide postoperative care:
    a. Assess respiratory status: Encourage and assist the patient to cough and deep-breathe every hour, and help him or her change position often.
    b. Avoid placing pressure on anastomoses and sutures.
    c. Irrigate the nasogastric tube and other tubes gently and only if prescribed: Withhold oral intake until GI function returns.

         d.   Inspect surgical incisions for inflammation, infection, and abscess formation.

         e.   Maintain aseptic technique when handling wound dressings.

G.   **Evaluation**

    1.   The patient reports only minimal discomfort.

    2.   The patient exhibits minimal or no respiratory compromise.

    3.   The patient maintains adequate nutritional status.

    4.   The patient exhibits improved skin and tissue integrity.

Bibliography

Berk, J. E. (ed.) (1985). *Gastroenterology* (Vol. 7). Philadelphia: W. B. Saunders.

Brunner, L. S., & Suddarth, K. S. (1988). *Textbook of medical-surgical nursing* (6th ed.). Philadelphia: J. B. Lippincott.

Brunner, L. S., & Suddarth, K. S. (1986). *The Lippincott manual of nursing practice* (4th ed.). Philadelphia: J. B. Lippincott.

Given, B. A., & Simmons, S. J. (1984). *Gastroenterology in clinical nursing*. St. Louis: C. V. Mosby.

Luckmann, J., & Sorenson, K. C. (1987). *Medical-surgical nursing: A psychophysiologic approach* (3rd ed.). Philadelphia: W. B. Saunders.

Moody, F. G. (1986). *Surgical treatment of digestive disease*. Chicago: Year Book Medical Publishers.

Ravenscroft, M. M., & Swan, D. H. J. (1984). *Gastrointestinal endoscopy and related procedures: A handbook for nurses and assistants*. Baltimore: Williams & Wilkins.

Schiff, L., & Schiff, E. R. (1987). *Diseases of the liver* (6th ed.). Philadelphia: J. B. Lippincott.

STUDY QUESTIONS

1. Bile is synthesized by which type of cell?
   a. enterocyte
   b. hepatocyte
   c. Kupffer cell
   d. Acinar cell

2. For which of the following reasons would a patient with jaundice develop the nursing diagnosis of High Risk for Impaired Skin Integrity?
   a. Jaundice is associated with decubitus formation.
   b. Jaundice impairs urea production, which produces pruritus.
   c. Jaundice produces pruritus due to impaired bile acid excretion.
   d. Jaundice leads to decreased tissue perfusion.

3. For which of the following reasons would the nurse explain placement of an esophageal-tamponade tube to a bleeding patient?
   a. to obtain cooperation and reduce fear
   b. to begin teaching for home care
   c. to have patient assist with tube insertion
   d. to maintain patient's level of anxiety

4. Which of the following nursing plans would be *most* helpful with a patient with chronic pancreatitis?
   a. Teach patient to modify protein in diet.
   b. Encourage patient to exercise daily.
   c. Allow patient to liberalize fluid intake.
   d. Counsel patient to stop alcohol consumption.

5. Which of these pancreatic fluids are secreted from the acinar exocrine cell?
   a. insulin
   b. glucagon
   c. trypsin
   d. pancreozymin

6. A patient with acute cholecystitis will usually demonstrate which of the following nutritional alterations?
   a. Nutrition Altered: Less Than Body Requirements related to poor oral intake due to anorexia
   b. Nutrition Altered: More Than Body Requirements related to decreased gastrointestinal losses
   c. Nutrition Altered: More Than Body Requirements related to decreased nutrient requirements
   d. Nutrition Altered: Less Than Body Requirements related to long-term malnutrition

7. Evaluation of the resolution of elevated direct or conjugated serum bilirubin generally indicates correction of which of the following?
   a. hepatocellular damage
   b. impaired bile excretion
   c. Kupffer cell damage
   d. hemolysis

8. Pancreatic lipase performs which of the following functions?
   a. breaks down fat into fatty acids and glycerol
   b. transports fatty acids into the brush border
   c. triggers cholecystokinin to contract the gallbladder
   d. breaks down protein into dipeptides and amino acids

9. After administering diuretic therapy to a patient with ascites, which of the following nursing actions most helps ensure safe care?
   a. Measure serum potassium for hyperkalemia.
   b. Assess the patient for hypervolemia.
   c. Measure body weight weekly.
   d. Document precise intake and output.

10. Which evaluation criteria would the nurse establish for a patient in hepatic coma?
    a. Patient is oriented to time, place, and person.
    b. Patient exhibits no ecchymotic areas.
    c. Patient increases oral intake to 2000 calories/day.

d. Patient exhibits increased serum albumin.

11. For a patient with a LeVeen or peritoneojugular shunt, the nurse should note presence of ascites because the shunt:

a. was placed to reduce portal hypertension

b. was placed to reduce ascites

c. diverts blood to the inferior vena cava

d. reduces bacterial ammonia production in the GI tract

12. When planning pain management for a patient following a pancreatoduodenectomy, the *best* plan for nursing care would be to

a. Hold pain medication because this operative procedure is minor.

b. Give pain medication regularly regardless of respiratory status.

c. Bypass assessment since the patient is unable to express pain with this procedure.

d. Administer pain medication frequently as prescribed.

13. Using the nursing diagnosis Knowledge Deficit about self-care activities at home following cholecystitis, the nurse would use the following criteria to evaluate the patient's understanding of an appropriate diet. The patient selects

a. low-carbohydrate food divided into six small meals

b. high-fat, high-carbohydrate meals

c. low-fat, high-carbohydrate meals

d. high-fat, low-protein meals

14. When caring for a patient following percutaneous transhepatic cholangiography, the nurse's evaluation of the patient would be that the patient demonstrates absence of

a. fever and chills

b. hypertension

c. bradycardia

d. nausea and diarrhea

15. In planning for home care of a patient with hepatitis A, which of the following preventive measures should the nurse emphasize to protect the patient's family?

a. Keep the patient in complete isolation.

b. Use good sanitation with dishes and shared bathroom.

c. Avoid contact with blood-soiled clothing or dressings.

d. Forbid sharing of needles or syringes.

16. Which of the following is the *most* important intervention for High Risk for Injury secondary to altered clotting mechanisms in a patient with hepatic cirrhosis?

a. Allow the patient complete independence of mobility.

b. Apply pressure to injection sites.

c. Administer antibiotics as prescribed.

d. Increase nutritional intake.

ANSWER KEY

1. **Correct response:b**
Hepatocytes (liver cells) synthesize and secrete bile into the canaliculi.
   a. Enterocytes are cells within the small intestine.
   c. Kupffer cells are the phagocytic cells of the liver.
   d. Acinar cells are the exocrine cells of the pancreas.
Knowledge/Physiologic/Assessment

2. **Correct response:c**
Pruritus occurs secondary to decreased bile acid excretion.
   a. Jaundice is not associated with decubitus formation; edema and hypoalbuminemia are.
   b and d. Jaundice itself does not impair urea production or lead to decreased tissue perfusion.
Comprehension/Safe care/Analysis (Dx)

3. **Correct response: a**
This tube is placed in critical situations; thus, the patient will be fearful.
   b. This tube is used only short term and is not indicated for home use.
   c. The tube is large and uncomfortable and would not be inserted by the patient.
   d. A patient's anxiety should be decreased, not maintained.
Application/Psychosocial/Implementation

4. **Correct response: d**
Continued alcohol consumption may cause recurrent attacks.
   a. Protein modification in the diet is not necessary for this patient.
   b. Exercise is helpful for health promotion but not most helpful for this patient.
   c. Liberalizing fluid intake may be helpful but not most helpful in this patient.
Analysis/Health promotion/Planning

5. **Correct response: c**
Trypsin is the proteolytic enzyme in pancreatic fluid.
   a and b. Insulin and glucagon are

pancreatic hormones secreted by the beta and alpha endocrine cells.
   d. Pancreozymin is released from the intestine and acts on the pancreas.
Knowledge/Physiologic/Assessment

6. **Correct response: a**
Anorexia, nausea, vomiting, or pain will lead to decreased oral intake.
   b. The patient may have increased GI losses with vomiting.
   c. As with an acute inflammatory process, nutrient requirements may increase.
   d. Cholecystitis generally is not associated with long-term malnutrition.
Comprehension/Physiologic/Analysis (Dx)

7. **Correct response: b**
Elevated direct bilirubin level indicates impaired bile excretion.
   a and c. Hepatocyte or Kupffer cell damage generally does not cause elevated bilirubin.
   d. Hemolysis leads to elevated indirect or unconjugated bilirubin levels.
Application/Physiologic/Evaluation

8. **Correct response: a**
Lipase hydrolyzes fat into fatty acids and glycerol.
   b. Lipase does not perform this transport function.
   c. Fat itself triggers cholecystokinin release.
   d. This is the function of trypsin, not lipase.
Comprehension/Physiologic/Assessment

9. **Correct response: d**
Careful intake and output measurement is essential for safe diuretic therapy.
   a. Hypokalemia, not hyperkalemia, commonly occurs with diuretic therapy.
   b. A patient should be assessed for hypovolemia after increased urine output.
   c. This patient should be weighed daily.
Analysis/Self care/Implementation

10. *Correct response: a*

With resolving hepatic coma, the patient should be able to express orientation to time, place, and person.

  b. Ecchymotic areas are related not to hepatic coma but to decreased synthesis of clotting factors.

  c. Although oral intake may be related to level of consciousness, oral intake or lack of it is more closely related to anorexia.

  d. Serum albumin does not indicate level of consciousness, but rather reflects hepatic synthetic ability.

Application/Self care/Evaluation

11. *Correct response: b*

This shunt diverts peritoneal ascites back into the venous system.

  a and c. The shunt does not reduce portal hypertension or divert blood.

  d. This shunt has no effect on bacterial growth or ammonia production.

Application/Self care/Implementation

12. *Correct response: d*

This is a major operative procedure generally done for a painful disorder; therefore, pain medication should be administered frequently.

  a. This is a long, major, extensive procedure.

  b. With analgesia administration, respiratory status should always be assessed.

  c. Because this procedure should not impair a patient's ability to express pain, pain should be assessed.

Application/Health promotion/Planning

13. *Correct response: c*

The patient should reduce fat intake and substitute fat calories with carbohydrates.

  a. Reducing carbohydrate intake would be contraindicated.

  b and d. A high-fat diet may lead to another attack of cholecystitis.

Application/Health promotion/Analysis (Dx)

14. *Correct response: a*

Fever and chills may indicate septicemia, a common postprocedure complication.

  b. Hypotension, not hypertension, is associated with septicemia.

  c. Tachycardia, not bradycardia, is most likely to occur.

  d. Nausea and diarrhea may occur but are not classic signs of sepsis.

Analysis/Physiologic/Evaluation

15. *Correct response: b*

Hepatitis A is transmitted through the fecal–oral route.

  a. Complete isolation is not required.

  c and d. These precautions are for hepatitis B, not hepatitis A.

Analysis/Health promotion/Planning

16. *Correct response: b*

With altered clotting mechanisms, prolonged application of pressure to injection or bleeding sites is important.

  a. Complete independence may increase potential for injury, because an unsupervised patient may injure himself or herself and bleed excessively.

  c and d. Antibiotics and good nutrition are important to promote liver regeneration; however, they are not most important for a patient with increased bleeding potential.

Analysis/Health promotion/Implementation

Renal and Urinary Disorders

18

I. **Anatomy and physiology**
   A. Structure
   B. Function

II. **Renal and urinary system overview**
   A. Assessment
   B. Laboratory studies and diagnostic tests
   C. Psychosocial implications
   D. Medications used to treat renal and urinary problems

III. **Urinary reflux**
   A. Description
   B. Etiology and incidence
   C. Pathophysiology
   D. Assessment findings
   E. Nursing diagnoses
   F. Planning and implementation
   G. Evaluation

IV. **Urinary retention**
   A. Description
   B. Etiology and incidence
   C. Pathophysiology
   D. Assessment findings
   E. Nursing diagnoses
   F. Planning and implementation
   G. Evaluation

V. **Urinary incontinence**
   A. Description
   B. Etiology
   C. Pathophysiology
   D. Assessment findings
   E. Nursing diagnoses
   F. Planning and implementation

   G. Evaluation

VI. **Neurogenic bladder dysfunction**
   A. Description
   B. Etiology
   C. Pathophysiology
   D. Assessment findings
   E. Nursing diagnoses
   F. Planning and implementation
   G. Evaluation

VII. **Urinary tract infection**
   A. Description
   B. Etiology and incidence
   C. Pathophysiology
   D. Assessment findings
   E. Nursing diagnoses
   F. Planning and implementation
   G. Evaluation

VIII. **Urolithiasis (renal calculi)**
   A. Description
   B. Etiology and incidence
   C. Pathophysiology
   D. Assessment findings
   E. Nursing diagnoses
   F. Planning and implementation
   G. Evaluation

IX. **Urinary tract cancer**
   A. Description
   B. Etiology and incidence
   C. Pathophysiology
   D. Assessment findings
   E. Nursing diagnoses
   F. Planning and implementation
   G. Evaluation

I.   Anatomy and physiology

    A. Structure

        1. The kidneys are paired organs located on either side of the ver-
            tebral column between the 12th thoracic and 3rd lumbar ver-
            tebrae in the posterior abdomen behind the peritoneum.

        2. Kidney components include (Fig. 18–1):

            a. Cortex: outer portion containing the glomerules, tu-
               bules, and part of the loop of Henle

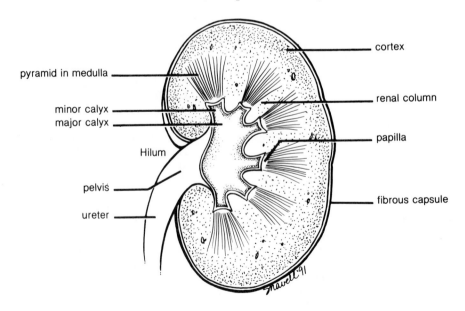

FIGURE 18–1.
Gross structure of a bisected kidney.

    b.   Medulla: middle portion containing part of the loop of Henle and the collecting ducts

    c.   Pelvis: inner portion where urine is collected; the narrowed portion becomes the proximal aspect of the ureter as it approaches the hilum

    d.   Hilum: area where nerves, blood vessels, and the ureter enter the kidney

    e.   Minor and major calyces: recesses of the pelvis that receive urine from papillae of collecting ducts

    f.   Renal column: cortical tissue between pyramids in the cortex

    g.   Pyramids: collecting ducts with bases on the border between the cortex and medulla; apices form papillae as they extend toward the pelvis

    h.   Papillae: apices of pyramids through which urine travels to the renal pelvis

    i.   Fibrous capsule: outer covering that adheres to the renal parenchyma

3.   The functional unit of the kidney, the nephron contains glomerulus and tubules; specific components include:

    a.   Glomerulus: beginning of the nephron; a tuft of capillaries supplied by afferent arterioles and drained by efferent arterioles within Bowman's capsule

    b.   Proximal tubule: convoluted portion with border of microvilli lining the lumen

    c.   Loop of Henle: narrows as it moves from the cortex to the medulla

    d.   Distal tubule: passes between afferent and efferent arterioles of glomerulus as it moves back into the cortex

    e.   Collecting duct: passes through the cortex and medulla receiving the terminal end of several nephrons

4.   Renal circulation involves (Fig. 18–2):

    a.   Renal artery, branching from the abdominal aorta

    b.   Interlobar arteries, whose subdivisions carry blood into the corticomedullary zone

    c.   Arcuate arteries, forming arches around bases of pyramids

    d.   Interlobular arteries, subdivisions of the arcuate arteries supplying the renal capsule

5.   Renal innervation is supplied through both sympathetic and parasympathetic nerves. Adrenergic fibers also are in proximity to juxtaglomerular apparatus.

6.   Urinary system components include:

    a.   Ureters, extending from the renal pelvis to the urinary bladder

    b.   Bladder, which serves as a reservoir for urine until it is excreted from the body

FIGURE 18–2.
Blood supply to the kidney. Renal artery branches from the abdominal aorta.

       c.   Urethras, extending from the base of the bladder to the urinary meatus; approximately 4 cm long in men, 20 cm long in women

   B.   **Function**

      1.   Table 18–1 gives a summary of major nephron component functions. Additional functions include:

         a.   Blood pressure regulation by renin secretion

         b.   Red blood cell production regulation by erythropoietin secretion

         c.   Metabolism of vitamin D

      2.   Ureters transport urine to the bladder via peristaltic waves of smooth muscle; the ureterovesical junction prevents back flow of urine (reflux).

      3.   Micturition (voiding) is under voluntary and involuntary control. The urge to void normally occurs when 150 to 300 cc urine has accumulated; the bladder normally contains no urine after voiding (residual urine).

II.   **Overview of renal and urinary function**

   A.   **Assessment**

      1.   The health history should focus on obtaining information about:

         a.   Usual voiding pattern

         b.   Changes in this pattern

         c.   Artificial orifice

         d.   Difficulty in starting or maintaining a urine stream

         e.   Feeling of urgency

TABLE 18-1.
Major Functions of Nephron Components

NEPHRON COMPONENT	MAJOR FUNCTIONS
Glomerulus	Filtration
Proximal tubule	65% Na^+ and H_2O reabsorbed (ADH not required) Glucose, K^+, amino acids reabsorbed HCO_3^- reabsorbed H^+ secreted Urea reabsorbed Filtrate leaves isotonic
Loop of Henle	Countercurrent multiplying and exchange mechanisms established between long, thin loops of Henle of juxtamedullary nephrons and adjacent vasa recta Filtrate leaves hypotonic
Distal tubule	Na^+ reabsorbed and K^+ secreted in presence of aldosterone; opposite occurs in absence of aldosterone Water reabsorbed with Na^+; ADH also influences water reabsorption Filtrate leaves hypotonic or isotonic
Collecting duct	Na^+ and K^+ regulated by aldosterone Acid–base regulation; H^+ secretion, HCO_3 reabsorption, NH_3 secretion, NH_4 excretion ADH determines final urine volume

    f.   Urine characteristics: odor, color, cloudy, or clear
    g.   Incontinence
    h.   Pain
    i.   History of disease process, surgical procedures, or trauma affecting the urinary system
    j.   Pertinent medication use (e.g., diuretics, antibiotics, narcotics, nephrotoxins, cholinergics, phenacetin)
    k.   Allergies

  2. Important physical examination steps include:
    a.   Inspecting for masses in the upper abdomen and flank area
    b.   Inspecting the external meatus for signs of discharge, cleanliness, location, and size
    c.   Palpating for the lower poles of the right and left kidney; note enlargement
    d.   Percussing above the symphysis pubis for a distended bladder
    e.   Auscultating for bruits over the renal arteries

B. **Laboratory studies and diagnostic tests**
  1. Urinalysis involves assessment of:
    a.   Color: normally yellow to amber
    b.   Opacity: normally clear

    c.   Odor: normally faintly aromatic

    d.   Specific gravity: normally 1.005 to 1.025

    e.   Osmolality: normally 300 to 900 mOsm/kg

    f.   pH: normally 4 to 8

    g.   Glucose, ketones, protein: normally negative

    h.   Red blood cells and white blood cells: normally none to trace amounts

    i.   Sediment (crystals or casts): normally none

    j.   Bacteria: normally none

    k.   Amount: normally 1500 to 2000 mL/24 hours

2.   Blood analysis includes:

    a.   Plasma creatinine: excellent indicator of renal function; normally 1 to 0.3 mg/dL, rises with renal failure

    b.   Blood urea nitrogen (BUN): normally 10 to 20 mg/dL; rises with renal failure and influenced by protein intake, catabolism, and bleeding

3.   Culture and sensitivity testing detects infective microorganisms; requires a midstream clean-catch urine specimen.

4.   Creatinine clearance evaluates glomerular filtration rate (GFR); increases as renal function diminishes.

5.   Vascular studies include:

    a.   Radionuclide tests: renal scan (provides anatomic information); renogram (provides information about renal blood flow, GFR, and tubular secretion)

    b.   Renal arteriography: outlines renal vasculature

    c.   Renal venography: outlines renal veins

6.   Plain roentgenogram of kidneys, ureters, and bladder (KUB) visualizes size, shape, and position of urinary structures.

7.   Ultrasound studies identify gross renal anatomy.

8.   Computed tomography scan detects renal masses, vascular disorders, and filling defects of the collecting system.

9.   Intravenous and retrograde pyelography (IVP) and cystourethrography provides information about the size, shape, and position of urinary tract structures and evaluates renal excretory function.

10.   Hemodynamic studies evaluate motor and sensory function of the bladder and micturition process.

11.   Cystoscopic examination allows direct endoscopic visualization of the entire urinary tract.

12.   Bladder and kidney biopsy determines the nature and extent of disease.

C.   Psychosocial implications

1.   A patient with a renal or urinary disorder may experience coping difficulty related to:

    a.   Chronic nature of the disorder

    b.   Progressive nature of symptoms

    c.   Fatigue
    d.   Fear of dying
    e.   Embarrassment (at incontinence)

2. The patient also may have self-concept concerns related to fear of:
    a.   Body image changes (with urinary diversion)
    b.   Altered sexual function
    c.   Role changes toward increased dependence

3. Lifestyle concerns may be related to potential changes in:
    a.   Physical activity
    b.   Work performance, with the possibility of job loss
    c.   Self-care ability

4. Disease-related changes in social interaction patterns may lead to:
    a.   Isolation
    b.   Hopelessness
    c.   Depression

D. **Medications used to treat renal and urinary problems**

1. *Adrenergic alpha receptor blocking agents*, such as phenoxybenzamine hydrochloride (Dibenzyline), are used to treat urinary reflux by decreasing the urinary sphincter's resistance to outflow.

2. Used to treat urinary tract infection, *antispasmodics* such as phenazopyridine hydrochloride (e.g., Pyridium) prevent spasms of the detrusor muscle and relieve pain.

3. *Broad-spectrum antibiotics* used to treat urinary tract infection include:
    a.   Trimethoprim-sulfamethoxazole (e.g., Bactrim, Septra)
    b.   Nitrofurantoin (e.g., Furadantin)
    c.   Sulfisoxazole (e.g., Gantrisin)
    d.   Ampicillin (e.g., Amcill)
    e.   Methenamine mandelate (e.g., Mandelamine)
    f.   Cephalexin monohydrate (e.g., Keflex)
    g.   Cephradine (e.g., Velosef)
    h.   Cefaclor (Ceclor)

4. *Drugs used to control calculi formation* include:
    a.   Aluminum hydroxide (e.g., Amphojel)
    b.   Allopurinol (e.g., Zyloprim)
    c.   Sodium cellulose phosphate (Calcibind)
    d.   Cholestyramine (Questran)

5. *Antineoplastic agents* used to treat renal and bladder cancer include:
    a.   Vinblastine sulfate (e.g., Velban)
    b.   MVC: methotrexate, vinblastine, cisplatin
    c.   CISCA: cisplatin, cyclophosphamide, doxorubicin

6. H_2 *receptor antagonists*, such as cimetidine (Tagamet), are used in the treatment of acute renal failure to prevent GI bleeding.

7. Immunosuppressive agents, administered after kidney transplantation to block the body's normal immune response to the graft, include:
   a. Azathioprine sodium
   b. Cyclosporine (Sandimmune)
   c. Prednisone (e.g., Panasol)
   d. ALG (antilymphocytic globulin)

III. Urinary reflux

A. Description: backward flow of urine from the bladder into the ureter and renal pelvis

B. Etiology and incidence
1. Reflux usually results from incompetency at the vesicoureteral junction but also can occur at the urethrovesical junction.
2. Factors commonly contributing to reflux include:
   a. Congenital malformations
   b. Urinary tract infection
   c. Neuromuscular dysfunction
   d. Bladder neck obstruction
3. Incidence is highest in boys during infancy and in girls between ages 3 and 7 years.

C. Pathophysiology
1. Reflux results in persistent residual urine, which commonly leads to urinary tract infection.
2. Chronic residual urine can alter detrusor muscle tone, increasing bladder capacity and raising the threshold for triggering the micturition reflex.
3. Prolonged reflux can lead to renal damage and infection, which may progress to renal failure.

D. Assessment findings
1. Common clinical manifestations include:
   a. Signs and symptoms of urinary tract infection (see Section VII.D)
   b. Residual urine detected on catheterization
   c. In later stages, signs of renal impairment (e.g., hypertension, anemia, lethargy)
2. Laboratory and diagnostic studies may reveal:
   a. Increased bacterial count, WBCs, RBCs, and pH detected on urinalysis
   b. Abnormal ureter structure or renal calyceals seen on IVP
   c. Elevated serum creatinine level in severe renal impairment
3. Voiding cystourethrography determines the degree of reflux.

E. Nursing diagnoses
1. High Risk for Infection
2. Knowledge Deficit

  3. Pain
  4. Urinary Retention

F. Planning and implementation

  1. Prepare the patient for surgical reimplantation of the ureter, if indicated.
  2. After surgery, provide routine postoperative care (see Chapter 24, Perioperative Nursing), and monitor ureteral catheter patency.
  3. Provide patient and family teaching, covering:
      a. Prescribed medication regimen and the importance of compliance
      b. The need for increased fluid intake, to 3 to 4 L/day
      c. The importance of frequent and complete bladder emptying
      d. Hygienic measures (e.g., wearing cotton panties, wiping from front to back, avoiding baths)
      e. The need to acidify urine with an acid–ash diet (i.e., increased intake of meats, cranberry juice)
      f. The importance of follow-up care

G. Evaluation

  1. The patient or a family member verbalizes understanding of the prescribed medication regimen.
  2. The patient or a family member verbalizes understanding of the need to drink 3 to 4 L of fluid daily.
  3. The patient demonstrates normal voiding pattern without residual urine.
  4. The patient or a family member states proper hygiene measures to adopt.
  5. The patient or a family member states foods that can help acidify urine.
  6. The patient or a family member schedules a follow-up appointment.

IV. Urinary retention

A. Description: retention of urine in the bladder in the presence of normal urine production, with the inability to release it even when the micturition reflex is activated

B. Etiology and incidence

  1. Common causes of retention in males include:
      a. Benign prostatic hypertrophy
      b. Urethral stricture
      c. Calculi or foreign body in the urethra
      d. Urethritis
      e. Tumor
      f. Phimosis

2. In females, possible causes include:
    a. Urethral obstruction secondary to stricture, calculi, vaginal cysts, tumor, edema
    b. Retroverted gravid uterus
3. Causes in both sexes include:
    a. Reflex spasm of sphincters following surgery of invasive procedures
    b. Trauma
    c. Neurogenic bladder dysfunction
    d. Medications (e.g., anticholinergics, antihistamines)
    e. Fecal impaction
    f. Psychogenic retention

C. Pathophysiology
1. Retention may be acute or chronic.
2. Chronic retention can lead to overflow incontinence or residual urine.
3. Other possible complications include urinary tract infection, bladder distention and damage, and hydronephrosis.
1. Common clinical manifestations include:
    a. Reports of inability to void, urgency, hesitancy, dribbling
    b. Lower abdominal pain or discomfort
    c. Restlessness, diaphoresis
    d. Visible or palpable bladder distention
    e. Dullness on bladder percussion
    f. Possibly signs and symptoms of lower urinary tract infection
2. Bladder catheterization commonly reveals residual urine.

E. Nursing diagnoses
1. High Risk for Infection
2. Pain
3. Urinary Retention

F. Planning and implementation
1. Facilitate bladder emptying through such actions as providing privacy, running water, having the patient assume a normal voiding position, and providing pain relief.
2. If the patient cannot void, perform intermittent catheterization to prevent overdistention of the bladder.
3. Administer prescribed medications to decrease sphincteric resistance to outflow (e.g., phenoxybenzamine) and reduce pain.
4. If indicated, prepare the patient for surgical intervention (e.g., dilation of urethra, cystoplasty).

G. Evaluation
1. The patient demonstrates a normal voiding pattern.

2. The patient displays no evidence of urinary tract infection.
3. The patient reports relief of pain related to urinary retention.

V. Urinary incontinence

A. Description

1. Incontinence refers to the inability of the urinary sphincters to control release of urine.
2. Types include:
   a. Enuresis (bedwetting): usually a childhood problem
   b. Stress incontinence: dribbling resulting from any kind of physical stress (e.g., coughing, sneezing, laughing; most commonly affects women)
   c. Urgency incontinence: inability to hold back urine flow when feeling the urge to void
   d. Paradoxical incontinence: urine retention with overflow, marked by involuntary voiding of small amounts
   e. Continuous incontinence: completely uninhibited micturition reflex, with an unpredictable voiding pattern

B. Etiology

1. Temporary episodes of incontinence can result from:
   a. Inflammation
   b. Stress
   c. Certain medications (e.g., narcotics, tranquilizers, sedatives, diuretics, antihistamines, antihypertensive drugs, atropinelike drugs)
2. Persistent or permanent incontinence may result from neuromuscular dysfunction due to such disorders as:
   a. Bladder lesions
   b. Spinal cord injury
   c. Multiple sclerosis
   d. Spinal cord tumor
   e. Complications of pelvic surgery
   f. Cerebrovascular accident
   g. Large bowel disease (e.g., spastic colon, diverticular disease)
3. Anatomic causes of incontinence include:
   a. Weak abdominal and perineal muscle tone due to obesity, sedentary lifestyle
   b. Sphincter weakness or damage from obstetric trauma, surgery, or congenital conditions
   c. Urethral deformity due to recurrent urinary tract infections, trauma, surgery, or estrogen-deficiency vulvitis
   d. Altered urethrovesical angle in women linked to previous pregnancies and perineal muscle weakness
4. In some persons, incontinence stems from psychosocial factors (e.g., rebellion, dependence, regression, anxiety, attention-getting behavior).

C. Pathophysiology

1. The embarrassment associated with incontinence often damages a person's self-esteem and can become an overwhelming negative factor in the person's life.
2. Incontinence is commonly viewed as an infantile behavior and may provoke feelings of helplessness, hopelessness, and frustration.

D. Assessment findings

1. Clinical manifestations of incontinence may include:
   a. Clothing or bedding wet with urine
   b. Reports of dribbling, urgency, hesitancy, or inability to get to the bathroom before voiding starts
2. The patient may exhibit or express anxiety, frustration, depression, poor self-esteem, or other psychologic effects of incontinence.

E. Nursing diagnoses

1. Anxiety
2. Body Image Disturbance
3. Knowledge Deficit
4. Powerlessness
5. Self-Concept Disturbance
6. Impaired Skin Integrity
7. Urinary Incontinence: Functional, Reflex, Stress, Total, Urge

F. Planning and implementation

1. Protect the patient's skin by keeping him or her dry; change clothing and bed linens as necessary.
2. Provide bladder training if indicated.
3. Encourage fluid intake of 2 to 2.5 L/day, if not contraindicated
4. If indicated, instruct the patient in perineal and Kegel exercises to help improve muscular control.
5. Check the patient's medication regimen for any drugs that could cause or contribute to incontinence.
6. Refer the patient for psychologic evaluation as appropriate.

G. Evaluation

1. The patient reports fewer episodes of incontinence.
2. The patient demonstrates skill at Kegel exercises by an ability to stop voiding in midstream.
3. The patient demonstrates application of bladder control training by a normal voiding pattern.
4. The patient verbalizes the need to drink at least 2 L of fluid daily.

VI. Neurogenic bladder dysfunction

A. Description: dysfunction of the bladder due to impaired neurologic control secondary to central or peripheral nervous system lesions

B. Etiology

    1. Major causes of neurogenic bladder include:

        a. Spinal cord injury

        b. Spinal cord tumor

        c. Herniated intervertebral disk

        d. Cerebrovascular accident and other cerebral disorders

        e. Neurologic disorders such as multiple sclerosis, diabetes mellitus, syphilis

        f. Congenital anomalies (e.g., spina bifida, myelomeningocele)

        g. Infection

    2. An upper motor neuron lesion causes spastic neurogenic bladder; a lower motor neuron lesion, flaccid neurogenic bladder.

C. Pathophysiology

    1. Spastic (reflex or autonomic) neurogenic bladder, the most common type, involves:

        a. Loss of conscious sensations and cerebral motor control

        b. Reduced bladder capacity and marked bladder wall hypertrophy

        c. A pattern of spontaneous, uncontrolled voidings

    2. In flaccid (atonic, nonreflex, areflexic, or autonomous) neurogenic bladder, the following sequence occurs:

        a. Inability of bladder musculature to contract allows the bladder to fill until it becomes grossly distended.

        b. When intrabladder pressure reaches a certain point, small amounts of urine dribble from the urethra.

        c. Sensory loss may make the patient unaware of incontinence.

        d. Extreme, prolonged bladder distension can result in damage to bladder musculature, urine stasis and infection, and renal infection.

    3. Mixed neurogenic bladder—usually associated with lesions at the conus–cauda equina junctions—involves a combination of spastic and flaccid dysfunction.

    4. Possible long-term complications of neurogenic bladder include:

        a. Urinary tract infection

        b. Hydronephrosis

        c. Urolithiasis

        d. Renal failure

D. Assessment findings

1. Clinical manifestations of neurogenic bladder vary widely depending on type and degree of neurologic damage; common signs and symptoms include:
   a. Residual urine detected on bladder catheterization
   b. Some degree of incontinence
   c. Bladder distension
   d. Restlessness

2. Pertinent laboratory and diagnostic studies include:
   a. BUN, creatinine clearance, and serum creatinine to evaluate renal function
   b. Cystography to detect vesicoureteral reflux
   c. Urethrography to detect urethral complications
   d. Urine pressure and flow studies
   e. Cystoscopy to assess muscle fiber status and perform tissue biopsy

E. Nursing diagnoses

1. Anxiety
2. Body Image Disturbance
3. Knowledge Deficit
4. Powerlessness
5. Self-Concept Disturbance
6. Impaired Skin Integrity
7. Altered Patterns of Urinary Elimination

F. Planning and implementation

1. Intervene as appropriate depending on the type and underlying cause of neurogenic bladder.
2. Provide bladder retraining, if indicated.
3. Perform bladder catheterization (continuous or intermittent) as appropriate.
4. If indicated, teach the patient self-catheterization techniques.
5. Encourage adequate fluid intake (2 to 2.5 L/day).

G. Evaluation

1. The patient demonstrates proper application of the bladder retraining program.
2. The patient demonstrates proper self-catheterization technique, if appropriate.
3. The patient verbalizes the need to drink at least 2 L of fluid daily.

VII. Urinary tract infection (UTI)

A. Description

1. Inflammation and infection of urinary tract structures is classified as upper UTI or lower UTI.
2. Upper UTIs include pyelonephritis (inflammation of the kidney).

3. Lower UTIs include:
   a. Ureteritis (inflammation of the ureter)
   b. Cystitis (inflammation of the bladder wall), the most common type
   c. Urethritis (inflammation of the urethra)

B. Etiology and incidence

1. UTIs result from pathogenic microorganisms in the urinary tract (e.g., *Escherichia coli*, *Proteus*, *Klebsiella*, *Enterobacter*).
2. Predisposing factors include:
   a. Loss of resistance to invading microorganisms
   b. Sexual intercourse
   c. Indwelling catheterization
   d. Urine stasis
   e. Urinary tract instrumentation
   f. Residual urine
   g. Urinary reflux
   h. Bladder overdistention
   i. Loss of intact mucosal lining
   j. Metabolic disorders
3. Women develop UTI more frequently than men because of their shorter urethras; approximately 25% of all women experience UTI at some time. Incidence in women increases with aging; incidence in men peaks after age 50.

C. Pathophysiology

1. Pyelonephritis commonly occurs secondary to urine reflux into the kidney.
2. In lower UTI, infection typically ascends from the urethra to the bladder and, possibly, to the ureter.
3. Other pathways of infection include blood and lymph.

D. Assessment findings

1. Common manifestations of acute pyelonephritis include:
   a. Flank pain
   b. Costovertebral angle tenderness
   c. Fever, chills
   d. Dysuria
   e. Frequency and urgency
   f. Malaise
   g. Possibly bloody or cloudy urine
   h. Urinalysis findings: elevated WBC count, white cell casts, bacteria
2. Lower UTI may be marked by:
   a. Frequency and urgency
   b. Burning on urination
   c. Nocturia
   d. Inflamed, swollen meatus in urethritis

            e.   Bacteriuria and RBCs in urine

            f.   Urine culture identifying the causative microorganism

E. Nursing diagnoses

1. High Risk for Fluid Volume Deficit
2. Knowledge Deficit
3. Pain
4. Altered Patterns of Urinary Elimination

F. Planning and implementation

1. Administer antispasmodic medication or antibiotics as prescribed.
2. Apply heat to the perineum to decrease discomfort.
3. Provide patient teaching, covering:
   a. Prescribed medication regimen and the importance of compliance
   b. The need to increase fluid intake to 3 to 4 L/day
   c. The importance of frequent and complete bladder emptying
   d. Hygienic measures (e.g., wearing cotton panties, wiping from front to back, avoiding tub baths)
   e. The importance of acidifying urine through an acid–ash diet (high in meats, cranberry juice)
   f. The need for follow-up care

G. Evaluation

1. The patient verbalizes understanding of the prescribed medication regimen.
2. The patient verbalizes understanding of the need to drink 3 to 4 L of fluid daily.
3. The patient demonstrates normal voiding pattern without residual urine.
4. The patient reports decreased pain and discomfort.
5. The patient states proper hygiene measures to adopt.
6. The patient states foods that can help acidify urine.
7. The patient schedules a follow-up appointment.

VIII. Urolithiasis (renal calculi)

A. Description: calculi in the urinary tract—bladder, ureters, and most commonly, kidneys

B. Etiology and incidence

1. Predisposing factors in calculi formation include:
   a. Immobility
   b. Hypercalcemia
   c. Urinary tract infection
   d. Urine stasis
   e. High urine specific gravity
   f. Genetic predisposition
2. Incidence peaks between ages 30 and 50 and is higher in men than in women.

C. **Pathophysiology**
  1. Calculi are formed by deposition of crystalline substances, including:
     a. Calcium oxalate
     b. Calcium phosphate
     c. Uric acid
  2. Most calculi contain calcium or magnesium in combination with phosphorus or oxalate.
  3. Calculi may pass through the urinary tract, or they may lodge and cause obstruction, leading to infection and possibly hydronephrosis.

D. **Assessment findings**
  1. Clinical manifestation vary with the location, size, and cause of calculi and may include:
     a. Acute, sharp, intermittent pain (ureteral colic)
     b. Dull, tender, ache in the flank (renal colic)
     c. Nausea and vomiting accompanying severe pain
     d. Fever and chills
     e. Hematuria
     f. Abdominal distention
     g. Pyuria
     h. Rarely, oliguria or anuria
  2. Laboratory and diagnostic studies may reveal:
     a. Visible calculi seen on KUB radiograph
     b. Mineral content of calculi detected on stone analysis
     c. Determination of calculi size and location using IVP
     d. Obstructive changes, such as hydronephrosis, detected on renal ultrasonography

E. **Nursing diagnoses**
  1. High Risk for Infection
  2. Knowledge Deficit
  3. Pain
  4. Altered Patterns of Urinary Elimination

F. **Planning and implementation**
  1. Intervene to control pain as indicated (e.g., narcotics, bedrest, relaxation techniques).
  2. Intervene to help prevent nausea and vomiting as needed.
  3. Facilitate calculus removal as indicated; interventions may include:
     a. Forcing fluids to encourage spontaneous passage
     b. Preparing the patient for surgical removal (lithotomy), lithotripsy, stone dissolution, or stone extraction
  4. After surgery, monitor for signs and symptoms of dehydration resulting from postobstructive diuresis; intervene as necessary to restore fluid balance.

5. Institute measures to help prevent stone recurrence, such as:
   a. Encouraging dietary modifications based on the stone's composition
   b. Increasing fluid intake to 3 to 4 L/day
   c. Promoting increased physical activity
   d. Monitoring urine pH
   e. Administering prescribed medications (see Section II.D.4)

G. **Evaluation**
   1. The patient reports relief of pain.
   2. The patient exhibits a normal voiding pattern without pain.
   3. The patient states appropriate foods in the prescribed diet to help prevent calculi formation.
   4. The patient verbalizes the need to drink 3 to 4 L of fluid daily.
   5. The patient expresses the intention to increase activity as tolerated.

IX. **Urinary tract cancer**
   A. **Description: neoplasms of the kidney, bladder, or elsewhere in the urinary system**
   B. **Etiology and incidence**
      1. The etiology of urinary tract cancer is unclear; known risk factors include:
         a. Long-term cigarette smoking
         b. Exposure to carcinogens (e.g., pesticides and various industrial chemicals)
         c. Familial predisposition
      2. Renal cancer affects men more often than women. Incidence of bladder cancer is two to three times greater in men than in women; peak incidence occurs between ages 50 and 70.
   C. **Pathophysiology**
      1. Kidney tumors include:
         a. Adenocarcinomas, accounting for about 90% of all renal tumors
         b. Renal cell carcinomas of the parenchyma
         c. Sarcomas of connective tissue
      2. Kidney cancer may metastasize readily to the other kidney and to the lung, bone, brain, and liver.
      3. Primary bladder tumors are papillomatous growths within the bladder lumen and possibly infiltrating the bladder wall.
      4. Bladder cancer tends to metastasize to the liver, bone, and lung.
      5. Malignant urethral neoplasms are uncommon but include squamous cell carcinomas and adenocarcinomas.

D. **Assessment findings**
1. Clinical manifestations vary with the site and type of cancer but may include:
    a. Gross, painless hematuria
    b. Dysuria
    c. Palpable mass in kidney or bladder
    d. Lower abdominal or flank (a late symptom)
    e. Fever
    f. Cachexia
    g. Fatigue
    h. Hypertension
2. Laboratory studies may reveal:
    a. Hypercalcemia
    b. Erythrocytosis
    c. Elevated ESR
    d. Abnormal liver function studies
3. Pertinent diagnostic procedures include:
    a. Urine cytology
    b. Excretory urography
    c. Cystoscopy
    d. Ultrasonography of the urinary tract

E. **Nursing diagnoses**
1. Anxiety
2. Fatigue
3. Knowledge Deficit
4. Pain
5. Self-Concept Disturbance
6. Altered Patterns of Urinary Elimination

F. **Planning and implementation**
1. Administer prescribed antineoplastic chemotherapy.
2. Prepare the patient for radiation therapy or surgery (e.g., cystectomy, nephrectomy) as ordered.
3. Teach the patient about self-care measures (e.g., catheter, stoma, drainage appliance, and skin care; nutritional and fluid intake; sexual activity).
4. Promote positive coping strategies, and encourage reliance on available support systems.
5. Help the patient and family work through the grieving process.

G. **Evaluation**
1. The patient verbalizes increased knowledge related to self-care.
2. The patient states possible side effects of chemotherapy or radiation therapy.
3. The patient demonstrates a willingness to seek support or help as appropriate.

4. The patient is able to express feelings and fears about the diagnosis, treatment, and prognosis.

X. Acute renal failure

A. Description

1. Acute renal failure is defined as sudden, rapid, potentially reversible deterioration of renal function.
2. It can be classified according to underlying cause as:
   a. Prerenal azotemia, stemming from decreased blood flow to kidneys
   b. Postrenal obstruction, involving obstruction to urine outflow
   c. Renal parenchymal failure, involving intrinsic damage to renal structures

B. Etiology and incidence

1. Causes of prerenal azotemia include factors that interfere with renal perfusion, such as:
   a. Hypovolemia (e.g., from hemorrhage, shock, burns)
   b. Increased intravascular capacity (e.g., due to sepsis, neurogenic shock)
   c. Cardiac disorders (e.g., myocardial infarction, dysrhythmias)
   d. Renal artery obstruction
   e. Hepatorenal syndrome
2. Possible causes of postrenal obstruction include:
   a. Ureteral obstruction due to calculi, strictures, trauma, or pregnancy
   b. Bladder obstruction (e.g., cancer, prostatic hypertrophy)
3. Renal parenchymal failure can result from:
   a. Acute tubular necrosis (ATN), which accounts for about 75% of all cases of acute renal failure
   b. Acute glomerulonephritis
   c. Acute pyelonephritis

C. Pathophysiology

1. Acute renal failure typically occurs in four phases:
   a. Onset phase: extending from the time of the precipitating event to the beginning of the oliguric–anuric phase
   b. Oliguric–anuric phase: marked by urine output <400 mL/day, volume overload, elevated BUN and creatinine, electrolyte abnormalities, metabolic acidosis, uremia
   c. Diuretic phase: extending from the time output becomes >400 mL/day to the time BUN stops rising and stabilizes in normal range; electrolyte and acid–base problems begin to normalize

        d.   Convalescent phase: extending from the time BUN stabilizes until the patient returns to normal activity; may take up to 2 years to regain 70% to 80% of normal function

   2.   Systemic effects of acute renal failure are widespread and may include:

        a.   Fluid and electrolyte imbalances

        b.   Acidosis

        c.   Increased susceptibility to infection

        d.   Anemia

        e.   Platelet dysfunctions

        f.   GI disturbances (e.g., anorexia, nausea, vomiting, diarrhea or constipation, stomatitis)

        g.   Pericarditis

        h.   Uremic encephalopathy

   1.   Clinical manifestations depend on the underlying condition; some of the most common include:

        a.   Altered urine output; may be oliguria, anuria, or (rarely) polyuria

        b.   Hypertension or hypotension

        c.   Tachypnea

        d.   Signs of fluid overload or extracellular fluid depletion

   2.   Laboratory studies may reveal the following:

        a.   Urine osmolality: in prerenal azotemia, >900 mOsm/kg; in postrenal obstruction, may be normal; in renal parenchymal failure, <250 mOsm/kg

        b.   Urine sodium: in prerenal azotemia, <20 mEq/L; in postrenal obstruction, may be normal; in renal parenchymal failure, >27 mEq/L

        c.   Elevated BUN, serum creatinine, and potassium levels

        d.   Decreased blood pH, bicarbonate, hemoglobin, and hematocrit

E. **Nursing diagnoses**

   1.   Fatigue

   2.   High Risk for Fluid Volume Deficit

   3.   High Risk for Fluid Volume Excess

   4.   High Risk for Infection

   5.   Knowledge Deficit

   6.   Impaired Physical Mobility

   7.   Altered Thought Processes

   8.   Altered Tissue Perfusion: Renal

   9.   Altered Patterns of Urinary Elimination

F. **Planning and implementation**

   1.   Provide prompt, aggressive interventions to manage the underlying problem.

2. During the oliguric–anuric phase:
   a. Assess fluid balance; restrict intake to urine output plus 500 mL/day.
   b. Monitor serum potassium, and assess for effects of hyperkalemia; restrict potassium in diet as necessary.
   c. Monitor for acidosis; administer an alkalinizing agent (e.g., Shohl's solution, sodium bicarbonate) as ordered.
   d. Assess for infection, especially respiratory and urinary tract; do not leave a urinary catheter in place; administer antibiotics as ordered.
   e. Monitor for hypocalcemia and hyperphosphatemia; administer phosphate-binding agents and calcium supplements as ordered.
   f. Monitor for anemia; administer blood transfusions as ordered.
   g. Prevent GI bleeding; administer an H_2 receptor antagonist (e.g., cimetidine) as ordered.
   h. Assess for central nervous system complications (e.g., drowsiness, confusion, delirium, coma, convulsions); administer short-acting barbiturates as ordered.
   i. Provide a high-calorie and low-protein diet, with hyperalimentation if the patient cannot eat.
   j. If indicated, prepare the patient for dialysis to correct hyperkalemia, fluid overload, acidosis, or severe uremia.
   k. Adjust dosages of drugs secreted by the kidney as necessary.
   l. Administer steroids, as prescribed, to decrease inflammation.

G. Evaluation
   1. The patient exhibits normal renal function, as evidenced by stabilized:
      a. Urine output
      b. Urine osmolality
      c. Urine sodium levels
      d. Blood pressure
      e. Fluid balance
   2. The patient demonstrates the ability to perform ADLs without undue fatigue.
   3. The patient verbalizes knowledge about the course of illness and required follow-up care.

XI. Chronic renal failure
   A. Description: the end result of progressive, irreversible loss of functioning renal tissue
   B. Etiology
      1. Chronic renal failure usually develops gradually (may take up

to several years); in some cases, it may occur rapidly because of an acute disorder (e.g., unresolved acute renal failure).

2. Major causes include:
   a. Hypertensive nephropathy
   b. Diabetic nephropathy
   c. Chronic glomerulonephritis
   d. Chronic pyelonephritis
   e. Lupus nephritis
   f. Polycystic kidney disease
   g. Chronic hydronephrosis

C. Pathophysiology
   1. Three basic stages of chronic renal failure have been identified:
      a. Decreased renal reserve: renal function 40% to 50% of normal; homeostasis maintained
      b. Renal insufficiency: renal function 20% to 40% of normal; GFR, clearance, and urine concentration decreased; homeostasis altered
      c. End-stage renal disease: renal function less than 10% to 15% of normal; all renal functions severely decreased; homeostasis significantly altered
   2. In chronic renal failure, end products of metabolism accumulate in blood instead of being excreted in urine. Retention of sodium and water leads to edema, congestive heart failure, and hypertension. Conversely, episodes of diarrhea and vomiting may lead to sodium and water depletion, exacerbating uremia and producing hypotension and hypovolemia.
   3. Metabolic acidosis occurs, interfering with the kidneys' ability to excrete hydrogen ions, produce ammonia, and conserve bicarbonate.
   4. Decreased GFR results in:
      a. Increased serum phosphate
      b. Decreased serum calcium
      c. Increased parathormone but depleted bone calcium, leading to bone changes (e.g., uremic bone disease, osteomalacia)
      d. Increased serum magnesium
   5. Erythropoietin production decreases, resulting in anemia.
   6. Neurologic complications develop, such as:
      a. Altered mental function
      b. Personality and behavioral changes
      c. Convulsions
      d. Coma
   7. Table 18–2 gives more information on the widespread pathologic effects of chronic renal failure.
   8. During the final stages of chronic renal failure, dialysis or kidney transplant is necessary to sustain life.

(text continued on page 528)

TABLE 18-2.
Systemic Manifestations of Chronic Renal Failure and Management

SYSTEM	MANIFESTATIONS	PATHOPHYSIOLOGIC BASIS	MANAGEMENT
Cardiovascular	Fluid overload; edema Congestive heart failure	Decreased excretion of water Fluid overload Hypertension	Restrict fluid in diet Restrict sodium in diet Restrict potassium in diet Alkaline medications (e.g., Shohl's Solution, Bicitra, Sodium Bicarbonate) Antihypertensive medications Correct electrolyte imbalances Dialysis
	Electrolyte imbalances Metabolic acidosis	Decreased excretion of electrolytes Decreased hydrogen ion secretion Decreased bicarbonate ion reabsorption and generation Retention of acid end products of metabolism Decreased ammonia synthesis and ammonium excretion	
	Hypertension	Fluid overload Increased sodium retention Inappropriate activation of the renin angiotensin system	
	Dysrhythmias	Electrolyte imbalances, especially hyperkalemia, hypocalcemia, and variations in sodium levels	
	Pericarditis, effusion, and tamponade	Uremic toxins Increased pericardial membrane permeability	
Hematopoietic	Anemia	Decreased erythropoietin secretion by kidneys Loss of red blood cells through the GI tract, mucous membranes, or dialysis Decreased red blood cell survival time due to uremic toxins Uremic toxins interfere with folic acid action	Iron supplements Folic acid supplements Androgens Blood transfusions Dialysis
	Alterations in coagulation Increased susceptibility to infection	Platelet dysfunction due to uremic toxins Decreased neutrophil phagocytosis and chemotaxis due to uremic toxins	
Integumentary	Pallor Yellowness Dryness	Uremic anemia Retained urochrome pigment is excreted through the skin Decreased secretions from oil and sweat glands due to uremic toxins	Bath oils and lotions Dialysis Correct hyperphosphatemia Teach self-care measures

(continued)

TABLE 18–2.
Systemic Manifestations of Chronic Renal Failure and Management (Continued)

SYSTEM	MANIFESTATIONS	PATHOPHYSIOLOGIC BASIS	MANAGEMENT
Integumentary (cont.)	Pruritus	Dry skin Calcium or phosphate deposits in the skin Uremic toxins effect on nerve endings	
	Purpura and ecchymosis Uremic frost (seen only in terminal or severely critically ill patients)	Increased capillary fragility Platelet dysfunction Urea or urate crystals are excreted through the skin	
Psychosocial	Decreased mentation, decreased concentration, and altered perceptions (even to the point of frank psychoses)	Uremic toxins produce a uremic encephalopathy Electrolyte imbalances Metabolic acidosis Tendency to develop cerebral edema	Dialysis Psychosocial counseling Patient and family education
Skeletal	Hypocalcemia and hyperphosphatemia	Hyperphosphatemia due to decreased renal excretion Decreased GI absorption of calcium due to decreased renal conversion of vitamin D	Dialysis Calcium supplements Vitamin D supplements Teach self-care measures
	Osteodystrophy	Increased osteoclastic activity in response to an increased secretion of parathyroid hormone	Phosphate-binding medications given with meals—Amphojel, Basaljel
	Metastatic calcifications	Deposition of calcium phosphate crystals in soft tissue and other structures	
Respiratory	Pulmonary edema	Fluid overload Increased pulmonary capillary permeability Left ventricular dysfunction	Restrict fluid intake Dialysis Treat cardiovascular problems Antibiotics
	Pneumonia or pneumonitis Kussmaul respirations	Thick tenacious oral secretions due to decreased fluid intake A weak, lethargic patient with a depressed cough reflex due to uremia Decreased pulmonary macrophage activity Fluid overload An increase in the rate and depth of the respirations to decrease the amount of carbon dioxide in the body to compensate for the metabolic acidosis.	Pulmonary hygiene (coughing and deep breathing exercises, oral care) Treat acidosis

(continued)

TABLE 18–2.
Systemic Manifestations of Chronic Renal Failure and Management (Continued)

SYSTEM	MANIFESTATIONS	PATHOPHYSIOLOGIC BASIS	MANAGEMENT
Neuromuscular	Drowsiness, confusion, coma, and irritability Tremors, twitching, and convulsions	Uremic toxins produce a uremic encephalopathy Metabolic acidosis Electrolyte imbalances Uremic toxins produce a uremic encephalopathy	Dialysis Seizure precautions Safety precautions during ambulation, exercise, and ADL
	Peripheral neuropathy Stage 1: restless leg syndrome and paresthesias Stage 2: motor involvement leading to footdrop Stage 3: paraplegia	Decreased nerve conduction, both motor and sensory, due to uremic toxins	
Gastrointestinal	Anorexia, nausea, and emesis	Uremic toxins Decomposition of urea in the GI tract releasing ammonia, which irritates the mucosa	Dialysis Oral hygiene Oral assessment Monitor hemoglobin and hematocrit Treat diarrhea or constipation Increase bulk in diet Exercise regimen Teach self-care measures
	Stomatitis and uremic halitosis	Uremic toxins Decomposition of the urea in the oral cavity releasing ammonia	
	Gastritis and bleeding	Uremic toxins Decomposition of urea in the GI tract releasing ammonia, which irritates the GI mucosa producing small ulcerations Increased capillary fragility	
	Bowel problems: diarrhea	Uremic toxins Hypermotility due to electrolyte imbalances, especially hyperkalemia	
	Constipation	Hypomotility due to electrolyte imbalances, decreased fluid intake, decreased activity, and decreased bulk in the diet	

D. Assessment findings
  1. Major clinical manifestations of chronic renal failure depend on the stage of the disorder:
    a. Decreased renal reserve: patient asymptomatic as long as he or she is not exposed to severe physiologic or psychologic stress

        b.   Renal insufficiency: polyuria and nocturia, signs and symptoms of mild anemia

        c.   End-stage renal disease: widespread systemic manifestations (see Table 18–2)

  2. Characteristic laboratory findings include:

        a.   Anemia

        b.   Elevated BUN, serum creatinine

        c.   Elevated serum phosphorus

        d.   Decreased serum calcium

        e.   Decreased serum proteins (particularly albumin)

        f.   Low blood pH

E. Nursing diagnoses

  1. Activity Intolerance

  2. Anxiety

  3. Ineffective Individual Coping

  4. High Risk for Fluid Volume Deficit

  5. High Risk for Fluid Volume Excess

  6. Knowledge Deficit

  7. Altered Nutrition: Less Than Body Requirements

  8. Impaired Skin Integrity

  9. Altered Patterns of Urinary Elimination

F. Planning and implementation

  1. Provide conservative therapy, as indicated, which may include:

        a.   Fluid control; daily fluid intake equaling 500 mL (insensible loss) plus the amount of the previous 24 hours' urinary output

        b.   Diet modifications: decreased protein intake (approximately 1 g/kg ideal body weight); this amount should be 85% to 90% high biologic value protein—containing complete essential amino acids (e.g., fish, poultry, eggs)—and 10% to 15% low biologic value protein—containing incomplete amino acids (e.g., nuts, cereals, breads); decreased sodium; decreased potassium; high-calorie foods of simple sugars and carbohydrates (e.g., candy and butter balls)

        c.   Medication administration (see Table 18-2)

        d.   Symptomatic treatment (see Table 18-2)

  2. Prepare the patient for peritoneal dialysis, if indicated. Assist with the procedure as instructed, maintaining septic technique and monitoring for signs and symptoms of peritonitis (e.g., rigid boardlike abdomen, fever, cloudy peritoneal fluid).

  3. Prepare the patient for and assist with hemodialysis, if indicated. Provide proper shunt care, and assess for possible complications (e.g., bleeding due to heparinization, hypovolemia and hypotension due to excessive water removal, dialysis disequilibrium syndrome [headache, confusion, seizures] due to rapid removal of urea from plasma).

4. Prepare the patient for kidney transplantation, if indicated. Provide postoperative care for any patient who has undergone major surgery (see Chapter 24, Perioperative Nursing), with special attention to catheter patency and adequacy, intake and output, fluid replacement, and protection from infection. Monitor for signs and symptoms of complications such as graft rejection (fever, elevated WBC, electrolyte abnormalities, abnormal renogram) and infection stemming from immunosuppressive therapy (sepsis pneumonia, wound infection, urinary tract infection).

G. Evaluation

1. The patient limits fluid intake to 500 cc plus amount equal to previous 24 hours' output.
2. The patient states foods allowed and prohibited in the prescribed diet.
3. The patient demonstrates reduced anxiety.
4. The patient exhibits the ability and desire to mobilize or identify resources to help with lifestyle adjustments.
5. The patient demonstrates the ability to participate in dialysis if it is to be done in the home setting.
6. The patient verbalizes ways to reduce the risk of infection.
7. The patient states the intention to adjust his or her activity level to reduce fatigue.

Bibliography

Brunner L. S., & Suddarth, D. S. (1988). *Textbook of medical-surgical nursing* (6th ed.). Philadelphia: J. B. Lippincott.

Brunner L. S., & Suddarth, D. S. (1986). *The Lippincott manual of nursing practice* (4th ed.). Philadelphia: J. B. Lippincott.

Luckmann, J., & Sorensen, K. C. (1987). *Medical-surgical nursing: A psychophysiologic approach* (3rd ed.). Philadelphia: W. B. Saunders.

STUDY QUESTIONS

1. Ms. Roberts' renal function has been deteriorating during her hospitalization. The nurse monitors for significant changes by focusing on which of the following laboratory tests?
   a. blood urea nitrogen (increase)
   b. serum creatinine (decrease)
   c. creatinine clearance (increase)
   d. serum potassium (decrease)

2. Acute tubular necrosis (ATN) is characterized by which of the following?
   a. oliguria (usually)
   b. gradual onset
   c. irreversibility
   d. glucosuria

3. Mr. Jabbar, a 55-year-old patient with chronic renal failure, should manage his fluid intake at home by
   a. subtracting the previous day's urine output from 500 mL and limiting intake to milk
   b. adding 500 mL to the previous day's urine output and dividing that amount over the next 24 hours
   c. consuming all of his fluid allowance during the day to prevent nighttime bladder distention
   d. weighing himself before each meal and drinking 500 mL of fluids four times a day

4. After the physician orders a culture and sensitivity test, why would the nurse instruct the patient to obtain a clean-catch midstream urine specimen?
   a. The urinary tract normally harbors some microorganisms.
   b. Microorganisms on the patient's external genitalia may contaminate the specimen.
   c. The nurse does not want to catheterize the patient.
   d. A midstream specimen obtains the largest number of microorganisms in the lower urinary tract.

5. Evaluation of normal kidney response to acidosis would be based on which of the following criteria?
   a. The kidneys secrete excess bicarbonate.
   b. The kidneys absorb hydrogen ions.
   c. The kidneys decrease ammonia production and ammonium excretion.
   d. The kidneys increase urine excretion.

6. Which of following interventions is important for the nurse to implement following kidney biopsy?
   a. Decrease fluid intake to less than 100 mL/day.
   b. Instruct the patient to ambulate as soon as possible after the procedure.
   c. Monitor vital signs closely.
   d. Perform neuro checks every 3 to 4 hours for the first 24 hours.

7. ATN may be caused by
   a. prolonged ischemia
   b. Goodpasture's syndrome
   c. ureteral calculi
   d. prostatic hypertrophy

8. The nursing diagnosis Knowledge Deficit related to the need for teaching to prevent pyelonephritis would *least* likely apply to which of following patients?
   a. a 25-year-old sexually active man
   b. a bedridden elderly patient with an indwelling (Foley) catheter
   c. an 18-month-old toddler with a history of vesicoureteral reflux
   d. a 55-year-old woman who has been treated for urinary retention

9. Why should the nurse plan to address malnutrition for a patient with renal failure?
   a. Anemia causes increased absorption of water-soluble vitamins.
   b. The patient requires increased carbohydrate intake.
   c. Increased anabolism occurs in renal failure.
   d. Anemia often causes anorexia, nausea, and vomiting.

10. After dietary instruction, evaluation of effective learning for a patient with chronic renal failure would reveal the

patient's understanding of what fact about high biologic value (HBV) proteins?

a. They contain the five essential amino acids in each food.
b. They are found in fish, poultry, and eggs.
c. They should compose only a small portion of a dialysis patient's total protein intake.
d. They are found in legumes, breads, and cereals.

11. A patient with chronic renal failure often experiences pruritus. To treat this problem, the nurse should teach the patient to perform which of these self-care measures at home?
a. increasing dietary intake of phosphate
b. increasing dietary intake of protein
c. applying glycerin to the skin
d. using superfatted soaps and lotions

12. Mary Jones, aged 16, has chronic renal failure. She reports taking a bath every day at home with soap even though she has been instructed against this practice. She states she doesn't care what she's told. ("What would my friends think if they knew I didn't bathe.") Based on this information, in this situation all the following nursing diagnoses would be appropriate *except*
a. High Risk for Impaired Skin Integrity

b. Impaired Adjustment
c. Decisional Conflict
d. Health-Seeking Behaviors

13. Causes of hypertension associated with chronic renal failure include
a. hypoaldosteronism
b. increased sodium and water retention
c. decreased renin production
d. decreased antidiuretic hormone production

14. On auscultating over the precordium of a patient with chronic renal failure, the nurse hears a pericardial friction rub. The nurse should promptly notify the physician because this finding is indicative of
a. pleural effusion
b. cardiac tamponade
c. ventricular dysrhythmias
d. anemic pericarditis

15. Ms. Black, an 18-year-old renal transplant patient, has expressed frustration at how alone she feels in her hospital room. "I wish I could be out in the waiting room visiting with my friends." Which of the following diagnoses is she demonstrating?
a. Ineffective Individual Coping
b. Self-Concept Disturbance
c. Social Isolation
d. Hopelessness

ANSWER KEY

1. **Correct response: a**
Decreased amounts of urea nitrogen are filtered in renal failure so plasma level increases.
   b, c, and d. Serum creatinine increases, creatinine clearance decreases, and serum potassium increases in renal failure.
Comprehension/Physiologic/Implementation

2. **Correct response: a**
Urine output is usually decreased in ATN.
   b and c. ATN has sudden onset and is usually reversible with treatment.
   d. Glucosuria is not commonly associated with ATN.
Knowledge/Physiologic/Assessment

3. **Correct response: b**
Insensible losses (500 mL) plus urine output determine intake in renal failure.
   a. This is an incorrect formulation.
   c. Fluid intake should be divided over a 24-hour period.
   d. This amount of fluid far exceeds the recommended allotment.
Analysis/Health promotion/Planning

4. **Correct response: b**
External genitalia normally harbor microorganisms.
   a. The urinary tract is considered sterile.
   c. Catheterization is not necessary for a culture and sensitivity specimen.
   d. This is an incorrect statement.
Comprehension/Safe care/Implementation

5. **Correct response: c**
Ammonia is produced in the renal tubule, and ammonium is excreted in response to acidosis.
   a and b. Bicarbonate is absorbed and hydrogen ions secreted in acidosis.
   d. Urine volume is not affected.
Comprehension/Physiologic/Evaluation

6. **Correct response: c**
Vital sign monitoring detects bleeding and shock.
   a. Fluid intake may be increased.
   b. The patient remains on bedrest for 6 to 8 hours.
   d. Neuro checks are unnecessary.
Application/Safe care/Implementation

7. **Correct response: a**
Ischemia is a common cause of ATN.
   b. Goodpasture's syndrome is glomerular disorder.
   c and d. Calculi and prostatic hypertrophy may cause hydronephrosis.
Knowledge/Physiologic/Assessment

8. **Correct response: a**
Kidney infections are caused by immobility, reflux, stasis, and debilitation. Women are more prone to UTI than men.
   b, c, and d. These patients all would be more prone to UTI than a yound adult man.
Analysis/Safe care/Analysis (Dx)

9. **Correct response: d**
Anorexia, nausea, and vomiting may lead to decreased intake and poor absorption of nutrients.
   a. Anemia may lead to decreased absorption of vitamins.
   b. Increased carbohydrate intake is important to provide energy.
   c. Catabolism commonly occurs in renal failure.
Analysis/Health promotion/Planning

10. **Correct response: b**
Fish, poultry, and eggs are good sources of HBV protein.
   a and c. HBV protein contains all essential amino acids and should compose the largest percentage of the total protein intake.
   d. Legumes, breads, and cereals contain low biologic value proteins.
Analysis/Health promotion/Evaluation

11. *Correct response: d*
    Superfatted soaps and lotion help keep skin moist and relieve pruritus.
    a. Excess phosphate in chronic renal failure contributes to skin problems.
    b. Dietary protein is decreased to help control the level of uremic toxins.
    c. Glycerin has a long-term drying effect.

Application/Health promotion/Planning

12. *Correct response: d*
    The scenario presents no evidence that this patient is exhibiting health-seeking behavior. Rather, her behavior is health-damaging because of the dry, scaly skin that results from uremic toxins. By continuing this behavior, she increases the risk of impaired skin integrity. Her behavior reflects both difficulty in adjusting to lifestyle changes and in making healthy decisions.
    a, b, and c. All of these nursing diagnoses could be appropriate for this patient.

Application/Psychosocial/Analysis (Dx)

13. *Correct response: b*
    The kidneys' inability to excrete sodium and water leads to increased vascular volume and increased blood pressure.

a and c. Renal failure may involve increased aldosterone and renin production.
    d. ADH is not commonly affected by renal failure.

Application/Physiologic/Assessment

14. *Correct response: d*
    Pericardial layers rub together due to inflammation from uremic toxins.
    a. Pleural effusion may lead to pleural friction rub.
    b. Pericardial friction rub would disappear with tamponade.
    c. Dysrhythmias are unrelated to pericardial friction rub.

Application/Safe care/Implementation

15. *Correct response: c*
    An immunosuppressed post-transplant patient is placed on mask isolation in a single room and protected from anyone with infection. She is reflecting social isolation.
    a, b, and d. This scenario offers no evidence that the patient has a disturbed self-concept, nor is there evidence of ineffective coping or hopelessness.

Application/Psychosocial/Analysis (Dx)

Hematologic Disorders

I. Anatomy and physiology

A. Structure

1. Whole blood consists of formed elements (blood cells) suspended in liquid component (plasma).

2. In an adult, total blood volume is approximately 5 L, constituting 7% to 8% of total body weight.

3. Whole blood contains three types of blood cells:

   a. Erythrocytes (red blood cells—RBCs); average number: 5 million/cubic mL of blood

   b. Leukocytes (white blood cells—WBCs); average total WBC count: 5000 to 10,000 cells per cubic mL of blood

   c. Thombocytes (platelets); normal platelet count: 150,000 to 450,000/cubic mL of blood

4. Erythrocytes, the major cellular element of circulating blood, are biconcave disks normally about 7 μm in diameter containing hemoglobin confined in a plasma membrane.

5. Reticulocytes, immature erythrocytes, may be released prematurely from marrow into circulation under conditions necessitating rapid blood cell production (compensatory mechanism).

6. Leukocytes are divided into two major types based on cell structure:

   a. Granular leukocytes, also called granulocytes or polymorphonuclear leukocytes

   b. Nongranular leukocytes, or mononuclear leukocytes

7. Produced in bone marrow, granulocytes normally comprise 70% of all WBCs. They are subdivided into three types based on staining properties: neutrophils, eosinophils, and basophils.

8. Mononuclear leukocytes are subdivided into:

   a. Lymphocytes, which are produced in bone marrow and undergo differentiation in lymph tissue; comprise 30% of total leukocytes

   b. Monocytes, which are produced in bone marrow and

transform into mature forms called macrophages on release into tissues; comprise 5% of total leukocytes

9. Thrombocytes are formed from fragmentation or breaking off
of parts of membrane and cytoplasm from very large cells in
bone marrow, lung, and spleen called megakaryocytes; normal
life span is 7 to 14 days.

10. Hematocrit refers to the percentage of total blood volume
comprised by cells; normal value is approximately 45%.

11. Hemoglobin, a protein, comprises about 95% of erythrocyte
mass. Hemoglobin has the ability to bind oxygen loosely and
reversibly; when combined with oxygen, it's called oxyhemo-
globin. Whole blood normally contains about 15 g of hemoglobin per 100 mL of blood.

12. Plasma, the liquid portion of whole blood remaining after
blood cells are removed, constitutes 55% of blood volume and
contains large quantities of organic and inorganic substances.

13. Serum is the fluid remaining when plasma is allowed to clot
(i.e., plasma minus fibrinogen and several clotting factors).

14. Plasma proteins consist primarily of:
    a. Albumin, the largest of plasma proteins, produced in
    the liver
    b. Globulins

15. Globulins are subdivided into:
    a. Gamma globulins, consisting mainly of antibodies
    known as immunoglobulins
    b. Alpha and beta fractions, including transport proteins
    and clotting factors, produced in the liver (Table 19–1)

B. Function

1. General blood functions include:
    a. Transporting oxygen absorbed from lungs and nutrients
    absorbed from gastrointestinal (GI) tract to body cells
    for cellular metabolism
    b. Transporting waste products from tissues to excretory
    organs
    c. Aiding in chemical, acid–base, and thermal regulation of
    body
    d. Transporting hormones and other substances internally
    secreted to their tissue sites of action
    e. Aiding in defense against infection through action of an-
    tibodies and phagocytes
    f. Aiding in regulation of extracellular fluid volume
    g. Promoting hemostasis: arrest of bleeding by blood clot
    formation, followed by clot dissolution

2. All blood cells originate from stem cells. Certain blood cells
derive from bone marrow but undergo differentiation and
maturation in various tissues (e.g., lymphocytes, monocytes).

3. Normal erythrocyte production (erythropoiesis), occurring in

TABLE 19–1.
Blood Coagulation Proteins

FACTOR	SYNONYMS	NORMAL PLASMA CONCENTRATIONS (mg/dL)
I	Fibrinogen	200–400
II	Prothrombin	10
III	Tissue thromboplastin, tissue factor	0
IV	Calcium ion	4–5
V	Proaccelerin, labile factor	1
VII	Serum prothrombin conversion accelerator (SPCA), stable factor	0.05
VIII	Antihemophilic factor	1–2
IX	Christmas factor	0.3
X	Stuart-Power factor	1
XI	Plasma thromboplastin antecedent (PTA)	0.5
XII	Hageman factor	3
XIII	Fibrin stabilizing factor (FSF)	1–2
Prekallikrein	Fletcher factor	5
High molecular weight kininogen	Fitzgerald, Flaujeac, Williams factor; contact activation cofactor	6

From Saito, H. (1984). *Disorders of Hemostasis*, Ratnoff, O. D. and Forbes, C. D. (eds.). Orlando, FL: Grune and Stratton.

the bone marrow, is stimulated by erythropoietin (a substance produced primarily by the kidneys) and requires several nutrients, notably iron, vitamin B, folic acid, pyridoxine (vitamin B), and ascorbic acid (vitamin C).

4. Erythrocytes transport oxygen from lungs to tissues. In active tissues, oxygen readily dissociates from hemoglobin; in venous blood, hemoglobin combines with hydrogen ions produced by cellular metabolism, buffering excess acid.

5. The average life span of a circulating erythrocyte is 120 days. Erythrocytes are removed by phagocytosis in the reticuloendothelial system, particularly the liver and spleen. Reticuloendothelial cells produce bilirubin, a pigment from hemoglobin released from destroyed erythrocytes excreted in bile.

6. Leukocytes defend the body against invasion by infectious and parasitic organisms through processes of phagocytosis (ingestion and destruction of invading organisms and foreign particles) and antibody production.

7. Neutrophils are phagocytic cells that arrive early at the site of inflammatory reaction but have a relatively short life span of only several days. Increased numbers (neutrophilia) occur with onset of infection, especially with pyogenic bacteria that augment the body's resistance. Infection also may produce a "shift to the left" (appearance of more immature forms of neutrophils in circulation, such as bands and metamyelocytes).

8. Eosinophils and basophils contain and release potent biologic materials (such as histamine, serotonin, and heparin), which alter blood supply to tissues and help mobilize the body's defense mechanisms.

9. Monocytes, the largest nongranular leukocytes, can phagocytize large foreign particles, cell fragments, and necrotic tissue.

10. Lymphocytes produce substances that aid in attack of foreign cells and substances. B lymphocytes produce antibodies; T lymphocytes kill foreign cells directly or release various lymphokines, substances that enhance activity of phagocytic cells.

11. Platelets help control bleeding by:
   a. Physically aggregating and adhering to sites of vascular injury, forming a patch or plug that temporarily stops bleeding
   b. Releasing biochemical substances that activate coagulation factors in plasma to form a stable fibrin clot

12. Approximately 10% to 15% of circulating platelets are continually being consumed in normal ongoing intravascular clot formation in repair of small vascular injuries.

13. Plasma provides a medium for circulation of blood cells. Various constituent substances contribute to acid–base balance, blood clot formation and clot lysis, fluid balance, transport of nutritional and hormonal substances, and immunologic defense and surveillance.

14. Capillary walls are impermeable to albumin, creating an osmotic force that maintains fluid volume within the vascular system. Albumin has the ability to bind several plasma substances for transport, such as fatty acids, drugs, metals, and bilirubin.

15. Coagulation or fibrin clot formation results from a complex series of reactions wherein inert plasma proteins are "activated" or transformed into enzymes in sequential manner, ending with thrombin-induced conversion of fibrinogen to fibrin (cascade theory).

16. Initial interactions of coagulation factors may be grouped into three separate pathways (Fig. 19–1); clot formation can occur by way of:
   a. Intrinsic and common pathways of coagulation, where triggering stimulus occurs within circulation (i.e., blood comes in contact with abnormal surface)
   b. Extrinsic and common pathways, when tissue injury releases thromboplastin into circulation

17. The fibrinolytic system is a plasma enzyme system responsible for blood clot removal after blood vessel integrity is restored.

18. Inert plasma protein—plasminogen—is activated into the enzyme plasmin, which digests fibrinogen and fibrin in a process called fibrinolysis.

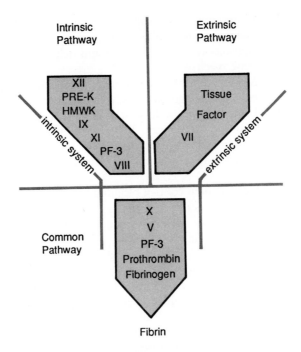

Intrinsic Pathway

Extrinsic Pathway

XII
PRE-K
HMWK
IX
XI
PF-3
VIII

intrinsic system

Tissue
Factor

VII

extrinsic system

Common Pathway

X
V
PF-3
Prothrombin
Fibrinogen

Fibrin

FIGURE 19–1.
Coagulation Pathways. (From Bithell, T. C. [1987]. In O.A. Thorup (Ed.), *Fundamentals of Clinical Hematology*. Philadelphia: W. B. Saunders.)

19. Fibrinolysis produces fibrin split products (FSP), also known as fibrin degradation products, which are removed from circulation by the reticuloendothelial system and liver and spleen; FSP normally is not present in circulation.

II. Hematologic system overview

A. Assessment

1. Inspection of skin and mucous membranes may reveal such color changes as:

    a. Pallor (paleness), occurring with decreased hemoglobin or decreased blood flow

    b. Cyanosis (bluish discoloration), occurring with increased circulating unoxygenated hemoglobin secondary to hypoxia

    c. Rubor (redness), occurring with increased visibility of normal oxyhemoglobin due to dilation of superficial blood vessels (e.g., fever) or with increased blood flow (e.g., inflammation)

    d. Jaundice (yellowish discoloration), resulting from increased bilirubin levels secondary to RBC hemolysis; appearing first in sclera, then mucous membranes, then generalized

2. Color changes are best assessed where capillary beds are superficial and pigmentation minimal (e.g., nailbeds, hard palate, lips, palms, soles, conjunctivae).

3. Skin and mucous membrane inspection also may reveal:
   a. Petechiae, small pinpoint hemorrhages on skin or mucous membranes, which most commonly occur with quantitative or qualitative platelet disorders; generally more numerous over bony prominences (increased trauma) or dependent areas (increased venous pressure)
   b. Ecchymoses, bluish-black macula, resulting from seepage of blood into skin or mucous membranes, often secondary to trauma
   c. Pruritus and malignant infiltrative skin lesions, occurring with certain hematologic malignancies (e.g., leukemias and lymphomas)
   d. Glossitis (inflammation of the tongue) and ulcerative lesions of oral cavity, which occur with certain anemias
   e. Gingival hypertrophy (enlargement of gums), common in monocytic leukemia due to leukemic cell infiltration

4. Palpation of the thorax and abdomen can detect:
   a. Splenomegaly (enlarged spleen), which occurs in various hematologic disorders, including several anemias and hematologic malignancies
   b. Hepatomegaly (enlarged liver), possibly indicating inflammation (as in hepatitis), venous congestion, or a hematologic malignancy

5. Detection of lymphadenopathy (enlarged lymph nodes) may point to regional or systemic infection or a hematologic malignancy.

B. **Laboratory studies**
   1. In bone marrow aspiration and biopsy, specimens of bone marrow and bone are obtained by introducing a needle with stylet into the iliac crest (the sternum may be used for aspiration in adults); purposes include:
      a. Diagnosing hematologic disorders through evaluating precursors of peripheral blood cells or iron content
      b. Evaluating effectiveness of treatment
      c. Diagnosing nonhematologic diseases (e.g., infectious diseases, certain granulomas) or staging solid tumor malignancies
   2. Complete blood count includes:
      a. Enumeration of the number of RBCs, WBCs, and platelets per cubic millimeter of venous blood
      b. Differential WBC count, or respective percentages of neutrophils, eosinophils, basophils, lymphocytes, and monocytes contributing to the total WBC count

3. Reticulocyte count detects the percentage of young (1 to 2 days old) non-nucleated erythrocytes in peripheral blood.

4. Red blood cell indices involve three calculated measurements of average RBC size and hematocrit and hemoglobin content; helpful in diagnosing and evaluating the severity of anemic disorders. Specific indices include:

   a. Mean corpuscular hemoglobin: average amount of hemoglobin contained within RBCs

   b. Mean corpuscular hemoglobin concentration: percentage representing the ratio of the weight of hemoglobin to the volume of an average RBC

   c. Mean corpuscular volume: value for average RBC size

5. Hemoglobin electrophoresis provides a means for identifying different hemoglobins (e.g., A, A2, F, S), based on the speed at which they travel when exposed to electrical current.

6. The sickling test detects characteristic sickling of RBCs occurring with sickle cell trait or disease by exposing blood to a reducing agent, thus depriving cells of oxygen.

7. Coombs' test determines the presence of immune globulin plasma (indirect Coombs'); used in diagnosing various hemolytic anemias.

8. Leukocyte alkaline phosphatase testing estimates the amount of this enzyme (normally present in high concentrations in neutrophils) through a special stain of peripheral blood.

9. Bleeding time involves measuring in minutes the time it takes for bleeding to stop after a standardized skin puncture, usually on the forearm; helps detect disorders of platelet function.

10. Platelet aggregation measures the time and completeness of platelet aggregate formation in a plasma sample after addition of a triggering agent.

11. Prothrombin time (PT) measures coagulation through extrinsic and common pathways; purposes include:

    a. Monitoring coumarin therapy

    b. Providing a screening test for liver disease and coagulation factor deficiencies

12. Partial thromboplastin time (PTT) evaluates coagulation through intrinsic and common pathways; purposes include:

    a. Monitoring heparin therapy

    b. Providing a screening test for coagulation factor deficiencies

13. Thrombin clotting time measures thrombin-induced conversion of fibrinogen to fibrin in the coagulation cascade; used to monitor heparin therapy.

14. Coagulation factor assay provides the definitive test for quantitative deficiency of coagulation factor. In this test, a sample of the patient's plasma is added to a sample of factor-deficient

plasma, then the amount of correction in PT and PTT is compared with correction by normal plasma (arbitrarily defined as 100% activity).

C. **Psychosocial implications**

1. The patient with a hematologic disorder may experience coping difficulty related to:
   a. Progressive nature of disease
   b. Disease chronicity
   c. Limitations imposed by treatments
   d. Fear of dying
   e. The need to learn much self-care information
   f. Ongoing follow-up care or lifelong preventive and therapeutic regimens
2. The patient also may have self-concept concerns related to fear of:
   a. Loss of self-esteem
   b. Body image changes related to the disorder and treatments
   c. Role changes toward increasing dependence
3. Disease-related lifestyle concerns may involve changes in:
   a. Physical ability
   b. Work performance, with potential for job loss
   c. Economic stability
   d. Family dynamics
4. The disease may lead to changes in social interaction patterns, possibly resulting in:
   a. Isolation
   b. Depression
   c. Helplessness
   d. Hopelessness

D. **Blood transfusion therapy**

1. This therapy involves transfusing whole blood or blood components (specific portion or fraction of blood lacking in patient).
2. One unit of whole blood consists of 450 mL of blood collected into 60 to 70 mL of preservative or anticoagulant. Whole blood stored for more than 6 hours does not provide therapeutic platelet transfusion, nor does it contain therapeutic amounts of labile coagulation factors (factors V and VIII).
3. Blood components include:
   a. Packed RBCs (100% of erythrocyte, 100% of leukocytes, and 20% of plasma originally present in one unit of whole blood), indicated to increase the oxygen-carrying capacity of blood with minimal expansion of blood volume

     b.   Leukocyte-poor packed RBCs, indicated for patients who have experienced previous febrile nonhemolytic transfusion reactions

     c.   Platelets, either HLA (human leukocyte antigen) matched or unmatched

     d.   Granulocytes (basophils, eosinophils, and neutrophils)

     e.   Fresh frozen plasma, containing all coagulation factors, including factors V and VIII (the labile factors)

     f.   Single donor plasma, containing all stable coagulation factors but reduced levels of factors V and VIII; the preferred product for reversal of coumadin-induced anticoagulation

     g.   Albumin, a plasma protein

     h.   Cryoprecipitate, a plasma derivative rich in factor VIII, fibrinogen, factor XIII, and fibronectin

     i.   Factor IX concentrate, a concentrated form of factor IX prepared by pooling, fractionating, and freeze-drying large volumes of plasma

     j.   Factor VIII concentrate, a concentrated form of factor VIII, prepared by pooling, fractionating, and freeze-drying large volumes of plasma

     k.   Prothrombin complex, containing prothrombin and factors VII, IX, X, and some factor XI

4.   Blood component therapy has the following advantages:

     a.   Avoids the risk of sensitizing the patient to other blood components

     b.   Provides optimal therapeutic benefit while reducing risk of volume overload

     c.   Increases availability of needed blood products to larger population

5.   Principles of blood transfusion therapy:

     a.   Whole blood transfusion: Generally indicated only for patients who need both increased oxygen-carrying capacity and restoration of blood volume when there is no time to prepare or obtain the specific blood components needed.

     b.   Packed RBCs: Should be transfused over 2 to 3 hours; if patient cannot tolerate volume over a maximum of 4 hours, it may be necessary for the blood bank to divide a unit into smaller volumes, providing proper refrigeration of remaining blood until needed. One unit of packed red cells should raise hemoglobin approximately 1%, hematocrit 3%.

     c.   Platelets: Administer as rapidly as tolerated (usually 4 units every 30 to 60 minutes). Each unit of platelets should raise the recipient's platelet count by 6000 to

10,000/mm³; however, poor incremental increases occur with alloimmunization from previous transfusions, bleeding, fever, infection, autoimmune destruction, and hypertension.

d. Granulocytes: May be beneficial in selected population of infected, severely granulocytopenic patients (less than 500/mm³) not responding to antibiotic therapy and who are expected to experience prolonged suppressed granulocyte production.

e. Plasma: Because plasma carries a risk of hepatitis equal to that of whole blood, if only volume expansion is required, other colloids (e.g., albumin) or electrolyte solutions (e.g., Ringer's lactate) are preferred. Fresh frozen plasma should be administered as rapidly as tolerated because coagulation factors become unstable after thawing.

f. Albumin: Indicated to expand blood volume of patients in hypovolemic shock and to elevate level of circulating albumin in patients with hypoalbuminemia. The large protein molecule is a major contributor to plasma oncotic pressure.

g. Cryoprecipitate: Indicated for treatment of hemophilia A, Von Willebrand's disease, disseminated intravascular coagulation (DIC), and uremic bleeding.

h. Factor IX concentrate: Indicated for treatment of hemophilia B; carries a high risk of hepatitis because it requires pooling from many donors.

i. Factor VIII concentrate: Indicated for treatment of hemophilia A; heat-treated product decreases the risk of hepatitis and HIV transmission.

j. Prothrombin complex: Indicated in congenital or acquired deficiencies of these factors.

III. Complications of blood transfusion

A. Overview

1. *Hemolytic transfusion reaction* is a life-threatening complication occurring from transfusion of donor blood that is incompatible with the recipient's blood.

2. In hemolytic transfusion reaction, antibodies in the recipient's plasma combine with antigens on donor erythrocytes, causing agglutination and hemolysis in circulation or in the reticuloendothelial system. Similarly, antibodies in donor plasma combine with antigen on the recipient's erythrocytes; however, complications from infusion of incompatible plasma are less severe than those associated with infusion of incompatible erythrocytes. The most rapid hemolysis occurs in ABO incompatibility; Rh incompatibility is often less severe.

3. *Delayed hemolytic transfusion reaction* occurs 1 to 2 weeks after

transfusion; erythrocytes hemolyzed by antibody are not detectible during crossmatch but are formed rapidly after transfusion. It generally is not dangerous, but subsequent transfusions may be associated with acute hemolytic reaction.

4. In hemolytic reaction, the severity of complications correlates with the amount of incompatible blood transfused; chances of fatal reaction are decreased if less than 100 mL of incompatible blood is infused.

5. *Febrile, nonhemolytic transfusion reaction*, the most common type of reaction, is commonly caused by sensitivity to leukocyte or platelet antigens.

6. *Septic reaction* is an often serious complication resulting from transfusion of a blood product contaminated with bacteria.

7. *Allergic reactions* may result from sensitivity to plasma protein or donor antibody, which reacts with recipient antigen.

8. *Circulatory overload* results from administration at a rate or volume greater than can be accommodated by the circulatory system, precipitating congestive heart failure or pulmonary edema.

9. Several *infectious diseases* can be transmitted through blood transfusion, including:
    a. Hepatitis B
    b. Non-A, non-B hepatitis
    c. Malaria
    d. Syphilis
    e. Acquired immunodeficiency syndrome (AIDS)

10. *Graft-versus-host (GVH) disease* results from engraftment of immunocompetent lymphocytes in bone marrow of immunosuppressed recipients, which triggers an immune response of the graft against the host.

11. *Reactions associated with massive transfusions* (>10 units of packed RBCs in 1 to 6 hours) include:
    a. Hypocalcemia, resulting from binding of recipient's circulating calcium to anticoagulant (citrate) in packed RBCs
    b. Citrate intoxication due to accumulation of citrate
    c. Hyperkalemia, in which stored red cells progressively increase extracellular potassium concentration
    d. Exacerbation of liver disease due to increased ammonia levels in stored blood
    e. Hypothermia, in which transfusion of cold blood (below 37°C) at rates >100 mL/min may produce dysrhythmias and cardiac arrest
    f. Aggregates of leukocytes and platelets in the lungs, resulting from accumulation of these aggregates during blood storage

      g.   Hemorrhage, resulting from excessive dilution of the re-
cipient's platelets and clotting factors

B.   **Assessment findings**

   1.   Clinical manifestations of transfusion complications vary depending on the precipitating factor.

   2.   Signs and symptoms of hemolytic transfusion reaction include:
      a.   Fever
      b.   Chills
      c.   Low back pain
      d.   Flank pain
      e.   Headache
      f.   Nausea
      g.   Flushing
      h.   Tachycardia
      i.   Tachypnea
      j.   Hypotension
      k.   Hemoglobinuria (cola-colored urine)
      l.   Abnormal bleeding

   3.   Clinical signs and laboratory findings in delayed hemolytic reaction include:
      a.   Fever
      b.   Mild jaundice
      c.   Gradual fall in hemoglobin
      d.   Positive Coombs' test

   4.   Febrile nonhemolytic reaction is marked by:
      a.   Temperature rise during or shortly after transfusion
      b.   Chills
      c.   Headache
      d.   Flushing
      e.   Anxiety

   5.   Signs and symptoms of septic reaction include:
      a.   Rapid onset of high fever and chills
      b.   Vomiting
      c.   Diarrhea
      d.   Marked hypotension

   6.   Allergic reaction may produce:
      a.   Hives
      b.   Generalized pruritus
      c.   Wheezing or anaphylaxis (rarely)

   7.   Signs and symptoms of circulatory overload include:
      a.   Dyspnea
      b.   Cough
      c.   Rales
      d.   Jugular vein distention

   8.   Manifestations of infectious disease transmitted through trans-

fusion may develop rapidly or insidiously, depending on the disease.

9. Characteristics of GVH disease include:
   a. Skin changes (e.g., erythema, ulcerations, scaling)
   b. Edema
   c. Hair loss
   d. Hemolytic anemia, with positive Coombs' test

10. Reactions associated with massive transfusion produce varying manifestations (see the appropriate chapter in this text for information on a specific condition).

C. **Nursing diagnoses**
   1. Ineffective Breathing Pattern
   2. Decreased Cardiac Output
   3. Fluid Volume Deficit
   4. Fluid Volume Excess
   5. Impaired Gas Exchange
   6. Hyperthermia
   7. Hypothermia
   8. High Risk for Infection
   9. High Risk for Injury
   10. Pain
   11. Impaired Skin Integrity
   12. Altered Tissue Perfusion

D. **Planning and implementation**
   1. Help prevent transfusion reaction by:
      a. Meticulously verifying patient identification beginning with type and crossmatch sample collection and labeling to double-check blood product and patient identification prior to transfusion
      b. Inspecting the blood product for any gas bubbles, clotting, or abnormal color before administration
      c. Beginning transfusion slowly (1 to 2 mL/min) and observing the patient closely, particularly during the first 15 minutes (severe reactions usually manifest within 15 minutes after the start of transfusion)
      d. Transfusing blood within 4 hours, and changing blood tubing every 4 hours to minimize the risk of bacterial growth at warm room temperatures
      e. Preventing infectious disease transmission through careful donor screening or performing pretests available to identify selected infectious agents
      f. Preventing GVH disease by ensuring irradiation of blood products containing viable WBCs (i.e., whole blood, platelets, packed RBCs, and granulocytes) before transfusion; irradiation alters ability of donor lymphocytes to engraft and divide

   g.   Preventing hypothermia by warming blood unit to 37°C before transfusion
   h.   Removing leukocyte and platelet aggregates from donor blood by installing a microaggregate filter (20- or 40-μm size) in the blood line to remove these aggregates during transfusion
2. On detecting any signs or symptoms of reaction:
   a.   Stop the transfusion immediately, and notify the physician.
   b.   Disconnect the transfusion set—but keep the IV line open with 0.9% saline to provide access for possible IV drug infusion.
   c.   Send the blood bag and tubing to the blood bank for repeat typing and culture.
   d.   Draw another blood sample for plasma hemoglobin, culture, and retyping.
   e.   Collect a urine sample as soon as possible for hemoglobin determination.
3. Intervene as appropriate to address symptoms of the specific reaction:
   a.   Treatment for hemolytic reaction is directed at correcting hypotension, DIC, and renal failure associated with RBC hemolysis and hemoglobinuria.
   b.   Febrile, nonhemolytic transfusion reactions are treated symptomatically with antipyretics; leukocyte-poor blood products may be recommended for subsequent transfusions.
   c.   In septic reaction, treat septicemia with antibiotics, increased hydration, steroids, and vasopressors as prescribed.
   d.   Intervene for allergic reaction by administering antihistamines, steroids, and epinephrine as indicated by the severity of the reaction. (If hives are the only manifestation, transfusion can sometimes continue but at a slower rate.)
   e.   For circulatory overload, immediate treatment includes positioning the patient upright with feet dependent; diuretics, oxygen, and aminophylline may be prescribed.

E. Evaluation
   1. The patient maintains normal breathing pattern.
   2. The patient demonstrates adequate cardiac output.
   3. The patient reports minimal or no discomfort.
   4. The patient maintains good fluid balance.
   5. The patient remains normothermic.
   6. The patient remains free of infection.

7. The patient maintains good skin integrity, with no lesions or pruritus.
8. The patient maintains or returns to normal electrolyte and blood chemistry values.

IV. Anemias: general considerations

A. **Description: a clinical condition (not a laboratory result) defined as decrease in hemoglobin content or red cell mass that impairs oxygen transport**

B. **Etiology and pathophysiology**

1. Anemia is one of the most common problems in clinical medicine; may be primary pathology or secondary to an underlying condition.
2. Anemia is classified according to either morphologic characteristics of erythrocytes or etiologic mechanisms resulting in decreased hemoglobin or red cell mass.
3. Morphologic characteristics refer to average red cell size and hemoglobin content. Average red cell size may be normal (normocytic), smaller than normal (microcytic), or larger than normal (hypochromic).
4. Physiologic mechanisms include:
   a. Decreased or ineffective red cell or hemoglobin production (bone marrow failure)
   b. Decreased or premature red cell destruction (hemolysis)
   c. Increased red cell loss (hemorrhage)
5. Bone marrow failure (i.e., reduced erythropoiesis) may result from nutritional deficiency, toxic exposure, invasion or replacement of marrow by tumor or fibrous tissue, or unknown causes.
6. Hemolysis may result from an intrinsic red cell defect incompatible with normal cell survival or from an extrinsic factor that promotes cell destruction.

C. **Assessment findings**

1. Clinical manifestations reflect deficient oxygenation of tissues and compensatory cardiopulmonary mechanisms regardless of the cause of anemia, and include:
   a. Pallor
   b. Susceptibility to fatigue
   c. Central nervous system manifestations: headache, dizziness, lightheadedness, slowing of thought processes, irritability, restlessness, and depression
   d. Effects of increased cardiac workload: tachycardia, palpitations, and angina pectoris or congestive heart failure in susceptible persons
   e. Tachycardia and dyspnea progressing from exertional to at rest

f. Complaints of feeling cold due to blood being shunted to areas of greater need

2. Severity of symptoms depends on:
    a. Whether anemia is of rapid or gradual onset (Generally, the more rapidly anemia develops, the more severe the symptoms.)
    b. Cardiopulmonary reserve
    c. Metabolic requirements
    d. Presence of other medical disorders
    e. Specific complications and features associated with the cause of anemia

3. Clinical and laboratory indices provide information regarding the site and nature of red cell hemolysis. Hemolysis generally occurs within phagocytic cells of reticuloendothelial system, especially liver and spleen.

4. Bilirubin formed within phagocyte by metabolism of hemoglobin, and released into blood stream, increasing plasma bilirubin concentration. (Levels above 1.5 mg/dL produce visible jaundice of sclera.)

5. Hemolysis may occur directly in the blood stream in some disorders, releasing hemoglobin into plasma (hemoglobinemia); initially hemoglobin binds to plasma protein—haptoglobin—but when haptoglobin saturated, hemoglobin diffuses through renal glomeruli and into urine (hemoglobinuria), giving the urine a cola-colored appearance.

6. Diagnostic evaluation to determine cause and type of anemia includes:
    a. Hemoglobin and hematocrit
    b. Red cell indices
    c. Examination of stained blood capacity
    d. Reticulocyte count
    e. Serum iron level
    f. Total iron binding capacity
    g. Serum ferritin
    h. Serum folate level
    i. Vitamin B_{12} level
    j. Hemoglobin electrophoresis
    k. Coombs' test
    l. White blood cell studies may include bone marrow aspiration and biopsy or studies to determine the source of any chronic blood loss

D. Nursing diagnoses
1. Activity Intolerance
2. Decreased Cardiac Output
3. Altered Nutrition: Less Than Body Requirements

E. Planning and implementation

1. Direct general management toward addressing the cause of anemia and replacing blood loss as needed to sustain adequate oxygenation.

2. Promote optimal activity and protect from injury:
   a. Encourage ambulation and participation in activities of daily living (ADLs) as tolerated; emphasize hazards of immobility (e.g., hypotension, muscle wasting).
   b. Assess the patient's subjective response to activity (e.g., complaints of fatigue, weakness, lightheadedness, breathlessness).
   c. Observe for dizziness or unsteady gait, and provide support as necessary.
   d. Provide for adequate rest periods, and defer or replan activities causing undue fatigue.
   e. Teach the patient to avoid sudden movement (e.g., rising from lying to standing or bending position) because the hypotensive effect may potentiate falling.

3. Reduce activities and stimuli that cause tachycardia and increased cardiac output:
   a. Monitor vital signs at rest and with activity.
   b. Encourage the patient to report palpitations, chest pain, or dyspnea experienced with activity or psychologic stress.
   c. Provide for a quiet environment and calm activity.
   d. For a patient experiencing dyspnea, elevate the head of the bed; avoid gas-forming foods (abdominal distention may aggravate dyspnea); oxygen therapy may be necessary.
   e. Observe and report signs of fluid retention (peripheral edema, neck vein distention, decreased urinary output).

4. Provide for nutritional needs:
   a. Provide high-protein and high-calorie foods and sufficient fruits and vegetables to assure essential nutrients for erythropoiesis.
   b. Discuss necessary dietary alterations with the patient and family.
   c. Administer any prescribed nutritional supplements (e.g., iron, vitamin B_{12}, folic acid, ascorbic acid).
   d. Promote small, frequent meals to help cope with problems of fatigue and anorexia.

F. Evaluation

1. The patient demonstrates normal activity tolerance.
2. The patient remains free from injury.
3. The patient follows a progressive schedule of rest, activity, and exercise.

4. The patient maintains normal cardiac output, as evidenced by:
    a. Vital signs within normal ranges
    b. No signs of fluid retention
5. The patient maintains adequate nutritional status.

V. Iron deficiency anemia

A. **Description: a type of anemia marked by below normal total body iron and inadequate hemoglobin production for body requirements**

B. **Etiology and incidence**

1. Iron deficiency anemia can result from:
    a. Chronic blood loss secondary to GI bleeding (e.g., from ulceration, tumor, hemorrhoids, hookworm infestation), excessive menstrual bleeding, multiple pregnancies
    b. Insufficient dietary iron intake
    c. Impaired GI absorption of iron secondary to gastrectomy or prolonged, severe diarrhea
    d. Increased iron requirements during periods of rapid body growth, pregnancy, or menstruation
2. It is the most common type of anemia in all age groups, affecting 10% to 30% of the adult population in the United States.

C. **Pathophysiology**

1. In iron deficiency anemia, body stores of iron decrease, as do stores of transferrin (which binds with and transports iron).
2. This leads to depletion of RBC mass, resulting in decreased hemoglobin concentration and decreased oxygen-carrying capacity of the blood.

D. **Assessment findings**

1. Iron deficiency anemia presents primarily with general manifestations of anemia (see Section IV.B).
2. Skin and mucous membrane manifestations may include fissuring at angles of mouth; smooth, sore tongue; and spoon-shaped, brittle nails.
3. Some patients may exhibit pica (craving to eat unusual substances such as clay and laundry starch) or extreme craving for ice.
4. Laboratory studies commonly reveal:
    a. Microcytic hypochromia: RBCs small and relatively devoid of pigment
    b. Hemoglobin proportionally lower than hematocrit and RBC count
    c. Serum iron concentration low, total iron binding capacity high, serum ferritin low (measure of iron stores)

E. **Nursing diagnoses**

1. Activity Intolerance

   2. Decreased Cardiac Output
   3. Altered Nutrition: Less Than Body Requirements

F. Planning and implementation

   1. Direct therapeutic goals at treating the underlying cause of anemia (e.g., GI bleeding) and correcting iron deficit through diet and supplemental iron preparations.
   2. Administer parenteral iron replacement as prescribed (commonly in patients with malabsorption, those who experience intractable GI side effects with oral preparations, or those with severe recurrent deficiency due to uncontrollable blood loss). Be alert for anaphylactic reaction following either intramuscular or IV injection of iron dextran.
   3. Advise the patient that despite the use of Z-track and air-lock injection techniques, intramuscular iron injection may produce skin discoloration and local pain.
   4. Teach the patient about oral iron replacement, if prescribed.
   5. Provide information on preventive measures including:
      a. Counseling and instruction to high-risk patients (e.g., menstruating and pregnant women)
      b. Reviewing foods high in iron (e.g., organ and other meats, cooked white beans, leafy vegetables, raisins, molasses)
      c. Encouraging taking a source of vitamin C with iron-rich foods to enhance absorption
      d. Advising that tannates (in tea) and carbonates hinder iron absorption
   6. Additional nursing interventions include those common to all anemias (see Section IV.F).

G. Evaluation

   1. The patient demonstrates normal activity tolerance.
   2. The patient remains free from injury.
   3. The patient follows a progressive schedule of rest, activity, and exercise.
   4. The patient maintains normal cardiac output, as evidenced by:
      a. Vital signs within normal ranges
      b. No signs of fluid retention
   5. The patient maintains adequate nutritional status.

VI. Megaloblastic anemia

A. Description

   1. Megaloblastic anemias are hematologic disorders characterized by the production and peripheral proliferation of large, immature, and dysfunctional RBCs.
   2. Types include:
      a. Vitamin B_{12} deficiency anemia (pernicious anemia)
      b. Folic acid deficiency anemia

B. Etiology
   1. Vitamin B_{12} deficiency can result from:
      a. Inadequate dietary intake (rare, except in strict vegetarians)
      b. Faulty absorption from the GI tract due to lack of secretion of intrinsic factor, normally produced by gastric mucosal cells
      c. Certain disorders of the small intestine that impair absorption
   2. Causes of folic acid deficiency anemia include:
      a. Inadequate dietary intake, especially of uncooked vegetables and fruits; may occur in patients on prolonged IV hyperalimentation
      b. Impaired absorption in the upper jejunum
      c. Increased requirements, common in alcoholism, pregnancy, chronic hemolytic anemias
      d. Impaired use from administration of drugs that act as folic acid antagonists (e.g., methotrexate)

C. Pathophysiology
   1. Both vitamin B_{12} and folic acid are essential for normal DNA synthesis and hematopoiesis; in a deficiency of either, RBCs cannot produce DNA, so normal nuclear maturation is arrested.
   2. Cytoplasmic maturation proceeds, however, resulting in abnormally large cells with increased membrane surface area.
   3. Because DNA metabolism is essential to formation of all cellular elements in bone marrow, WBCs and platelets are diminished.

D. Assessment findings
   1. Both types of megaloblastic anemia present with common general signs and symptoms of anemia (see Section IV.D).
   2. Other manifestations may include:
      a. Smooth, sore tongue
      b. Diarrhea
      c. Paresthesias
      d. Impaired coordination and position sense
      e. Confusion, behavioral changes
   3. Diagnostic tests may reveal:
      a. Low serum and red cell folate levels and serum vitamin B_{12} level
      b. Blood smear showing marked variation in size and shape of cell and a variable number of abnormally large cells with normal hemoglobin concentration
      c. Impaired vitamin B_{12} absorption seen on Schilling test

E. Nursing diagnoses
   1. Activity Intolerance

2. Decreased Cardiac Output
3. Altered Nutrition: Less Than Body Requirements

F. Planning and implementation

1. Instruct the patient in the need for lifelong replacement of vitamin B_{12} using intramuscular injection for pernicious anemia.
2. Explain oral folic acid replacement (or possibly intramuscular injection if malabsorption is a problem) for folic acid deficiency, reassuring the patient that therapy can cease when hemoglobin returns to normal.
3. Institute general interventions common to all anemias (see Section III.F).

G. Evaluation: those common to all anemias (see Section IV.G)

VII. Sickle cell anemia

A. Description: a severe, chronic, incurable hemolytic anemia resulting from an inherited defective hemoglobin molecule (hemoglobin S) and marked by episodic painful crises

B. Etiology and incidence

1. Sickle cell anemia results from homozygous inheritance of the hemoglobin S-producing gene.
2. Incidence is highest in persons of tropical African descent; about 10% of African-Americans carry the abnormal gene (sickle cell trait), and 1 in 600 African-American infants are born with the disease.
3. Significant incidence of sickle cell anemia is also found in the Middle East, the Mediterranean area, India, South America, and the Caribbean islands.

C. Pathophysiology

1. The hemoglobin S molecule acquires its characteristic sickle shape when exposed to low oxygen tension.
2. Hemoglobin S is significantly less soluble than normal hemoglobin when it gives up its oxygen; deoxygenated hemoglobin S turns into a firm gel, deforming RBC shape.
3. Hemoglobin S-containing RBCs have a decreased survival time and adhere to vascular endothelium, causing anemia and vascular occlusion.
4. A high concentration of misshapen cells during sickling crises makes blood abnormally viscous, resulting in sluggish circulation and sludging of sickled cells, especially within microcirculation.
5. Occlusion in microcirculation increases hypoxia, which in turn triggers sickling in other RBCs, perpetuating the cycle.
6. The organs most vulnerable to infarction and necrosis include:
   a. Brain
   b. Kidneys
   c. Bone marrow and spleen

7. If ischemia or infarction occurs, the patient experiences severe pain, possibly with swelling and fever—known as *painful crisis*. Precipitating factors for painful crises include:
   a. Dehydration
   b. Infection
   c. Fatigue
   d. Menstruation
   e. Alcohol use
   f. Emotional stress
   g. Acidosis
8. *Aplastic crises* associated with infection and decreased RBC can cause a precipitous, life-threatening drop in hemoglobin.
9. Increased hemolysis (*hyperhemolytic crises*) can occur with infection, with increased bilirubin levels predisposing to gallstone formation (bilirubin stones).
10. *Sequestration crises* (most common in infants) are characterized by rapid onset of splenomegaly (from blood pooling) and a precipitous drop in hemoglobin.
11. The various types of crises often occur in combination rather than as isolated events.
12. Crises typically become less frequent and severe with aging; risk of death from crisis is greatest in children under age 5 years.
13. In persons with sickle cell anemia, premature death commonly results from the infection or from the effects of recurrent occlusion of microcirculation (e.g., cerebrovascular accident).

D. **Assessment findings**
   1. Chronic manifestations of sickle cell anemia include:
      a. Jaundice
      b. Progressively impaired kidney function
      c. Signs and symptoms secondary to hemolysis and thrombosis
      d. Enlarged facial and skull bones
      e. Susceptibility to infections, especially osteomyelitis and pneumonia
      f. Leg ulcers, usually secondary to trauma
      g. Gallstones
      h. Splenomegaly
      i. Cardiomegaly
      j. Tachycardia, flow murmurs
      k. Growth retardation
      l. Delayed puberty
      m. In adulthood, characteristic "spiderlike" body habitus (elongated extremities, narrow shoulders and hips, barrel chest, curved spine, elongated skull)
   2. Painful crisis may be marked by:
      a. Severe abdominal, chest, back, muscle, or bone pain

        b.   Increased jaundice

        c.   Dark urine

        d.   Low-grade fever

   3.   Aplastic crisis may produce:

        a.   Pallor

        b.   Dyspnea

        c.   Lethargy, stupor, possibly coma

   4.   Acute sequestration crisis is characterized by:

        a.   Pallor

        b.   Lethargy

        c.   If untreated, signs and symptoms of hypovolemic shock

   5.   Diagnosis of sickle cell anemia is confirmed by:

        a.   A stained blood smear exhibiting sickle cells

        b.   Serum electrophoresis showing hemoglobin S

E. **Nursing diagnoses**

   1.   High Risk for Infection

   2.   Knowledge Deficit

   3.   Pain

F. **Planning and implementation**

   1.   Direct management at preventing crises and controlling symptoms.

   2.   Provide pain relief:

        a.   Have the patient rest and support affected joints as indicated.

        b.   Administer and monitor effectiveness of analgesics; acute, severe pain may necessitate oral or parenteral narcotics.

        c.   Monitor narcotic administration closely to avoid impairing respiration and decreasing oxygenation.

        d.   Encourage patient-controlled analgesia, when appropriate, which may decrease the patient's anxiety concerning timely administration of pain medication and provide excellent pain relief using lower total narcotic doses.

        e.   Administer fluids (to dilute blood and reverse sludging of cells), and monitor hydration.

   3.   Provide information to assist patient and family adjustment to disease, its treatment, and prevention of crises:

        a.   Instruct in measures to prevent crises: avoid infections, dehydration, strenuous physical activity or emotional stress, tight or restrictive clothing, high altitudes.

        b.   Folic acid replacement may be indicated to support erythropoiesis.

        c.   Simple red cell or exchange transfusion may be indicated for aplastic crises, severe painful crisis unresponsive to other therapies, preoperatively to dilute the amount of sickled blood, during the final trimester of pregnancy to prevent crises, or to treat leg ulcers unresponsive to therapy.

    d. Review genetic implications, and refer for counseling as necessary.

    e. Encourage participation in support groups.

  4. Institute infection prevention measures:

    a. Encourage appropriate dental care and prompt treatment for breaks in skin integrity.

    b. Review immunization schedule with patient and family.

    c. Instruct the patient and family to observe for fever; cough; tachypnea; urinary symptoms; and any reddened, painful, or open areas and to seek prompt medical attention if they develop.

G. Evaluation

  1. The patient reports minimum or no pain.

  2. The patient and family verbalize understanding of sickle cell disorder, its causes, and signs and symptoms of crisis.

  3. The patient demonstrates appropriated self-care measures to prevent or manage infection.

VIII. Leukemias

A. Description

  1. Leukemias are malignant disorders of blood-forming tissues characterized by uncontrolled proliferation of WBCs in bone marrow, replacing normal marrow elements, and in the liver, spleen, lymph nodes, and nonhematologic organ systems (skin, kidney, GI tract, and central nervous system).

  2. Leukemias are classified according to:

    a. Specific cell line(s) involved: lymphocytic, myelocytic, monocytic

    b. Maturity of malignant cells: acute (immature cells) and chronic (differentiated cells)

  3. Types include:

    a. Acute nonlymphocytic leukemia (ANLL)

    b. Acute lymphocytic leukemia (ALL)

    c. Chronic myelogenous leukemia (CML)

    d. Chronic lymphocytic leukemia (CLL)

B. Etiology and incidence

  1. Etiology is unknown, but certain factors are associated with increased incidence, including:

    a. Exposure to radiation

    b. Chemical agents (e.g., benzene, alkylating chemotherapeutic agents)

    c. Infectious agents (viruses implicated in animal models)

    d. Genetic variables (increased incidence reported in patients with Down's syndrome; some reports of increased familial incidence)

2. Incidence varies with type:
    a. ANLL: most common in adults; incidence increases with age
    b. ALL: most common in children (85% of all cases); accounts for 90% of leukemias in children
    c. CML: uncommon before age 20; incidence rises with age
    d. CLL: the most common type of leukemia in persons age 50 and older

C. Pathophysiology

1. Acute leukemias are rapidly progressive diseases usually characterized by uncontrolled proliferation of very immature cells (blasts) in bone marrow and peripheral tissue.
2. Leukemic blast cells in marrow suppress differentiation and proliferation of normal hemopoietic cells, predisposing to severe anemia, thrombocytopenia (hemorrhage), and granulocytopenia (infection). Acute leukemias typically prove rapidly fatal if untreated.
3. ANLL affects cells committed to granulocytic, monocytic, megakaryocytic, and erythrocytic stem cell lines; typically, aberration in growth of one cell type predominates. The most common types of ANLL involve maturational arrest and proliferation of cells in myeloblastic and monoblastic stages of development.
4. ALL affects lymphoid-committed stem cell lines and is characterized by proliferation of immature lymphoid cells (lymphoblasts) in bone marrow.
5. CML involves malignancy of myeloid stem cells, with more mature cells present than in acute forms and symptoms generally not as severe as in acute forms (i.e., terminal phase of disease involves progression to less differentiated, or blastic, phase). Onset typically is gradual and insidious.
6. CLL is characterized by marked increase in mature lymphocytes in circulation and lymphoid tissue. The disease may be relatively asymptomatic over many years; progressive anemia and thrombocytopenia may result from bone marrow infiltration, immune destruction, or hypersplenism.

D. Assessment findings

1. Clinical manifestations may include:
    a. Petechiae, ecchymoses, epistaxis, gingival bleeding, retinal hemorrhages, or frank bleeding from any body orifice secondary to thrombocytopenia
    b. Gingival hypertrophy (most commonly in AML)

       c.   Pallor, fatigue, dyspnea secondary to anemia

       d.   Fever, signs and symptoms of infection due to neutropenia

       e.   Lymphadenopathy, splenomegaly, hepatomegaly due to tissue invasion

       f.   Bone pain, arthralgias secondary to pressure from rapidly proliferating cells in marrow

       g.   Neurologic effects secondary to leukemic infiltration of central nervous system

  2. Laboratory studies typically reveal:

       a.   Peripheral WBC count varying widely (1000 to >100,000/mm^3) but always including immature cells (ANLL/ALL)

       b.   Elevated leukocyte count (CML)

       c.   Low leukocyte alkaline phosphatase (CML)

       d.   Elevated leukocyte count, possibly exceeding 100,000/mm^3 (CLL)

       e.   Decreased erythrocytes, granulocytes, and platelets (CLL)

       f.   A large percentage (60% to 90%) of bone marrow's nucleated cells identified as blasts (which normally comprise up to only 5% of normal marrow elements), with reduced erythroid precursors, mature cells, and megakaryocytes (ANLL/ALL)

       g.   Philadelphia chromosome present in bone marrow cells in over 90% of patients (CML)

E. **Nursing diagnoses**

  1. Activity Intolerance

  2. Ineffective Individual Coping

  3. Fluid Volume Deficit

  4. High Risk for Infection

  5. Altered Nutrition: Less Than Body Requirements

  6. Pain

F. **Planning and implementation**

  1. Monitor temperature, and report elevation.

  2. Assess for and report other signs and symptoms of infection.

  3. Recognize that the patient is at high risk for infection when absolute neutrophil count falls below 1000/mm^3 and at grave risk when count is 500/mm^3 or less.

  4. Obtain cultures and initiate empiric IV antibiotic therapy as prescribed.

  5. Be aware that classic signs of infection may not be apparent in a patient with leukemia.

  6. Maintain a protective environment as indicated.

  7. Maintain integrity of skin and mucous membranes.

8. Teach the patient and family signs and symptoms of infection and preventive techniques.
9. Institute measures to prevent bleeding, and monitor for bleeding.
10. Provide information on scheduled treatments:
    a. For ANLL and ALL: initial combination chemotherapy, allogenic bone marrow transplantation, consolidation therapy, and intermittent long-term maintenance chemotherapy for several years
    b. For CML: initial single-agent chemotherapy, followed by long-term, low-dose maintenance therapy; in acute exacerbation phase (blast crisis), possibly bone marrow transplantation
    c. For CLL: possibly no treatment for asymptomatic patients; for symptomatic patients, initially single-agent chemotherapy, followed by combination chemotherapy and possibly splenectomy for refractory thrombocytopenia
11. Promote positive coping mechanisms to help the patient and family deal with stressors related to the disease and its treatment.
12. Provide pain relief as needed and as prescribed.
13. Promote activity in accordance with the patient's strength and tolerance. Alternate period of rest and activity as needed.
14. Teach the patient safety measures (see Section IV.F).
15. Ensure adequate nutrition and hydration.

G. Evaluation
1. The patient remains free of infection, or infection is minimized.
2. The patient exhibits minimal or no bleeding.
3. The patient demonstrates positive coping skills.
4. The patient reports minimal or no discomfort.
5. The patient maintains an activity level compatible with blood value changes.
6. The patient maintains adequate nutritional intake.
7. The patient exhibits adequate fluid balance.

IX. Lymphomas
A. Description:
1. Lymphomas are neoplastic diseases of cells of lymphoreticular system; lymphocytes and histiocytes (fixed, nonmotile macrophages).
2. Classification of lymphomas is based on:
   a. Predominant malignant cell type (i.e., lymphocytic lymphomas, histiocytic lymphomas, or Hodgkin's disease)

      b.   Degree of malignant cell differentiation (i.e., well-differentiated, poorly differentiated, or undifferentiated)

    3. Lymphomas usually are divided into two large subgroups based on morphologic appearance of involved lymph nodes:

      a.   Hodgkin's disease

      b.   Non-Hodgkin's lymphomas

    4. Mycosis fungoides is a rare, chronic cutaneous T-cell lymphoma producing skin lesions closely resembling those of Hodgkin's disease in lymph nodes and viscera.

B.   **Etiology and incidence**

    1. The etiology of lymphomas is unknown.

    2. Hodgkin's disease most commonly affects young adults; incidence is higher in males than in females and peaks in two age groups: age 15 to 38 and after age 50.

    3. Non-Hodgkin's lymphomas are two to three times more common in men than in women and affect all age groups, with incidence increasing with age.

    4. Mycosis fungoides is rare; peak incidence is between age 40 and 60.

C.   **Pathophysiology**

    1. Lymphomas usually originate in lymph nodes and may originate in or involve lymphoid tissue throughout body (e.g., spleen, tonsils, stomach wall, liver, bone marrow). They commonly spread to extralymphatic tissue (e.g., lungs, kidneys).

    2. The pathognomonic malignant cell of Hodgkin's disease is Reed-Sternberg cell, a gigantic atypical tumor cell of unique morphology and uncertain origin.

    3. Different histopathologic subtypes are associated with varying prognoses:

      a.   Lymphocyte predominant: most favorable prognosis

      b.   Nodular sclerosing: next best prognosis

      c.   Mixed cellularity: characteristically more aggressive than either nodular sclerosing or lymphocyte-predominant subtypes

      d.   Lymphocyte depleted: most unfavorable prognosis

    4. Hodgkin's disease usually shows highly predictable pattern of spread through lymphatic channels to contiguous nodes. It also may spread via hematogenous route to extranodal sites (e.g., GI tract, bone marrow, skin, and other organs).

    5. The clinical pattern at presentation determines the all-important stage (extent) of disease (Table 19–2) and strongly correlates with histologic subtype.

    6. In non-Hodgkin's lymphomas, the major determinants of clinical patterns of disease and of prognosis are:

      a.   Cell type of origin (state of differentiation)

TABLE 19–2.
Ann Arbor Staging Classification

Stage I	Involvement of a single lymph node region (I) or of a single extralymphatic organ or site (IE)
Stage II	Involvement of two or more lymph node regions on the same side of the diaphragm (II) or localized involvement of extralymphatic organ or site and of one or more lymph node regions on the same side of the diaphragm (IIE). Optional recommendation: number of node regions involved indicated by superscript (e.g., II3)
Stage III	Involvement of lymph node regions on both sides of the diaphragm (III), which may also be accompanied by localized involvement of extralymphatic organ or site (IIIE), or the spleen (IIIS), or both (IIISE)
Stage IV	Diffuse or disseminated involvement of one or more extralymphatic organs or tissues with or without associated lymph node enlargement. The reason for classifying the patient as Stage IV should be identified further by defining site by symbols
Systemic symptoms	Each stage is subdivided into A and B categories; B for those with defined symptoms and A for those without. The B classification will be given to those with (1) unexplained weight loss of more than 10% body weight in the 6 months before admission, (2) unexplained fever with temperatures above 38°C, (3) night sweats
Staging criteria	Clinical (CS) when based solely on physical examination and laboratory results. Pathologic (PS) when based on biopsies

From Williams W., et al. (Eds.). (1990). *Hematology* (4th ed.). New York: McGraw-Hill. Used by permission.

b. Pattern of growth within involved lymph nodes (follicular or diffuse)

7. Diagnostic terminology has been clarified in a major comparative study. According to the working formulation, three broad groups may be defined (Table 19–3):
   a. Low-grade or favorable group: has less aggressive cell types or possesses follicular (also called nodular) growth pattern
   b. Intermediate-grade group: has either aggressive cell types in follicular patterns or diffuse patterns of cells, many or all of which appear aggressive
   c. High-grade or unfavorable group: pattern of growth diffuse and cell type appears highly malignant

8. Non-Hodgkin's lymphomas are more likely than Hodgkin's to involve generalized lymph node disease or extranodal disease at time of diagnosis. Bone marrow invasion, with associated anemia and thrombocytopenia, and immune dysfunction, with associated infections, are evident with these lymphomas.

TABLE 19–3.
A Working Formulation of Non-Hodgkin's Lymphoma for Clinical Use: Recommendations of an Expert International Panel; Comparisons to the Rappaport Scheme

WORKING FORMULATION	RAPPAPORT TERMINOLOGY
Low Grade	
A. Malignant lymphoma Small lymphocytic consistent with chronic lymphocytic leukemia plasmacytoid	Diffuse well-differentiated lymphocytic

B. Malignant lymphoma, follicular, predominantly small cleaved cell
  diffuse areas
  sclerosis
	Nodular poorly differentiated lymphocytic

C. Malignant lymphoma, follicular mixed, small cleaved and large cell
  diffuse areas
  sclerosis
	Nodular mixed lymphocytic histiocytic

Intermediate grade	

D. Malignant lymphoma, follicular
Predominately large cell
  diffuse areas
  sclerosis
	Nodular histiocytic

E. Malignant lymphoma, diffuse small cleaved cell	Diffuse poorly differentiated lymphocytic

F. Malignant lymphoma, diffuse mixed, small and large cell
  sclerosis
  epithelioid cell component
	Diffuse mixed lymphocytic-histiocytic

G. Malignant lymphoma, diffuse
large cell
  cleaved cell
  noncleaved cell
  sclerosis
	Diffuse histiocytic

High grade	

H. Malignant lymphoma
large cell, immunoblastic
  plasmacytoid
  clear cell
  polymorphous
  epithelioid cell component
	Diffuse histiocytic

I. Malignant lymphoma
lymphoblastic
  convoluted cell
  nonconvoluted cell
	Diffuse lymphoblastic

J. Malignant lymphoma
small noncleaved cell
  Burkitt's
  follicular areas
	Diffuse undifferentiated

From DeVita, V., et al. (1985). *Cancer: Principles and Practice of Oncology* (2nd ed.). Philadelphia: J. B. Lippincott.

9. Mycosis fungoides commonly begins in skin as pruritic, red rash, and months or years later manifests with mushroomlike growths (lymphoma) varying in size from 1 to 5 cm. Disease eventually spreads to lymph nodes, spleen, liver, and lungs.

D. Assessment findings

1. Common clinical manifestations of lymphomas include:
    a. Palpable lymph nodes, especially cervical, axillae, or groin
    b. Fatigue
    c. Weight loss
    d. Mild to high fever, often exhibiting Pel-Ebstein fever pattern
    e. Chills, night sweats
    f. Pruritus

2. The disease also may produce signs and symptoms secondary to encroachment of enlarged mediastinal and retroperitoneal lymph nodes, including:
    a. Dyspnea secondary to pressure against trachea
    b. Dysphagia secondary to pressure against esophagus
    c. Laryngeal paralysis and brachial, lumbar, or sacral neuralgias secondary to pressure on nerves
    d. Edema in extremities or effusions into pleura or peritoneum due to pressure on veins
    e. Signs of obstructive jaundice from pressure on the common bile duct
    f. Splenomegaly
    g. Hepatomegaly

3. Diagnosis and staging of Hodgkin's disease involves:
    a. Lymph node biopsy to identify histologic features
    b. Chest radiograph to identify any mediastinal, hilar, or intrapulmonary disease
    c. CT scan to evaluate lymph node involvement
    d. Bone marrow biopsy
    e. Liver function tests and liver scan
    f. Lymphangiography to detect abdominal lymph node involvement, which may not be seen on CT scan
    g. Surgical staging laparotomy with splenectomy, liver and multiple lymph node biopsies to identify disease in spleen and lymph nodes below the diaphragm

4. Procedures involved in diagnosis and staging of non-Hodgkin's lymphomas include:
    a. Lymph node biopsy
    b. Bone marrow aspirate and biopsy
    c. Liver and renal function tests
    d. CT scan
    e. Laparotomy

5. Diagnosis of mycosis fungoides involves:
   a. Biopsy of skin lesions
   b. Biopsies of lymph nodes, bone marrow, liver

E. Nursing diagnoses
   1. Ineffective Individual Coping
   2. High Risk for Infection
   3. Altered Nutrition: Less Than Body Requirements
   4. Pain

F. Planning and implementation
   1. Maintain optimal skin hydration and protection to decrease pruritus.
   2. Care for skin reactions in radiation treatment fields as prescribed by radiation oncology center.
   3. Treat fever symptomatically with antipyretics once infection is ruled out.
   4. Administer analgesics as needed to relieve painful encroachment of enlarged lymph nodes.
   5. Ensure adequate nutrition and hydration.
   6. Protect the patient from infection.
   7. Instruct the patient and family about treatment protocols:
      a. For Hodgkin's disease: depending on stage, symptoms, and cell type, radiation therapy and combination chemotherapy; in disease resistant to conventional chemotherapy or in relapse, possibly intensive therapy with autologous bone marrow transplant rescue
      b. For non-Hodgkin's lymphomas: depending on staging and histopathologic classification, radiation therapy (possibly curative with localized disease) or combination chemotherapy (for widespread disease); in patients with relapsed or refractory disease after initial intensive therapy, possibly autologous (or less commonly, allogeneic) bone marrow transplantation
      c. For mycosis fungoides: based on clinical staging, topical chemotherapy (nitrogen mustard) or corticosteroids for skin manifestations, radiation therapy, systemic chemotherapy, or a combination of topical chemotherapy, radiation therapy, and systemic chemotherapy
   8. Provide emotional and psychologic support during extensive diagnostic testing and treatments.

G. Evaluation
   1. The patient reports decreased discomfort.
   2. The patient maintains adequate nutritional intake.
   3. The patient remains free of infection or exhibits only minor infection.
   4. The patient demonstrates effective coping with diagnosis and effects of treatment.

X. Multiple myeloma

A. Description: a malignant disease of plasma cells that infiltrates bone, soft tissues, lymph nodes, liver, spleen, and kidneys

B. Etiology and incidence

1. The etiology of multiple myeloma is unclear.
2. Incidence is highest in men older than age 40.

C. Pathophysiology

1. Widespread proliferation of immature plasma cells takes place mainly in bone marrow throughout the skeletal system.
2. Plasma cells derived from B lymphocytes normally produce immunoglobulins. Malignant plasma cells produce large quantities of abnormal immunoglobulin or fragments of immunoglobulin protein (Bence Jones protein) that can usually be detected in serum and urine by immunoelectrophoresis.
3. Plasma cell tumors can infiltrate extraskeletal sites such as the skin, mouth, kidneys, and pleura.
4. Osteolytic bone lesions often are associated with hypercalcemia; pathologic fractures are common, especially in vertebrae and ribs.

D. Assessment findings

1. Characteristic clinical manifestations include:
   a. Severe bone pain
   b. Signs and symptoms of anemia secondary to marrow replacement with plasma cells
   c. Weight loss
   d. Signs and symptoms of renal failure due to precipitation of immunoglobulin in tubules, hypercalciuria, increased uric acid, or infiltration of kidney with plasma cells
   e. Signs and symptoms of infection secondary to impaired antibody production
2. Diagnostic studies include:
   a. Bone marrow aspiration or biopsy demonstrating increased numbers of plasma cells
   b. Serum electrophoresis showing abnormal globulins appearing as monoclonal "spikes"; fragments of these globulins excreted in urine as Bence Jones protein
   c. Radiographs and bone scans revealing numerous osteolytic bone lesions; generalized demineralization of skeleton (osteoporosis) is common

E. Nursing diagnoses

1. Ineffective Individual Coping
2. High Risk for Infection
3. Injury: High Risk for Trauma
4. Pain

F.   Planning and implementation

1. Provide pain relief as indicated (e.g., analgesics, back brace).
2. Assess for focal sites of pain that may be palliated with radiation therapy.
3. As indicated, prepare the patient for combination chemotherapy to decrease malignant cell mass and relieve pain.
4. As indicated, prepare the patient for radiation therapy to palliate bone pain and reduce the size of extraskeletal plasma cell tumors.
5. Protect the patient from injury: Teach measures to prevent pathologic fractures, avoid immobilization (unless ambulation is contradicted due to risk of cord compression with spinal lesion), monitor for and report signs and symptoms of spinal cord compression (e.g., motor weakness or dysfunction, paresthesias or sensory loss, bladder or bowel dysfunction).
6. Ensure good hydration; avoid dehydration, which can precipitate acute renal failure.
7. Monitor serum calcium levels, and assess for signs and symptoms of hypercalcemia:
   a. Restlessness
   b. Confusion
   c. Lethargy
   d. Decreased muscle tone
   e. Cardiac dysrhythmias
8. Protect the patient from infection.
9. Provide psychosocial and emotional support.

G.   Evaluation

1. The patient reports relief of bone pain.
2. The patient exhibits increased ambulation.
3. The patient participates in the planned regimen to prevent injury.
4. The patient remains free of infection, or infection is minimized.
5. The patient exhibits positive coping skills to deal with the diagnosis and effects of treatment.

XI.   Bleeding disorders

A.   Description

1. This term refers to various disorders of impaired hemostasis—the physiologic processes involved in terminating abnormal bleeding.
2. Specific disorders include:
   a. Thrombocytopenia, a quantitative platelet disorder
   b. Idiopathic thrombocytopenic purpura (ITP), a group of bleeding disorders of unknown etiology
   c. Clotting factor defects (hemophilia A and B)

d.   Von Willebrand's disease

e.   DIC

B.   Etiology and incidence

1.   Thrombocytopenia, the most common cause of generalized bleeding, can result from:

   a.   Decreased production of platelets by marrow (e.g., infiltrative diseases of marrow such as leukemia; myelosuppressive therapy; myelofibrosis; drug effects)

   b.   Increased platelet destruction (e.g., infection, immune disorders)

   c.   Abnormal distribution or sequestration (e.g., hypersplenism)

   d.   Loss of platelets from blood stream (e.g., excessive bleeding without replacement, extracorporeal circulation)

2.   The etiology of ITP is unknown.

3.   Clotting factor defects result from inherited (sex-linked recessive) deficiency of individual coagulation factors.

   a.   Hemophilia A involves deficiency of factor VIII (antihemophilic factor); it is the most common inherited disorder of coagulation, affecting approximately 1 in 10,000 of the male population.

   b.   Hemophilia B involves deficiency of factor IX (Christmas factor); incidence is 5 to 10 times lower than for hemophilia A.

4.   Von Willebrand's disease is a common bleeding disorder of either autosomal dominant or recessive inheritance.

5.   DIC always occurs secondary to an underlying disease or condition, including:

   a.   Septicemia

   b.   Obstetrical complications

   c.   Disseminated malignancies

   d.   Massive tissue injury (burns and trauma)

   e.   Hemolytic transfusion reaction

   f.   Shock

   g.   Anaphylaxis

6.   Other acquired coagulation defects include:

   a.   Coumarin drug toxicity, which interferes with synthesis of vitamin-K-dependent coagulation factors by the liver; excessive doses or administration with other drugs that interfere with metabolism can produce prothrombin deficiency

   b.   Heparin administration, which interferes with thrombin-induced conversion of fibrinogen to fibrin

   c.   Clotting factor deficiencies resulting from impaired synthesis by the liver

       d.   Massive transfusion creating a dilutional clotting factor deficiency, unless all coagulation factors included in blood components are transfused

C. Pathophysiology

1.   Hemostasis (arrest of bleeding) involves three sequential events:

       a.   Vascular reaction: immediate vasoconstriction of injured vessels

       b.   Formation of platelet plug (normally within 5 minutes of vessel injury), which effectively stops bleeding in small vessels and provides temporary protection in larger injuries

       c.   Activation of the clotting cascade, resulting in formation of more permanent, stable fibrin clot

2.   Other mechanisms can contribute to hemostasis, including:

       a.   Hemorrhage from large wound slowed by abrupt lowering of arterial blood pressure (shock), reducing rate of blood flow throughout body

       b.   Hematoma formation or tissue swelling at site of injury, which may slow bleeding by compressing affected vessel

3.   A fibrin clot eventually will be lysed by another plasma protein system—the fibrinolytic system—once tissue repair of the vascular endothelium has occurred.

4.   Bleeding disorders can result from defects in vessels, platelets, coagulation factors, or the fibrinolytic system.

5.   Vascular disorders involve spontaneous rupture of small vessels that are defective or injured; they may be localized or widespread, and result from:

       a.   Vascular injury secondary to drug reactions, allergic disorders, collagen-vascular diseases, bacterial infections

       b.   Alteration in the connective tissue framework supporting blood vessels due to vitamin C deficiency, adrenocortical hormone excess, senile purpura

6.   Thrombocytopenia is marked by a deficient number of circulating platelets. Because platelets play a vital role in coagulation, thrombocytopenia poses a serious threat to hemostasis.

7.   ITP involves immune destruction of platelets and production of antiplatelet antibodies, which markedly shorten platelet life span.

8.   Bleeding associated with clotting factor defects, which may be very severe, characteristically manifests with large, spreading bruises and bleeding into muscles and joints with even minor trauma. Recurrent joint hemorrhages can result in such severe damage that chronic pain or ankylosis (fixation) of joint occurs.

9.   The risk of bleeding correlates with coagulation factor assay results:

a. Severe bleeding diathesis (high risk of spontaneous bleeding), with 5% or less of circulating factor VIII or IX

b. Moderate bleeding diathesis (minimal to moderate risk of spontaneous bleeding but high risk of profuse bleeding with surgery or trauma), with 5% to 25% circulating factor VIII or IX

c. Mild bleeding diathesis (rare spontaneous bleeding, abnormal bleeding with surgery or trauma), with 25% to 40% circulating factor VIII or IX

10. Von Willebrand's disease is characterized by mild deficiency of factor VIII (15% to 50% of normal) with impaired platelet function. This results in such manifestations as nosebleeds, menorrhagia, prolonged bleeding from cuts, and postoperative bleeding; massive soft tissue and joint hemorrhages are absent.

11. DIC is characterized by widespread clotting in microcirculation, leading to consumption of coagulation factors and platelets and ultimately resulting in bleeding. Bleeding can range from minimal occult internal bleeding to profuse hemorrhaging from all orifices. The clinical picture is a complex combination of thrombosis and bleeding; acute renal failure may result from fibrin deposition in renal microcirculation.

D. Assessment findings

1. Signs and symptoms of bleeding disorders vary with the particular defect (Table 19–4).

2. Vascular abnormalities usually manifest as local bleeding into

TABLE 19–4.
Clinical Distinction Between Disorders of Vessels and Platelets and Disorders of Blood Coagulation

FINDINGS	DISORDERS OF COAGULATION	DISORDERS OF PLATELETS OR VESSELS ("PURPURIC DISORDERS")
Petechiae	Rare	Characteristic
Deep dissecting hematomas	Characteristic	Rare
Superficial ecchymoses	Common; usually large and solitary	Characteristic; usually small and multiple
Hemarthrosis	Characteristic	Rare
Delayed bleeding	Common	Rare
Bleeding from superficial cuts and scratches	Minimal	Persistent; often profuse
Sex of patient	80%–90% of hereditary forms occur only in males	Relatively more common in females
Positive family history	Common	Rare

From Wintrobe M. M., et al. (1981). *Clinical Hematology* (8th ed.). Philadelphia: Lea and Febiger.

the skin; the term *purpura* refers to extravasation of blood into skin and mucous membranes.

3. Platelet defects, either quantitative or qualitative, usually produce:

   a. Petechiae

   b. Easy bruising

   c. Bleeding that generally stops with local pressure and does not recur when pressure is released

4. Coagulation factor defects usually present with:

   a. Deep tissue bleeding after minor trauma, such as intramuscular hematomas and hemarthroses (bleeding into joint spaces)

   b. Usually, no petechiae or superficial hemorrhages

   c. Recurrence of external bleeding several hours after pressure is removed

5. Abdominal, flank, or joint pain may indicate internal bleeding.

6. Hypotension, tachycardia, chest pain, pallor, cool clammy skin, tachypnea, or altered responsiveness may indicate internal bleeding associated with hypovolemia.

7. Headache and altered neurologic signs and symptoms may indicate cerebral hemorrhage.

8. Vision changes may indicate retinal hemorrhage.

9. Dyspnea, respiratory distress, hemoptysis, cyanosis, or rales may indicate interstitial hemorrhage in lungs.

10. Laboratory findings in thrombocytopenia may include:

    a. Platelet deficiency secondary to underlying disease, generally diagnosed by bone marrow aspiration and biopsy

    b. Platelet deficiency due to increased destruction, as evidenced by marrow showing increased megakaryocytes and normal platelet production

11. In ITP, laboratory studies may indicate:

    a. Abnormalities in platelet size or morphologic appearance

    b. Increased levels of immunoglobulins (IgG) or complement components identified on platelet surface

12. Findings in hemophilia A and B commonly include:

    a. Abnormal coagulation factor assay

    b. Prolonged PTT

13. Von Willebrand's disease may be marked by:

    a. Abnormal coagulation factor assay

    b. Normal platelet count

    c. Prolonged bleeding time

    d. Slightly prolonged PTT

14. Laboratory studies in DIC may reveal:

    a. Decreased platelet count

    b. Decreased fibrinogen

      c.   Prolonged PT and PTT
      d.   Increased FSP
      e.   Schistocytes (red cell fragments) on peripheral smear

E. Nursing diagnoses
1. Fear
2. High Risk for Injury
3. Knowledge Deficit
4. Pain

F. Planning and implementation
1. Observe location of petechiae and ecchymoses (e.g., presence of petechiae in the conjunctive of the eye may be a clinical indication of a tendency toward spontaneous bleeding, as opposed to petechiae over bony prominences or areas subjected to trauma).
2. Note color of ecchymoses to distinguish old versus new bleeding (purple or purplish blue, fading to green, yellow and brown with time).
3. Observe for frank bleeding from any orifice: mouth (gums), nose, vagina, rectum, urethra. Also look for bleeding from suture lines and venous access sites.
4. Test all drainage and excreta for occult blood (feces, urine, emesis, gastric drainage).
5. Assess joints for swelling, mobility limitation, and pain.
6. Assess color and temperature of skin (e.g., pale, cool, clammy); note tachypnea, hypotension, tachycardia, palpitations, altered responsiveness, or decreased urine output; these findings may indicate inadequate tissue oxygenation or decreased blood volume.
7. Measure blood loss; weigh linens, bandages, and note saturation of pads during menses.
8. Monitor for orthostatic changes in blood pressure and pulse.
9. Minimize invasive procedures; avoid injections or, if injection is essential, use small gauge needles with Z-track technique, and apply firm pressure up to 5 minutes.
10. Avoid increasing intracranial pressure with Valsalva maneuver in a patient with a platelet count $<20,000/mm^3$ due to increased risk of cerebral bleed. Symptomatically treat cough, constipation, chills, nausea, and vomiting; instruct the patient to avoid strenuous activity, forceful nose blowing, and other such actions.
11. Warn the patient to avoid alcohol and medication containing aspirin, which interfere with platelet function.
12. Instruct the patient in general preventive measures, including:
    a.   Using an electric shaver instead of a razor
    b.   Using a soft or sponge-tipped toothbrush for oral hygiene

     c.   Maintaining rigorous dental prophylaxis

     d.   Avoiding contact sports

     e.   Avoiding use of rectal thermometers, suppositories, enemas, and vaginal tampons

13.   Intervene to control bleeding, as indicated, which may include:

     a.   In thrombocytopenia, prophylactic platelet transfusions, steroids or other immune modulation, hormonal control of menstrual periods

     b.   In ITP, corticosteroids, gamma globulin, preparation for splenectomy, immunosuppression therapy (e.g., vincristine, cyclophosphamide, azathioprine)

     c.   In hemophilia A or B, appropriate replacement therapy (factor VIII or IX concentrates) to prevent or treat bleeding

     d.   In Von Willebrand's disease, cryoprecipitate, which contains factor VIII, fibrinogen, and factor XIII

     e.   In DIC, transfusion of red cells, platelets, or cryoprecipitate; IV heparin to slow coagulation process

     f.   In coumarin toxicity, oral or parenteral vitamin K to correct prothrombin deficiency; if urgent replacement needed, transfusion of single donor plasma or prothrombin complex concentrates

     g.   To correct excess heparin dosage, protamine sulfate administration

     h.   For factor deficiencies from liver disease, transfusion of fresh frozen plasma, fresh whole blood, or factor IX concentrate

14.   Promote comfort with analgesics, orthopedic devices, and a bed cradle as indicated.

15.   Provide psychologic support to the patient and family members. Assess their anxiety level and understanding of the disorder and its treatment; encourage verbalization of questions and fears.

16.   Provide information to facilitate the patient's participation and control in the preventive and therapeutic regimens; emphasize safe physical activities along with realistic restrictions.

17.   Provide information to assist the patient and family members with adjustment to the disease process, including:

     a.   Signs and symptoms in relation to disease pathophysiology

     b.   Rationale for interventions

     c.   Measures to prevent and control bleeding

     d.   Rehabilitative measures (e.g., mobilization and physiotherapy subsequent to hemarthrosis)

     e.   Genetic implications of the bleeding disorder as appropriate

    18. Refer the patient and family members to counseling or support groups as indicated.

G. **Evaluation**

    1. The patient reports minimal or no pain and an acceptable comfort level.

    2. The patient regains or maintains adequate tissue perfusion.

    3. The patient verbalizes understanding of the cause and treatment of the blood disorder.

    4. The patient demonstrates positive coping with the diagnosis and therapeutic regimen.

Bibliography

Brunner, L. S., & Suddarth, D. S. (1988). *Textbook of medical-surgical nursing* (6th ed.). Philadelphia: J. B. Lippincott.

Brunner, L. S., & Suddarth, D. S. (1986). *The Lippincott manual of nursing practice* (4th ed.). Philadelphia: J. B. Lippincott.

DeVita, Jr., V. T., Hellman, S., & Rosenberg, S. A. (1989). *Cancer: Principles and practice of oncology* (3rd ed.). Philadelphia: J. B. Lippincott.

Doenges, M. E., Jeffries, M. F., & Moorhouse, M. F. (1984). *Nursing care plans, nursing diagnoses in planning patient care*. Philadelphia: F. A. Davis.

Fishback, D. P., & Fogdall, R. P. (1981). *Coagulation: The essentials*. Baltimore: Williams & Wilkins.

Leavell, B. S., & Thorp, Jr., O. A. (1987). *Leavell and Thorp's fundamentals of clinical hematology* (5th ed.). Philadelphia: W. B. Saunders.

Luckmann, J., & Sorenson, K. C. (1987). *Medical-surgical nursing: A psychophysiologic approach* (3rd ed.). Philadelphia: W. B. Saunders.

Powers, L. W. (1989). *Diagnostic hematology: Clinical and technical principles*. St. Louis: C. V. Mosby.

Wintrobe, M. M., Lee, G. R., & Bogg, D. R. (1981). *Clinical hematology* (8th ed.). Philadelphia: Lea & Febiger.

Yasako, J. M. (1983). *Guidelines for cancer care: Symptom management*. Reston, VA: Reston Publishing.

STUDY QUESTIONS

1. The most common sign of thrombocytopenia is
   a. petechiae
   b. hemostasis
   c. melena
   d. hemarthrosis

2. Transfusion of which of the following blood components would therapeutically provide all of the coagulation factors?
   a. cryoprecipitate
   b. random donor platelets
   c. fresh frozen plasma
   d. stored whole blood

3. Which of the following clinical signs and symptoms would suggest an anemia secondary to vitamin deficiency rather than folic acid deficiency?
   a. smooth, sore tongue
   b. palpitations
   c. paresthesias
   d. dizziness

4. Mr. Andrews has a diagnosis of ITP. A CBC from today shows WBC 5000/mm³, Hgb 12.9 g/dL, and platelet count 7000/mm³. Which of the following measures should be implemented in caring for this patient?
   a. cough and deep breathe every 4 hours to prevent infection
   b. platelet transfusions to maintain platelet count above 20,000/mm³
   c. aspirin as needed to control temperature or chills
   d. stool softeners as needed to prevent constipation

5. Patient teaching about self-management of the fatigue associated with anemia should include instructions to
   a. Continue bedrest to conserve energy.
   b. Participate in all usual ADLs.
   c. Follow a progressive ambulatory program.
   d. Exercise to increase heart rate and respiratory rate to build greater endurance.

6. Which of the following would most likely be a contributing factor in the development of infection in a patient with acute leukemia?
   a. myelosuppressive effects of chemotherapy
   b. granulocytopenia
   c. immature WBCs
   d. neutrophilia

7. Ms. Kane, aged 36, has been diagnosed with iron deficiency anemia and started on a prescribed iron supplement, ferrous sulfate. Which of the following statements by Ms. Kane would lead the nurse to include the nursing diagnosis Knowledge Deficit on the patient problem list?
   a. "I take my iron supplements with food to enhance their absorption."
   b. "I know that the gastrointestinal side effects that I'm experiencing are common with ferrous sulfate."
   c. "I eat organ meats weekly because they are a good dietary source of iron."
   d. "I take vitamin C tablets to enhance iron absorption."

8. Signs and symptoms of infection in a severely neutropenic patient would most likely include
   a. chills without fever
   b. chills with fever
   c. altered mental status
   d. skin abscess

9. Ms. Hopkins, aged 26, is receiving 1 unit of packed RBCs. Her baseline vitals before transfusion were temperature, 98°F; BP, 136/72 mmHg; pulse rate, 100 beats per minute; respiratory rate, 22 breaths per minute. A routine check of vital signs 1 hour into transfusion now reveals the following changes: temperature, 101°F; BP, 140/76 mmHg; pulse rate, 104 beats per minute; and respiratory rate, 20 breaths per minute. Based on these findings, which of the following would be the most appropriate initial nursing intervention?

a. Continue the transfusion, and monitor every 15 minutes for development of further signs and symptoms.
b. Stop the transfusion immediately, and notify the physician.
c. Continue infusion, and administer aspirin for fever.
d. Slow the rate of transfusion, and continue monitoring.

10. Mr. and Mrs. Wilson's infant son has been newly diagnosed with hemophilia A. Which of the following parental actions would indicate their effective adjustment to their son's illness?
   a. They request counseling regarding family planning.
   b. They request teaching on the procedure for IV administration of factor VIII.
   c. They verbalize feelings of guilt.
   d. They discourage their child's participation in sports.

11. Ms. Burton, aged 47, has been diagnosed with multiple myeloma. Which of the following actions might indicate a knowledge deficit regarding the disease?
   a. She decreases ambulation with bone pain.
   b. She increases fluid intake.
   c. She avoids heavy lifting.
   d. She monitors her serum calcium levels.

12. Laboratory findings for Mr. Peterson, aged 57, include WBC, 10,800/mm³; Hgb, 11.2 g/dL; platelet count, 100,000/uL; and differential showing neutrophils 4%, bands 0, lymphocytes 94%, monocytes 1%, and eosinophils 1%. Based on these data, the priority nursing diagnosis for Mr. Peterson would be High Risk for
   a. Fluid Volume Deficit related to bleeding with thrombocytopenia
   b. Infection related to neutropenia
   c. Injury related to anemia
   d. Injury related to leukocytosis

13. Which of the following diseases or conditions is *least* likely to be associated with increased potential for bleeding?
   a. metastatic liver cancer
   b. gram-negative septicemia
   c. pernicious anemia
   d. iron deficiency anemia

14. Ms. Lawrence, aged 39, has been diagnosed with DIC and transferred to the medical intensive care unit (ICU) subsequent to an acute bleeding episode. In the ICU, continuous heparin drip therapy is initiated. Which of the following assessment findings would indicate a positive response to heparin therapy?
   a. increased platelet count
   b. decreased fibrinogen
   c. decreased fibrin split products
   d. decreased bleeding

15. Steven Soles, aged 17, was recently diagnosed with Hodgkin's disease. After staging, therapy is planned to include combination radiation therapy and systemic chemotherapy with MOPP (nitrogen mustard, vincristine (Oncovin), prednisone, and procarbazine). In planning care for Steven, the nurse should anticipate which of the following effects to contribute to a sense of altered body image?
   a. cushingoid appearance
   b. alopecia
   c. temporary or permanent sterility
   d. pathologic fractures

16. Which of the following would be an appropriate item to include in planning care for a severely neutropenic patient?
   a. Transfuse neutrophils (granulocytes) to prevent infection.
   b. Exclude raw vegetables from the diet.
   c. Avoid administering rectal suppositories.
   d. Prohibit vases of fresh flowers and plants in the patient's room.

ANSWER KEY

1. **Correct response: a**
    Petechiae are characteristic of quantitative or qualitative platelet defects since platelets are primarily responsible for cessation of bleeding in small vessels.
    b and c. Although these findings may occur with thrombocytopenia, they are not characteristic.
    d. Hemarthrosis is characteristic of coagulation factor deficiencies.
    Knowledge/Physiologic/Assessment

2. **Correct response: c**
    Fresh frozen plasma contains all the coagulation factors, including the labile factors (V and VIII).
    a. Cryoprecipitate contains factor VIII, fibrinogen, and factor XIII.
    b. Random donor platelets contain large amounts of platelets in a minimum (nontherapeutic) amount of plasma.
    d. Stored whole blood does not include the labile coagulation factors.
    Application/Physiologic/Implementation

3. **Correct response: c**
    Vitamin B_{12} is essential for nervous system function, and the neurologic manifestations of B_{12} deficiency are not seen in folic acid deficiency.
    a. A smooth, sore tongue may be seen with either B_{12} or folic acid deficiency.
    b and d. Palpitations and dizziness are general manifestations of anemia and can be observed in either deficiency.
    Application/Physiologic/Assessment

4. **Correct response: d**
    This patient is at risk of spontaneous bleeding. Preventing constipation decreases the risk of intracerebral bleeding secondary to increased intracranial pressure with Valsalva maneuver.
    a. Coughing increases intracranial pressure.
    b. Platelets are not transfused prophy-
    lactically in patients with ITP (cells are destroyed and produce little therapeutic benefit).
    c. Aspirin is contraindicated in bleeding disorders since it interferes with platelet function. Nonaspirin antipyretics should be used instead.
    Analysis/Safe care/Implementation

5. **Correct response: c**
    The patient should gradually increase activity and endurance, alternating periods of rest with periods of activity.
    a. Immobility is associated with muscle wasting and hypotension.
    b. Participation in the usual ADLs should be as tolerated, with activities causing undue fatigue replanned or deferred.
    d. Care should be directed toward decreasing activities that necessitate increased cardiac output—like exercise—until the anemia improves.
    Application/Health promotion/ Implementation

6. **Correct response: d**
    Neutrophilia, an increase in circulating mature neutrophils, occurs in healthy persons as a compensatory response to the onset of bacterial infection.
    a. Suppression of marrow production of WBCs due to chemotherapy puts the patient at profound risk of "nadir" sepsis.
    b. Decreased production of mature granulocytes due to chemotherapy and the disease process places the patient at risk of infection.
    c. Immature WBCs, although perhaps present in large numbers, are not functional.
    Comprehension/Health promotion/ Evaluation

7. **Correct response: a**
    Adequate iron absorption requires an acid environment; therefore, supplements should be taken between meals.
    b. Various GI side effects are common

(e.g., nausea, heartburn, abdominal cramping).

   c. Organ meats are one of the best food sources of iron.

   d. Vitamin C enhances iron absorption and is included in several iron preparations.

Application/Health promotion/Analysis (Dx)

8. **Correct response: d**

Abscess formation may not be observed in a patient with an absolute neutrophil count less than 1000/mm³ because purulent exudate is formed by the influx of WBCs at the site of inflammation.

   a and b. Infection commonly produces chills, with or without fever.

   c. Altered mental status is a common early sign of infection.

Knowledge/Physiologic/Assessment

9. **Correct response: b**

Temperature elevation may indicate a hemolytic transfusion reaction; therefore, the transfusion must be stopped and the physician and blood bank notified.

   a. If hemolytic transfusion reaction is suspected, the transfusion must be stooped immediately.

   c. Antipyretics may be administered subsequent to physician's order only if the medical diagnosis is febrile, nonhemolytic transfusion reaction.

   d. This is incorrect because the transfusion must be stopped to enable the physician to rule out hemolytic versus nonhemolytic transfusion reaction (due to leukocyte or platelet antigens).

Analysis/Safe care/Implementation

10. **Correct response: d**

Contact sports should be avoided, but noncontact sports (e.g., swimming) are acceptable activities and can contribute to the child's independence and self-esteem. Preventing the child from engaging in safe physical activity may indicate overprotective behavior.

   a. Seeking this knowledge is a positive coping strategy and indicates an understanding of the genetic implications of the disease.

   b. This request indicates an interest in participating in the therapeutic regimen, which is essential in adjusting to illness.

   c. Guilt is a common parental reaction to genetically based illnesses; identifying feelings facilitates coping.

Analysis/Psychosocial/Evaluation

11. **Correct response: a**

Immobilization should be avoided because ambulation prevents further bone resorption and hypercalcemia. Analgesics should be administered to relieve pain and help maintain mobility.

   b. This action indicates knowledge that adequate hydration prevents renal failure.

   c. This precaution is appropriate to protect against pathologic fracture.

   d. This action reflects the patient's understanding regarding predisposition to hypercalcemia due to lytic bone lessons.

Comprehension/Health promotion/Evaluation

12. **Correct response: b**

Although the patient's total WBC count is 10,800, only 4% of these cells are neutrophils, placing him at grave risk of infection (i.e., absolute neutrophil count less than 500/mm³).

   a. Although the platelet count is below normal, generally there is no significant risk of bleeding until the count falls to 50,000/mm³ or below.

   c. The patient's Hgb is near normal.

   d. The WBC count is only slightly above normal; it is the interpretation of the differential that's important.

Analysis/Safe care/Analysis (Dx)

13. **Correct response: c**

Pernicious anemia results from vitamin B₁₂ deficiency due to lack of intrinsic factor.

a. Because nearly all the coagulation factors are synthesized in the liver, any liver disease predisposes to bleeding disorders.
b. Gram-negative septicemia predisposes to DIC.
d. Bleeding is a common cause of iron deficiency anemia.

Application/Physiologic/Planning

14. **Correct response: b**
Effective heparin therapy should stop the process of intravascular coagulation, which should result in increased fibrinogen.
a. Platelet count would increase in effective therapy, due to decreased thrombus formation.
c. Lysis of thrombi should decrease.
d. Bleeding should cease due to the increased availability of platelets and coagulation factors.

Analysis/Physiologic/Evaluation

15. **Correct response: d**
Pathologic fractures are not common to

the disease process or its treatment though osteoporosis may be a potential complication of steroid use.
a. Cushingoid appearance may result from steroid therapy.
b. Alopecia is a potential side effect of chemotherapy.
c. Temporary or permanent sterility may result from the chemotherapeutic regimen.

Comprehension/Psychosocial/Planning

16. **Correct response: a**
Granulocyte transfusion is not indicated to prevent infection.
b. Raw vegetables should be avoided to provide a low-bacterial diet.
c. Rectal temperatures, suppositories, and enemas are contraindicated in order to maintain integrity of mucous membranes.
d. Flower vases and plants should be avoided since stagnant water provides a favorable medium for bacterial growth.

Application/Safe care/Planning

Infectious Disorders

I. **Anatomy and physiology**
   - A. Infectious process and chain of infection
   - B. Trends in infectious diseases

II. **Overview of infectious disorders**
   - A. Assessment
   - B. Psychosocial implications
   - C. Medications used to treat infections

III. **General nursing interventions for persons with infectious disorders**
   - A. Treat and prevent further infection
   - B. Promote comfort
   - C. Resolve any fluid volume deficit
   - D. Improve gas exchange
   - E. Provide information regarding causes, prevention, and treatment of infection
   - F. Reduce elevated body temperature
   - G. Resolve impairment in tissue integrity
   - H. Minimize social isolation

IV. **General nursing interventions to prevent infectious disorders in health care facilities**
   - A. Reduce host susceptibility
   - B. Prevent nosocomial infections
   - C. Practice proper handwashing procedures
   - D. Institute appropriate isolation procedures

V. **General nursing interventions to prevent spread of infectious disease in communities**
   - A. Perform case finding and reporting
   - B. Provide individual and community teaching
   - C. Participate in community immunization programs as possible

VI. **Septicemia and septic shock**
   - A. Description
   - B. Etiology and incidence
   - C. Pathophysiology
   - D. Assessment findings
   - E. Nursing diagnoses
   - F. Planning and implementation
   - G. Evaluation

VII. **Gonorrhea: sexually transmitted disease (STD)**
   - A. Description
   - B. Etiology and incidence
   - C. Pathophysiology
   - D. Assessment findings
   - E. Nursing diagnoses
   - F. Planning and implementation
   - G. Evaluation

VIII. **Staphylococcal infections: specific bacterial infection**
   - A. Description
   - B. Etiology
   - C. Pathophysiology
   - D. Assessment findings
   - E. Nursing diagnoses
   - F. Planning and implementation
   - G. Evaluation

IX. **Tuberculosis (TB): specific bacterial infection**
   - A. Description
   - B. Etiology and incidence
   - C. Pathophysiology
   - D. Assessment findings

I.   Anatomy and physiology

   A.   Infectious process and chain of infection

   1.   Infectious agents are defined as organisms capable of causing disease.

   2.   Organisms that normally inhibit body to maintain homeostasis (normal flora) can cause opportunistic diseases.

   3.   Not all infections (presence of organisms within a host) cause a pathologic process or disease.

   4.   Types of infectious organisms include:

      a.   Bacteria

      b.   Viruses

      c.   Rickettsia

    d.   Protozoa

    e.   Fungi

    f.   Heminths

5. Virulence refers to an organism's degree of pathogenicity (ability to cause disease).

6. Sources and reservoirs of infection include:

    a.   Communicable disease: infectious disease that can be transmitted from an infected person, animal, or object to an uninfected person

    b.   Nosocomial infection: infection acquired within a health care facility

    c.   Opportunistic infection: infection that occurs in immunocompromised hosts (e.g., elderly persons, organ transplant recipients) caused by microbes that rarely cause infection in hosts with normal immune systems

    d.   Reservoirs: commonly moist, warm environments (e.g., sewage, stagnant water)

7. Factors that increase a host's susceptibility to infection include:

    a.   Damaged or inadequate defense mechanisms

    b.   Debilitation and stress (such as in many hospitalized patients)

    c.   Invasive procedures that provide a route of access for microorganisms (e.g., urinary catheterization)

    d.   Therapies that cause immunosuppression (e.g., corticosteroids, chemotherapy)

8. The most common sites of infection are:

    a.   Urinary tract

    b.   Surgical wounds

    c.   Respiratory tract

9. Four modes of transmission to host exist:

    a.   Contact (e.g., sexually transmitted diseases [STDs])

    b.   Common source of transmission (e.g., shared foods or drinks)

    c.   Airborne (e.g., droplet nuclei resulting in tuberculosis, histoplasmosis)

    d.   Vector borne (e.g., mosquitos carrying malaria)

10. Portals of entry—the points at which infectious agents enter the host's body—include:

    a.   Skin: by organisms burrowing into skin (e.g., hookworm larvae) or through injection by insect bite (e.g., malaria)

    b.   Gastrointestinal (GI) tract: typically via contaminated foods and drinks (e.g., cholera)

    c.   Respiratory tract: via airborne droplet nuclei (e.g., tuberculosis, influenza)

     d.   Genitourinary tract: sometimes via contamination from GI tract, route for STDs

     e.   Placenta: rare, although syphilis spirochete passes through this portal

     f.   Blood: through invasive procedures (e.g., venipuncture) or via insect bites

11.   Portals of exit from the host—routes by which infectious agents leave the host body—also include the skin, GI tract, respiratory tract, genitourinary (GU) tract, placenta, and blood.

12.   Identifying the portal of exit for a specific microorganism guides interventions to prevent disease transmission (e.g., wearing gown and gloves when bathing and changing bed linen for a patient with hepatitis A because the virus leaves the host by way of the feces).

13.   The severity of infection and infectious disease depends on both host factors (e.g., susceptibility, amount of exposure) and organism factors (e.g., virulence).

14.   Exposure can result in one of four conditions:

     a.   Exposure with no infection

     b.   Subclinical infection

     c.   Disease limited by host responses (resolves without treatment)

     d.   Severe disease requiring treatment

B. Trends in infectious diseases

1.   Deaths from infectious diseases have declined greatly in industrialized nations.

2.   Infectious diseases continue to be a major cause of death in developing countries.

3.   "New" infectious diseases—such as acquired immune deficiency syndrome (AIDS)—plague both industrialized and developing nations.

II. Overview of infectious disorders

A. Assessment

1.   Nursing health history should focus on obtaining information about:

     a.   Possible recent exposure to infectious disease due to contact with a person who has a known or suspected infection or may be a carrier of infectious disease, or from travel to a place where certain infections are endemic

     b.   Current immunization status

     c.   Other medical problems that may compromise defenses (e.g., cancer, diabetes mellitus)

     d.   Systemic symptoms such as fever and chills, dysuria, arthralgias, myalgias, generalized weakness, anorexia

      e.   Signs and symptoms of local infection: redness, swelling, pain, warmth

      f.   Medication use, particularly corticosteroids, antibiotics, cancer chemotherapy

      g.   Exposure to insect or animal bites

      h.   Sexual practices

      i.   Sensitivities, allergies

2.   Significant physical assessment findings include:

      a.   Lesions of skin or mucous membranes

      b.   Skin rashes

      c.   Abnormal drainage from open lesions or body orifices

      d.   Lymph node enlargement

      e.   Altered nutritional status

      f.   Altered vital signs (e.g., elevated temperature, tachycardia, blood pressure changes)

      g.   Respiratory abnormalities (e.g., cough, breathing difficulties, changes in lung sounds)

3.   Important laboratory studies and diagnostic tests may include:

      a.   Microbiologic specimens: urine, blood, sputum, wound exudate, feces, mucous membrane secretions

      b.   White blood cell count: elevated in infection

      c.   Serology: presence of antigens or antibodies to specific diseases

B.   **Psychosocial implications**

    1.   The patient with an infectious disease may experience coping difficulties related to:

      a.   Fear of rejection based on the perceived cause of infection (e.g., unconventional sexual practices)

      b.   Uncertainty about recovery and long-term manifestations or complications

      c.   Concern about contagion

    2.   The patient also may have self-concept concerns related to fear of:

      a.   Body image changes

      b.   Rejection as a sexual partner

    3.   Disease-related lifestyle concerns may be associated with potential changes in:

      a.   Physical ability

      b.   Activity level

      c.   Work performance, with potential for job loss

    4.   Infectious disease can result in social isolation, possibly leading to:

      a.   Isolation

      b.   Depression

C.   **Medications used to treat infections**

    1.   *Inotropics and vasopressors*, used to treat septicemia and septic

shock by improving cardiac output and tissue perfusion, include:
   a.   Digoxin (e.g., Lanoxin)
   b.   Norepinephrine bitartrate (Levophed)
   c.   Nitroprusside sodium (e.g., Nipride)
2. *Antimicrobials*, used to control bacterial or fungal infections, include:
   a.   Nafcillin sodium (e.g., Nafcil, Unipen)
   b.   Cefazolin sodium (e.g., Ancef, Kefzol)
   c.   Carbenicillin disodium (e.g., Geopen)
   d.   Chloramphenicol (e.g., Chloromycetin)
   e.   Gentamicin sulfate (e.g., Garamycin)
3. *Antibiotics* include:
   a.   Penicillins
   b.   Amoxicillin trihydrate (e.g., Amoxil, Polymox)
   c.   Tetracycline hydrochloride (e.g., Achromycin)
   d.   Ceftriaxone sodium (Rocephin)
   e.   Spectinomycin hydrochloride (Trobicin)
4. *Antituberculosis agents* include:
   a.   Isoniazid (e.g., Hyzyd, Rolazid)
   b.   Rifampin (e.g., Rifadin)
   c.   Ethambutol hydrochloride (Myambutol)
5. *Antiviral agents* include amantadine hydrochloride (Symmetrel).
6. *Antipruritic agents*, used to reduce itching in skin and mucous membrane infections, include diphenhydramine hydrochloride (e.g., Benadryl).
7. *Antifungal agents* include:
   a.   Nystatin (e.g., Mycostatin, Nystex)
   b.   Clotrimazole (e.g., Lotrimin, Mycelex)
   c.   Miconazole nitrate (e.g., Monistat)
   d.   Ketoconazole (Nizoral)
   e.   Amphotericin B (Fungizone)

III. General nursing interventions for persons with infectious disorders
   A. Treat and prevent further infection (see Sections IV and V).
   B. Promote comfort.
      1. Administer analgesics as ordered.
      2. Reposition the patient as needed.
      3. Use nonpharmacologic pain control methods when appropriate, such as:
         a.   Guided imagery, distraction
         b.   Relaxation techniques
         c.   Hypnosis
         d.   Massage

    4. Provide prompt treatment for infection.

C. **Resolve any fluid volume deficit.**
    1. Assess for signs and symptoms:
        a. Postural hypotension
        b. Poor skin turgor
        c. Tachycardia
        d. Weight loss
        e. Oliguria
        f. Weakness
        g. Decreased urine specific gravity
        h. Flat neck veins
    2. Encourage oral fluid intake.
    3. Administer IV fluids if indicated.
    4. Monitor intake and output, vital signs.

D. **Improve gas exchange.**
    1. Assess for signs and symptoms of impaired gas exchange:
        a. Dyspnea
        b. Increased respiratory rate and depth
        c. Signs of hypoxia, hypercapnia
        d. Restlessness, confusion, somnolence
        e. Decreased lung sounds, rales, rhonchi, expiratory wheezes
    2. Administer oxygen therapy for hypoxia.
    3. Reposition the patient to increase lung expansion, perfusion, and ventilation.
    4. Encourage good pulmonary hygiene, including:
        a. Coughing and deep breathing exercises
        b. Diaphragmatic breathing
        c. Cessation of smoking, maintaining a smoke-free environment
    5. Facilitate mobilization of secretions through:
        a. Ensuring good hydration
        b. Promoting rest and comfort
        c. Splinting the patient's chest during coughing to minimize discomfort
        d. Administering prescribed aerosol treatments
        e. Encouraging ambulation as tolerated

E. **Provide information regarding causes, prevention, and treatment of infection.**
    1. Assess what the patient and family already know.
    2. Give brief explanations; clarify when necessary.
    3. Use audiovisual aids when available.
    4. Teach:
        a. Methods of preventing infectious disease (e.g., prophylaxis, good personal health)

    b.   Ways to prevent disease transmission

    c.   Sources of infectious diseases

    d.   Treatment for specific infectious disease

    e.   Possible complications and reportable symptoms

F. Reduce elevated body temperature.

1. Assess vital signs frequently to monitor the pattern and severity of febrile episodes.
2. Keep in mind that not every infection is accompanied by fever, and conversely, fever does not always indicate infection. In some patients, fever may be an adaptive response; thus, antipyretic measures are not always indicated.
3. In cases where antipyretic measures are indicated, provide appropriate interventions, which may include:
   a. Administering antipyretics (e.g., aspirin [*Note:* Do not give to children—may cause Reye's syndrome], acetaminophen)
   b. Removing heavy or restrictive garments and excess bed linens
   c. Sponging the patient's body with tepid water—avoid cold water or direct application of ice
   d. Applying cool compresses to areas of increased blood supply—axilla, groin, face
   e. Using a hypothermia blanket if indicated
4. Encourage increased fluid intake to replace losses from sweating.
5. Promote rest and comfort.
6. Administer antimicrobial therapy to eliminate the cause of fever.

G. Resolve impairment in tissue integrity.

1. Monitor for:
   a. Changes in skin color (e.g., blanched or reddened)
   b. Changes in turgor suggesting dehydration or edema
   c. Open lesions
2. Maintain optimal nutrition.
3. Maintain good personal hygiene.
4. Culture any draining lesions.
5. Administer appropriate topical agents.
6. Change dressings as appropriate.

H. Minimize social isolation.

1. Explain the rationale for isolation procedures to the patient and support persons.
2. Encourage the maximum social contact possible while under isolation.
3. Schedule regular periods to talk with the patient.
4. Interact with the patient in a caring, nonjudgmental manner.

5. Encourage the patient to express anxieties and emotions.
6. Discontinue isolation as soon as possible.
7. Work with the patient to devise means of reducing boredom.
8. Teach the patient stress-reduction techniques.

IV. General nursing interventions to prevent infectious disorders in health care facilities

A. Reduce host susceptibility.

1. Improve host nutritional and fluid status.
2. Administer prescribed medical therapy to treat immunodeficiencies.
3. Teach the patient about the importance of immunizations and about immunization methods.
4. Prevent damage to host defenses (e.g., avoid invasive procedures when possible).

B. Prevent nosocomial infections.

1. To prevent urinary tract infections (UTIs):
   a. Avoid urinary catheterization whenever possible.
   b. Use aseptic technique during catheterization.
   c. Maintain asepsis of urinary drainage systems.
   d. Remove urinary catheters as soon as possible.
   e. Avoid irrigating catheters.
2. To prevent surgical wound infections:
   a. Maintain asepsis intraoperatively.
   b. Use aseptic technique during dressing changes.
   c. Avoid preoperative hair removal when possible; if hair removal is necessary, use clippers or depilatories instead of razors, and remove hair immediately before surgery.
   d. Limit personnel movement into and out of the operating room (OR) during surgical procedures.
   e. Change dressings over closed wounds only when wet or if signs and symptoms of infection develop.
3. To prevent respiratory tract infections:
   a. Use only properly disinfected and sterilized respiratory equipment.
   b. Perform respiratory therapies (e.g., tracheal suctioning) using aseptical technique.
   c. Assist the patient in maintaining good respiratory hygiene through deep breathing and coughing exercises.
4. To prevent bacteremias (bacterial infections of blood):
   a. Limit invasive procedures whenever possible.
   b. Maintain aseptic technique during invasive procedures.
   c. Change IV and intra-arterial fluids and tubing at recommended intervals.
   d. Assess IV catheter sites for signs of infection.
   e. Alternate IV catheter sites at recommended intervals.

    f.   Prevent and treat infections at other body sites; microbes from other sites can gain access to vasculature.

C. **Practice proper handwashing procedures. (Thorough handwashing is the most important nursing action to decrease spread of infection.)**

  1. To wash hands:
    a.   Remove jewelry.
    b.   Use regular soap for routine patient care.
    c.   Wash for 10 to 15 seconds under briskly running water for routine patient care.
    d.   Keep nails short, and always scrub around and under them.
    e.   Use an antimicrobial product to kill organisms when working with immunocompromised patients or before invasive procedures.

  2. Be sure to wash your hands:
    a.   Following intense, prolonged patient contact
    b.   Before any invasive procedure
    c.   Before caring for susceptible patients (e.g., newborns, elderly persons)
    d.   Before and after touching mucous membranes, body fluids, secretions, or excretions—even if gloves were worn
    e.   After contact with objects that likely are contaminated (e.g., urine measuring devices)
    f.   Before entering high-risk units (e.g., intensive care nursery)
    g.   Between direct contacts with different patients

D. **Institute appropriate isolation procedures.**

  1. Category-specific isolation includes:
    a.   Strict
    b.   Contact
    c.   Respiratory
    d.   Tuberculosis
    e.   Enteric
    f.   Drainage or secretion
    g.   Blood or body

  2. Disease-specific isolation includes:
    a.   Salmonellosis
    b.   Hepatitis
    c.   Herpes zoster

  3. Take universal precautions:
    a.   Expand original body and fluid precautions.
    b.   Encourage use of gloves and other barriers when contacting blood-containing patient body fluids.

4. Ensure a private room for:
   a. Patients with certain highly communicable or virulent infections (e.g., active tuberculosis)
   b. Patients with poor personal hygiene, who are likely to contaminate the environment
5. Wear a mask, gown, and gloves when coming in contact with a patient in strict isolation (and with other patients as indicated) to prevent transmission of infection from nurse to patient.

V. General nursing interventions to prevent spread of infectious disease in communities
   A. Perform case finding and reporting.
   B. Provide individual and community teaching.
   1. Teach about methods to improve host defenses, including:
      a. Maintaining good nutrition
      b. Keeping immunizations current
   2. Teach the importance of chemoprophylaxis (e.g., taking chloroquine when traveling in malaria-infested regions).
   3. Teach ways to maintain:
      a. Good hygiene
      b. Proper sanitation
      c. Safe meal preparation
      d. Proper food storage
   4. Teach guidelines for "safe sex" to prevent STDs.
   C. Participate in community immunization programs as possible.

VI. Septicemia and septic shock
   A. Description
   1. Septicemia, or sepsis, is a systemic infection of the blood stream producing clinically apparent manifestations.
   2. Septic shock is a life-threatening form of shock resulting from uncontrolled septicemia.
   B. Etiology and incidence
   1. Septicemia most commonly results from gram-negative bacteria, including *Escherichia coli, Klebsiella, Enterobacter, Pseudomonas aeruginosa, Proteus, Neisseria meningitidis*, and *Bacteroides fragilis*. Gram-positive bacteria—*Staphylococcus aureus* and *Streptococcus pneumoniae*—have been implicated in some cases.
   2. Septicemia can produce septic shock in persons with compromised defenses; approximately 40% of cases of septic shock lead to septicemia.
   3. Risk factors include:
      a. Hospitalization
      b. Invasive procedures
      c. Immunodeficiency
      d. Advanced age

      e.   Trauma

      f.   Burns

      g.   Disorders that result in debilitation

C. **Pathophysiology**

1. The pathophysiology of septic shock is incompletely understood.
2. It is thought that shock results in reaction to an endotoxin that triggers release of chemical mediators and hormones.
3. These mediators and hormones cause cardiovascular changes and cellular injury.
4. Arteriolar and venous spasms cause pooling of blood in pulmonary, renal, splanchnic, and peripheral tissues, leading to tissue anoxia and acidosis.
5. Intense vasoconstriction increases peripheral resistance, decreases cardiac output, and diminishes blood flow to major organs.
6. Activation of factor XII of the intrinsic coagulation system can produce intravascular coagulation and fibrinolysis.
7. Death may occur from vascular collapse.
8. Septic shock typically occurs in two phases: hyperdynamic and hypodynamic.

D. **Assessment findings**

1. Septicemia commonly produces:
   a. Fever
   b. Chills
   c. Prostration
   d. Pain, headache
   e. Nausea
   f. Diarrhea
2. Clinical manifestations of septic shock depend on the stage of shock, causative organism, and patient's condition.
3. Common findings in the hyperdynamic phase include:
   a. Warm, flushed skin
   b. Normal or high urine output
   c. Mild hypotension
   d. Tachycardia
   e. Edema (due to capillary leakage)
4. Manifestations of the hypodynamic phase include:
   a. Marked hypotension
   b. Cold, dry skin
   c. Oliguria or anuria
   d. Edema
   e. Respiratory abnormalities (e.g., apnea, tachypnea)
   f. Restlessness, confusion secondary to hypoxia
   g. Altered level of consciousness

5. Laboratory studies may reveal:
   a. Causative organism identified on blood cultures
   b. Metabolic acidosis, indicated by decreased PCO_2, PO_2, HCO_3, and pH
   c. Clotting abnormalities
   d. Anemia

E. Nursing diagnoses
1. Decreased Cardiac Output
2. Impaired Verbal Communication
3. Ineffective Individual Coping
4. Fluid Volume Excess
5. Impaired Gas Exchange
6. High Risk for Infection
7. Sleep Pattern Disturbance
8. Altered Tissue Perfusion: Cardiopulmonary

F. Planning and implementation
1. Administer medications and fluids as prescribed to improve cardiac output and tissue perfusion; therapy may include:
   a. IV fluid replacement
   b. Inotropics and vasopressors (e.g., norepinephrine, sodium nitroprusside, digitalis)
   c. Antimicrobials to combat infection
   d. Diuretic agents
   e. Packed red blood cells, platelets
2. Take steps to improve gas exchange (see Section IV.D).
3. Explain all procedures to the patient to help relieve anxiety.
4. Encourage the patient and family members to communicate feelings and concerns regarding the disorder, its treatment, and possible outcome.
5. Intervene as indicated to limit blood loss due to clotting abnormalities, including:
   a. Protecting the patient from trauma that could cause hemorrhage (e.g., bumps, falls)
   b. Avoiding venipuncture and other invasive procedures whenever possible
   c. Using small-gauge needles when injections and venipuncture are unavoidable
   d. Applying firm pressure to venipuncture sites for 3 to 7 minutes; for prolonged bleeding, applying sandbags
   e. Preventing the patient from coughing, vomiting, or straining with bowel movements
   f. Providing assistance with activities of daily living or teaching the patient to avoid shaving, brushing with a hard-bristled toothbrush, and flossing
6. Assist an intubated patient with communications as needed.

7. Help the patient maintain as normal a sleep pattern as possible; keep the room quiet and dimly lit; promote rest and relaxation; cluster necessary procedures to minimize disturbances.
8. Treat and prevent further infection (see Sections V and VI).

G. **Evaluation**
1. The patient exhibits adequate cardiac output and tissue perfusion, as evidenced by:
   a. Normal blood pressure
   b. Warm skin, normal skin color
   c. Normal mentation
   d. Adequate urinary output
2. The patient maintains normal fluid balance, as evidenced by:
   a. Good skin turgor
   b. Normal blood pressure and heart rate
   c. Absence of venous distention and edema
3. The patient maintains adequate gas exchange, as indicated by:
   a. Normal respiratory rate and depth
   b. Normal arterial blood gas values
   c. No dyspnea
4. The patient demonstrates the ability to communicate needs, feelings, and concerns.
5. The patient is able to sleep uninterrupted for prolonged periods.
6. The patient exhibits minimal blood loss.
7. The patient remains free from infection.

VII. **Gonorrhea: STD**
A. **Description: a common infection of the genitourinary tract**
B. **Etiology and incidence**
1. The infectious agent is the *Neisseria gonorrhoeae* bacterium.
2. Transmission may occur through:
   a. Sexual intercourse
   b. Oral–genital contact
   c. Anal–genital contact
3. Infection also may be acquired by a newborn during vaginal delivery.
4. Gonorrhea is the most common reported communicable disease in the United States; incidence is highest in persons aged 15 to 24.
C. **Pathophysiology**
1. Gonorrhea has a short incubation period, which permits rapid spread.
2. Many disease carriers are asymptomatic.
3. The bacterium generally affects selected epithelial mucous membranes, causing inflammation:
   a. Urethritis

        b.   Cervicitis

        c.   Proctitis

  4. Coinfection with other STDs commonly occurs:

        a.   AIDS

        b.   Chlamydia

        c.   Genital herpes

        d.   Syphilis

  5. Uncomplicated gonorrhea, arthritis, hepatitis, or pelvic inflammatory disease (women) occurs.

D. **Assessment findings**

  1. Common genitourinary manifestations include:

        a.   In men: dysuria, urethral discharge, prostatitis, urethritis

        b.   In women: urinary frequency, dysuria, vaginal discharge, pelvic inflammatory disease

  2. GI manifestations (most common in homosexual males) may include:

        a.   Anal itching and irritation

        b.   Rectal bleeding

        c.   Diarrhea

        d.   Painful defecation

  3. Oral involvement may produce:

        a.   Sore throat

        b.   Lip ulcers

        c.   Inflamed gingivae

        d.   Oropharyngeal vesicles

  4. Systemic effects (in disseminated gonorrhea) may include:

        a.   Bacteremia

        b.   Hemorrhagic skin rash

        c.   Arthritis

        d.   Fever

  5. Diagnostic tests include:

        a.   In men: urethral, pharyngeal, anal cultures; gram stain of urethral smears

        b.   In women: endocervical, anal, pharyngeal cultures

E. **Nursing diagnoses**

  1. High Risk for Infection

  2. Noncompliance with Treatment and Follow-Up Regimen

  3. Pain

  4. Altered Sexuality Patterns

  5. Social Isolation

  6. Impaired Tissue Integrity

  7. Altered Patterns of Urinary Elimination

F. **Planning and implementation**

  1. Obtain a complete sexual history, ensuring the patient's privacy and covering:

           a.   Types of sexual activity engaged in

           b.   Number of sexual partners

           c.   Previous STDs or exposure to STDs

2. Minimize social isolation (see Section IV.H).

3. Minimize discomfort through prompt treatment, which may include:

    a.   Penicillin, amoxicillin, or ampicillin plus probenecid

    b.   Tetracycline

4. Treat oral or rectal lesions, pharyngitis by:

    a.   Instituting prompt antibiotic therapy, as prescribed, with proper follow-up monitoring

    b.   Teaching the patient to keep affected areas clean

5. Manage dysuria by instituting prompt antimicrobial therapy and proper follow-up care.

6. Assist the patient in maintaining intimacy with sexual partners through "safe sex" methods such as:

    a.   Mutual masturbation

    b.   Body massage, hugging

    c.   Using condoms (not 100% effective)

7. Help minimize noncompliance by:

    a.   Teaching the patient reasons for strictly adhering to the treatment and follow-up regimens

    b.   Treating the patient with respect and dignity

    c.   Ensuring privacy

    d.   Arranging follow-up appointments at convenient times for the patient

8. Teach the patient how to prevent spread of disease through:

    a.   Using forms of safe sex

    b.   Limiting the number of sex partners and learning the sexual history of potential partners before engaging in sexual contact

    c.   Referring sex partners for evaluation and treatment

    d.   Being aware of the high incidence of coinfection with other STDs

    e.   Seeking follow-up assessment after treatment to prevent recurrence

    f.   Having periodic check-ups, if sexually active, to identify STDs early

    g.   Being aware that pregnant women can pass the disease to infants during delivery

G. Evaluation

1. The patient maintains social contacts without transmitting disease.

2. The patient exhibits prompt and complete elimination of symptoms through proper treatment and follow-up.

3. The patient demonstrates compliance with the treatment regimen.
4. The patient avoids recurrence and other STDs.

VIII. Staphylococcal infections: specific bacterial infection

A. Description: infections caused by pathogenic species of *Staphylococcus*, a gram-positive bacteria; types include bacteremia, pneumonia, enterocolitis, osteomyelitis, food poisoning, and skin infections

B. Etiology
   1. The most common causative bacteria are:
      a. *Staphylococcus aureus*
      b. *Staphylococcus epidermidis*
   2. Modes of transmission include:
      a. Direct contact
      b. Common source
      c. Animal
   3. Persons at greatest risk include those with:
      a. Impaired skin integrity
      b. Newborns
      c. Prosthetic heart valves or joints

C. Pathophysiology
   1. Staphylococci are part of normal flora of the skin and mucous membranes.
   2. Staphylococci also are widely distributed in air, dust, and fomites.
   3. Local involvement may cause skin infections such as:
      a. Boils
      b. Abscesses
   4. Systemic involvement may produce:
      a. Bacteremias
      b. Toxic shock syndrome (TSS), associated with menstruation and tampon use
      c. Endocarditis
   5. Staphylococci are a common cause of nosocomial infections.
   6. *Staphylococcus epidermidis* is a common cause of infected intravascular devices.

D. Assessment findings
   1. Skin infection may be manifested by:
      a. Cellulitis
      b. Painful abscesses
      c. Boils
      d. Other skin lesions
   2. Signs and symptoms of food poisoning may include:
      a. Nausea and vomiting
      b. Abdominal cramps
      c. Diarrhea

          d.   Anorexia

3.   Invasive infection may produce signs and systems of systemic infections such as:

      a.   Endocarditis
      b.   Meningitis
      c.   Arthritis
      d.   UTIs

4.   TSS is commonly marked by:

      a.   High fever
      b.   Diarrhea
      c.   Peripheral edema, hypotension, renal failure
      d.   Desquamation of skin, especially on soles and palms
      e.   Myalgias

5.   Diagnosis is based on culture, gram stain.

E. Nursing diagnoses

1.   High Risk for Altered Body Temperature
2.   Diarrhea
3.   High Risk for Infection
4.   High Risk for Injury
5.   Pain
6.   Altered Skin Integrity
7.   Altered Tissue Perfusion: Cerebral, Cardiopulmonary, Renal
8.   Altered Patterns of Urinary Elimination

F. Planning and implementation

1.   Intervene to treat fever as indicated (see Section IV.F).
2.   Intervene as appropriate to manage effects of systemic infection (see information on specific infectious disorders in other chapters of this book).
3.   Intervene as appropriate to minimize pain (see Section IV.B).
4.   Minimize damage to tissue integrity (see Section IV.G).
5.   Intervene as necessary to maintain adequate tissue perfusion (see Section VII.D).
6.   Help minimize transmission of nosocomial infections (see Section V.B).
7.   Limit any blood losses due to clotting abnormalities (see Section VII.D).

G. Evaluation

1.   The patient maintains temperature within normal range without complications.
2.   The patient maintains a normal elimination pattern.
3.   The patient reports no or minimal pain.
4.   The patient maintains or regains integrity of skin and mucous membranes.
5.   The patient maintains adequate tissue perfusion, as evidenced by:

        a.   Adequate blood pressure, urine output

        b.   Normal mentation

        c.   Warm, dry skin of normal color

   6.   The patient exhibits minimal blood loss.

   7.   The patient demonstrates decreased incidence of nosocomial infections.

IX. Tuberculosis (TB): specific bacterial infection

A. Description: a chronic granulomatous infection that usually affects the pulmonary system but also may invade other organs and tissues

B. Etiology and incidence

   1.   Infectious agents include:

        a.   *Mycobacterium tuberculosis*

        b.   *Mycobacterium bovis* (rarely)

   2.   Transmission occurs through inhalation or ingestion of infected droplets from a person with active disease.

   3.   Incidence is greatest in crowded, poverty-stricken environments.

   4.   Those at greatest risk include immunocompromised or debilitated persons and persons with a history of previous infection.

C. Pathophysiology

   1.   Inhaled infected droplets travel to the pulmonary alveoli.

   2.   Here, the bacilli form lesions known as tubercles.

   3.   Tubercles may heal, leaving scar tissue, or may continue as granuloma, which may heal and may be reactivated later.

   4.   Granulomas may produce necrosis, liquefaction, sloughing, and cavitation of lung tissue.

   5.   The initial lesion may disseminate bacilli to other tissues (e.g., kidneys, bones, lymph nodes).

D. Assessment findings

   1.   In early stages, TB often is asymptomatic.

   2.   Manifestations of advanced TB include:

        a.   Fatigue, weight loss

        b.   Cough, initially dry, later productive of mucopurulent sputum

        c.   Hemoptysis

        d.   Fever and chills

   3.   Diagnostic tests include:

        a.   Tuberculin skin test to detect infection

        b.   Chest radiograph, sputum sample analysis to identify active disease

        c.   Follow-up sputum cultures every 2 to 4 weeks

E. Nursing diagnoses

   1.   High Risk for Altered Body Temperature

   2.   Ineffective Breathing Pattern

   3. High Risk for Infection
   4. Knowledge Deficit
   5. Noncompliance with Treatment Regimen

F. Planning and implementation

   1. Take steps to prevent disease transmission, including:
      a. Teaching the patient to cover his or her mouth and nose with thick tissue when coughing or sneezing
      b. Ensuring proper disposal of soiled tissues
      c. Emphasizing the importance of handwashing
      d. Instituting TB precautions if the patient is hospitalized
   2. Provide patient and family teaching, covering:
      a. The prescribed medication regimen (typically a 9- to 18-month course of isoniazid and rifampin plus ethambutol or streptomycin) and the need for compliance
      b. The importance of long-term treatment and follow-up care
      c. Possible complications and reportable symptoms (e.g., hemorrhage, pleurisy)
      d. The need to avoid factors that may exacerbate symptoms (e.g., smoking, asbestos, silicone exposure)
      e. The importance of skin testing for family members to identify disease in household contacts
   3. Encourage compliance with the prescribed treatment regimen by:
      a. Adapting the medication schedule to fit the patient's routine as possible
      b. Being sensitive to the patient's sociocultural environment
      c. Consulting social services to ensure insurance coverage and proper follow-up care
      d. Helping the patient minimize medication side effects
      e. Scheduling follow-up appointments at convenient times and places
      f. Treating the patient with dignity and respect
   4. Treat fever as indicated (see Section IV.F).
   5. Intervene to maintain an effective breathing pattern (see Section IV.D).

G. Evaluation

   1. The patient and family members verbalize measures to help prevent disease transmission.
   2. The patient and family members verbalize knowledge of:
      a. Medication regimen
      b. Prevention of disease spread
      c. Recognition of possible complications (e.g., hemorrhage, pleurisy)

3. The patient demonstrates compliance with the medication regimen and follow-up care schedule.
4. The patient maintains normal body temperature.
5. The patient maintains an effective breathing pattern, as evidenced by:
   a. Normal respiratory rate
   b. Regular, nonlabored breathing pattern
   c. Arterial blood gas values within normal ranges

X. Influenza: specific viral infection

A. **Description: an acute, highly contagious respiratory tract infection**

B. **Etiology and incidence**
   1. Influenza results from one of three different types of *Myxovirus influenzae*, an RNA myxovirus: Type A, Type B, or Type C.
   2. It usually occurs seasonally in epidemics.
   3. Persons at high risk include:
      a. Young children
      b. Elderly persons
      c. Persons with chronic diseases
      d. Health care workers

C. **Pathophysiology**
   1. Infection occurs via droplet transmission from an infected person or by indirect contact (e.g., drinking from a contaminated glass).
   2. The infection invades the respiratory tract epithelium, causing inflammation and desquamation; symptoms typically appear after an incubation period of 24 to 72 hours.
   3. Usually a self-limiting disorder, influenza can cause life-threatening complications (e.g., pneumonia) in high-risk persons.

D. **Assessment findings**
   1. Respiratory manifestations of influenza may include:
      a. Sinusitis
      b. Dyspnea
      c. Sore throat
      d. Nasal stuffiness
      e. Nasal discharge
      f. Dry cough
   2. Other common signs and symptoms include:
      a. Fever
      b. Chills
      c. Malaise
      d. Headache
      e. Myalgias

E. **Nursing diagnoses**
1. Activity Intolerance
2. High Risk for Altered Body Temperature
3. Ineffective Breathing Pattern
4. High Risk for Infection

F. **Planning and implementation**
1. Provide patient and family teaching, covering:
   a. Infection prevention measures (see Sections III, IV, and V)
   b. The importance of annual vaccination for persons at high risk
2. Intervene to treat fever when indicated (see Section III.F).
3. As prescribed, administer amantadine to high-risk persons as prophylaxis for influenza A.
4. Take steps to improve breathing patterns, which may include:
   a. Helping the patient relax and positioning him or her properly to ease breathing
   b. Providing room vaporization and administering antitussive agents for cough and administering decongestants for nasal stuffiness and secretions
   c. Encouraging increased fluid intake to thin secretions (and to replace fluid losses from fever)
5. Encourage adequate rest periods.

G. **Evaluation**
1. The patient avoids infection.
2. The patient maintains normal body temperature.
3. The patient exhibits normal breathing pattern.
4. The patient regains normal activity tolerance.

XI. **Rocky Mountain spotted fever: specific rickettsial infection**

A. **Description: a potentially fatal tick-borne infectious disease marked by fever and skin rash and possibly leading to shock and renal failure**

B. **Etiology and incidence**
1. The infectious agent—*Rickettsia rickettsii*—is transmitted by the dog tick (*Dermacentor variabilis*), wood tick (*Dermacentor andersoni*), and other tick species in the United States.
2. Common reservoirs include dogs and rodents and other wild animals.
3. Incidence is highest in the south-central and south Atlantic regions of the United States and peaks in early summer.

C. **Pathophysiology**
1. The infectious agent reproduces in the endothelium of small and medium-sized blood vessels, causing widespread swelling and degeneration.

2. This generalized vasculitis produces disease symptoms, which may involve multiple body organs and systems.

D. Assessment findings
1. Clinical manifestations include:
    a. Malaise, lethargy, stupor
    b. Severe headache
    c. Photophobia
    d. Anorexia
    e. High, continuous fever with chills
    f. Rash on extremities, spreading medially (usually occurring on the third to fifth day after onset)
    g. Possible skin necrosis, especially of the ear lobes, scrotum, toes, and fingers
    h. Generalized edema
    i. Myalgia, arthralgia, abdominal pain
    j. Splenomegaly
2. Laboratory findings may include:
    a. Thrombocytopenia
    b. Coagulation defects
    c. Serologic confirmation of infection

E. Nursing diagnoses
1. High Risk for Altered Body Temperature
2. High Risk for Infection
3. Pain
4. Impaired Skin Integrity

F. Planning and implementation
1. Teach preventive measures, including:
    a. Inspecting the skin frequently for ticks when in high-risk areas
    b. Tick removal (flicking an unattached tick off the skin; removing an attached tick with tweezers, grasping it close to the attachment point)
    c. Washing hands and the attachment site immediately after tick removal
2. Administer medications as prescribed, which may include:
    a. Tetracycline
    b. Chloramphenicol
3. Intervene to reduce fever as indicated (see Section III.F).
4. Intervene as appropriate to minimize pain (see Section III.B).
5. Intervene to minimize damage to skin (see Section III.G).

G. Evaluation
1. The patient verbalizes knowledge of appropriate preventive measures.
2. The patient maintains body temperature within normal range.
3. The patient reports minimal or no discomfort.

4.   The patient exhibits resolution of rash without complications.

XII.   Candidiasis: specific fungal infection

A.   **Description: a variable fungal infection producing superficial mucocutaneous and, less commonly, serious systemic manifestations**

B.   **Etiology**
1.   Infectious agents are those of the *Candida* genus (e.g., *Candida albicans, Candida tropicalis*).
2.   These organisms commonly are part of the normal flora of the GI tract, vagina, mouth, and skin.
3.   They can cause infection when some change in the body triggers proliferation or systemic invasion; such factors may include:
     a.   Immunosuppression
     b.   Invasive procedures
     c.   Use of broad-spectrum antibiotics
     d.   Hyperglycemia
     e.   Debilitation
4.   A mother with vaginal candidiasis can pass the infection on to her infant during vaginal delivery.

C.   **Pathophysiology**
1.   Candidiasis usually is a mild, superficial infection affecting the skin, mucous membranes, or nails.
2.   Rarely, organisms enter the bloodstream and invade deep organs (e.g., meninges, lungs, endocardium), causing serious infection that possibly can lead to shock and death.

D.   **Assessment findings**
1.   Manifestations of oral candidiasis (thrush) include:
     a.   Creamy, white, curdlike patches on tongue, oral mucosa
     b.   Painful, bleeding lesions, especially if patches are scraped
2.   Candida esophagitis is marked by:
     a.   Painful swallowing, feeling of obstruction with swallowing
     b.   Substernal chest discomfort
     c.   Nausea and vomiting
3.   Signs and symptoms of candida vaginitis include:
     a.   Discharge: scanty to moderate amount, thick, white, curdlike
     b.   Severe vulvar pruritus
     c.   Vaginal and labial erythema
     d.   Symptoms of secondary urethral infection
4.   Manifestations of disseminated candidiasis commonly include high fever, chills, hypotension, prostration, and possibly rash; other signs and symptoms depend on the site of infection:
     a.   Pulmonary: hemoptysis, cough

b. Renal: flank pain, dysuria, hematuria, pyuria
c. Brain: headache, nuchal rigidity, seizures, focal neurologic deficits
d. Endocardium: heart murmur, chest pain
e. Eye: blurred vision, pain, scotoma, exudate
5. Diagnosis is based on:
   a. Tissue culture
   b. Histologic examination of biopsy specimen

E. Nursing diagnoses
1. Decreased Cardiac Output
2. High Risk for Infection
3. Altered Nutrition: Less Than Body Requirements
4. Altered Oral Mucous Membrane
5. Pain
6. Impaired Tissue Integrity
7. Altered Tissue Perfusion

F. Planning and implementation
1. Alleviate pain as indicated (see Section III.B).
2. Relieve pruritus, as necessary, by:
   a. Administering antipruritic medication (e.g., diphenhydramine)
   b. Applying cool compresses to affected areas
   c. Keeping affected areas clean, dry, and open to air (if possible)
3. Institute measures to prevent infection: oral, esophageal, disseminated (see Section IV.A–D).
4. Teach patient to prevent vaginal candidiasis by:
   a. Encouraging her to have sex partners checked for infection and to use condoms to prevent transmission
   b. Avoiding tight-fitting underwear and pants
   c. Avoiding synthetic underwear; wear cotton ones instead
   d. Practicing good perineal hygiene
5. Promote good nutrition by:
   a. Assessing for signs and symptoms of undernutrition: malaise, fatigue, nausea, vomiting (risk factors); physical and biochemical indices of malnourishment
   b. Observing for decrease in intake or loss of interest in food
   c. Encouraging a high-calorie, high-protein diet
   d. Monitoring weight
   e. Encouraging small, frequent meals, especially if the patient is fatigued or nauseated
   f. Administering antiemetics as necessary
   g. Administering total parenteral nutrition or tube feedings, if indicated

6. Help the patient maintain oral mucosal integrity by:
   a. Promoting frequent, thorough mouth care
   b. Instructing the patient to avoid alcohol-containing mouthwashes, which dry the mucosa and can cause pain
   c. Administering topical antifungal agents as needed
   d. Observing for signs of disseminated infection
7. Promote good skin integrity by:
   a. Applying topical antifungal agents as prescribed
   b. Keeping affected areas clean, dry, and open to air, if possible
   c. Observing for signs of disseminated infection
8. Intervene as necessary to maintain adequate cardiac output and tissue perfusion.
9. Administer prescribed medications, which may include:
   a. For mucocutaneous candidiasis: nystatin, clotrimazole, miconazole, ketoconazole
   b. For disseminated or deep organ candidiasis: amphotericin B

G. Evaluation
1. The patient reports minor or no discomfort.
2. The patient reports reduced pruritus.
3. The patient avoids infection or reinfection and doesn't spread infection to others.
4. The patient maintains adequate nutritional status.
5. The patient displays intact oral mucosa that returns to normal state without complications.
6. The patient maintains intact skin that returns to normal state without complications.
7. The patient maintains adequate tissue perfusion and cardiac output.

XIII. Malaria: specific protozoan infection

A. Description: a serious infectious disease caused by protozoa transmitted to the blood stream through mosquito vectors

B. Etiology and incidence
1. Malaria is caused by protozoa of the genus *Plasmodium*; species include *Plasmodium falciparum*, *Plasmodium vivax*, *Plasmodium malariae*, and *Plasmodium ovale*.
2. The organism usually is transmitted to humans through the bite of the female *Anopheles* mosquito.
3. Other modes of transmission include:
   a. Transfusion of infected blood
   b. Parenteral inoculation (e.g., sharing contaminated needles)
   c. Placental leak during delivery
4. Malaria affects over 300 million people worldwide; it is endemic in tropical and subtropical climates.

C. Pathophysiology

1. After injection, *Plasmodium* sporozoites migrate through the blood stream to parenchymal liver cells.
2. Cystlike structures are formed; these contain merozoites, which invade erythrocytes, engulf hemoglobin, and eventually cause cell rupture.
3. Erythrocyte rupture releases heme (malaria pigment), cell debris, and more merozoites that, unless destroyed by phagocytosis, enter other erythrocytes.
4. An infected person then becomes a reservoir of malaria whose blood can transmit the disease to others through mosquito vectors.
5. Hepatic parasites may persist for years, producing a chronic carrier state.
6. Prognosis is good with treatment; if untreated, however, malaria can prove fatal—most commonly from disseminated intravascular coagulation or other serious complications.

D. Assessment findings

1. Common clinical manifestations include:
   a. Fever and chills, usually following a characteristic pattern of recurrence every 48 to 72 hours (depending on protozoan species)
   b. Diaphoresis
   c. Effects of pancytopenia
2. Uncomplicated malaria also may produce such signs and symptoms as:
   a. Nausea
   b. Fatigue
   c. Malaise
   d. Dizziness
   e. Headache
   f. Myalgias accompanying recurrent fever
3. Severe infections (usually associated with *P. falciparum*) may be marked by:
   a. Anemia
   b. Jaundice
   c. Renal insufficiency
   d. Adult respiratory distress syndrome (ARDS)
   e. Hemoglobinuria
   f. Diarrhea
   g. Coma
4. Relapses are common and may recur periodically for several years.
5. Diagnosis is confirmed by identification of *Plasmodium* parasites in peripheral blood.

E. Nursing diagnoses
1. High Risk for Altered Body Temperature
2. High Risk for Infection
3. Knowledge Deficit
4. Pain

F. Planning and implementation
1. Teach prevention techniques to persons traveling to areas where malaria is endemic, including:
    a. Remaining in screened areas whenever possible and using mosquito nets when outdoors
    b. Using insect repellent
    c. Staying indoors during mosquitos' most active feeding period (dusk until dawn)
    d. Taking a prophylactic antimalarial agent (e.g., chloroquine, doxycycline)
    e. Wearing clothing that covers most of the body
2. Teach strategies for prevention of disease spread, such as:
    a. Urging travelers to high-risk areas to seek prompt medical advice for flulike symptoms
    b. Instructing travelers to malaria-ridden areas to refrain from donating blood for up to 3 years following exposure
3. Teach about prescribed drug therapy, including the agent, dosage schedule, duration (usually 3 to 14 days depending on the agent), and possible side effects.
4. Provide other nursing interventions to reduce fever, minimize discomfort, and address other symptoms (see Section III).

G. Evaluation
1. The patient states appropriate measures to prevent exposure to or infection with the malaria parasite.
2. The patient verbalizes understanding of early signs and symptoms and treatment of malaria.
3. The patient maintains normal body temperature.
4. The patient reports minimum or no discomfort.
5. The patient verbalizes understanding of measures to prevent transmission of infectious disease to other persons.

XIV. Ascariasis: specific helminthic infections
A. Description: a parasitic infection caused by roundworm infestation
B. Etiology and incidence
1. The infectious organism is *Ascaris lumbricoides*, a large roundworm (15 to 35 cm long).
2. Infection is transmitted by ingesting ova contained in contaminated food, water, or soil. Direct person-to-person transmission does not occur.

    3.   Ascariasis has a worldwide distribution but is most common in tropical regions with poor sanitation and in Asia, where many farmers use human feces for crop fertilization.

C. **Pathophysiology**

    1.   After ingestion, *A. lumbricoides* ova hatch and release larvae, which penetrate the intestinal wall and travel through the blood stream to the lungs and heart.

    2.   In the lungs, larvae penetrate alveoli and move up the respiratory tree to the pharynx.

    3.   From the pharynx, larvae are swallowed; they then travel through the GI tract back to the small intestine, where they mature into worms. This entire process takes about 3 months.

    4.   The life span of *A. lumbricoides* is approximately 1½ years.

    5.   Heavy infestation can cause obstruction of the trachea, intestine, bile duct, pancreatic duct, or appendix, producing severe pain and other symptoms.

D. **Assessment findings**

    1.   Some infections are asymptomatic.

    2.   Large numbers of worms in the intestine may produce:
        a.   Severe cramping pain
        b.   Nausea and vomiting

    3.   Invasion of the lungs is commonly marked by:
        a.   Dyspnea
        b.   Fever and chills
        c.   Cough
        d.   Pneumonia

    4.   Eosinophilia commonly occurs during the larval stage.

    5.   Ascariasis is diagnosed by identifying ova or adult worms in stool.

E. **Nursing diagnoses**

    1.   Impaired Gas Exchange

    2.   High Risk for Infection

    3.   Altered Nutrition: Less Than Body Requirements

    4.   Pain

F. **Planning and implementation**

    1.   Teach preventive measures to people traveling to high-risk areas, including:
        a.   Practicing good personal hygiene
        b.   Avoiding ingestion of contaminated food or water

    2.   Intervene to minimize discomfort, improve gas exchange, and improve nutrition (see Section III).

    3.   Administer prescribed medications, which may include:
        a.   Piperazine citrate
        b.   Mebendazole
        c.   Pyrantel pamoate

G. **Evaluation**
1. The patient avoids or exhibits resolution of roundworm infection.
2. The patient states the importance of early identification and prompt treatment of infection.
3. The patient reports minor or no discomfort.
4. The patient demonstrates adequate gas exchange.
5. The patient maintains adequate nutrition.

Bibliography

American Hospital Association (1989). Management of HIV infection in the hospital. *American Journal of Infection Control, 17*(4), 24A–41A.

Brunner, L. S., & Suddarth, D. S. (1988). *Textbook of medical-surgical nursing* (6th ed.). Philadelphia: J. B. Lippincott.

Brunner, L. S., & Suddarth, D. S. (1986). *The Lippincott manual of nursing practice* (4th ed.). Philadelphia: J. B. Lippincott.

Garner, J. S. (1985). CDC guidelines for the prevention and control of nosocomial infections: Guideline for prevention of surgical wound infections. *American Journal of Infection Control, 14*(2), 71–82.

Garner, J. S., & Favero, M. S. (1986). CDC guidelines for the prevention and control of nosocomial infections: Guidelines for handwashing and hospital environmental control. *American Journal of Infection Control, 14*(3), 110–129.

Luckmann, J., & Sorenson, K. C. (1987). *Medical-surgical nursing: A psychophysiologic approach* (3rd ed.). Philadelphia: W. B. Saunders.

Lynch, P., & Jackson, M. M. (1986). Infection control: Medical asepsis. In K. C. Sorensen & J. Luckmann, *Basic nursing: A psychophysiologic approach* (2nd ed.). Philadelphia: W. B. Saunders.

Mandell, G. L., Douglas, R. G., & Bennett, J. E. (Eds.) (1990). *Principles and practices of infectious disease* (3rd ed.). New York: John Wiley & Sons.

STUDY QUESTIONS

1. The nurse discovers a sputum sample at a patient's bedside. The sample is dated with today's date, along with the patient's name and identification number, but there is no time marked on it. What should the nurse do in this situation?
   a. Send the sample to the clinical laboratory immediately.
   b. Discard the sample, and collect another one as soon as possible.
   c. Send the sample to the clinical laboratory immediately, but call the laboratory to tell them that the collection time is unknown.
   d. Refrigerate the sample, and call the clinical laboratory to pick up the specimen as soon as possible.

2. Because of the impact of STD transmission on relationships, the nurse must proceed carefully when assessing a person with suspected STD, covering all the following topics *except*
   a. previous history of STDs
   b. names of sexual partners
   c. presence of dysuria
   d. sexual history

3. When planning care for a patient in a health care facility, the nurse must be aware that a nosocomial infection
   a. occurs only in immunocompromised hosts
   b. occurs in at least 30% of patients in a given hospital
   c. usually is present within a community but is not always clinically apparent
   d. is acquired in a health care facility

4. Ms. Helms, aged 27, has just been admitted to the intensive care unit with a medical diagnosis of toxic shock syndrome. All the following nursing diagnoses likely would be appropriate for this patient *except*
   a. Altered Patterns of Urinary Elimination
   b. High Risk for Injury
   c. High Risk for Impaired Skin Integrity

   d. Altered Tissue Perfusion: Peripheral

5. All of the following interventions are recommended to prevent nosocomial wound infections *except*
   a. Avoiding hair removal when possible.
   b. Changing dressings on closed wounds only when they become wet or if signs of infection occur.
   c. If hair removal is necessary, using a clean, sharp-edged razor.
   d. Maintaining asepsis during surgery by limiting personnel movement in and out of the OR.

6. In a neonatal intensive care unit, which of the following actions should the nurse perform before caring for patients?
   a. Wash hands using a new bar of soap.
   b. Soak all rings in isopropyl alcohol for 5 minutes.
   c. Don sterile gloves instead of washing hands.
   d. Scrub around and under nails.

7. Which of the following likely would be a major nursing diagnosis for a person in the hypodynamic phase of septic shock requiring prompt intervention?
   a. Ineffective Individual Coping
   b. Altered Patterns of Urinary Elimination
   c. Decreased Cardiac Output
   d. High Risk for Infection

8. A patient with septicemia is at risk for coagulation defects. Thus, one goal of nursing intervention is to minimize the patient's blood loss. Specific indicators of successful attainment of this goal would include all the following *except*
   a. The patient displays blood pressure of 130/78 mmHg.
   b. The patient exhibits a hematocrit level of 37.
   c. The patient exhibits CVP of 8 cm H_2O.
   d. The patient demonstrates a heart rate of 135 beats per minute.

9. Mr. Gordon, aged 80, has come to a health maintenance organization for an annual physical examination during a regional flu epidemic. The nurse's evaluation that Mr. Gordon's preventive measures to protect himself against the illness are appropriate would be based on which of the following behaviors?
   a. He covers his nose and mouth with a handkerchief when he sneezes or coughs.
   b. He takes prophylactic antibiotics.
   c. He receives the appropriate flu vaccine each year.
   d. He asks to have a throat culture done to detect infection.

10. Which of the following instructions should the nurse give to a person planning a backpacking trip in an area known to have ticks that carry organisms causing Rocky Mountain spotted fever?
    a. Inspect the face and hands frequently for presence of ticks.
    b. When an unattached tick is found on the skin, flick it off.
    c. When an attached tick is found, remove it by crushing it between your fingernails.
    d. When an attached tick is found, remove it by rubbing soap on it.

11. Which of the following statements would indicate that a patient has the knowledge necessary to prevent recurrent vaginal candidiasis?
    a. "I douche regularly with a vinegar preparation."
    b. "I now wear only cotton underwear."
    c. "I have stopped using oral contraceptives."
    d. "My boyfriend now wears a condom when we have vaginal intercourse."

12. While on a trip to a malarious tropical region, the nurse determines that her traveling companion is at risk for malaria because she
    a. takes prophylactic chloroquine

    b. wears long-sleeved shirts and pants
    c. seems to nap often
    d. takes frequent evening walks

13. Ms. Taylor, aged 68, has just been admitted with uncontrolled diabetes and congestive heart failure. What actions should the nurse take to minimize this patient's risk of nosocomial infection?
    a. Insert a urinary catheter as soon as possible.
    b. Monitor PO_2 and other arterial blood gas values every 30 minutes.
    c. Change IV catheter sites only when they become infected.
    d. Teach and assist the patient to perform coughing and deep breathing exercises frequently.

14. The problem described by which one of the following nursing diagnoses would *least* likely result in creating a reservoir for infection?
    a. Functional Urinary Incontinence
    b. Impaired Skin Integrity
    c. Ineffective Breathing Pattern
    d. Fluid Volume Deficit

15. When assessing a person with suspected ascariasis, which of the following findings would the nurse *not* expect to find?
    a. fever and chills
    b. abdominal pain
    c. history of exposure to animal bites
    d. dyspnea and cough

16. Ms. Roberts, a 23-year-old single mother of two young children, comes sporadically to the infectious disease clinic for follow-up treatment of tuberculosis. The nurse knows that she is on antidepressive medication because last week at the clinic she dropped her pills and the nurse happened to pick them up. To ensure proper treatment and follow-up, all the following interventions would be appropriate *except*
    a. Arrange to have Ms. Roberts meet with the social worker to discuss insurance benefits.
    b. Schedule Ms. Roberts' appointments during her lunch break from work.

c. Tell Ms. Roberts that you understand how hard it is to comply with treatment when she is feeling blue.
d. Keep crayons and paper in the waiting room so that her children can occupy themselves while they wait.

ANSWER KEY

1. **Correct response: b**
   Prompt delivery and analysis of micro-biologic specimens is essential. Because the specimen had set for an unknown period, it must be discarded.
   a, c, and d. These actions would be inappropriate; another sample must be obtained.
   Application/Safe care/Planning

2. **Correct response: b**
   It is inappropriate to ask for names in the assessment phase. Should the patient be found to have an STD, instruct the person to notify sex partners and encourage them to be assessed and treated, if necessary.
   a and c. Sexual history and previous STD history is important information to assess the current and future risk of contracting STDs.
   d. Dysuria is a common symptom of STDs.
   Analysis/Psychosocial/Assessment

3. **Correct response: d**
   Nosocomial infections are those that are acquired during hospitalization.
   a. Nosocomial infections can occur in immunocompromised persons as well as in persons with normal immune systems.
   b. Although there can be multiple cases of nosocomial infections within an institution, they can also occur in a single patient.
   c. An endemic infection is one that is usually present within a community but is not always clinically apparent.
   Knowledge/Physiologic/Planning

4. **Correct response: a**
   Dysuria is not a symptom of TSS (it does, however, accompany UTIs caused by staphylococcal bacteria) although oliguria may be.
   b. Thrombocytopenia occurs with TSS, resulting in clotting abnormalities and excessive bleeding.
   c. Impaired skin integrity occurs with rash and subsequent desquamation of skin on palms and soles.
   d. Inadequate tissue perfusion occurs because of decreased systolic blood pressure.
   Analysis/Physiologic/Analysis (Dx)

5. **Correct response: c**
   If hair removal is necessary, depilatories or clippers are suggested.
   a, b, and d. Avoiding hair removal except when absolutely necessary, changing dressing only when necessary, and maintaining asepsis are all appropriate interventions.
   Knowledge/Safe care/Implementation

6. **Correct response: d**
   Proper handwashing includes scrubbing the nails thoroughly.
   a. In special care units, an antimicrobial cleanser should be used instead of plain soap.
   b. Jewelry should be removed before washing hands.
   c. Wearing gloves is not a substitute for handwashing.
   Application/Safe care/Planning

7. **Correct response: c**
   Although ineffective coping may occur, especially in earlier stages of septicemia, the hypodynamic phase represents a grave situation, one in which the patient may be obtunded or comatose. The septicemia may have begun as a urinary tract infection, but at the hypodynamic stage, the UTI is not likely to be a major problem. Oliguria is the probable alteration in urinary elimination. Although the septic patient is at risk for potential, additional infections, the major problem is the sequelae from the existing infection.
   a, b, and d. These diagnoses, al-

though possibly pertinent, likely would not be as high a priority as Decreased Cardiac Output for this patient.

Comprehension/Physiologic/Analysis (Dx)

8. **Correct response: d**
Tachycardia may result from blood loss with a resultant increase in heart rate to maintain cardiac output.
   a, b, and c. The other three answers are all normal values, indicating stable cardiovascular and hematologic status.

Application/Physiologic/Evaluation

9. **Correct response: c**
Vaccination is the best method of protecting against infection.
   a. Covering his nose and mouth when sneezing or coughing will protect others if he has the flu but will not protect the patient from getting it himself.
   b. Antibiotics, which work against bacteria, will not be effective against the influenza virus.
   d. Submitting to diagnostic procedures will not prevent the patient from contracting influenza.

Application/Health promotion/Evaluation

10. **Correct response: b**
Unattached ticks should be removed by flicking them off the skin.
   a. Ticks are most likely to burrow into skin in warm, moist areas of the body, including the scalp. The face and hands are less likely areas of burrowing.
   c. Attached ticks should never be crushed because crushing may expose broken skin to contaminated tick secretions. Rather, they should be removed with tweezers.
   d. Rubbing soap on an attached tick will not help remove it.

Comprehension/Health promotion/ Implementation

11. **Correct response: a**
Douches have not been shown to be effective against recurrent vaginitis.
   b. Cotton underwear are recommended because cotton is more absorbent than synthetic fabrics and thus keeps the perineal area drier.
   c. Since oral contraceptive use is associated with increased incidence of recurrent candidiasis, many practitioners recommend alternative birth control.
   d. Condom use lessens the chance of transmitting the fungus between sexual partners.

Application/Health promotion/Evaluation

12. **Correct response: d**
Because mosquitos feed at night, being out after dusk increases the risk of acquiring the disease.
   a. Prophylactic chloroquine is an appropriate intervention to prevent infection.
   b. Wearing clothes that cover most of the body helps prevent infection.
   c. Fatigue is a symptom of infection but does not indicate increased risk for infection.

Analysis/Health promotion/Assessment

13. **Correct response: d**
This intervention prevents nosocomial pneumonias.
   a. For this patient, urinary catheterization should be avoided whenever possible.
   b. Frequent invasive procedures increase risk of nosocomial bacteremias.
   c. IV sites should be changed at regular intervals and when signs of infection occur.

Application/Physiologic/Implementation

14. **Correct response: d**
Reservoirs are likely to be moist, warm environments either within the body or in the external environment, such as described in responses a, b, and c. (Ineffective breathing patterns will likely result

in the use of a respirator, with the tubing providing a moist environment.)

a, b, and c. These nursing diagnoses describe situations at high risk for creating reservoirs for infection.

Comprehension/Safe care/Analysis (Dx)

15. *Correct response: c*

Ascariosis is not transmitted through animal bites.

a, b, and d. Presence of fever, chills, abdominal pain, dyspnea, and cough are all signs and symptoms of this infectious disease, which is transmitted through contaminated food, water, or soil, not animal bites.

Analysis/Physiologic/Assessment

16. *Correct response: c*

If Ms. Roberts does not volunteer information about her depression, it would be inappropriate to discuss it with her and in fact would be an invasion of her privacy.

a. Learning about her health care benefits likely would alleviate Ms. Roberts' anxiety about expensive medical treatments.

b. Ms. Roberts would be more likely to keep appointments made at convenient times. A lunch time appointment will minimize lost income due to time away from work.

d. Ms. Roberts may have to bring her children with her to some appointments. Providing a pleasant environment to wait may reduce missed appointments.

Analysis/Psychosocial/Implementation

Cancer Nursing

619

I. Overview of cancer

A. Description

1. Cancer is the general name given to a large group of diseases characterized by:
   a. Uncontrolled growth and spread of abnormal cells
   b. Proliferation: rapid reproduction by cell division
   c. Invasion: growth of primary tumor into surrounding tissue
   d. Metastasis: spread or transfer of cancer cells from one organ or part to another not directly connected
2. Many cancers are now theorized to be multifocal or systemic (e.g., breast cancer).
3. The metastatic process may be divided into three stages:
   a. Invasion of neoplastic cells from primary tumor into surrounding tissue with penetration of blood or lymph; occurs because cells are not encapsulated
   b. Spread of tumor cells through lymph or circulation or by direct expansion
   c. Establishment and growth of tumor cells at secondary site; either in lymph filter (lymph nodes) or in organs from venous circulation

B. Theory of pathogenesis

1. Healthy cells are transformed by unknown mechanisms on exposure to certain etiologic agents, including:
   a. Viruses (e.g., Epstein-Barr, herpes simplex type II, cytomegalovirus, papillomavirus, hepatitis B)
   b. Chemical carcinogens (e.g., chromium, cobalt, tar, soot, asphalt, nitrogen mustards, certain plastics, aniline dyes, hydrocarbons in cigarette smoke, air pollutants from industry, crude paraffin oil, fuel oils, nickel, asbestos, and arsenicals)
   c. Physical stressors (e.g., excessive exposure to sunlight or radiation, chronic irritation)
   d. Hormonal factors (e.g., imbalance of endogenous or exogenous hormones, such as estrogen or diethylstilbestrol [DES])
   e. Genetic factors (e.g., abnormal chromosome patterns, such as Burkitt's lymphoma, chronic myelogenous or acute leukemia, and skin cancers, or familial predisposition, such as in breast, endometrial, colorectal, stomach, and lung cancer)
2. Development of cancer often is closely linked to immune system failure, as evidenced by:
   a. Increased incidence of malignancy in organ transplant recipients who receive immunosuppressive therapy

b. Increased risk for development of second malignancies in patients receiving long-term chemotherapy to treat a primary malignancy

3. Cancer occurrence typically reflects a combination of genetic inheritance, host mechanisms, and environmental influences; environmental factors are thought to contribute 80% to 90% of all cancers.

II. Neoplasms
A. Proliferative patterns

1. Benign and malignant cells display different characteristics of cellular growth; the degree of differentiation (anaplasia) determines cells' malignant potential.

2. *Hyperplasia* involves an increase in the number of cells in a tissue; may be a normal or an abnormal cellular response.

3. *Metaplasia* refers to the conversion of one type of cell in a tissue to another type not normal for that tissue. It results from an outside stimulus affecting parent stem cells and may be reversible or progress to dysplasia.

4. *Dysplasia* refers to a change in size, shape, or arrangement of normal cells into bizarre cells; may precede an irreversible neoplastic change.

5. *Anaplasia* involves a change in the structure of cells and in their orientation to one another, characterized by a loss of differentiation and a return to a more primitive form. The resulting poorly differentiated, irregularly shaped cells are nearly always malignant.

6. *Neoplasia* refers to abnormal cell growth; may be benign or malignant:
   a. Benign neoplasm: usually harmless and not infiltrative of other tissues
   b. Malignant neoplasm: always harmful; may spread or metastasize to tissues sometimes far removed from the site of origin

B. Characteristics of normal cells

1. The replicative cell cycle is divided into the following intervals:
   a. GO: resting phase
   b. GI: cellular production of RNA and protein in preparation for DNA synthesis; length of phase dependent on cell type
   c. S: synthesis of DNA and proteins; phase length typically 6 to 8 hours
   d. G2: RNA synthesis in preparation for mitosis; lasts only a few hours
   e. M: mitosis (cell division), resulting in two daughter cells; duration ranges from one to several hours

2. Differentiation refers to the process by which cells develop specialized structures and functions.
3. Normal cells spread until they make contact with other cells, at which point growth stops (contact inhibition).
4. Normal cells contribute in some way to homeostasis.

C. Characteristics of neoplastic cells
1. Neoplastic cells typically appear larger than normal cells, with bigger nuclei. They may bear little resemblance to the normal tissue cells.
2. These cells exhibit uncontrolled proliferation with no contact inhibition.
3. Neoplastic cells serve no homeostatic function.

D. Characteristics of neoplastic tumors
1. Neoplastic tumors are disorganized, irregular nests or sheets or neoplastic cells.
2. They tend to flourish in antagonistic physical, chemical, hormonal, and viral environments.
3. Tumors contain a high percentage of proliferating cells.
4. Approximately 20 doublings of tumor cells must occur to produce a 1-mm tumor—the smallest mass clinically detectable.
5. Some tumors have the ability to metastasize—spread from the original site to distant organs. Certain types of tumors are more likely to metastasize to certain sites.

III. Epidemiology

A. Incidence
1. The number of reported cancer cases has increased steadily since 1900; factors contributing to this rise include:
   a. Increasingly precise diagnostic methods
   b. More sophisticated gathering, analysis, and publication of statistics
   c. Increased life span (Elderly persons are more vulnerable to cancer because of accumulated years of exposure to carcinogens.)
2. Currently in the United States, more that 1 million new cases of cancer are diagnosed annually.
3. Cancer affects every age group, but more than 50% of cancers occur in persons older than age 65.
4. Men experience a higher overall incidence than women.
5. Cancer incidence is higher in industrialized nations of the world and in industrial sectors of more developed countries.

B. Mortality
1. Cancers are second only to cardiovascular diseases as the leading cause of death in the United States.
2. In order of frequency, leading causes of cancer deaths include:
   a. In men: cancers of the lung, colon or rectum, and prostate

      b.   In woman: cancers of the lung, breast, and colon or rectum

C. Survival

  1. A person exhibiting no evidence of disease for at least 5 years after diagnosis usually is considered cured; however, some cancers may require longer periods of scrutiny.

  2. Generally, 5-year survival rates have increased steadily since the 1940s.

  3. Current statistics reveal encouraging survival trends in certain cancers, including:

      a. Acute lymphocytic leukemia in children

      b. Hodgkin's disease

      c. Burkitt's lymphoma

      d. Ewing's sarcoma

      e. Wilms' tumor

      f. Rhabdomyosarcoma

      g. Choriocarcinoma

      h. Testicular cancer

      i. Ovarian cancer

      j. Osteogenic sarcoma

  4. Unfortunately, survival rates have not improved significantly for some major cancers (e.g., lung and colon).

IV. Prevention and detection of cancer

A. Early detection

  1. Recognizing early signs and symptoms and seeking prompt treatment can significantly reduce morbidity and mortality of several types of cancer.

  2. Cancer's seven early warning signals include:

      a. *Change in bowel or bladder habits*

      b. *A sore that does not heal*

      c. *Unusual bleeding or discharge*

      d. *Thickening of lump in breast or elsewhere*

      e. *Indigestion or difficulty in swallowing*

      f. *Obvious change in wart or mole*

      g. *Nagging cough or hoarseness*

B. Primary prevention

  1. Cancer prevention focuses on reducing risk factors—factors in the external and internal environment that increase a persons' susceptibility to cancer development.

  2. General factors that influence cancer incidence and mortality include:

      a. Sex

      b. Age

      c. Geographic location

      d. Socioeconomic status

      e.   Ethnic or cultural background

      f.   Personal habits

      g.   Occupation

      h.   Personal and family health histories

3.   Specific risk factors vary with the type of cancer and include:

      a.   Breast cancer: age, familial history in mother or sisters, precancerous condition on breast biopsy, obesity, first pregnancy after age 30, nulliparous status

      b.   Colorectal cancer: colorectal polyps, family history of colorectal cancer, inflammatory bowel disease, high-fat and low-fiber diet

      c.   Lung cancer: cigarette smoking, involuntary smoke inhalation, occupational exposures such as asbestos

      d.   Cervical cancer: early age at first intercourse, multiple sexual partners, human papilloma virus (HPV) infection (condyloma or warts), smoking

      e.   Endometrial cancer: obesity, prolonged use of unopposed postmenopausal estrogens, hypertension, diabetes

      f.   Urinary tract or bladder cancer: smoking, exposure to chemical carcinogen, personal history of bladder cancer

      g.   Oral cancer: smoking and alcohol use, use of smokeless tobacco

      h.   Prostate cancer: no known risk factors

      i.   Skin cancer: fair skin, sun exposure, severe sunburn in childhood, and familial conditions such as dysplastic nevus syndrome (ACS, 1989)

4.   Risk reduction involves specific actions aimed at decreasing (but not eliminating) the risk of cancer development.

5.   The American Cancer Society (ACS) has issued the following nutritional guidelines to reduce the risk of many types of cancer:

      a.   Avoiding obesity

      b.   Decreasing total dietary fat intake

      c.   Eating more high-fiber foods, such as whole grain cereals, fruits, and vegetables

      d.   Including foods rich in vitamins A and C in the daily diet

      e.   Including cruciferous vegetables (e.g., cabbage, broccoli, brussels sprouts, kohlrabi, cauliflower) in the diet

      f.   Consuming alcoholic beverages only in moderation

      g.   Consuming salt-cured, smoked, and nitrite-cured foods only in moderation

6.   Other accepted risk-reduction measures include:

      a.   Avoiding tobacco use (Cigarette smoking accounts for approximately 83% of lung cancer cases and 30% of all cancer deaths; use of smokeless tobacco increases the risk of mouth, laryngeal, throat, and esophageal cancers.)

    b.   Avoiding excessive sun exposure, particularly between 10 A.M. and 3 P.M. (Almost all cases of nonmelanoma skin cancers are considered sun related; sun exposure also is a major factor in development of melanomas.)

    c.   Avoiding exposure to industrial agents known to increase cancer risk (e.g., nickel, chromate, asbestos, vinyl chloride)

C. Secondary prevention

    1.   Secondary prevention involves detection and case-finding efforts to achieve early diagnosis.

    2.   After early detection, prompt intervention may halt the cancerous process in some cases.

V. Cancer diagnosis

A. Early detection

    1.   Early cancer detection commonly hinges on thorough, accurate:

        a.   Familial and environmental history

        b.   Physical examination

        c.   Evaluation of laboratory data and test findings

    2.   ACS guidelines for early detection of breast cancer include:

        a.   Monthly breast self-examination (BSE) by all women age 20 and older

        b.   Physical examination every 3 years from ages 20 to 40 and every year thereafter

        c.   Mammography every year for asymptomatic women age 50 and over, with baseline between ages 35 and 39

        d.   Mammography every 1 to 2 years for women age 40 to 49 depending on physical and mammographic findings

    3.   ACS guidelines for early detection of colorectal cancer include:

        a.   Digital rectal examination every year after age 40

        b.   Stool examination for occult blood every year after age 50

        c.   Proctosigmoidoscopy every 3 to 5 years after age 50 following two negative annual exams

    4.   ACS guidelines for early detection of cervical cancer include:

        a.   Annual Papanicolaou (Pap) test until two consecutive satisfactory tests are negative, then once every 3 years (less effective for endometrial cancer)

        b.   More frequent Pap tests for women with high risk factors

    5.   The ACS has not promulgated guidelines for early detection of lung cancer.

B. Tumor staging
1. Cancer staging is based on:
    a. Characteristics of primary tumor (both clinical and histologic)
    b. Involvement of lymph nodes
    c. Evidence of metastasis
2. The TNM system (T = tumor, N = node, M = metastasis) is the most commonly used staging method; designations include:
    a. TO = no evidence of primary tumor
    b. TS = carcinoma in situ (neoplasm that remains confined to site of origin, potentially invasive if not surgically removed)
    c. T1, T2, T3, T4 = progressive increase in tumor size and involvement
    d. NO = regional lymph nodes not demonstrably abnormal
    e. N1, N2, N3 = increasing degrees of demonstrable abnormality of regional lymph nodes
    f. MO = no evidence of distant metastasis
    g. M1, M2, M3 = ascending degrees of distant metastasis, including metastasis to distant lymph nodes
3. Other staging systems in widespread use include:
    a. Duke's for colon cancer
    b. Clark's for malignant melanoma

C. Tumor grading
1. Performed by a pathologist, grading involves evaluating the extent to which tumor cells differ from their normal precursors, then assigning a corresponding numerical value to reflect this differentiation.
2. Low numerical grades reflect well-differentiated tumors that deviate minimally from normal cells.
3. High numerical grades reflect poorly differentiated tumors that deviate substantially from normal cells; the highest grades are assigned to the most aberrant tumors.

D. Classification of malignant neoplasms (Table 21–1)

E. Cancer management
1. Major treatment modalities for cancer include:
    a. Surgery
    b. Radiation therapy
    c. Chemotherapy
2. Other treatments that may be useful in certain cancers include:
    a. Immunotherapy
    b. Biologic response modifiers
    c. Bone marrow transplantation

TABLE 21-1.
Classification of Neoplasms

PARENT TISSUE	BENIGN TUMOR	MALIGNANT TUMOR
Epithelium		
Skin and mucous membrane	Papilloma	Squamous cell carcinoma
	Polyp	Basal cell carcinoma
		Transitional cell carcinoma
Glands	Adenoma	Adenocarcinoma
	Cystadenoma	
Endothelium		
Blood vessels	Hemangioma	Hemangioendothelioma
		Angiosarcoma
Lymph vessels	Lymphangioma	Lymphangiosarcoma
Bone marrow		Multiple myeloma
		Ewing's sarcoma
		Leukemia
		Lymphosarcoma
		Lymphangioendothelioma
Lymphoid tissue		Reticular cell sarcoma (difficult to classify because of cell embryology)
		Lymphatic leukemia
Connective tissues		
Embryonic fibrous tissue	Myxoma	Myxosarcoma
Fibrous tissue	Fibroma	Fibrosarcoma
Adipose tissue	Lipoma	Liposarcoma
Cartilage	Chondroma	Chondrosarcoma
Bone	Osteoma	Osteogenic sarcoma
Synovial membrane	Synovioma	Synovial sarcoma
Muscle tissue		
Smooth muscle	Leiomyoma	Leiomyosarcoma
Striated muscle	Rhabdomyoma	Rhabdomyosarcoma
Nerve tissue		
Nerve fibers and sheaths	Neuroma	Neurogenic sarcoma
	Neurinoma (neurilemmoma)	
	Neurofibroma	Neurofibrosarcoma
Ganglion cells	Ganglioneuroma	Neuroblastoma
Glial cells	Glioma	Glioblastoma
		Spongioblastoma
Meninges	Meningioma	

(continued)

TABLE 21–1.
Classification of Neoplasms (Continued)

PARENT TISSUE	BENIGN TUMOR	MALIGNANT TUMOR
Pigmented neoplasms		
Melanoblasts	Pigmented nevus	Malignant melanoma
		Melanocarcinoma
Miscellaneous		
Placenta	Hydatidiform mole	Choriocarcinoma
	Dermoid cyst	Embryonal carcinoma
		Embryonal sarcoma
		Teratocarcinoma

3. Selection of recommended treatment depends on such factors as:
   a. Cancer type and stage
   b. Site
   c. Sensitivity to anticancer drugs
   d. Previous treatments
   e. Concurrent organ system dysfunction

VI. Cancer management: surgery

A. Description: surgical removal of tumors, the most commonly used treatment modality for cancer

B. Objectives

1. Preventive or prophylactic surgery involves removing precancerous lesions (e.g., unusual skin growth, colorectal polyps, cervical cancer in situ).
2. Diagnostic surgery is done to confirm or rule out malignancy from analysis of tissue samples obtained from incisional, excisional, or needle biopsies.
3. Curative surgery, the most widely used cancer treatment modality, is a localized intervention with the goal of removing all tumor tissue while limiting structural and functional impairment.
4. Reconstructive surgery aims to improve the patient's quality of life by restoring maximal function and appearance; this is possible to various degrees, depending on the cancer site and extent of surgery.
5. Palliative surgery is done to:
   a. Retard tumor growth
   b. Decrease tumor size
   c. Relieve distressing manifestations of cancer when cure is no longer possible

C. Nursing diagnoses: Basic nursing diagnoses applying to general preoperative and postoperative patient care also apply to care of patients undergoing cancer surgery (see Chapter 24, Perioperative Nursing).

D. Planning and implementation: Basic principles of preoperative and postoperative nursing care also apply to cancer surgery (see Chapter 24, Perioperative Nursing).

E. Evaluation: Evaluation criteria for patients undergoing cancer surgery are similar to those for all surgical patients (see Chapter 24, Perioperative Nursing).

VII. **Cancer management: radiation therapy (RT)**

    A. Description and overview

        1. RT involves directing high-energy ionizing radiation to destroy malignant tumor cells without harming surrounding tissues.

        2. Types of ionizing radiation include:

            a. Radiographs

            b. Gamma rays

            c. Electrons

            d. Beta particles

        3. Generally, RT is used as localized treatment for solid tumors; approximately 50% of cancer patients receive RT at some point during the course of disease.

        4. RT interrupts cellular growth by damaging cellular DNA. The degree of cellular DNA damage from RT depends on such factors as:

            a. Cellular division rate (Rapidly dividing cells are more radiosensitive.)

            b. Phase of the cell cycle (Cells undergoing DNA synthesis and mitosis are most sensitive.)

            c. Cell oxygenation level (Well-oxygenated cells are more sensitive.)

            d. Degree of cell differentiation (Poorly differentiated cells may be more sensitive than well-differentiated cells.)

        5. Damage may occur at time of treatment or later, when cells attempt to divide.

        6. Each body organ can receive only a specific, limited amount of radiation before irreparable damage to normal tissue occurs. Tissue damage can be minimized through:

            a. Fractionation (dividing total radiation dose into small, frequent doses) tumor cells less able to repair than normal cells

            b. Alternating sites of entry (ports) of radiation so that normal tissue receives only portion of total dose

            c. Using customized blocks and shields, whenever possible, to protect normal tissues

B. **Objectives**
1. Curative therapy aims to eradicate all evidence of disease and give the patient the same life expectancy as a person who never had cancer. RT is often curative for such cancers as:
   a. Hodgkin's disease
   b. Testicular seminomas
   c. Localized cancers of the head and neck
   d. Cervical cancers
2. RT also may be used as a control or an adjunct to other therapy, with the goal of prolonged and improved survival without disease eradication; examples include:
   a. Preoperative RT to shrink a tumor
   b. Postoperative RT to eradicate microscopic disease
   c. RT in conjunction with chemotherapy to prevent leukemic infiltration to the brain and spinal cord
3. RT may be used as palliative therapy in advanced cancer to relieve symptoms of metastatic disease (e.g., pain, obstruction, bleeding, pathologic fractures).

C. **Sources of radiation therapy**
1. External RT (teletherapy) usually is administered by high-energy radiograph machines (e.g., betatron, linear accelerator) or machines containing a radioisotope (e.g., Cobalt 60). Patients receiving external RT do not retain radioactivity after therapy.
2. Internal radiation therapy (brachytherapy) involves placing specially prepared radioisotopes directly into or near the tumor itself or into systemic circulation. Sources include:
   a. Sealed source: isotopes placed in applicators, needles, seeds, ribbons, or catheters before placement into malignant tumor or cavities; removed when exposure time is adequate or may be left in tumor permanently (depends on half-life of source)
   b. Unsealed source: used in systemic therapy and administered intravenously or orally (e.g., Phosphorus 32, Iodine 131)

D. **Principles of radiation protection**
1. Close contact with persons receiving internal radiation therapy provides exposure to small amounts of radiation.
2. The nurse should follow calculated safe time and distance parameters specified by the radiation physicist.
3. Protection from exposure to excessive radiation depends on:
   a. Time (The less time spent close to a radiation source, the less the exposure.)
   b. Distance (The greater the distance maintained from the source, the less the exposure.)

c. Shielding (Using lead or other materials to absorb energy helps reduce exposure in some cases; the type of rays emitted determines the radioactive precautions specified by the radiation safety officer.)

E. Radiation therapy side effects
1. Side effects are directly related to the body site being irradiated.
2. The severity of side effects depends on:
   a. Radiation dosage (daily or fractionated dose and total dose)
   b. Type of radiation
   c. Proximity of tumor to skin surface
   d. Size of treatment field
3. When counseling a patient about possible side effects, be sure to emphasize the positive benefits of therapy.

F. Nursing diagnoses
1. Diarrhea
2. Fatigue
3. High Risk for Infection
4. High Risk for Injury
5. Altered Nutrition: Less Than Body Requirements
6. Pain
7. High Risk for Impaired Skin Integrity
8. Social Isolation
9. Impaired Tissue Integrity

G. Planning and implementation
1. Never refer to radiation skin reactions as burns.
2. Supplement teaching about skin care as necessary, covering:
   a. Keeping the treatment area dry
   b. Washing with water only, patting skin dry
   c. Never applying ointment, powder, lotion, heat, ice, or other substances to the treatment field unless prescribed by the radiotherapist
   d. Avoiding washing off marks made by the radiotherapist
   e. Shaving with an electric razor only in the treatment area
   f. Avoiding clothes that rub or bind
   g. Avoiding sun exposure to the treatment site
3. Monitor WBC count, and notify the radiotherapist if it drops below 2000/μL.
4. Teach the patient with depressed WBC count signs and symptoms of infection to watch for and report.
5. Monitor platelet count, and notify the radiotherapist if it drops below 100,000/mm³.
6. Teach the patient with depressed platelet count to:
   a. Avoid physical trauma and aspirin products
   b. Report signs of hemorrhage

      c.   Avoid parenteral injections

7.   Reassure the patient that fatigue commonly results from RT and is not an indicator of worsening disease.

8.   Teach the patient to conserve energy for priority activities; encourage adequate rest.

9.   Promote a high-protein, high-calorie diet (if the patient is not a diabetic).

10.   Provide a bland diet as indicated.

11.   Monitor the oral cavity daily for signs of stomatitis.

12.   Encourage the patient to avoid smoking and alcohol ingestion.

13.   Monitor fluid and electrolyte balance, and record daily weights.

14.   Promote increased fluid intake—up to 3000 mL/day, if not contraindicated.

15.   Encourage oral hygiene only as prescribed by the radiotherapist, warning the patient to avoid commercial mouthwashes.

16.   Offer artificial saliva or sugarless candy to increase salivation if xerostomia (dryness due to salivary changes) occurs.

17.   Monitor stools for diarrhea; if indicated, reinforce a low-residue diet and high fluid intake, and administer antidiarrheal medication as prescribed.

18.   If the patient complains of nausea, administer antiemetics as prescribed, and plan rest periods before and after meals.

19.   Assess for central nervous system (CNS) changes; report any significant findings to the radiotherapist.

20.   Assess the patient's compliance with the prescribed medication regimen (e.g., steroids).

21.   Encourage the patient to express feelings and concerns related to potential hair loss secondary to RT.

22.   Suggest covering the head with a wig, scarf, or hat to reduce embarrassment.

23.   Promote gentle hair care to minimize loss (see Section VIII.J.55–61 for more information).

24.   Monitor for urinary system complications (e.g., hematuria, dysuria, frequency).

25.   Reinforce radiation safety precautions.

26.   Promote measures to reduce social isolation, such as:
    a.   Frequent telephone calls to friends and relatives
    b.   Television, radio, puzzles, hobbies depending on mobility
    c.   Frequent staff checks on the patient, with time to talk with him or her whenever possible

H.   **Evaluation**

1.   The patient shows no evidence of altered skin integrity secondary to RT.

2.   The patient demonstrates proper skin care techniques.

3. The patient displays no evidence of infection related to RT.
4. The patient exhibits no evidence of bleeding related to platelet depression.
5. The patient verbalizes understanding of the need to alter activities to adjust to weakness and fatigue.
6. The patient maintains a normal bowel elimination pattern.
7. The patient maintains dietary intake sufficient to meet nutritional needs.
8. The patient reports no pain related to complications from RT.
9. The patient interacts with others appropriately to reduce social isolation.

VIII. Cancer management: chemotherapy

A. **Description and overview**
1. Chemotherapy involves administering antineoplastic drugs to promote tumor cell death by interfering with cellular functions and reproduction.
2. It is a systemic cancer intervention for widespread disease or when the risk of undetectable disease is high.
3. Chemotherapy is administered to eradicate neoplastic cells, allowing the body's immune system to destroy remaining tumor cells.
4. Each exposure to chemotherapy destroys a percentage of tumor cells (20% to 90%), depending on dosage (cell-kill theory).
5. Repeated doses over a prolonged period are necessary to achieve tumor regression.

B. **Objectives**
1. *Curative therapy* involves early, aggressive treatment aimed at eradicating disease. Cure is considered to be achieved when the patient exhibits no evidence of disease; reference points of 5- and 10-year survival rates are used. After cure, the patient would have the same expected life span as age- and sex-matched persons without cancer.
2. A second attempt at curative intervention when disease recurs is known as *salvage therapy.*
3. *Control therapy* aims to cause or sustain tumor regression and diminish symptoms to extend and improve the patient's quality of life when cure is no longer possible.
4. *Palliative treatment* is given to relieve or diminish distressing symptoms such as pain, obstruction, pleural effusions, or hypercalcemia.

C. **Treatment methods**
1. *Combination chemotherapy* consists of two or more drugs (used effectively as single agents) administered simultaneously or in sequence to treat specific cancer and reduce the likelihood of drug resistance.

2. *Adjuvant chemotherapy* involves administering chemotherapeutic agents in combination with surgery or radiation therapy. This therapy may eradicate possible micrometastasis before it becomes clinically apparent.

D. Pharmacologic action

1. Anticancer drugs directly or indirectly disrupt reproduction of cells by altering essential biochemical processes.
2. Agents are classified according to their mechanism of action.
3. *Antimetabolites* inhibit cell reproduction by interfering with manufacture of protein; agents include:
   a. Methotrexate
   b. 5-fluorouracil (5FU)
   c. Cytosine arabinoside
   d. 6 mercaptopurine
   e. 6-thioguanine
4. *Alkylating agents* interfere with DNA replication; types include:
   a. Cyclophosphamide
   b. Thiotepa
   c. Mechlorethamine
   d. Chlorambucil
   e. Carmustine
   f. Lomustine
   g. Semustine
   h. Busulfan
   i. Phenylalanine mustard
   j. Cisplatin
   k. Decarbazine
5. *Antineoplastic antibiotics* interfere with or inhibit DNA or RNA synthesis; agents include:
   a. Actinomycin-D
   b. Mithramycin
   c. Doxorubicin
   d. Daunorubicin
   e. Bleomycin
   f. Mitomycin-C
   g. Streptozocin
6. Vinca alkaloids inhibit cell division at metaphase
   a. Vincristine
   b. Vinblastine
   c. Vindesine
7. Various *hormones and steroidal agents* may influence processes related to RNA-to-protein synthesis; these include:
   a. Adrenocortical steroids
   b. Androgens
   c. Estrogens
   d. Antiestrogens

e.   Progestins
8.   *Miscellaneous* chemotherapeutic agents with various modes of action include:
    a.   Hydroxyurea
    b.   Procarbazine
    c.   Hexamethylmelamine
    d.   Methyl-gag
    e.   L-asparaginase
9.   Chemotherapy administration may be coordinated with the cell cycle.
10. *Cell-cycle-specific agents* are effective against actively dividing cells only during certain phases of the cell cycle.
11. *Cell-cycle-nonspecific agents* act during all phases of the cell cycle.
12. Selection of specific agents depends on:
    a.   Stage of disease
    b.   Site of disease (primary site)
    c.   Sensitivity to anticancer drugs
    d.   Prior therapy
    e.   Performance status
    f.   Concurrent organ system dysfunction

E. **Administration of chemotherapy**
    1.   Administration route varies depending on the properties of the medication and the purpose of therapy.
    2.   Dosage is based primarily on total body surface area, previous therapies, and physical status.
    3.   Special care must be taken during administration of vesicant agents (e.g., dactinomycin, daunorubicin, nitrogen mustard, mithramycin, mitomycin, vinblastine, vincristine, vindesine, and streptozocin) since extravasation can cause tissue necrosis and damage to underlying tendons, nerves, and blood vessels. Only specially trained physicians and nurses should administer vesicants.
    4.   Systemic administration routes include:
        a.   Oral
        b.   Intramuscular
        c.   Subcutaneous
        d.   Intravenous
        e.   Long-term central venous catheter or implantable infusion device (may be necessary if frequent, prolonged administration of vesicants is anticipated)
    5.   Regional administration, which allows high concentrations of drugs to be directed to a localized tumor, include:
        a.   Topical (e.g., nitrogen mustard preparation used for mycosis fungoides)
        b.   Intrathecal (instillation into CNS using lumbar puncture or an Ommaya reservoir placed in a ventricle)

      c.   Intracavitary, which instills medication directly into areas such as the abdomen, bladder, or pleural space

      d.   Intraarterial, which allows major organs or tumor sites to receive maximal exposure with limited serum levels of drugs, reducing systemic side effects

      e.   Intraperitoneal chemotherapy, used to treat colorectal and ovarian cancers

F.   Limitations of chemotherapy

1. Over time, drug resistance may develop, involving emergence of a line of malignant cells resistant to specific drugs.
2. Excessive intervals between treatments can allow tumor cell population to exceed the original population.
3. Administering inadequate doses of antineoplastic drugs results in ineffective chemotherapy.
4. Development of severe nonhematologic toxicity necessitates discontinuation of the drug(s) to which tumor cells appear responsive; examples include:
   - a. Cardiotoxicity from doxorubicin
   - b. Pulmonary fibrosis from bleomycin
5. Other potential problems of chemotherapy include:
   - a. Inability of drugs to reach certain body tissues (e.g., brain because of the blood–brain barrier)
   - b. Hematologic toxicity; bone marrow suppression
   - c. Natural resistance to cytotoxic drugs due to genetic variations

G.   Considerations for safe administration of chemotherapy

1. Never use chemotherapeutic agents to test vein patency.
2. Stop infusion any time vein patency is in question.
3. Anticipate possibility of extravasation and hypersensitivity reactions, and review management procedures before administration.
4. Administer drugs in a quiet, relaxed environment.
5. Monitor the patient closely throughout administration.
6. Anticipate anaphylactic reactions as for any drug; if generalized or local reactions occur, stop infusion, and maintain venous access with normal saline or sterile distilled water.

H.   Chemotherapy toxicity and side effects

1. Cells with rapid turnover (e.g., epithelium of GI tract and oral cavity, bone marrow, hair follicles) are more susceptible to damage.
2. Planning a chemotherapeutic regimen should involve risk–benefit assessment to ensure that expected benefits outweigh apparent risks.
3. Most anticancer agents depress bone marrow function, resulting in decreased blood cell production.

4. Myelosuppression is the most common reason for limiting dosages of chemotherapeutic drugs; WBCs and platelets are most vulnerable.

I. Nursing diagnoses
1. Activity Intolerance
2. Ineffective Individual Coping
3. High Risk for Injury
4. Altered Nutrition: Less Than Body Requirements
5. Altered Oral Mucous Membrane
6. Impaired Tissue Integrity

J. Planning and implementation
1. Monitor laboratory results for reduced leukocytes, erythrocytes, and platelets; report abnormal findings.
2. Observe for evidence of infection and bleeding; during menses, record pad count, and note amount of saturation.
3. Assess for pallor, dizziness, rapid pulse, ringing in ears, or anginal pain.
4. Explain the patient's increased vulnerability to infection; caution him or her to guard against exposure to upper respiratory and other infections.
5. Observe the patient's skin frequently for ecchymoses, petechiae.
6. Instruct the patient to avoid cuts, bruises, or other trauma; tell him or her to shave with an electric razor and keep nails short.
7. Avoid administering parenteral injections; if they are unavoidable, apply pressure to the injection site after administration.
8. Encourage frequent handwashing and overall cleanliness.
9. Caution the patient regarding overexertion; suggest frequent rest periods.
10. Reassure the patient that fatigue and blood transfusions do not indicate disease progression.
11. Instruct the patient to avoid use of alcohol or medications that may alter platelet production and function, including:
    a. Aspirin products
    b. Anticoagulants
    c. Phenothiazines
12. Monitor emesis, urine, and stool daily for occult blood.
13. Promote adequate hydration and mobility to prevent constipation.
14. Instruct the patient to avoid using enemas and straining during bowel movements.
15. Assist the patient with self-care as needed.
16. Administer prescribed antiemetics before chemotherapy sessions, and assess their effectiveness.

17. Adjust the patient's diet before and after treatment according to patient preference. Experiment with sour foods; avoid sweet, fatty, or spicy foods.
18. Provide cold or room-temperature foods to minimize food odors, which can trigger nausea.
19. Offer clear liquids to be sipped slowly.
20. Eliminate unpleasant sights, odors, and sounds from the patient's environment.
21. Provide fresh air if possible.
22. Provide frequent mouth care.
23. Use distraction, relaxation techniques, and imagery before, during, and after chemotherapy.
24. Monitor frequency of vomiting and the amount and character of emesis.
25. Weigh the patient daily, noting any weight loss.
26. Assess skin turgor frequently.
27. Maintain accurate intake and output records.
28. Make provisions for calorie counting and diet history.
29. Monitor laboratory values that help evaluate nutritional status, including:
    a. Serum protein
    b. Transferrin
    c. Iron
    d. Hemoglobin
    e. Hematocrit
    f. Lymphocyte levels
    g. Urinary creatinine levels
30. Provide refreshing mouth care before meals.
31. Serve high-protein and high-carbohydrate food; allow the patient to choose foods, but guide his or her selection.
32. Present small portions as attractively as possible in a pleasant setting.
33. Ensure physical comfort, and encourage company during mealtimes.
34. Keep in mind that cancer or cancer treatment may contribute to altered taste and food preferences.
35. Assess the patient's oral cavity daily, and report changes in sensation, appearance, or taste.
36. Provide instruction for an oral care regimen following meals and at bedtime.
37. Instruct the patient to:
    a. Avoid lemon and glycerin products and all commercial mouthwashes; these promote drying and irritation.
    b. Gargle with a solution of baking soda and water (1 tsp in 500 mL) or salt (½ tsp), baking soda (1 tsp), and water (1000 mL).

    c.   Use a soft toothbrush or "toothette."

    d.   Remove dentures except for eating.

    e.   Avoid extremely hot or cold foods, spices, citrus juices.

    f.   Avoid smoking and alcohol intake.

    g.   Keep lips moist with K-Y Jelly or another water-based lip balm.

38. Instruct the patient to report:

    a.   Any discomfort, areas of redness

    b.   Open lesions

    c.   Decreased tolerance to temperatures of food

39. Administer systemic or topical analgesics as prescribed.

40. Assist the patient in coping with alopecia by:

    a.   Informing him or her if hair loss is expected and when

    b.   Explaining that the hair that regrows may differ in color or texture

    c.   Suggesting gradual and regular cutting of hair length to minimize the shock of hair loss and reduce early loss due to weight and pulling on hair

    d.   Suggesting that occasional wig wearing before hair loss may ease the adjustment process and helping him or her obtain a hairpiece before hair loss begins

    e.   Taking an honest, gentle, caring approach, encouraging him or her to express fears and feelings of loss

    f.   Realizing that hair loss may become so difficult that the patient may refuse to accept treatment

    g.   Arranging for contact with another person who has experienced hair regrowth after chemotherapy

    h.   Never communicating that hair loss is an insignificant problem compared to life-threatening alternatives; the patient's emotional needs may be at least as great as his or her physical needs

41. Advise a patient with alopecia to:

    a.   Use a mild, protein-based shampoo every 3 to 5 days, avoid excessive shampooing, rinse thoroughly, and gently pat hair dry

    b.   Avoid using hair dryers, electric curlers, curling irons, hair clips, elastic bands, barrettes, bobby pins, hair spray, dye, and permanents—all of which may increase fragility of hair

    c.   Sleep on a satin pillowcase to decrease hair trauma and tangles

    d.   Avoid excessive brushing and combing of hair; comb only with a wide-tooth comb

    e.   Wear a hairnet to minimize shedding of hair onto the bed or clothing

    f.   Covering the head when outdoors to prevent body heat loss or sunburn

42. Allow and encourage verbalization of anger, sadness, or resentment by the patient and significant others.

43. Convey sincere concern by listening, pointing out other attributes, appropriate touching to convey acceptance, and so forth

44. Assess intensity and patterns of fatigue; aggravating and alleviating factors.

45. Assess the impact of fatigue on the patient's lifestyle.

46. Monitor laboratory values for the presence of anemia.

47. Help the patient cope with fatigue by:
    a. Providing for rest periods during the day, especially before and after priority activities
    b. Helping him or her rearrange daily schedule and organize activities to conserve energy
    c. Teaching that fatigue is an expected side effect of chemotherapy that will resolve after treatment is completed
    d. Encouraging him or her to ask for assistance with necessary chores

48. Assess for pain and anxiety.

49. Assess for signs and symptoms of depression:
    a. Irritability
    b. Withdrawal
    c. Apathy
    d. Tearfulness
    e. Decreased ability to make decisions
    f. Impaired concentration or memory
    g. Increasing insomnia
    h. Suicidal ideas

50. Provide adequate protein and calorie intake; give dietary supplements as needed.

51. Encourage fluid intake of 3000 mL/day, unless contraindicated, to prevent accumulation of cellular waste products.

52. Administer blood products as prescribed.

53. Provide pain management as needed.

54. Assess the patient's specific stressors.

55. Evaluate the patient's perception of stressors and beliefs about their causes.

56. Determine available resources and support systems.

57. Provide for consistent, uninterrupted time with the patient; encourage verbalization of concerns.

58. Design strategies; gather agency support to address concerns about:
    a. Equipment
    b. Prostheses
    c. Home care

59. Assist the patient in mastering self-care to the maximum level possible.

60. Explain the importance of staying involved in normal routines.
61. Encourage the patient to generate good options for solving problems.
62. Identify unsuccessful coping behaviors, and make referrals to mental health professionals or clergy as indicated.

K. Evaluation
1. The patient displays no evidence of infection from myelosuppression.
2. The patient displays no evidence of bleeding from myelosuppression.
3. The patient maintains sufficient nutritional intake to prevent dietary imbalance.
4. The patient remains free of stomatitis.
5. The patient demonstrates positive adaptation to body image changes related to alopecia.
6. The patient alters activity pattern in response to changes in physical ability and energy level.
7. The patient demonstrates appropriate coping mechanisms in adapting to the disease.
8. The patient makes use of agency support as needed for home care.

IX. Bone marrow transplantation

A. Description and overview
1. This procedure involves aspirating bone marrow cells from a compatible donor and infusing them into the recipient.
2. Bone marrow transplantation is a complex therapy with a high risk of complications.
3. Types of transplantation include:
   a. Autologous: The marrow donor is the recipient; marrow is harvested during a period of disease remission, treated, and stored for later infusion.
   b. Syngeneic: The marrow donor is the recipient's identical twin.
   c. Allogeneic: The marrow donor is a family member whose HLA type matches that of the recipient.

B. Objective
1. Cure
2. Complete marrow recovery within 6 to 8 weeks
3. Proliferation of donor cells in marrow, leading to release of functional blood cells into circulation

C. Indications
1. Acute lymphoblastic leukemias
2. Acute myelogenous leukemias
3. Lymphomas

D. Nursing diagnoses
1. Fatigue

   2. Fear
   3. High Risk for Infection
   4. Altered Nutrition: Less Than Body Requirements
   5. Pain
   6. Social Isolation
   E. **Planning and implementation**
      1. Ensure thorough pretransplantation preparation, including:
         a. Complete histocompatibility studies of all possible donors and the recipient
         b. Thorough assessment of recipient and donor to determine physical and psychosocial factors that may influence transplantation
         c. Large doses of chemotherapy or radiation to the recipient to eradicate any viable marrow
      2. Monitor for signs and symptoms of infection.
      3. Assess for signs and symptoms of graft-versus-host (GVH) disease, a syndrome induced by donor T lymphocytes acting against host tissues (see Section III of Chapter 19, Hematologic Disorders, for more information on GVH disease).
      4. Explain to the patient that fatigue is a common effect of transplantation and does not indicate disease exacerbation. Teach energy conservation measures, and encourage adequate rest.
      5. Instruct the patient to:
         a. Avoid physical injury and aspirin-containing products
         b. Promptly report signs of hemorrhage or infection
         c. Avoid parenteral injections if platelet count is depressed
      6. Promote measures to reduce social isolation, including:
         a. Frequent telephone calls
         b. Television, radio, hobbies, other activities
         c. Regular patient–staff contact
   F. **Evaluation**
      1. The patient exhibits no signs of infection, GVH disease, or hemorrhage.
      2. The patient verbalizes necessary precautions to prevent complications.
      3. The patient states energy conservation measures to reduce fatigue.
      4. The patient maintains adequate nutritional status.
      5. The patient interacts with others to prevent social isolation.
X. **Investigational approaches**
   A. **Immunotherapy**
      1. This treatment uses the body's own immune mechanisms to combat and overcome cancer.
      2. Through the administration of chemical or microbial agents, immunotherapy aims to challenge and induce mobilization of immune defenses.

3. The resultant delayed hypersensitivity response can be directed against cancer cells.

4. In *active immunotherapy*, the patient is injected with antigen that stimulates development of antibodies; may be specific or nonspecific:

   a. Specific: The patient is vaccinated with tumor-associated antigen to stimulate immune response.

   b. Nonspecific: Injected materials have no relationship to the tumor but increase the patient's overall immune capacity.

5. *Passive immunotherapy* involves direct transfer of antitumor antibodies, immunologically competent lymphocytes, or immune lymphoid cells from a donor (a person cured of cancer or in remission) to a patient with an active neoplasm; it provides short-term immunity.

6. *Adoptive immunotherapy* involves transferring passive immunity to a patient, who later develops and maintains active immunity. Cells with antitumor reactivity to the patient with cancer are administered; the patient adopts the immunity from the cells and then incorporates it into his or her own immune system.

7. *Adjunctive immunotherapy* is a combination of the above immunotherapeutic approaches with other cancer modalities (surgery, radiation therapy, chemotherapy).

B. Biologic response modifiers (BRMs)

1. This investigational therapy involves agents or treatment methods that have the ability to alter the immunologic relationship between tumor and host in a therapeutically beneficial way.

2. The goal is destruction or cessation of malignant growth.

3. The basis of BRM treatment lies in:

   a. Restoration

   b. Stimulation

   c. Augmentation of natural immune defenses

4. Types of BRMs include:

   a. Immunomodulating agents: Bacille Calmette-Guerin and Corynebacterium Parvum (C. Parvum)

   b. Interferons

   c. Interleukins

   d. Monoclonal antibodies

   e. Lymphokines and cytokines

C. Nursing considerations with investigational therapies

1. Keep in mind that these approaches may be viewed as "last chance" efforts at cure.

2. When caring for a patient receiving such therapy, be sure to gain familiarity with each agent given and potential adverse effects.

3. Careful documentation is essential for all aspects of data collection and nursing care.

Bibliography

American Cancer Society (1989). *Cancer facts and figures*. Atlanta: Author.

Brunner, L. S., & Suddarth, D. S. (1988). *Textbook of medical-surgical nursing* (6th ed.). Philadelphia: J. B. Lippincott.

Brunner, L. S., & Suddarth, D. S. (1986). *The Lippincott manual of nursing practice* (4th ed.). Philadelphia: J. B. Lippincott.

Luckman, J., & Sorenson, K. C. (1987). *Medical-surgical nursing: A psychophysiologic approach* (3rd ed.). Philadelphia: W. B. Saunders.

McNally, J. C., Stair, J. C., & Somerville, E. T. (Eds.) (1985). *Guidelines for cancer nursing practice*. Orlando, FL: Harcourt Brace Jovanovich.

Phipps, W. J., Long, B. C., & Woods, N. F. (Eds.) (1987). *Medical-surgical nursing: Concepts and clinical practice* (3rd ed.). St. Louis: C. V. Mosby.

Snyder, C. C. (1986). *Oncology nursing*. Boston: Little, Brown.

Yasko, J. M. (Ed.) (1986). *Nursing management of symptoms associated with chemotherapy* (rev. ed.). Columbus, OH: Adria Laboratories.

Ziegfeld, C. R. (Ed.) (1987). *Core curriculum for oncology nursing*. Philadelphia: W. B. Saunders.

STUDY QUESTIONS

1. Which of the major treatment modalities for cancer is the most frequently used?
   a. bone marrow transplantation
   b. chemotherapy
   c. radiation
   d. surgery

2. Ms. Bowen, a 35-year-old blonde woman with a family history of dysplastic nevus syndrome, has been advised that sun exposure puts her at great risk for developing skin cancer. She states that she's careful and won't get skin cancer but continues to sunbathe from 1 to 3 P.M. every other day and has a deep tan next time she comes in for an appointment. Her actions demonstrate which of the following diagnoses?
   a. Knowledge Deficit related to causes of skin cancer
   b. Dysfunctional Grieving
   c. Ineffective Denial
   d. Anxiety

3. For a person experiencing low-grade fever, chronic cough with hemoptysis, hoarseness, weight loss, and foul-smelling stools, all the following nursing diagnoses represent warning signals of cancer *except*
   a. Ineffective Airway Clearance
   b. Diarrhea
   c. High Risk for Altered Body Temperature
   d. Impaired Verbal Communication

4. Which of the following factors are believed to contribute to 80% to 90% of all cancers?
   a. environmental
   b. genetic
   c. socioeconomic
   d. geographic

5. Ms. Carman, a 30-year-old airline stewardess, was admitted following seizure activity. CT of the head revealed an enhancing lesion, and stereotactic needle biopsy obtained tissue identifying the lesion as a glioma. When Ms. Carman asks the nurse what kind of treatment she will have to undergo, the nurse should explain that the most likely treatment would be
   a. chemotherapy
   b. treatment for a benign lesion
   c. radiation therapy
   d. immunotherapy

6. Although radiation therapy (RT) carries potentially serious side effects, it provides site-specific, often effective treatment for certain cancers. General nursing diagnoses for patients receiving RT should include all the following *except*
   a. Fatigue
   b. High Risk for Infection
   c. Ineffective Thermoregulation
   d. High Risk for Impaired Skin Integrity

7. Mr. Russell, aged 70, is receiving RT to treat pituitary cancer. He tells the nurse that he has lost the mouth care instructions that were given to him at the first treatment session. Which of the following measures should the nurse instruct him to take until he can obtain complete instructions from the radiation nurse?
   a. "Gargle with Listerine several times daily."
   b. "Don't eat or drink until you're sure it's O.K."
   c. "Brush your teeth vigorously, and use a good mouthwash."
   d. "Drink lots of fluids, and avoid smoking."

8. Mr. James, aged 46, is undergoing daily RT for a glioblastoma. When caring for him, the nurse should be alert for which of the following side effects?
   a. fatigue, nausea and vomiting, and headache
   b. fatigue, diarrhea, and stomatitis
   c. severe diarrhea and headache
   d. cystitis, diarrhea, and alopecia

9. Mr. Marston, a 60-year-old accountant, is undergoing RT for painful prostatic

metastasis of the lumbosacral spine. During treatment, he tells the nurse, "I'm going to beat this disease." The nurse's best response to this statement would be

a. "Once cancer gets in the bones, there is nothing to be done."

b. "Many cancers are curable with radiation."

c. "Have you considered trying a macrobiotic diet?"

d. "You may obtain very good pain relief from the radiation."

10. Secondary prevention of cancer refers to

a. prevention of second malignancies

b. detection and screening efforts to achieve early diagnosis and prompt intervention

c. prevention of genetic cancer inheritance

d. avoiding smoking and sun exposure

11. For early detection of breast cancer, the American Cancer Society's guidelines recommend

a. mammograms every other year for women age 35 and older

b. mammograms every year for women past age 40

c. mammograms every other year for women past age 50

d. monthly self-breast examinations by all women age 20 and over

12. Which of the following statements about bone marrow transplantation is true?

a. It is performed when cure is impossible.

b. It is now fairly risk-free because of improved methods of marrow harvesting.

c. It requires thorough physical and psychosocial assessment of both donor and recipient.

d. The donor must always be a family member.

13. Ms. Allen has recently been diagnosed with ovarian cancer and is scheduled to receive aggressive chemotherapy. The physician has written the order for nitrogen mustard, a potent vesicant with serious side effects, including myelosuppression, stomatitis, alopecia, and nausea and vomiting. The plan of care for this patient should include all the following *except*

a. identifying a nurse or physician with training in chemotherapy administration

b. checking laboratory values for reduced number of leukocytes, erythrocytes, and platelets

c. establishing a mouth care regimen

d. communicating that hair loss is insignificant compared to potentially life-threatening complications

14. Mr. Taylor's lung tumor has been staged as T3, N1, M1. This indicates

a. a measurable tumor with regional nodes and metastasis involved

b. a well-differentiated tumor

c. a tumor that cannot be treated

d. the tumor markers

15. Mr. Patrick, aged 54, has just received brachytherapy to his tongue. His family asks the nurse how they can protect themselves after he is discharged. From this question, the nurse would determine that the family

a. needs further teaching

b. understands about brachytherapy

c. has had no teaching

d. is unable to understand simple instructions

ANSWER KEY

1. **Correct response: d**
   Surgery is the most frequently used major modality.
   a. Bone marrow transplantation is not a major treatment modality.
   b and c. Chemotherapy and radiation therapy are major modalities but not the most frequently used.
   Comprehension/Safe care/Planning

2. **Correct response: c**
   Even though the patient is aware of the risk, she still refuses to limit cancer risk activities.
   a. The patient understands the risk and preventive measures.
   b and d. There is no evidence that she is either anxious or grieving.
   Knowledge/Psychosocial/Analysis (Dx)

3. **Correct response: c**
   Chronic cough, unusual bleeding, hoarseness, and change in bowel habits are warning signals of cancer. Low grade fever and weight loss are not included in the warning signals.
   a, b, and d. These diagnoses all represent warning signs of cancer.
   Application/Physiologic/Analysis (Dx)

4. **Correct response: a**
   Environmental factors are thought to contribute to 80% to 90% of all cancers.
   b. Genetic factors combine with host mechanisms and environmental influences.
   c and d. Socioeconomics and geographics are predisposing factors.
   Comprehension/Safe care/Evaluation

5. **Correct response: b**
   Gliomas are benign lesions.
   a and c. Chemotherapy and radiation therapy are indicated only for neoplastic disease.
   d. This scenario offers no evidence that the patient's immune system is compromised.
   Application/Physiologic/Implementation

6. **Correct response: c**
   Thermoregulation is not an expected side effect of RT.
   a, b, and d. These are all potential side effects of RT.
   Application/Physiologic/Analysis (Dx)

7. **Correct response: d**
   Increased fluid intake helps soothe irritated tissue and moisturize mucous membranes; smoking is an irritant.
   a. Commercial mouthwashes contain alcohol and promote further drying of mucous membranes.
   b. A high-protein, high-calorie diet is essential to facilitate healing of normal epithelial tissue.
   c. RT may cause mouth ulcers; vigorous brushing is contraindicated.
   Application/Health promotion/Implementation

8. **Correct response: a**
   Fatigue is an expected result of RT; nausea and vomiting are possible because of increased intracranial pressure resulting from brain irradiation.
   b, c, and d. Side effects of RT are directly related to the body site being irradiated. Brain irradiation would not result in diarrhea or stomatitis; headache is possible. Alopecia is expected.
   Analysis/Physiologic/Planning

9. **Correct response: d**
   The nurse should reinforce the positive effects of therapy for metastatic disease.
   a. Reclassification may occur from radiation to bony metastasis; the nurse should avoid destroying hope with negative responses.
   b. Metastatic disease dictates the goal of palliation.
   c. Macrobiotic diet is an unproved treatment method.
   Analysis/Psychosocial/Implementation

10. **Correct response: b**
    This answer is the definition of secondary cancer prevention.

648

a. General cancer prevention measures apply to any malignancy.

c. There is no known way to prevent genetic tendencies.

d. Avoiding smoking and sun exposure are primary prevention measures.

Application/Health promotion/ Implementation

11. *Correct response: d*

All women aged 20 and older should perform self-breast examination at least monthly.

a, b, and c. The ACS recommends a baseline mammogram between age 35 and 39. For women age 40 to 49, the recommended interval is every 1 to 2 years; for asymptomatic women age 50 and older, every year.

Knowledge/Health promotion/Assessment

12. *Correct response: c*

Thorough assessment of recipient and donor is required to determine physical and psychosocial factors that may influence bone marrow transplant.

a. Cure is the singular goal of bone marrow transplant.

b. Bone marrow transplant involves high risks.

d. In autologous transplants, the marrow donor is also the recipient.

Analysis/Health promotion/Assessment

13. *Correct response: d*

It is not a good idea to minimize emotional concerns.

a. Only specially trained physicians and nurses should be involved in the administration of vesicants to prevent extravasation.

b. Adequate counts must exist before therapy can begin.

c. Good oral care is essential.

Application/Safe care/Planning

14. *Correct response: a*

Staging systems specify tumor characteristics, lymph node involvement, and evidence of metastasis.

a. Grading, not staging, provides information about differentiation.

c. Staging systems do not specify the treatability of tumors.

d. Many malignancies are associated with specific cancer markers (laboratory values) that seem to indicate tumor progression or regression.

Analysis/Physiologic/Assessment

15. *Correct response: a*

This statement indicates that the family does not know that sealed sources placed in tissue in a container are removed before discharge; further teaching is indicated.

b, c, and d. The nurse should never jump to conclusions about a person's ability to understand information imparted. A patient and family members typically receive much information that is scary and completely foreign; reinforcement and clarification often are necessary. Remember, these are not simple issues to people who are frightened and who have been told horrible "stories" about radiation.

Analysis/Safe care/Evaluation

Gerontologic Nursing

I. Aging and older adults
- A. Life span changes
- B. Stereotypes of older adults
- C. Modification of age-related changes
- D. Selected theories of aging

II. Overview of gerontologic nursing
- A. Health history
- B. Physical assessment
- C. Mental status examination
- D. Assessment of functional capacity
- E. Environmental assessment
- F. Special considerations for nursing intervention
- G. Psychosocial implications

III. Dementias
- A. Description
- B. Etiology and incidence
- C. Pathophysiology
- D. Assessment findings
- E. Nursing diagnoses
- F. Planning and implementation
- G. Evaluation

IV. Osteoporosis
- A. Description
- B. Etiology and incidence
- C. Pathophysiology
- D. Assessment findings
- E. Nursing diagnoses
- F. Planning and implementation
- G. Evaluation

V. Pressure sores (decubitus ulcers)
- A. Description
- B. Etiology and incidence
- C. Pathophysiology
- D. Assessment findings
- E. Nursing diagnoses
- F. Planning and implementation
- G. Evaluation

VI. Falls
- A. Etiology
- B. Pathophysiology
- C. Assessment findings
- D. Nursing diagnoses
- E. Planning and implementation
- F. Evaluation

VII. Dehydration
- A. Description
- B. Etiology
- C. Assessment findings
- D. Nursing diagnoses
- E. Planning and implementation
- F. Evaluation

VIII. Constipation
- A. Description
- B. Etiology and incidence
- C. Assessment findings
- D. Nursing diagnosis
- E. Planning and implementation
- F. Evaluation

IX. Hearing deficit
- A. Description
- B. Etiology
- C. Assessment findings
- D. Nursing diagnoses
- E. Planning and implementation
- F. Evaluation

X. Visual deficit
- A. Description
- B. Etiology and incidence and pathophysiology
- C. Assessment findings
- D. Nursing diagnoses

Note: This chapter is not meant to provide comprehensive coverage of health of older adults. Other important health problems are presented elsewhere in this text; see particularly:

▶ Chapter 6, Respiratory Disorders (chronic obstructive lung disease, pneumonia)
▶ Chapter 8, Peripheral Vascular Disorders (hypertension)
▶ Chapter 9, Gastrointestinal Disorders (hiatal hernia)
▶ Chapter 10, Endocrine and Metabolic Disorders (diabetes mellitus)
▶ Chapter 14, Neurologic Disorders (cerebrovascular accident)
▶ Chapter 16, Musculoskeletal Disorders (osteoarthritis, fractures)
▶ Chapter 18, Renal and Urinary Disorders (incontinence)

I. Aging and older adults
A. Life span changes
1. Aging encompasses life span changes common to all people.
2. These changes involve biologic, social, and psychologic components.
B. Stereotypes of older adults
1. Refuting the stereotype of invariable progressive physical and mental decline with aging, more than 80% of older adults live in the community.
2. The elderly population is very heterogeneous and diverse.
3. Other inaccurate myths about older adults include:
   a. Most are inactive and unproductive.
   b. Most are abandoned by their families.
   c. Most have no sex life.
   d. Most are rigid and inflexible.
C. Modification of age-related changes
1. Age-related changes are modified by environment, heredity, and time-related pathologic events.
2. A person's chronologic age is not always indicative of biologic age.
3. The rate of aging may differ for various organ systems.
4. Physiologic changes that may be intrinsic to aging include:
   a. Gray hair

     b.   Decreased basal metabolic rate

     c.   Slowed reaction time

     d.   Decreased deep tendon reflexes

     e.   Delayed pancreatic insulin release

     f.   Body composition changes: decreased bone and muscle mass, decreased total body water, increased body fat, decreased subcutaneous fat, increased anteroposterior chest diameter

5. Examples of age-related changes associated with pathology likely to be found in a representative sample of the elderly population include:

     a.   Decreased height

     b.   Decreased cardiac output

     c.   Increased peripheral vascular resistance

     d.   Decreased stroke volume

     e.   Decreased heart rate response to stress

     f.   Decreased renal blood flow

     g.   Reduced creatinine clearance

6. Race, ethnicity, or culture affect many age-related changes because of such variables as:

     a.   Genetic traits

     b.   Modification of disease risk factors

7. Aging and disease are not synonymous; many pathologic changes can be treated and possibly reversed.

8. Various diseases of older adults have adverse effects on function and behavior, including:

     a.   Atherosclerosis

     b.   Cancer

     c.   Osteoarthritis

     d.   Hiatal hernia

     e.   Diverticulosis

     f.   Cataracts

     g.   Adult-onset diabetes

     h.   Stroke

     i.   Presbycusis

9. Certain reversible effects of disuse and physical deconditioning may result from prolonged bedrest and inactivity.

D. Selected theories of aging (not likely a single cause)

   1. Biologic theories include:

     a.   Cellular

     b.   Autoimmune

     c.   Neuroendocrine

   2. Psychosocial theories encompass:

     a.   Disengagement

     b.   Activity

     c.   Continuity

     d.   Developmental stages

II. Overview of gerontologic nursing

A. Health history

1. When obtaining a health history from an elderly adult, the nurse should determine the person's ability to comprehend the questions and allow sufficient time for him or her to respond.
2. The history should include the following parameters:
   a. Previous illness
   b. Lifestyle, including usual daily routine
   c. Diet and fluid intake
   d. Medication use
   e. Sources of income, financial status
   f. Social network
   g. Presence of a confidant
   h. Living arrangements
   i. Personal perception of health status
   j. Satisfaction with activity level
   k. Available sources of health care and psychosocial support
3. The nurse should collect data in more than one session if the person shows signs of tiring.
4. The nurse should be alert for atypical disease presentation that can occur in elderly persons (e.g., painless myocardial infarction).

B. Physical assessment

1. During physical assessment of an elderly person, the nurse should pay special attention to positioning, comfort, and mobility.
2. The nurse should compare findings on both sides of the body when norms for elderly persons are absent.
3. Insufficient normative data commonly interfere with accurate evaluation of laboratory test results.

C. Mental status examination

1. Altered mental status may be due to physical problems such as infection and heart failure.
2. The patient may feel threatened when the nurse assesses memory, orientation, reasoning, calculation ability, and judgment.
3. To put the patient at ease, the nurse should demonstrate kindness and empathy, and progress from simple to more complex questions.
4. A person with dementia may exhibit superficial social skills, creating a false impression of adequate mental function.

D. Assessment of functional capacity

1. The nurse should evaluate both activities of daily living (ADL) and instrumental activities of daily living (IADL; e.g., managing money, telephone use, shopping, use of transportation).

    2. Assessment findings will be influenced by pain, motivation, and environment, as well as by the patient's functional ability.

    3. A patient's prior performance is a good predictor of current ability.

E. **Environmental assessment**

    1. Assessment of the patient's environment should cover:

        a. Cleanliness

        b. Temperature regulation

        c. State of repair

        d. Presence of smoke alarms

        e. Food storage and preparation facilities

        f. Safety features to reduce the risk of injury (e.g., adequate lighting, handrails, absence of throw rugs)

        g. Presence of stairs

        h. Medication storage

        i. Furniture with sharp edges or obstructing pathways

    2. This assessment also should evaluate the patient's community for safety and for availability of:

        a. Public transportation

        b. Home health services

        c. Respite care

        d. Meals on wheels

        e. Home maintenance assistance

        f. Senior centers

        g. Health care facilities

F. **Special considerations for nursing intervention**

    1. Pay special attention to both functional status and specific medical problems.

    2. Emphasize the patient's strengths; do not focus only on problems.

    3. Always consider restorative potential or maintenance of function when setting goals for the patient.

    4. Consider altered pharmacokinetics in the elderly when evaluating drug effects.

    5. Recognize that the patient may have increased susceptibility to disease due to:

        a. Impaired immunity

        b. Multiple disease states

        c. Chronic illness

    6. Recognize the decreased adequacy of body's response to stress.

    7. Provide support and information to caregivers, family, and significant others; suggest self-help groups.

    8. Establish mutually satisfactory means of communication, considering vision and hearing deficits.

    9. Incorporate the multidisciplinary team into the care process.

10. Provide for continuity of care in unit transfers, among different levels of care, and by various service providers.

11. Recognize that Medicare and Medicaid legislation has a significant effect on care delivery and reimbursement of health professionals caring for older adults.

G. **Psychosocial implications**
1. Elderly persons are particularly susceptible to cumulative effects of loss and associated grief on:
   a. Social interactions: spouse, family, friends
   b. Self-concept: job, health
   c. Financial security: income, home, possessions
2. The elderly patient may have difficulty coping with age-related lifestyle changes, leading to:
   a. Economic and psychologic stresses
   b. Feelings of loss of control and independence
3. The elderly patient's coping ability may be overwhelmed quickly if past successful strategies are not encouraged.

III. **Dementias**
A. **Description: a group of chronic, progressive, organic mental disorders; the most common are Alzheimer's disease and multi-infarct dementia**
B. **Etiology and incidence**
1. The cause of Alzheimer's disease is unknown.
2. Multi-infarct dementia results from cerebrovascular disease producing multiple small cerebral infarctions.
3. Alzheimer's disease accounts for more than 50% of dementias and affects 2% to 4% of persons over age 65. Incidence increases with age, particularly after age 75.
4. Multi-infarct dementia accounts for about 15% of cases of dementia; incidence is greater in males than females, and onset generally is earlier than in Alzheimer's disease.
C. **Pathophysiology**
1. Alzheimer's disease is characterized by specific neurologic and biochemical changes, including:
   a. Neurofibrillary tangles, granulovacuolar degeneration of neurons, and senile or neuritic plaques, primarily in the cerebral cortex
   b. Brain atrophy, with widened cortical sulci and enlarged cerebral ventricles
   c. Decreased acetylcholine production
2. Typically of insidious onset, Alzheimer's disease produces multifaceted intellectual deficits (e.g., memory, abstract thought, judgment, and higher cortical functions) and personality and behavioral changes.
3. Pathologic changes in multi-infarct dementia include multiple

areas of extensive localized softening, along with various changes in cerebral vessels.

4. Multi-infarct dementia is marked by an uneven decline in mental function due to cerebral damage. The pattern of deficits is patchy, depending on the areas of damage; some cognitive functions may be affected early, whereas others may remain relatively intact.

D. **Assessment findings**

1. Clinical manifestations of Alzheimer's disease are highly variable and may include:

   a. Early, subtle changes such as forgetfulness, recent memory loss, and poor concentration, which the patient may be able to hide

   b. Later, more overt signs of impaired cognition (e.g., severe memory loss and forgetfulness; inability to hold a conversation, think abstractly, or formulate concepts; poor hygiene and grooming and inappropriate dress; inability to perform IADLs)

   c. Behavioral changes, such as depression, anxiety, wandering, impulsive behavior, catastrophic reactions, imitation, emotional lability, and withdrawal

2. Common signs and symptoms of multi-infarct dementia include:

   a. Dizziness, headaches

   b. Confusion

   c. Patchy memory loss

   d. Hallucinations, delusions

   e. Focal neurologic signs (e.g., muscle weakness, dysreflexia, dysarthria)

3. Laboratory and diagnostic studies to evaluate dementias include:

   a. Computed tomography (CT) scan

   b. Electroencephalography (EEG)

   c. Positron emission tomography (PET)

   d. Blood chemistries

E. **Nursing diagnoses**

1. Bowel Incontinence
2. Impaired Verbal Communication
3. Ineffective Family Coping: Compromised
4. Altered Health Maintenance
5. Impaired Home Maintenance Management
6. High Risk for Injury
7. Impaired Physical Mobility
8. Altered Nutrition: Less Than Body Requirements
9. Self-Care Deficit: Bathing/Hygiene, Dressing/Grooming, Feeding, Toileting

10. Sleep Pattern Disturbance
11. Altered Thought Processes
12. Functional Urinary Incontinence
13. High Risk for Violence

F. **Planning and implementation**
   1. On admission:
      a. Record the patient's usual daily routine as well as words and behaviors used to communicate ADL needs; validate this information with a reliable informant in separate interview; chart words and techniques that "get through" to the patient.
      b. Request that a family member or other person stay with the patient if the patient wanders or cannot be sent to diagnostic tests by himself or herself; avoid sedation and restraints whenever possible.
      c. Assign the patient to a room that maximizes the potential for observation and is not next to an exit or stairwell (if the patient is prone to wandering).
      d. Orient the patient to the room and the unit; mark the room and bedside area with familiar belongings.
      e. Attach an ID bracelet; alert others to wandering (special clothing, care plan, posted notice).
   2. Maximize effective communication by:
      a. Using short sentences, simple words, gestures, and written or pictorial cues, if needed; explain and repeat instructions unless this increases distress
      b. Maintaining a calm demeanor and a consistent approach
      c. Avoiding excessive questioning and confrontation
      d. Breaking down instructions into simple components
      e. Supporting the anxious or depressed patient
      f. Attempting to analyze behavior for meaning
   3. Maximize environmental safety by:
      a. Installing alarms on stairwells
      b. Instituting injury, fire, and poisoning precautions
      c. Providing adequate lighting in all rooms
      d. Keeping the bed in low position or placing the mattress on the floor (Siderails may pose a hazard.)
   4. Intervene as necessary to manage evening agitation ("sundowning"): provide a night light, soft music, and supervision.
   5. If indicated, create a limited-access, safe unit to obviate activity restriction and decrease the need for supervision.
   6. Promote optimum functioning through:
      a. Fitting daily diagnostic and therapeutic procedures into the patient's usual schedule as possible
      b. Assigning consistent caregivers
      c. Establishing a daily routine for care, maintaining the pa-

tient's preadmission sleep–wake cycle if possible and desirable

  d. Providing a clock, calendar, and daily schedule in the room (but avoiding pressuring the patient for accuracy)

  e. Prompting for ADLs with memory aids and verbal cues and encouraging performance within the limits of ability (avoiding pressure for performance, which could trigger catastrophic reaction)

  f. Focusing the patient on simple, repetitive, and purposeful activities

  g. Monitoring for adverse effects of drug therapy

  h. Encouraging ambulation and other exercise

  i. Ensuring good grooming and personal hygiene

  j. Using distraction to alter undesirable behavior, break episodes of preservation, or remove from harm

  k. Intervening as necessary to calm an agitated patient

  l. Limiting stimuli (e.g., noise, people, caffeine)

  m. Regularly assessing the skin, gums, teeth, and feet for breakdown and infection, and providing good skin and mouth care

  n. Maximizing opportunities for social interaction

  o. Providing touch, respect, affection, praise, and the opportunity for choice

7. Optimize nutrition and fluid balance by:

  a. Monitoring food and fluid intake, noting increased or decreased hunger and thirst

  b. Reminding the patient to eat regularly

  c. Providing small, frequent meals with high-calorie supplements if appropriate

  d. Matching food consistency to the patient's chewing and swallowing ability

8. Optimize elimination by:

  a. Making sure the patient knows where the bathroom is to encourage its use

  b. Monitoring bowel elimination patterns

  c. Preventing constipation

  d. Giving periodic reminders to urinate

  e. Scheduling toileting based on voiding pattern

  f. Providing protective pants as indicated

9. Provide discharge planning:

  a. Begin discharge planning on the patient's admission to the hospital.

  b. Determine whether the patient will be discharged to home alone, to live with family, or to a nursing home; evaluate whether independent living could be hazardous to the patient.

   c.   As indicated, assist the patient's family in arranging for a nursing home, day care, or respite care.
   d.   Refer the patient and family to community agencies, legal and financial counseling, and disease-specific groups (e.g., the Alzheimer Disease and Related Disorder Association).
   e.   Encourage regular health care following discharge.
   f.   Document all patient information on transfer forms to promote continuity of care.
   g.   Teach home caregivers to assist the patient with ADLs as needed and to provide any special care required.

G. Evaluation
   1.   The patient demonstrates the ability to perform ADLs and IADLs to the maximum extent possible.
   2.   The patient is included in social interactions with family, friends, and groups.
   3.   The patient maintains adequate nutrition and hydration.
   4.   The patient receives protection of rights and respect.
   5.   The patient and family verbalize understanding of the disorder.
   6.   The patient maintains adequate elimination patterns or control of incontinence as appropriate.
   7.   The patient remains free from injury and infection.
   8.   The patient receives analysis of words and behavior for meaning.
   9.   The patient and family receive information about respite care, community services, and support organizations.
   10. The patient exhibits good personal hygiene.
   11. The caregiver verbalizes understanding of the cause of behavioral problems and methods of calming the patient.
   12. The caregiver maintains health and social contacts, using respite care when appropriate.

IV. Osteoporosis

   A. Description: a disorder of bone metabolism making bones abnormally prone to fracture

   B. Etiology and incidence
   1.   Osteoporosis may be iatrogenic or secondary to other disorders.
   2.   Predisposing factors include:
      a.   Postmenopausal status
      b.   Nutritional deficiency or malabsorption
      c.   Catabolic hormone excess (e.g., Cushing's disease)
      d.   Long-term corticosteroid use
      e.   Prolonged immobilization
      f.   Chronic disorders (e.g., liver disease)
   3.   Osteoporosis affects approximately one fourth of all older

adults; incidence is greatest in white females between ages 50 and 70.

C. Pathophysiology

1. In osteoporosis, the rate of bone loss (resorption) exceeds bone formation, resulting in a decrease in total bone mass.
2. Bones affected by osteoporosis lose calcium and phosphate salts.
3. As a result, they become porous, brittle, and susceptible to fracture.
4. Osteoporosis primarily affects weight-bearing vertebrae; severe, advanced disease can affect ribs, long bones, and the skull.

D. Assessment findings

1. Common clinical manifestations include:
    a. Fractures, particularly vertebral compression fractures, hip fractures, and long bone fractures
    b. Pain
    c. Visible deformity (e.g., kyphosis)
    d. Loss of height
    e. Constipation
2. Diagnostic evaluation includes:
    a. Radiographic and bone density studies showing loss of bone density, deformity
    b. Serum calcium, phosphorous, and alkaline phosphatase levels within normal ranges

E. Nursing diagnoses

1. Constipation
2. High Risk for Injury
3. Impaired Physical Mobility
4. Pain

F. Planning and implementation

1. Encourage regular moderate exercise regimen (e.g., walking).
2. Teach knee flexion and muscle relaxing exercises.
3. Instruct the patient to perform range-of-motion exercises at least twice daily.
4. Teach the patient to move the trunk as a unit and maintain good posture and body mechanics.
5. Encourage increased intake of foods high in calcium (e.g., milk, cheese, salmon, spinach, broccoli, rhubarb), vitamin D, fiber, and protein.
6. Teach safety measures to prevent injury from falling.
7. Use caution when turning, lifting, and transferring the patient to prevent fracture.
8. If indicated, apply a lumbosacral corset to promote spinal stability; avoid appliances that can decrease mobility.
9. Instruct the patient to sleep on a firm, nonsagging mattress.

10. Teach the patient about the disease process and prevention of progression.
11. Administer medications as prescribed (e.g., analgesics, stool softeners, calcium, vitamin D, 1,25-dihydroxycholecalciferol, estrogen in postmenopausal women).
12. Monitor for medication side effects:
    a. Calcium: gastrointestinal (GI) distress, constipation, renal calculi
    b. Estrogen: vaginal bleeding, embolism

G. **Evaluation**
1. The patient maintains or improves mobility and physical function.
2. The patient modifies lifestyle to include increased exercise, use of safety precautions, and independent ADLs within limitations of condition.
3. The patient reports reduced discomfort and pain.
4. The patient sustains no new fractures.
5. The patient identifies and verbalizes plans to increase consumption of foods high in fiber, calcium, protein, and vitamin D.

V. **Pressure sores (decubitus ulcers)**
A. **Description: localized areas of cellular necrosis on the skin and subcutaneous tissue**
B. **Etiology and incidence**
1. As the name implies, pressure sores result from excessive pressure on body areas, particularly over bony prominences.
2. Older adults are especially susceptible due to:
    a. Decreased skin thickness
    b. Decreased vascularity of dermal layer
       owed tissue repair and healing capacity
3. Major risk factors include:
    a. Decreased or limited activity, immobility
    b. Malnutrition
    c. Incontinence
    d. Impaired circulation and sensation
    e. Sensory deficits
    f. Cognitive dysfunction
4. Other risk factors from related conditions may include:
    a. Fever with diaphoresis
    b. Radiation therapy
    c. Anemia
    d. Dehydration
C. **Pathophysiology**
1. Excessive pressure on the skin interrupts normal circulatory function by constricting cutaneous and subcutaneous blood vessels.

2. Impaired circulation leads to tissue anoxia, necrosis, and ulceration.

3. Ulcer severity depends on the intensity and duration of pressure.

4. Ulcers are classified in four stages:
   a. Stage I: area with unresolved erythema, skin intact
   b. Stage II: blister, superficial skin break
   c. Stage III: involving the dermis through subcutaneous tissue with necrotic tissue, eschar, exudate
   d. Stage IV: involving subcutaneous tissue, fascia, and possibly muscle, joint, or bone with undermining sinus tract formation

5. Necrotic tissue is susceptible to bacterial invasion and infection.

D. Assessment findings

1. Pressure ulcers are marked by variable skin lesions, ranging from superficial erythema to small blisters or erosions to marked ulcerations.

2. Signs of local infection may be apparent.

3. Wound culture or biopsy may identify infective organisms and guide choice of antimicrobial therapy.

E. Nursing diagnoses

1. High Risk for Infection
2. Pain
3. Impaired Tissue Integrity

F. Planning and implementation

1. Relieve pressure by:
   a. Turning the patient at least every 2 hours
   b. Avoiding positioning the patient on the ulcerated side
   c. Teaching wheelchair push-ups if appropriate
   d. Using pressure-relieving devices (e.g., egg crate mattress, convoluted foam, air-fluidized therapy) as necessary

2. Prevent skin friction by:
   a. Using anatomic pads when necessary
   b. Using a lift sheet to prevent dragging across the bed

3. Prevent shearing force on the skin by:
   a. Elevating the head of the bed 30 degrees when not contraindicated
   b. Providing a footboard to prevent sliding downward in bed
   c. Helping the patient maintain appropriate body position and alignment

4. Keep skin clean and dry; if necessary, apply a fecal incontinence bag or external urine collection device.

5. Apply pressure sore dressings according to lesion stage:
   a. Stage I: transparent dressings
   b. Stage II: transparent or hydrocolloid dressing
   c. Stage III: hydrocolloid dressing for clean wound
6. Avoid occlusive dressings.
7. Use normal saline solution for dressing changes; avoid Betadine and Dakin's solution.
8. Promote wound healing through:
   a. Pressure relief
   b. Nutritional support
   c. Mechanical debridement with wet-to-dry dressing, if indicated
   d. Preparation for surgical debridement, if indicated
   e. Protection of the skin around ulcers
   f. Administration of antibiotics or blood transfusions as prescribed
9. Teach the patient and family:
   a. Measures to help prevent recurrence
   b. Wound care and infection control measures
   c. Sources of supplies and community resources

G. Evaluation

1. The patient exhibits resolution of pressure sores, as evidenced by:
   a. Granulation tissue
   b. No drainage or bleeding
   c. Decrease in size and depth
   d. Intact skin around ulcers
   e. No maceration
2. The patient verbalizes understanding of measures to promote healing and prevent further damage.
3. The patient or caregiver correctly demonstrates wound care using occlusive dressing or other appropriate method.
4. The patient acknowledges the need for turning or pressure-relieving devices.

VI. Falls

A. Etiology

1. Falling results from the inability of the body's postural mechanism to sustain an upright position because of internal or external destabilization.
2. Predisposing factors to falls in elderly patients include:
   a. Neuromuscular and cardiovascular problems
   b. Sensory deficits
   c. Environmental hazards
   d. Drug effects (e.g., diuretics, sedatives, hypnotics, cardiac glycosides, antiarrhythmics, antihypertensives)

B. **Pathophysiology**
 1. A fall can produce various musculoskeletal traumas, including:
    a. Fractures, particularly hip fracture
    b. Dislocations
    c. Sprains
 2. It also can cause:
    a. Head injury
    b. Neurologic damage
    c. Tissue trauma

C. **Assessment findings**
 1. Clinical manifestations of injuries due to falls vary and may include:
    a. Pain
    b. Visible deformity
    c. Loss of movement
    d. Sensory changes
    e. Tissue damage (e.g., bruising, laceration, swelling)
 2. Diagnostic tests to evaluate damage due to falls include:
    a. Radiographs
    b. CT scans

D. **Nursing diagnoses**
 1. High Risk for Injury
 2. Impaired Physical Mobility
 3. Pain
 4. Self-Care Deficit
 5. Impaired Skin Integrity: High Risk for
 6. Social Isolation

E. **Planning and implementation**
 1. Provide appropriate emergency management, which may include:
    a. Wound care and repair
    b. Immobilization of affected limb
    c. Hemorrhage control
    d. Tetanus toxoid as prescribed
 2. Institute preventive measures, such as:
    a. Identifying a patient at risk for falling
    b. Observing the patient frequently
    c. Monitoring for side effects of drugs
    d. Assessing for orthostatic hypotension
    e. Taking safety precautions (e.g., keep bed in low position with siderails up; place call light within reach; provide a night light; apply a posey vest or seat belt or restraints if necessary)
 3. Provide follow-up care as necessary, which may include:
    a. Limiting activity

b. Providing pain relief with prescribed medications and, if applicable, nonpharmacologic measures
c. Assessing for impaired circulation and nerve damage
d. Referring for radiographic and medical treatment

4. Develop a unit procedure for fall prevention and action plans to reduce the risk of injury.
5. Teach the patient about the importance of:
   a. Safety precautions (e.g., wearing nonskid shoes, using adaptive devices, installing night lights, eliminating safety hazards)
   b. Avoiding sudden or rapid position changes
   c. Reporting falls and injuries promptly

F. Evaluation
1. The patient exhibits diminished incidence of falling.
2. The patient states the need for safety precautions to reduce the risk of falling.
3. The patient identifies medications that affect balance.
4. The patient calls for assistance as needed.

VII. Dehydration

A. Description: excessive loss of water from body tissues

B. Etiology
1. Dehydration may result from fluid volume depletion related to:
   a. Marked decrease in water intake, enteral nutrition
   b. Diminished sense of thirst
   c. Age-related changes in body composition
   d. Incontinence
   e. Drug reactions
2. It also may be associated with medical problems such as:
   a. Diabetes mellitus
   b. Excessive fluid loss from fever, vomiting, or diarrhea

C. Assessment findings
1. Manifestations of dehydration include:
   a. Poor skin turgor
   b. Dry skin and mucous membranes, cracked lips and tongue
   c. Behavioral changes: delirium, apathy, confusion
   d. Oliguria
   e. Sunken cheeks, weight loss
   f. Hypotension
   g. Tachycardia
   h. Weakness
   i. Fever
2. Laboratory studies may reveal:
   a. Elevated blood urea nitrogen (BUN)
   b. Elevated hematocrit

      c.   Elevated serum sodium

      d.   Elevated urine specific gravity

D. Nursing diagnoses

  1. Activity Intolerance

  2. Constipation

  3. Fluid Volume Deficit

  4. Altered Oral Mucous Membrane

  5. Impaired Skin Integrity

  6. Altered Thought Processes

E. Planning and implementation

  1. Offer electrolyte supplements, as indicated, if the patient is conscious.

  2. Administer IV therapy as prescribed; monitor for fluid overload.

  3. Measure intake and output; weigh daily.

  4. Assess skin turgor and hydration of the buccal mucosa and tongue every shift.

  5. Monitor vital signs.

  6. Monitor laboratory study results.

  7. Assess mental status and level of consciousness.

  8. Teach the patient about:

      a.   The need for adequate fluid intake

      b.   Affects of certain drugs on fluid balance (e.g., diuretics)

      c.   Signs of dehydration to watch for and report

      d.   The need to wear proper clothing and avoid excessive exposure to heat and sunlight

F. Evaluation

  1. The patient remains alert and oriented.

  2. The patient demonstrates the ability to drink adequate fluids.

  3. The patient exhibits moist oral mucosa and tongue, elastic skin turgor.

  4. The patient displays vital signs and laboratory study results within acceptable ranges.

  5. The patient verbalizes understanding of the need to wear appropriate clothing and avoid excessive heat and sun exposure.

VIII. Constipation

A. Description: abnormal delay in defecation or infrequent passage of dry, hard stool

B. Etiology and incidence

  1. An elderly patient is at increased risk for constipation because of a tendency for decreased intake of roughage and fluids or decreased mobility.

  2. Other contributing factors may include:

      a.   Inability to recognize or neglecting the defecation urge

      b.   Chronic enema or laxative use

      c.   Neurologic degeneration

   d. Loss of abdominal muscle tone
   e. Environmental changes
   f. Emotional stress
   g. Effects of medication (e.g., narcotics, anticholinergics)
   h. Organic disorders (e.g., tumors, hypothyroidism, hemorrhoids)

C. Assessment findings
   1. The patient may report infrequent defecation. (*Note:* Keep in mind that bowel regularity is quite subjective; what the patient perceives as constipation may in fact be a normal elimination pattern.)
   2. Clinical manifestations of constipation may include:
       a. Abdominal distention and pain
       b. Absent or sluggish bowel sounds
       c. Stool-filled rectum on rectal examination
       d. Infrequent passage of dry, hard stool

D. Nursing diagnosis: constipation

E. Planning and implementation
   1. Encourage the patient to:
       a. Increase roughage in diet unless contraindicated
       b. Increase fluid intake to greater than 2 L/day
       c. Perform regular, moderate exercise as possible
   2. Establish a regular bowel evacuation schedule; provide privacy and assistance to the toilet or commode (if the patient is able to use these) or with using a bedpan.
   3. Encourage ingestion of hot liquids after a large meal to stimulate gastrocolic reflex.
   4. Teach the patient about the causes and management of constipation.
   5. Administer stool softeners, bulk-forming agents, laxatives, suppositories, and enemas as prescribed; monitor for side effects such as nausea, vomiting, diarrhea, and electrolyte imbalances.
   6. Keep in mind that severe constipation may lead to fecal impaction, which necessitates manual extraction of stool before initiating other treatments.

F. Evaluation
   1. The patient passes soft, formed stools regularly.
   2. The patient states an intention to incorporate methods to prevent constipation into daily routine.

IX. Hearing deficit

A. Description: hearing deficit associated with aging involves either sensorineural loss—presbycusis, progressive, and bilateral—or conductive loss (see Chapter 15, Eye, Ear, Nose, Sinus, and Throat Disorders, for more information)

B. Etiology
   1. Presbycusis results from disturbances of inner ear neural struc-

tures (e.g., cochlear nuclei, nerve pathways leading to the brain).

  2. Conductive loss or transmission deafness results from disturbances of the sound transmission mechanism of the external or middle ear, which prevents sound waves from entering the inner ear. Older adults commonly suffer from conductive hearing loss due to impacted cerumen in the ear canal.

C. **Assessment findings: See Chapter 15, Sections IX, X, and XI.**

D. **Nursing diagnoses**

  1. Impaired Verbal Communication

  2. Sensory and Perceptual Alteration: Auditory

  3. Social Isolation

E. **Planning and implementation**

  1. Keep in mind that a hearing-impaired elderly patient may be inaccurately labeled as demented because of impaired communication. Be sure to record the patient's hearing deficit on the chart and care plan.

  2. Instruct the patient in proper ear hygiene.

  3. Work with the patient to develop a means of communication that is effective and mutually satisfying (e.g., lip reading, writing).

  4. When talking to the patient, speak slowly and distinctly in a low-pitched, clear voice; minimize background noise; and use nonverbal cues.

  5. Instruct the patient in the use and care of a hearing aid, if indicated.

  6. Assist the patient in obtaining assistive devices (e.g., amplifying mechanisms) as necessary.

  7. Evaluate the impact of hearing loss on the patient's lifestyle (social isolation) and safety.

  8. Teach the patient about environmental changes to promote independence and safety (e.g., installing a flashing light on the doorbell and telephone).

F. **Evaluation**

  1. The patient demonstrates effective communication using the technique or equipment of choice.

  2. The patient identifies potential safety hazards related to hearing loss.

  3. The patient maintains social contacts and avoids isolation.

X. **Visual deficit**

A. **Description: visual deficits commonly associated with aging include:**

  1. Presbyopia, caused by thickening and hardening of the lens, which leads to decreased accommodation

  2. Cataract: clouding or opacity of normally transparent crystalline lens, which results in blurred vision and decreased visual acuity

668

B. Etiology and incidence and pathophysiology: See Chapter 15, Sections I through VII.

C. Assessment findings: See Chapter 15, Sections II and VII.

D. Nursing diagnoses
1. Sensory and Perceptual Alteration: Visual
2. High Risk for Injury
3. Social Isolation

E. Planning and implementation
1. Encourage the use of magnifying eyeglasses as indicated.
2. Use large, bold letters for written patient education materials and signs. Avoid muted colors, especially in the blue and green spectrum; a sharp color contrast from background promotes readability.
3. Protect the patient from injury: keep paths clear of obstacles, provide adequate lighting, avoid glare.
4. Identify yourself when approaching the patient.
5. Insert a notation regarding the patient's visual deficit in the care plan.
6. Keep the patient's belongings and essential equipment in consistent locations within his or her visual field.
7. Help the patient obtain assistive devices (e.g., magnifying lenses, large-print books) as necessary.
8. Teach the patient the importance of annual eye examinations.
9. Encourage cataract extraction when visual deficit interferes with desired activities.
10. Following cataract extraction, help the patient obtain special glasses or lenses and provide instruction regarding necessary adjustments to cope with altered depth perception, abnormal magnification, and loss of peripheral vision.

F. Evaluation
1. The patient identifies potential safety hazards related to vision loss.
2. The patient states an intention to modify lifestyle and environment as necessary to maximize functional abilities.
3. The patient participates in desired social activities.
4. The patient receives appropriate medical follow-up.

Bibliography

American Psychiatric Association (1987). *Diagnostic and statistical manual of mental disorders (DSM-III-R)* (3rd ed.—rev.). Washington, DC: Author.

Bartol, M. (1979). Nonverbal communication in patients with Alzheimer's disease. *Journal of Gerontological Nursing, 5*(4), 21–31.

Brunner, L. S., & Suddarth, D. S. (1988). *Textbook of medical-surgical nursing* (6th ed.). Philadelphia: J. B. Lippincott.

Brunner, L. S., & Suddarth, D. S. (1986). *The Lippincott manual of nursing practice* (4th ed.). Philadelphia: J. B. Lippincott.

Burnside, I. (1988). *Nursing and the aged: A self-care approach*. New York: McGraw-Hill.

Calkins, E., Davis, P., & Ford, A. (1986). *The practice of geriatrics*. Philadelphia: W. B. Saunders.

Lewis, S., & Collier, I. (1987). *Medical-surgical nursing: Assessment and management of clinical problems*. New York: McGraw-Hill.

Luckmann, J., & Sorenson, K. C. (1987). *Medical-surgical nursing: A psychophysiologic approach* (3rd ed.). Philadelphia: W.B. Saunders.

Matteson, M., & McConnell, E. (1988). *Gerontological nursing: Concepts and practice*. Philadelphia: W. B. Saunders.

Phipps, W., Long, B., & Woods, N. (1987). *Medical-surgical nursing: Concepts and clinical practice*. St. Louis: C. V. Mosby.

STUDY QUESTIONS

1. Which of the following statements about the aging process is correct?
   a. Age-related physiologic changes are distinct from those reflecting disease.
   b. Aging rate is consistent for various organ systems.
   c. A stereotype of progressive physical and mental decline is associated with aging.
   d. The effects of disuse and physical deconditioning caused by inactivity in the older adult are usually irreversible.

2. Which of the following likely would be the most successful approach when intervening for a patient with dementia who will not sit and eat at mealtime?
   a. Demonstrate putting food in the mouth and eating. Have finger foods available so that the patient can eat while pacing.
   b. Keep repeating the request to sit and eat until the patient does so. Guide the patient back into the chair when he or she rises.
   c. Restrain the patient in the chair; place a tray in front of the patient, and explain that it contains food.
   d. Question the patient about preferred mealtimes and favorite foods; adapt foods and mealtimes to stated preferences.

3. Which of the following patient statements would indicate successful learning regarding bowel management?
   a. "I will take a laxative every day."
   b. "I will walk two blocks once each week."
   c. "I will drink 2 quarts of fluid every day."
   d. "I will eat bran cereal once each week."

4. Which of the following would be an appropriate goal for a patient with osteoporosis?
   a. Maintain a sedentary lifestyle.

   b. Demonstrate awareness of lifting safely.
   c. Verbalize knowledge of cure for the disease.
   d. Increase intake of dietary estrogen.

5. Which of the following is the most important consideration regarding history taking in elderly patients?
   a. Obtain information as quickly as possible, avoiding long interviews.
   b. Traditional historical information will provide adequate data.
   c. Adjust the method and pace of information gathering for sensory deficits and physical condition.
   d. Start the history with a mental status examination to validate reliability of informant.

6. Mrs. Walesea, aged 76, has just been diagnosed with Alzheimer's disease. Discharge planning to a home-alone living situation for Mrs. Walesea requires
   a. no community agency referrals because of the patient's mild impairment (Discussing available services may provoke anxiety for the patient and family members.)
   b. referrals for meals on wheels and adult care because of diagnosis of Alzheimer's disease; family respite needs to begin early
   c. arrangements for a visiting nurse to assess the home environment and link the patient with appropriate community services
   d. discouraging home living and planning for posthospital nursing home admission because of the progressive decline expected with this diagnosis

7. Which of the following sets of assessment data would most likely lead the nurse to believe that a patient's nursing diagnosis of Altered Thought Processes could be reversed?
   a. depression, history of multiple strokes, known vitamin B deficiency
   b. subdural hematoma, pneumonia, digoxin toxicity

c. brain tumor, intoxication, and dehydration

d. urinary tract infection, AIDS, history of head trauma

8. Mrs. Simpson, an 84-year-old white woman, was admitted to a medical unit from a nursing home at 3 P.M. Her regular physician was out of town until the next day, but he wrote that she was being admitted for occult GI bleeding. Laboratory studies revealed a hemoglobin of 8 and a positive stool guaiac. Mrs. Simpson's transfer form noted blindness and deafness but no functional deficits except the need for assistance with bathing. It did not specify her mental status and means of communication. Assessment findings included body weight of 96 lb (representing a gradual loss of 15 lb) and frail appearance. Activity orders stated "up with assistance." Admission data from the nurse and intern noted failed attempts at communication and that Mrs. Simpson was asking where she was. Mrs. Simpson was placed in bed. At 11 P.M., Mrs. Simpson was reported to have been incontinent twice since admission. It was also noted that she had been placed in a posey vest because of attempts to get out of bed. After reviewing Mrs. Simpson's chart, the night nurse determined that Mrs. Simpson's incontinence was most likely

a. total incontinence related to dementia because she is old and had been admitted from a nursing home

b. transient physiologic incontinence related to her current poor physical condition

c. urge incontinence because she had not used the nurse call system for assistance to the bathroom

d. functional incontinence caused by restraints and inability to find the bathroom

9. At 12:30 A.M., the night nurse decided to check on Mrs. Simpson's need to urinate. She noticed that Mrs. Simpson turned toward her when she spoke near her left ear and asked, "What did you say?" Based on this incident and the information on Mrs. Simpson's chart, the nurse might best attempt to assist Mrs. Simpson concerning elimination by the following.

a. Touch her arm to gain attention; speak with simple words directly toward her and try each ear at close distance, varying tone, to explain that she will be assisted to the bathroom. Then help her up and guide her hand to touch the side of the bed, furniture, wall, and door on way to the toilet, and then to touch bathroom fixtures. Repeat this procedure in 2 hours.

b. Touch her arm and, speaking very loudly, tell her that she will be assisted to the bathroom. Help her sit on the side of the bed, then take her arm and guide her to the toilet. Touch her hand to the toilet seat and guide her to a sitting position. Repeat this procedure in 2 hours.

c. Touch her arm and, facing her directly and speaking loudly, ask whether she needs to use the bathroom. If she doesn't respond, have her touch the bedpan (because it is nighttime); if she still doesn't respond positively, repeat in 2 hours.

d. Touch her arm, then take her hand and move it over the call button, demonstrating how to press the button. Next, touch her hand to the nurse's arm, then to the bedpan, and place her on the bedpan if she responds positively. Wait for her to use the call light to signal the need for the next toileting.

10. The nursing home staff confirmed that Mrs. Simpson did not have dementia, could understand simple conversation in her left ear, and was up independently prior to transfer. Based on this and previously known information, the nurse would best promote continence and safety for Mrs. Simpson by

a. scheduling toileting, using the bathroom, every 2 hours; continuing to use a posey vest at night for safety; not relying on Mrs. Simpson's ability to locate and use the call light

b. removing restraints; orienting her to the room and bathroom environments; placing the bed in a low position without siderails up; allowing her to ambulate freely; and monitoring the room periodically

c. removing restraints; placing the bed in a low position without siderails up; instructing her to use the call light to summon the nurse, who will provide assistance with ambulation; placing the call light within easy reach and keeping it in the same place

d. removing restraints; putting siderails up to prevent her from getting out of bed alone; scheduling regular toileting using a bedpan because of weakness; not relying on her ability to locate and use the call light

11. Findings from ongoing assessment and diagnostic tests reveal iron deficiency anemia due to bleeding associated with a hiatal hernia. No surgery is recommended at this time, and Mrs. Simpson is discharged to the nursing home on appropriate medications and diet. Which of the following would represent the best measure of successful outcome of Mrs. Simpson's hospital nursing care?

a. no injury from falling; no development of urinary tract infection

b. evaluation for hearing aid; no reduction in functional independence during hospital stay

c. hemoglobin increased; understands diet appropriate for hiatal hernia

d. infrequent episodes of incontinence; no gastric pain

12. Which of the following interventions would be appropriate to reduce the risk of constipation in a 79-year-old patient hospitalized following a hip fracture?

a. Limit fluid intake to less than 2 L/day.

b. Avoid administering narcotic analgesics.

c. Perform range-of-motion exercises daily.

d. Administer daily enemas.

13. Which of the following nursing diagnoses would most likely lead the nurse to believe that a postmenopausal patient is at risk for progression of osteoporosis?

a. Altered Nutrition: More Than Body Requirements

b. Urinary Incontinence, Stress

c. Altered Patterns of Sexuality

d. Impaired Physical Mobility

14. Which of the following nursing interventions would be most appropriate to incorporate when working with a hearing-impaired patient?

a. Provide nonverbal cues to augment communication.

b. Discourage reliance on amplifying devices.

c. Speak in a high-pitched voice.

d. Discourage attempts by the patient to perform ear hygiene.

15. Mr. Smithson, aged 80 and with a history of left hip fracture, is admitted with a 48-hour history of vomiting, diarrhea, and weight loss. Based on this information, the nurse should monitor Mr. Smithson closely for

a. hypokalemia

b. decreased serum creatinine level

c. hypertension

d. anasarca

16. Which of the following would represent the best evaluation criteria reflecting successful outcome of treatment for dehydration?

a. The patient exhibits no signs or symptoms of CVA, dysrhythmia, or hyperproteinemia.

b. The patient exhibits no signs or symptoms of shock, circulatory overload, or hypokalemia.

c. The patient exhibits no signs or symptoms of renal failure, pressure sores, or hypoproteinemia.

d. The patient exhibits no signs or symptoms of congestive heart failure, polyuria, or hyperkalemia.

ANSWER KEY

1. **Correct response: c**
   Many stereotypes and myths about older adults alter our view of their capabilities.
   a. Aging changes are often difficult to distinguish from those reflecting disease.
   b. Aging rate can differ among various organ systems.
   d. Disuse and physical deconditioning effects are often reversible.
   Knowledge/Physiologic/Assessment

2. **Correct response: a**
   This approach provides nonverbal information and avoids questioning or explaining, which may not be understood or can be too stimulating.
   b, c, and d. Verbal instructions may not be understood or may be overstimulating. Food intake is possible without forcing the patient to sit.
   Application/Physiologic/Implementation

3. **Correct response: c**
   Adequate fluid intake is essential for normal bowel function.
   a. Daily laxative use leads to physiologic dependence.
   b. Walking 2 blocks once a week is insufficient exercise.
   d. Fiber must be consumed daily to have a beneficial effect on bowel function.
   Comprehension/Physiologic/Evaluation

4. **Correct response: b**
   A patient with osteoporosis is at risk for fracture; understanding of safe movement is essential.
   a. Regular, moderate exercise has a role in prevention and treatment of osteoporosis.
   c. There is no cure for osteoporosis.
   d. Estrogen cannot be ingested through the diet.
   Analysis/Health promotion/Planning

5. **Correct response: c**
   The rate and method of information exchange must be adjusted to enhance the patient's ability to respond.
   a. A too rapid pace could confuse the patient and interfere with accurate data collection.
   b. Besides traditional health history information, history taking in elderly patients should include more detailed information in areas such as social supports, living arrangements, functional capacity, and drug-taking practices.
   d. Mental status examination is often perceived as threatening and thus should be done at the end of the assessment session.
   Comprehension/Psychosocial/Assessment

6. **Correct response: c**
   A visiting nurse can assess the appropriateness of home living and suggest modifications and referrals to enhance home care.
   a. The patient and family need to be informed about available community services.
   b. This may not be appropriate; the family may want to provide some services in early stages to hold down long-term expenses.
   d. Home living may be possible if hazards can be removed and necessary support systems provided.
   Application/Safe care/Planning

7. **Correct response: b**
   These problems are all potentially reversible causes of altered thought processes.
   a, c, and d. These responses all contain at least one cause of dementia; cognitive problems resulting from dementia do not have as high a likelihood of reversibility as do cognitive problems resulting from other causes.
   Analysis/Physiologic/Analysis (Dx)

8. *Correct response: d*
Because Mrs. Simpson's transfer form does not note major functional deficits or prior incontinence and dementia, functional causes should be suspected.

   a, b, and c. Based on the assessment data, neither total incontinence, transient physiologic incontinence, nor urge incontinence are likely diagnoses.

Analysis/Physiologic/Analysis (Dx)

9. *Correct response: a*
The nurse should promote understanding by using clear, simple speech, possibly directed to the ear with the best hearing, and orient the patient to the environment through touch.

   b. The nurse should avoid loud speech.

   c and d. The patient should not use a bedpan because she can ambulate with assistance.

Application/Safe care/Implementation

10. *Correct response: c*
These interventions provide some safety precautions but do not limit her independence.

   a, b, and d. These interventions either discourage independence or rely on the patient's ability to use the call light (which may be difficult because of her blindness).

Application/Safe care/Implementation

11. *Correct response: b*
The overall goal of care of older adults is to promote optimum function.

   a, c, and d. These goals may be important, but the nurse's major responsibility is to maintain functional level.

Analysis/Health promotion/Evaluation

12. *Correct response: b*
A major side effect of narcotic and analgesics is constipation.

   a. Fluid intake more than 2 L/day is recommended to promote bowel function.

   c. Range-of-motion exercise once each day is insufficient exercise.

   d. Use of daily enemas fosters dependence.

Application/Health promotion/Planning

13. *Correct response: d*
Weight-bearing exercise is important in stabilization of osteoporosis.

   a, b, and c. These nursing diagnoses do not represent risk factors for progression of osteoporosis.

Knowledge/Health promotion/Analysis (Dx)

14. *Correct response: a*
Using nonverbal cues would facilitate communication with a hearing-impaired client.

   b, c, and d. These interventions would discourage or hamper independence and facilitation of hearing.

Application/Psychosocial/Implementation

15. *Correct response: a*
As vomiting persists, fluid and essential electrolytes are lost, which may lead to circulatory failure.

   b, c, and d. These problems are not specifically associated with this patient's clinical profile.

Comprehension/Safe care/Assessment

16. *Correct response: b*
A patient with inadequate treatment may develop shock. Aggressive fluid replacement may lead to circulatory overload and congestive heart failure. Inappropriate administration of potassium replacement may led to either hypokalemia or hyperkalemia.

   a, c, and d. These complications are not specifically associated with dehydration.

Analysis/Physiologic/Evaluation

Emergency Nursing

Note: This chapter covers emergency conditions not discussed elsewhere in this text. See appropriate chapters for information on these common emergency conditions:

▶ Chapter 7, Cardiovascular Disorders (cardiac arrest, myocardial infarction)
▶ Chapter 12, Immunologic Disorders (anaphylaxis)
▶ Chapter 13, Integumentary Disorders (burns)
▶ Chapter 14, Neurologic Disorders (head injuries, spinal cord injury)
▶ Chapter 16, Musculoskeletal Disorders (fractures)
▶ Chapter 20, Infectious Disorders (food poisoning)

I. Overview of emergency nursing

A. Roles and functions of emergency room nurse

1. Provide care to patients with urgent and critical physiologic or psychologic needs.
2. Understand that the perceptions of the ill or injured person or his or her family define a situation as an emergency.
3. Treat the patient and family with understanding, and respect the anxiety they are experiencing. Keep in mind that emergency patients often feel out of control because the suddenness of their problem leaves little or no time for coping and adjusting; also remember that family members or significant others need personal consideration.
4. Practice triage, a system for setting priorities of patient care; steps in nursing process from assessment through evaluation conducted rapidly with emphasis on assessing and intervening in order to save life and limb (Table 23–1).

B. Practice settings

1. Emergency department
2. A mobile unit
3. Freestanding emergency unit
4. Suicide prevention center

TABLE 23–1.
Priorities for Emergency Care

1. Assess respirations.
2. Ensure a patient airway, and ventilate if necessary.
3. Assess cardiovascular function.
4. Maintain adequate blood pressure.
5. Apply pressure to any bleeding sites.
6. Assess level of consciousness.
7. Reassess vital physical parameters continually.
8. Splint all suspected fractures.
9. Apply sterile dressings to wounds.

II. Airway obstruction
A. Description and etiology
1. Airway obstruction refers to any mechanical impediment to oxygen delivery or absorption in the lungs.
2. Food is the most common cause of obstruction in a conscious person; the tongue, in an unconscious person.

B. Assessment findings
1. A patient with *complete* airway obstruction is unable to breathe or speak, becomes cyanotic, and collapses.
2. A patient with *incomplete* obstruction appears anxious, uses accessory muscles to breathe, may have stridor and flared nostrils, and usually is able to speak.

C. Nursing diagnosis: Ineffective Airway Clearance
D. Planning and implementation
1. Keep in mind that airway obstruction takes priority over any other injury or emergency problem.
2. In partial obstruction, instruct the conscious patient to cough forcefully; if this does not dislodge the object, perform the Heimlich maneuver (subdiaphragmatic abdominal thrusts).
3. In complete obstruction in a conscious patient, immediately perform the Heimlich maneuver.
4. In partial or complete obstruction in an unconscious patient, follow these steps:
   a. Position the patient on his or her back.
   b. Use the head-tilt–chin-lift technique to open the airway. (Use the jaw thrust technique if cervical spine injury is suspected.)
   c. Attempt to ventilate the patient.
   d. Perform the Heimlich maneuver.
   e. Perform a finger sweep.
   f. Attempt ventilation again.
   g. Continue until the obstruction is removed.
5. If indicated, assist with cricothyroidotomy (puncture of the cricothyroid membrane with an 11-gauge needle) to establish an airway.

E. Evaluation
1. The patient maintains a patent airway.
2. The patient resumes spontaneous respirations.

III. Near-drowning
A. Description: the pathologic state of a person who has survived events that nearly led to drowning
B. Assessment findings
1. Near-drowning is commonly marked by:
   a. Cyanosis
   b. Pulmonary edema

        c.   Possible hypothermia
        d.   Possible cardiac arrest
    2.   Laboratory studies may reveal:
        a.   Severe hypoxia
        b.   Metabolic acidosis

C. Nursing diagnoses
    1.   Ineffective Airway Clearance
    2.   Hypothermia

D. Planning and implementation
    1.   Initiate vigorous, purposeful CPR.
    2.   Ventilate with 100% oxygen and positive end expiratory pressure.
    3.   Insert an IV line, a central venous line, an indwelling urinary catheter, or a nasogastric tube as ordered.
    4.   Initiate cardiac monitoring.
    5.   Begin internal rewarming (e.g., warm peritoneal dialysis, warm aerosol inhalation) and external rewarming (e.g., hyperthermia blanket) if necessary.
    6.   Monitor vital signs, level of consciousness, electrocardiogram (ECG) findings, central venous pressure (CVP), intake and output, arterial blood gases (ABGs), and serum electrolytes.
    7.   Admit the patient to the ICU.

E. Evaluation
    1.   The patient resumes spontaneous respirations and pulse.
    2.   The patient exhibits stable vital signs.
    3.   The patient registers temperature above 97°F.
    4.   The patient is alert and responsive.

IV. Hemorrhage

A. Description: rapid, massive blood loss, either internally or externally

B. Etiology and pathophysiology
    1.   Possible causes of hemorrhage include:
        a.   External: penetrating trauma, lacerations
        b.   Internal: blunt or penetrating trauma, blood dyscrasias, ruptured aortic aneurysm
    2.   Severe hemorrhage may result in hypovolemic shock from blood loss and necessitates immediate emergency intervention.

C. Assessment findings
    1.   Clinical manifestations of hemorrhage include:
        a.   Obvious bleeding from wound or orifices
        b.   Signs of internal bleeding (e.g., ecchymoses, occult or frank blood in urine or stool)
        c.   Cold, moist, pale skin
        d.   Apprehension
        e.   Hypotension

> f. Tachycardia
> g. Oliguria
>
> 2. Guaiac testing of stool may detect occult blood.

D. Nursing diagnosis: Fluid Volume Deficit

E. Planning and implementation

1. Apply pressure over bleeding area or involved artery (external bleeding).
2. Elevate and immobilize the injured body part (external bleeding), and position the patient supine.
3. Start a peripheral IV for blood replacement, and administer fluids, blood products as ordered.
4. Apply medical antishock trousers (MAST) as indicated.
5. Prepare the patient for surgery, and continue to monitor vital signs, ABGs, CVP, and level of consciousness.
6. Apply a tourniquet *only as a last resort* to stop bleeding.

F. Evaluation

1. The patient shows no evidence of obvious bleeding.
2. The patient maintains vital signs, ABGs, ECG waveforms, and urine output all within normal ranges.

V. Chest trauma

A. Description and etiology

1. Causes of blunt chest trauma include:
   a. Falls
   b. Blows
   c. Automobile accidents
2. Common penetrating chest injuries include:
   a. Gunshot wounds
   b. Stab wounds

B. Pathophysiology

1. Patients with blunt chest injuries require careful and complete assessment to detect hidden injuries such as:
   a. Tears of major blood vessels, causing internal hemorrhage
   b. Lung or heart contusions, which can develop into serious cardiorespiratory emergencies
2. Patients with penetrating chest wounds often require emergency nursing care that focuses on management of pneumothorax (accumulation of air in pleural space) that may result in partial or complete collapse of affected lung.
3. Patients with pneumothorax are at risk for life-threatening tension pneumothorax.

C. Assessment findings

1. Blunt chest trauma may be marked by:
   a. Tachypnea
   b. Stridor

        c.   Cyanosis
        d.   Assymmetric chest expansion
        e.   Signs and symptoms of hypovolemia and shock
        f.   Abrasions, bruises, and other signs of injury

    2.   Penetrating chest trauma may produce:
        a.   Dyspnea and tachycardia accompanied by sudden sharp chest pain
        b.   Diminished or absent breath sounds on the affected side
        c.   Tympanic notes on chest percussion

    3.   Tension pneumothorax may cause mediastinal shift, resulting in:
        a.   Shock
        b.   Tracheal shifting from midline
        c.   Severe respiratory distress

D. **Nursing diagnoses**
    1.   Ineffective Breathing Pattern
    2.   Decreased Cardiac Output
    3.   Pain

E. **Planning and implementation**
    1.   For a patient with a blunt chest injury:
        a.   Report abnormal findings immediately.
        b.   Monitor vital signs, ECG, level of consciousness, ABGs.
        c.   Auscultate breath sounds, and assess for respiratory difficulty.
        d.   Maintain airway, ventilation, and oxygenation if necessary.
        e.   Treat shock as indicated.
        f.   Prepare the patient for surgery if necessary.

    2.   For penetrating chest injury:
        a.   Position the patient in high-Fowler's position, and administer oxygen as necessary.
        b.   Prepare the patient for insertion of a chest tube or mushroom chest catheter (McSwain's dart) as indicated.
        c.   Monitor respirations, vital signs, level of consciousness, and ABGs.

F. **Evaluation**
    1.   The patient maintains vital signs, ABGs, and level of consciousness within normal ranges.
    2.   The patient maintains a patent airway and displays no evidence of tracheal shift.

VI. **Abdominal trauma**
  A. **Description and etiology**
    1.   Abdominal injuries may be:
        a.   Blunt, due to falls, blows to the abdomen, or automobile accidents

        b.   Penetrating (e.g., gunshot wounds, stab wounds)
2. Patients with blunt abdominal wounds require careful and complete assessment because hidden injuries often are not easily detected.

B. Assessment findings
1. Findings in a patient sustaining abdominal injury may include:
    a.   Visible bruises, lacerations, penetrating wounds, etc.
    b.   Abdominal distention, pain, tenderness
    c.   Absent or diminished bowel sounds
    d.   Hypotension and other signs of impending shock
2. Guaiac testing of stool may detect occult blood.

C. Nursing diagnoses
1. High Risk for Fluid Volume Deficit
2. Impaired Tissue Integrity

D. Planning and implementation
1. Perform CPR if necessary.
2. Maintain the patient on bedrest with knees flexed (to decrease abdominal pain).
3. Instruct the patient to lie still; explain that movement may dislodge the clot, causing hemorrhage.
4. Apply pressure to external bleeding wounds.
5. Keep the patient NPO.
6. Insert a nasogastric tube, an IV catheter, and an indwelling urinary catheter as indicated.
7. Cover any exposed viscera with sterile normal saline solution dressings.
8. Administer prophylactic antibiotics and tetanus toxoid as directed.
9. Monitor vital signs, CVP, and intake and output.
10. Auscultate bowel sounds.
11. Prepare the patient for peritoneal lavage or surgery, if indicated.

E. Evaluation
1. The patient exhibits no signs of infection or abdominal distention.
2. The patient reports decreased pain.
3. The patient displays audible bowel sounds.
4. The patient maintains vital signs within normal ranges.

VII. Poisoning with ingested agents
A. Description: the condition resulting from accidental or deliberate ingestion of poisonous substances
B. Etiology
1. Commonly ingested alkaline agents include:
    a.   Lye
    b.   Drain and oven cleaners

      c.   Bleach

      d.   Clinitest

2. Acidic substances that may be ingested include:
   a. Toilet bowl cleaners
   b. Battery acid
   c. Rust removers

C. Assessment findings

1. Depending on the agent ingested, the patient may experience:
   a. Burning pain in the mouth and throat
   b. Dysphagia
   c. Vomiting
   d. Drooling
   e. Respiratory distress
   f. Altered level of consciousness
2. Possible laboratory studies include ABGs, CBC, blood urea nitrogen (BUN), creatinine, and electrolyte levels.

D. Nursing diagnoses

1. Ineffective Airway Clearance
2. Pain
3. Impaired Swallowing
4. Impaired Tissue Integrity

E. Planning and implementation

1. Open the airway, and provide ventilation and oxygenation if needed.
2. Position the patient on his or her side with the head down.
3. Suction as needed to prevent aspiration of gastric contents into respiratory tract.
4. Remove or inactivate poison before absorption occurs, through:
   a. Syrup of Ipecac—only for an alert patient who has ingested a noncorrosive substance
   b. Gastric lavage
   c. Specific antidote to neutralize poisonous substance
   d. Milk or water for dilution if the patient can swallow
5. Do *not* induce vomiting.
6. Obtain a blood sample for analysis as ordered.
7. Monitor neurologic status, noting:
   a. Seizure activity
   b. Mentation
   c. Central nervous system (CNS) depression
8. Insert an indwelling urinary catheter as ordered.
9. Before discharge, provide the patient or parents with poisoning prevention guidelines.
10. Refer the patient for psychiatric consultation if poisoning was a suicide attempt. (Admission to the hospital may be necessary.)

F. Evaluation
1. The patient exhibits good mucous membrane integrity.
2. The patient reports decreased pain and discomfort.
3. The patient states an interest in psychologic counseling if poisoning was a suicide attempt.

VIII. Substance abuse
A. Description
1. Substance abuse refers to misuse of specific substances intended to alter mood or behavior.
2. Commonly abused substances include:
   a. Alcohol
   b. Narcotics
   c. Hallucinogens
   d. Amphetamines
   e. Barbiturates
   f. Aspirin
3. Be aware that drug abusers often misuse more than one substance at same time.

B. Assessment findings
1. Clinical manifestations of substance abuse vary widely, depending on the substance and the amount ingested.
2. Common signs and symptoms include:
   a. Signs of CNS depression or stimulation
   b. Altered temperature (hypothermia or hyperthermia)
   c. Respiratory depression or tachypnea
   d. Hallucinations
   e. Seizure activity
   f. Abnormal pupil size and response
   g. Nausea and vomiting
   h. Altered renal function, marked by oliguria or polyuria, abnormal BUN, serum creatinine, and serum electrolyte levels
   i. Abnormal ABG values, indicating acidosis or alkalosis

C. Nursing diagnoses
1. Ineffective Breathing Pattern
2. Sensory and Perceptual Alterations
3. High Risk for Violence

D. Planning and implementation
1. Treat the patient suffering from drug overdose, focusing on:
   a. Respiratory and cardiovascular support
   b. Elimination of drug(s) from the body
2. Control airway, ventilation, and oxygenation. (Insertion of a cuffed endotracheal tube may be necessary.)
3. Develop a supportive, empathic rapport, and attend the patient at all times.

4. Start IV fluid infusion as indicated.
5. Remove ingested drug from the stomach with Ipecac or gastric lavage as ordered; prevent aspiration in a patient with absent gag or cough reflexes by first intubating patient.
6. Administer specific drug antidote; for example:
   a. Narcan for narcotic overdose
   b. Activated charcoal only after emesis or lavage
7. Assist with hemodialysis or peritoneal dialysis as indicated.
8. Treat hypothermia or hyperthermia as appropriate (see Sections IX and X).
9. Transfer an unconscious patient to the ICU.
10. Arrange consultation with psychiatrist or drug or alcohol treatment program before discharge.

E. **Evaluation**
   1. The patient exhibits effective respirations.
   2. The patient maintains stable vital signs, ABG values, and ECG findings.
   3. The patient is alert and oriented.
   4. The patient maintains serum electrolytes, creatinine, BUN, and urinary output within normal ranges.

IX. Hypothermia and frostbite

A. **Description and etiology**
   1. Hypothermia refers to abnormally low core body temperature (below 34.4°C or 94°F) resulting from exposure to cold environmental temperatures.
   2. Frostbite involves damage to tissue and blood vessels due to exposure to extreme cold.

B. **Assessment findings**
   1. Manifestations of hypothermia may include:
      a. Subnormal body temperature
      b. Altered level of consciousness: apathy, drowsiness, coma
      c. Weak or undetectable peripheral pulses
      d. Cardiac dysrhythmias, possibly cardiac arrest
      e. Signs and symptoms of hypoxia and acidosis
   2. In frostbite, the affected body part may be:
      a. Cold
      b. Hard
      c. White to bluish white
      d. Numb or painful
      e. Blistered
      f. Edematous

C. **Nursing diagnoses**
   1. Hypothermia
   2. Impaired Skin Integrity
   3. Altered Tissue Perfusion

D. **Planning and implementation**
   1. Initiate CPR if indicated.
   2. Rewarm the patient with:
      a. Hyperthermia blanket (external)
      b. Warmed humidified oxygen
      c. Warmed IV fluids (internal)
   3. Monitor vital signs, CVP, ECG, ABGs, intake and output.
   4. Administer IV fluids and sodium bicarbonate as ordered.
   5. For frostbite:
      a. Protect the affected area from injury; handle it gently, use a protective cradle if indicated, and maintain strict aseptic technique.
      b. Rewarm the body part (e.g., in a warm whirlpool).
      c. Elevate the body part.

E. **Evaluation**
   1. The patient maintains body temperature above 97°F.
   2. The patient maintains vital signs and ABG values within normal ranges.
   3. The patient is alert and oriented.
   4. The patient with frostbite maintains good skin integrity and exhibits palpable pulses in affected extremities.

X. **Hyperthermia (heat stroke)**
   A. **Description: abnormally high body temperature due to heat stress**
   B. **Etiology and pathophysiology**
      1. Hyperthermia occurs when the body's heat-regulating mechanisms fail.
      2. Risk factors include:
         a. Exposure to high humidity heat waves
         b. Age extremes
         c. Debilitating disease
         d. Impaired self-care ability
         e. Certain drugs (e.g., major tranquilizers, anticholinergics, diuretics, propranolol)
   C. **Assessment findings**
      1. Common clinical manifestations of hyperthermia include:
         a. Hyperpyrexia
         b. Altered level of consciousness: confusion, delirium, or coma
         c. Hot, dry skin with absence of sweating
         d. Tachycardia
         e. Tachypnea
         f. Hypotension
         g. Possibly vomiting and diarrhea
      2. Laboratory studies may reveal grossly elevated SGOT, LDH, and CPK values.

D. Nursing diagnosis: Hyperthermia
E. Planning and implementation
    1. Reduce body temperature rapidly by:
        a. Immersing the patient in cool water
        b. Sponging with cool water
        c. Using a hypothermia blanket
        d. Administering iced saline lavage
    2. Monitor vital signs, ECG findings, level of consciousness, CVP, and intake and output.
    3. Massage the patient to promote circulation.
    4. Initiate IV fluids and oxygen therapy as indicated.
    5. Admit the patient to the ICU.
F. Evaluation
    1. The patient maintains body temperature below 100°F.
    2. The patient maintains vital signs, level of consciousness, ECG, and intake and output within normal parameters.

Bibliography

Brunner, L. S., & Suddarth, D. S. (1988). *Textbook of medical-surgical nursing* (6th ed.). Philadelphia: J. B. Lippincott.

Brunner, L. S., & Suddarth, D. S. (1986). *The Lippincott manual of nursing practice* (4th ed.). Philadelphia: J. B. Lippincott.

Luckmann, J., & Sorenson, K. C. (1987). *Medical-surgical nursing: A psychophysiologic approach* (3rd ed.). Philadelphia: W. B. Saunders.

STUDY QUESTIONS

1. Which of the following statements describes why patients with emergencies are unique?
   a. The families of patients with emergencies are also in need of special attention.
   b. All the steps in the nursing process must be performed when caring for a patient with an emergency.
   c. Emergency patients often feel an intense sense of anxiety because of the suddenness of the illness or injury.
   d. The psychosocial needs of patients with emergencies are necessarily neglected.

2. After rapid assessment, the nurse categorizes emergency patients by priority nursing diagnoses. Based on the following diagnoses, which patient should be given priority attention?
   a. High Risk for Trauma: Injury: a 14-year-old with a suspected fractured femur
   b. High Risk for Suffocation: Injury: a 60-year-old with burns of the face and neck
   c. Impaired Skin Integrity: a 25-year-old with a lacerated finger
   d. Anxiety: a 50-year-old complaining of "feelings of panic"

3. Which of the following nursing interventions would *not* be appropriate when planning care for the family of an emergency patient?
   a. encouraging the family members to verbalize their anxieties
   b. informing the family frequently about the care the patient is receiving
   c. discouraging any feelings of anger the family feels about the situation
   d. handling the family's feelings of denial by preparing the family for the reality of the patient's condition

4. Nursing care of a patient who has ingested a poison always includes which of the following nursing interventions?

   a. immediately administering an emetic to prevent further absorption of the poison
   b. placing the patient in high-Fowler's position to facilitate respirations
   c. referring for psychiatric consultation before discharge
   d. performing ongoing assessment of neurologic and cardiorespiratory status

5. Symptoms of a partial airway obstruction include which of the following?
   a. stridor
   b. respiratory arrest
   c. inability to speak
   d. complete collapse

6. The emergency department nurse prepares to insert a nasogastric (NG) tube in a near-drowning victim. The purpose of the NG tube is to
   a. Obtain gastric contents for analysis.
   b. Establish a vehicle for medication administration.
   c. Prevent aspiration of any swallowed water.
   d. Establish a route for nutritional supplements.

7. Which of the following evaluation criteria represent successful resolution of internal bleeding?
   a. The patient demonstrates an absence of hypertension and bradycardia.
   b. The patient demonstrates an absence of hypotension and tachycardia.
   c. The patient demonstrates an absence of pyrexia and flushing.
   d. The patient demonstrates an absence of lethargy and drowsiness.

8. Which of the following nursing interventions would be appropriate for the patient who has arrived in the emergency room with a head injury?
   a. Immobilize the spine.
   b. Place the patient in modified Trendelenburg position.

c. Restrain the patient's arms.

d. Infuse IV fluids rapidly.

9. Mr. Jones comes to the emergency department complaining of chest pain and shortness of breath. The nurse repeatedly reassures him and explains all procedures. The nurse's actions would be in response to which of the following nursing diagnoses?

a. Self-Concept Disturbance

b. Sensory and Perceptual Alteration

c. Fear

d. Altered Thought Processes

10. The nurse should use which of the following techniques to open the airway in a patient with a suspected cervical spine injury?

a. head tilt

b. jaw thrust

c. finger sweep

d. Heimlich maneuver

11. Which of the following should the emergency nurse include in a teaching plan for the patient with frostbite of the toes?

a. Elevate the foot on pillows.

b. Massage the foot with lotion.

c. Apply lotion to toes daily.

d. Walk briskly twice a day.

12. To evaluate the effectiveness of fluid replacement for the patient in hemorrhagic shock, the emergency department nurse would look for a return to normal range of

a. hemoglobin

b. pulse rate

c. temperature

d. blood pressure

13. A 25-year-old patient comes into the emergency department complaining of sudden shortness of breath after being hit accidentally in the right chest. Which of the following assessment findings would lead the nurse to suspect an emergency situation?

a. an abrasion on the right chest wall

b. right-sided chest pain

c. tracheal shift to the left side

d. anxiety

ANSWER KEY

1. **Correct response: c**
   Patients with emergencies often have not had time to accept the traditional patient role. This leads to a loss of control and increased anxiety and fear.
   a and b. These statements are true for all patients.
   d. This is an untrue statement.
   Knowledge/Psychosocial/Assessment

2. **Correct response: b**
   The nurse should always suspect an inhalation injury with facial burns. Inhalation injury may cause an airway obstruction. Maintaining a patent airway is always a first priority.
   a, c, and d. These all necessitate emergency care but are not prioritized before an airway obstruction.
   Analysis/Physiologic/Analysis (Dx)

3. **Correct response: c**
   The family's feelings of anger should be handled with understanding because anger is often a way of expressing anxiety. The nurse also should allow the patient to express anger.
   a, b, and d. These are all part of the special considerations necessary for the emergency patient's family.
   Comprehensive/Health promotion/Planning

4. **Correct response: d**
   A poisoning patient needs careful monitoring to detect subtle changes in status, which can develop quickly.
   a. Induced vomiting is unsafe if the patient has ingested a corrosive substance.
   b. High-Fowler's position is unsafe; rather, the patient should be sidelying with head down to prevent aspiration in the event of vomiting.
   c. A psychiatric consultation is necessary only if the poisoning was a deliberate suicide attempt.
   Application/Safe care/Implementation

5. **Correct response: a**
   An incomplete airway obstruction often causes stridor.
   b, c, and d. These are signs of complete airway obstruction.
   Knowledge/Physiologic/Assessment

6. **Correct response: c**
   Near-drowning victims frequently swallow large amounts of water, which may be aspirated during resuscitation.
   a, b, and d. These measures would be unnecessary at this time.
   Comprehensive/Safe care/Planning

7. **Correct response: b**
   Decreased blood pressure and tachycardia are cardinal signs of shock.
   a. Hypertension and bradycardia are not associated with shock.
   c. This is incorrect; the patient's skin would be pale and cool.
   d. This is incorrect; shock is manifested by restlessness, not lethargy.
   Comprehensive/Physiologic/Evaluation

8. **Correct response: a**
   A patient with a head injury should be treated as a possible cervical spine injury until proven otherwise.
   b, c, and d. These measures would be unsafe because they may cause increased intracranial pressure.
   Analysis/Safe care/Implementation

9. **Correct response: c**
   Fear frequently occurs in the emergency patient with chest pain because of the sense of experiencing a catastrophic event.
   a, b, and d. These answers are incorrect; this nurse's actions are not directed at these diagnoses.
   Analysis/Psychosocial/Analysis (Dx)

10. **Correct response: b**
    The jaw thrust can be done without extending the neck and without causing further spinal injury.
    a. The head tilt could possibly cause further spinal injury.

c and d. The finger sweep and Heimlich maneuver are used when a foreign object other than the tongue is thought to be obstructing the airway.

Application/Safe care/Implementation

11. *Correct response: a*
    Elevating the part will prevent further swelling.

    b, c, and d. These actions would cause further damage to the tissues.

Application/Health promotion/Planning

12. *Correct response: d*
    Adequate fluid replacement expands the fluid volume in the intravascular space and will raise the blood pressure.

a. Hemoglobin measures red blood cell replacement, not overall fluid replacement.

b and c. Pulse rate and temperature are only indirectly related to fluid status.

Analysis/Physiologic/Evaluation

13. *Correct response: c*
    A tracheal shift away from the affected side is indicative of mediastinal shift—a life-threatening complication if untreated.

    a, b, and d. These findings would be expected, considering this patient's history, but are not imminently life threatening.

Analysis/Physiologic/Assessment

Perioperative Nursing

I. Perioperative nursing overview

A. General

1. The perioperative period encompasses a patient's total surgical experience, including the preoperative, intraoperative, and postoperative phases.

2. Perioperative nursing refers to activities performed by the professional nurse during these phases.

B. Operative phases

1. The preoperative phase begins with the decision to perform surgery and ends with the patient's transfer to the operating room (OR) table.

2. The intraoperative phase begins when the patient is received in

the OR and ends with his or her admission to the postanesthesia recovery room (PARR) or postanesthesia care unit (PACU).

3. The postoperative phase begins when the patient is admitted to PARR or PACU and extends through follow-up home or clinic evaluation.

C. Categories of surgery

1. Optional surgery is done totally at the patient's discretion (e.g., cosmetic surgery).
2. Elective surgery refers to procedures that are scheduled at the patient's convenience (e.g., cyst removal).
3. Required surgery is warranted for conditions necessitating intervention within a few weeks (e.g., cataract surgery).
4. Urgent or imperative surgery is indicated for a problem requiring intervention within 24 to 48 hours (e.g., some cancers).
5. Emergency surgery describes procedures that must be done immediately to sustain life or maintain function (e.g., repair of a ruptured aortic aneurysm).

D. Types of anesthesia

1. General anesthesia refers to drug-induced depression of the central nervous system that produces analgesia, amnesia, and unconsciousness (affects whole body); stages include:
   a. Stage I—beginning
   b. Stage II—excitement
   c. Stage III—surgical anesthesia
   d. Stage IV—danger
2. Regional anesthesia suspends sensation and motion in a body region or part; the patient remains awake. Continuous monitoring is required in the event the block is not totally effective and the patient experiences pain or reactions to blocking agents occur (e.g., nausea, cardiovascular collapse).
3. Regional anesthesia differs in terms of location and size of the anatomic area anesthetized and the volume and type of anesthetic agent used.

E. General surgical considerations

1. The patient meets with the surgical team (e.g., surgeon, OR nurse, anesthesiologist, surgical technicians, surgical first assistants, radiographic or cardiovascular technicians) before surgery.
2. An anesthesiologist or nurse anesthetist makes a preoperative assessment to plan the type of anesthesia to be administered and to evaluate the patient's physical status.
3. A professional registered OR nurse makes preoperative nursing assessments and documents the intraoperative patient care plan.
4. All persons in OR are required to don specific, clean, attire, with the goal of "shedding" the outside environment. Specific clothing requirements are prescribed and standardized for all ORs.

5. Hair must be completely covered; shoes have special covers; masks are worn at all times in the OR and are changed between operations or more often, if necessary.
6. Any personnel who harbor pathogenic organisms (e.g., those with colds or infections) must report themselves unable to be in the OR to protect the patient from outside pathogens.

F. **Principles of surgical asepsis**
1. All items used in the OR must be sterile.
2. All personnel must perform a surgical scrub and wear a sterile mask, gown, and gloves.
3. Sterile scrubbed personnel should touch only sterile items.
4. Sterile gown and sterile drapes have defined borders of sterility.
5. That which is used for one patient must be discarded or, in some cases, resterilized.
6. The circulator and unsterile personnel must stay at the periphery of the sterile operating area in order not to contaminate the sterile area.
7. Sterile supplies are unwrapped and delivered by the circulator following specific standard protocol so as not to cause contamination.
8. The utmost caution and vigilance must be used when handling sterile fluids to prevent splashing or spillage.
9. OR personnel must practice strict blood and body substance isolation techniques.

II. **Preoperative period**
A. Assessment
1. Identify any obvious risk factors for surgery-related complications, including:
   a. Age (The very young and old are at risk for increased stress from the surgical experience.)
   b. Nutritional status (Compromised nutritional status has a negative effect on recovery and wound healing.)
   c. Obesity (An obese patient presents certain technical problems during surgery; is at greater risk for postoperative pulmonary complications such as hypoventilation and hypoxia; and is more likely to have coexisting cardiac, hepatic, biliary, or endocrine or metabolic problems that could complicate surgery.)
2. Assess respiratory status, including history of pulmonary problems to identify risk factors for postoperative complications, such as:
   a. Dyspnea, complaints of shortness of breath
   b. Upper respiratory infection
   c. Cough, wheezing
   d. Copious mucus or expectorate

e. Chest pain
f. Clubbed fingers
g. History of smoking

3. Assess cardiovascular status, noting:
   a. Blood pressure
   b. Pulse rate
   c. ECG tracings
   d. Presence and amplitude of peripheral pulses

4. Assess for and report evidence of fluid and electrolyte imbalance, including:
   a. Dehydration
   b. Hypovolemia
   c. Prolonged vomiting, diarrhea, or bleeding
   d. Abnormal serum potassium, sodium, magnesium, calcium, or pH level

5. Assess hepatic and renal function, noting:
   a. History of liver disease (e.g., cirrhosis, chronic alcoholism)
   b. Complaints of dysuria, oliguria or anuria, or urinary tract infections
   c. Urinalysis results

6. Examine the patient's record for any endocrine or metabolic problems that could affect the patient's response to surgery (e.g., poorly controlled diabetes mellitus).

7. Assess immunologic and hematologic function, noting:
   a. History of allergies
   b. Previous reactions to blood transfusion
   c. Immunosuppressed status

8. Assess neurologic function, noting:
   a. History of seizures or other neurologic disorders (e.g., Parkinson's disease, myasthenia gravis)
   b. Unsteady gait
   c. Unequal pupils

9. Evaluate medication history for drugs that could increase operative risk by affecting coagulation time or interacting with anesthetics, such as:
   a. Steroids
   b. Diuretics
   c. Phenothiazines
   d. Antidepressants
   e. Antibiotics
   f. Anticoagulants

10. Assess the patient's and family's knowledge base to guide the preoperative teaching program.

11. Consider psychosocial factors that could affect the patient's response to surgery, including:
    a. Anxiety and fear

   b.   Defense mechanisms (e.g., regression, denial, intellectuali-
        zation)
   c.   Self-esteem and body image concerns
B. Nursing diagnoses
   1.   Anxiety
   2.   Body Image Disturbance
   3.   Fear
   4.   Knowledge Deficit
   5.   Self-Esteem Disturbance
C. Planning and implementation
   1.   Teach the patient:
        a.   Deep breathing and coughing exercises
        b.   Relaxation techniques
        c.   Postoperative exercises of extremities
        d.   Turning and moving techniques
        e.   Pain control techniques
        f.   Incentive spirometry use
   2.   Perform preoperative skin preparation as appropriate, which may
        include:
        a.   Shaving the skin in and around the surgical area (*Note:*
             Shaving is somewhat controversial; generally, the longer
             the interval between shaving and surgery, the increased risk
             of postoperative infection.)
        b.   Using an electric razor or a depilatory cream as an alterna-
             tive to a razor, if possible
        c.   Having the patient take a cleansing shower with antimicro-
             bial scrub solution
   3.   Provide gastrointestinal preparation as prescribed, which may in-
        clude:
        a.   Restricting solid food and fluid for 8 to 10 hours before
             surgery (to reduce the risk of aspiration)
        b.   Posting an NPO sign at the patient's bedside
        c.   Administering an enema and inserting a nasogastric tube
             as prescribed
   4.   Make sure the patient or a responsible family member has pro-
        vided informed consent for surgery. Verify that an operative per-
        mit is signed and witnessed, with informed consent based on un-
        derstandable explanation from the surgeon about what will be
        done and risks involved. Make sure that the patient signs the
        permit if he or she is an emancipated minor or adult and is men-
        tally competent to give valid consent. If these requirements can-
        not be met, a responsible relative or guardian should sign for the
        patient. State laws govern situations when a relative or guardian
        is not available.
   5.   Perform standard preoperative procedures (using a checklist to
        ensure completeness, if desired):

       a. Take and record vital signs.

       b. Verify any allergy, identification, or diabetic bands.

       c. Validate NPO status.

       d. Complete and record medical preoperative orders.

       e. Remove all jewelry and nail polish.

       f. Have the patient void and don a clean hospital gown.

       g. Remove dentures, eyeglasses, and hearing aids, or send labeled containers with the patient to the OR for safe placement in case removal becomes necessary.

       h. Administer preanesthetic medications, and instruct the patient to stay in bed.

       i. Document any patient condition requiring OR staff attention (e.g., musculoskeletal or sensorineural problems).

    6. Ensure safe transport of the patient to the surgical suite (e.g., check for a stretcher with siderails, safety strap, and warm blankets).

D. Evaluation

    1. The patient demonstrates knowledge of postoperative exercises according to criteria.

    2. The patient states effects of preoperative medication.

    3. The patient uses relaxation techniques and imagery preoperatively and states the intention of using them postoperatively.

    4. The patient exhibits and reports decreased anxiety.

    5. The patient receives appropriate preoperative standards of care, as evidenced by a completed preoperative checklist.

    6. The patient verbalizes understanding of postoperative pain relief, including how to use devices such as patient-controlled analgesia pumps if appropriate.

III. Intraoperative period

A. Assessment

    1. Classify the patient's physical status for anesthesia:

       a. No organic or systemic disturbance present

       b. Mild disturbance (e.g., mild cardiac disease, mild diabetes mellitus)

       c. Severe systemic disturbance (e.g., poorly controlled diabetes mellitus, pulmonary complications)

       d. Life-threatening systemic disease (e.g., severe renal or cardiac disease)

       e. Moribund—little chance of survival (e.g., ruptured aortic aneurysm)

    2. Assess the patient's record for current signed consent; completed history and physical assessment record; recent laboratory and diagnostic reports; and evaluation of the patient's overall physiologic, emotional, and psychologic status.

    3. Specifically ask the patient if he or she has any allergies.

4. Verify patient identification and correct surgery scheduled.
5. Assess for any special surgical considerations (e.g., locations where an electric grounding plate can be safely placed on the patient, avoiding areas where metal or a prosthesis is present) and precautions (e.g., shielding with a lead apron if radiation is involved).
6. Assess the patient's risk for accidental hypothermia or malignant hyperthermia during anesthesia administration and surgery.

B. Nursing diagnoses
   1. High Risk for Fluid Volume Deficit
   2. High Risk for Fluid Volume Excess
   3. Hyperthermia
   4. Hypothermia
   5. High Risk for Infection
   6. High Risk for Injury
   7. Altered Tissue Perfusion

C. Planning and implementation
   1. Ensure the patient's safety in the OR; for example:
      a. Set room temperature and humidity to prevent hypothermia.
      b. Remove any potential contaminants.
      c. Curtail unnecessary room traffic.
      d. Keep room noise and talk at a minimum.
      e. Recheck electrical equipment for proper operation.
      f. Make sure that necessary equipment and supplies are available.
      g. Ensure that instruments, sutures, and dressings are ready.
      h. Count and record sutures, needles, instruments, and sponges.
      i. Make sure that staff call the patient by name and provide individualized attention.
      j. Assist in transferring the patient to the OR table.
      k. Cover the patient with a warm blanket, and attach the safety strap.
      l. Remain at the patient's side during anesthesia induction.
      m. Verify proper patient positioning to protect nerves, circulation, respiration, and skin integrity.
      n. Ensure that newly requested items are quickly supplied to the anesthesia or scrub team by the circulating nurse.
   2. Perform other actions as appropriate:
      a. Act in the role of patient advocate: provide privacy, protect from harm.
      b. Follow established procedures and protocols.
      c. Document all OR care.
      d. Help coordinate health team activities.

e.   Promote ethical behaviors (e.g., respect, confidentiality).

f.   Monitor blood, fluid, and other drainage output.

D.   Evaluation

1.   The patient remains free of any operative injury due to electrical, chemical, or physical hazards related to surgery.

2.   The patient maintains satisfactory body temperature between 96° and 100°F on completion of surgery.

3.   The patient remains free of injury linked to positioning during surgery, as evidenced by no complaints of numbness, paralysis, or abrasions.

4.   The patient arrives safely in the recovery area and exhibits adequate respiratory effort and good skin color.

IV.   Immediate postoperative period

A.   Assessment

1.   Perform assessment immediately on the patient's admission to the PARR or PACU to obtain baseline data.

2.   Position the patient before assessment to ensure an adequate airway; most commonly, lateral Sims' position for an unconscious patient unless contraindicated.

3.   Priorities for assessment include:

a.   Respiratory: airway patency, skin color

b.   Cardiovascular: vital signs

4.   The verbal report from the OR nurse and anesthesiologist or nurse-anesthetist to the PACU nurse should describe:

a.   The patient's age and general condition

b.   Any intraoperative problems encountered

c.   Medical diagnosis, pathology

d.   Fluids administered, blood loss and replacement, tubings and drains present

e.   Specific individual problems or deficits: hearing, vision, and mental status; and any symptoms that might need to be immediately reported to the surgeon

B.   Nursing diagnoses

1.   Ineffective Airway Clearance

2.   Ineffective Breathing Pattern

3.   High Risk for Fluid Volume Deficit

4.   High Risk for Infection

5.   Impaired Physical Mobility

6.   Pain

7.   Impaired Tissue Integrity

8.   Altered Tissue Perfusion: Cardiopulmonary and Peripheral

9.   Altered Pattern of Urinary Elimination

C.   Planning and implementation

1.   Document the patient's condition on the recovery room scoring guide.

2.   Assess at least every 15 minutes (or more frequently depending on the patient's status):

a. Airway
b. Vital signs
c. General appearance
d. Level of consciousness and reflexes
e. Pain level
f. Urine output
g. Intravenous or central line patency
h. Drain or catheter patency
i. Operative site and dressings for signs of hemorrhage or abnormal drainage
j. Functioning of cardiac and O_2 monitors

3. Maintain airway patency and optimum respiratory function; position the patient on side until he or she awakens, and administer oxygen as necessary.
4. Promote patient comfort by:
   a. Administering prescribed analgesics or narcotics
   b. Repositioning for comfort as indicated
   c. Encouraging postoperative exercises as tolerated
5. Maintain safety precautions.
6. Offer emotional support and reassurance.
7. Be alert for signs and symptoms of hypovolemic shock, a potential postoperative complication stemming from loss of blood and plasma during surgery.

D. Evaluation (for discharge from recovery room)
1. The patient performs deep breathing and coughing and exhibits clear lungs on auscultation.
2. The patient can lift his or her head off the pillow and hold it up.
3. The patient moves all extremities (unless contraindicated by surgery, physician's order, or previous physical condition).
4. The patient's dressings remain dry or have only light drainage apparent.
5. The patient's urinary output remains at least 30 mL/hour.
6. The patient maintains blood pressure and vital signs at stable levels and within normal ranges for the patient's situation.
7. The patient reports pain relief with adequate dosages of pain medication.
8. The patient can be safely transferred to a clinical unit for further care.
9. The patient scores at least seven out of 10 possible points on a postanesthesia scoring chart by the time of discharge to a clinical unit.

V. Intermediate and extended postoperative period
A. Assessment
1. Perform a head-to-toe physical assessment on the patient's admission to the clinical unit.
2. Monitor overall condition and blood pressure, pulse, and respira-

tions every 15 minutes for the first 2 hours, every 30 minutes for the next 2 hours, and, if stable, every 4 hours thereafter.
3. Assess respiratory status, including:
    a. Rate, depth, and pattern
    b. Character of breath sounds
    c. Airway patency
4. Assess circulatory status in extremities.
5. Observe level of consciousness and responsiveness.
6. Inspect surgical wounds, dressings, and drains; note signs of healing or infection, patency, and drainage characteristics.
7. Assess comfort level, noting:
    a. Time of last pain medication
    b. Any current pain; its location, nature, and intensity
    c. Position of maximum comfort
    d. Complaints of nausea or vomiting
    e. Body temperature
    f. Constrictive or irritating casts, dressings, traction
8. Evaluate urinary status, noting:
    a. Last voiding and amount
    b. Presence of indwelling catheter.
9. Explore pychosocial concerns related to such factors as:
    a. The nature of patient's surgical diagnosis and prognosis.
    b. Available support systems
    c. The patient's need for rest and quiet
10. Assess safety aspects, such as:
    a. The need for side rails on the bed
    b. Correct IV infusion rate
    c. Splinting of IV site
    d. Call bell kept within easy reach
    e. Ambulation status and the need for assistance
    f. Condition of all equipment
B. **Nursing diagnoses**
    1. Common nursing diagnoses applying to postsurgical patients include:
        a. Ineffective Airway Clearance
        b. Anxiety
        c. Constipation
        d. High Risk for Fluid Volume Deficit
        e. High Risk for Infection
        f. High Risk for Injury
        g. Impaired Physical Mobility
        h. Altered Nutrition: Less Than Body Requirements
        i. Pain
        j. Impaired Tissue Integrity
        k. Altered Tissue Perfusion: Peripheral
        l. Altered Patterns of Urinary Elimination

     2. More individualized diagnoses addressing psychosocial concerns related to the patient's particular condition and the nature of the surgery could include:

        a. Body Image Disturbance

        b. Hopelessness

        c. Powerlessness

        d. Spiritual Distress

C. Planning and implementation

     1. Promote lung expansion and help prevent atelectasis and pneumonia by:

        a. Encouraging coughing, deep breathing, and turning

        b. Using an incentive spirometer, as indicated

        c. Encouraging ambulation as tolerated.

     2. Monitor for signs and symptoms of postoperative complications, including:

        a. Hypovolemia

        b. Hemorrhage

        c. Pulmonary embolism

        d. Allergic drug reactions

        e. Cardiac dysrhythmias

     3. Provide appropriate pain relief measures, which may include:

        a. Prescribed analgesics, possibly patient-controlled analgesia units

        b. Nonpharmacologic pain relief measures (e.g., relaxation, guided imagery)

     4. Promote adequate fluid intake and monitor electrolyte balance.

     5. Provide adequate nutrition; resume oral feeding as soon as gastric and bowel motility return, or provide IV hyperalimentation as indicated.

     6. Auscultate for bowel sounds to detect the return of peristalsis. (Paralytic ileus may occur after abdominal or bowel surgery.)

     7. As indicated, minimize abdominal distention resulting from decreased peristalsis (typically persisting 3 to 4 days postoperatively) through exercise, ambulation, decreased narcotic dosage, or rectal tube placement.

     8. Assess for urinary retention after bladder catheter removal, particularly in patients who have undergone surgery involving the pelvic or rectal area. (See Chapter 18, Renal and Urinary Disorders, for more information on retention.)

     9. Promote normal voiding patterns through such measures as:

        a. Providing privacy

        b. Running tap water or providing other stimuli to induce urination

        c. Increasing fluid intake

        d. Relieving pain

    10. Assess for and report unrelieved nausea and vomiting; administer antiemetics as prescribed, and decrease the risk of aspirating vomitus through proper positioning.

11. Reduce the risk of nosocomial infection by maintaining medical and surgical asepsis. Classify the original surgical wound as clean, clean-contaminated, contaminated, or infected; observe for complications of a nonhealing wound. (See Chapter 20, Infectious Disorders, for more information.)

12. Respond quickly to evisceration (rupture of wound with coils of intestines pushed out, preceded by a gush of serosanguineous fluid) by:
    a. Staying with and attempting to calm the patient
    b. Positioning to decrease abdominal strain
    c. Applying moist, sterile saline dressings to cover exposed intestine
    d. Notifying the surgeon, who will need to perform reclosure surgery as soon as possible

13. Encourage movement and ambulation, as indicated. Have the patient gradually increase exercise from lying, to sitting, to standing, to ambulating. Provide assistance and encouragement; maintain safety precautions.

14. Minimize the risk of deep vein thrombosis (DVT) by:
    a. Assessing for early signs (e.g., redness, swelling, tenderness along vein, positive Homans' sign)
    b. Applying elastic hose, applying a sequential compression device, or administering low-dose heparin, as precribed
    c. Teaching measures to prevent vessel constriction. (See Chapter 8, Peripheral Vascular Disorders, for more information on DVT.)

15. Intervene as appropriate to prevent postoperative depression, disorientation, or psychosis; measures include:
    a. Providing preoperative teaching and information
    b. Orienting the patient postoperatively
    c. Providing prescribed medication, close supervision, and consultation with mental health personnel as required

16. Teach the patient and family members to assess for and report signs or symptoms of complications, such as:
    a. DVT
    b. Wound infection
    c. Wound dehiscence

17. Teach the patient and family members about:
    a. Prescribed medications
    b. Treatments
    c. Diet
    d. Activity level
    e. Planned follow-up care

18. Discuss postoperative depression and ineffective coping with the

patient and family members; teach them about the grieving process and refer them to support groups as appropriate.

19. As necessary, refer the patient and family to social services to arrange for such services as:
    a. Home care
    b. Meals on Wheels
    c. Visiting nurse
    d. Transportation assistance
    e. Special equipment (e.g., wheelchair, walker, oxygen equipment)

D. **Evaluation**
1. The patient maintains optimum respiratory function, as evidenced by:
   a. Performing deep breathing exercises four times daily for the first 48 hours postoperatively
   b. Demonstrating clear breath sounds on auscultation
   c. Turning, exercising, and ambulating as instructed
   d. Coughing effectively to expectorate secretions and sputum
2. The patient maintains optimum cardiovascular function, as evidenced by:
   a. No signs or symptoms of cardiac dysrhythmias
   b. Good capillary refill and normal skin color
   c. Normal body temperature and vital signs within acceptable ranges
   d. No signs of hemorrhage or hematoma
3. The patient reports adequate pain control.
4. The patient maintains optimum fluid and electrolyte status.
5. The patient maintains optimum nutritional status.
6. The patient demonstrates optimum bowel elimination pattern.
7. The patient demonstrates optimum urine elimination pattern.
8. The patient displays optimum wound healing, as evidenced by:
   a. No abnormal wound drainage
   b. Afebrile state with normal white blood cell count
   c. Intact wound with no breakdown, redness, or signs of dehiscence or evisceration.
9. The patient attains optimum mobility and self-care ability by time of discharge.
10. The patient exhibits optimum psychological functioning, as evidenced by:
    a. Absence of psychotic or disoriented behavior
    b. Ability to communicate needs to health care team
    c. Asking appropriate questions related to operation and sexual matters
    d. Reporting feelings of depression
    e. Appropriate eye contact
    f. Good grooming and personal hygiene (as ability allows)

704

11. The patient or family members discuss assessment of potential complications and the importance of reporting symptoms.
12. The patient or family members verbalize understanding of prescribed medications, diet, activity, and other therapies.
13. The patient or family states appropriate arrangements made for home care.

Bibliography

Baeles, B. (1989). Perioperative nursing research, Part IV: Intraoperative phase. *AORN Journal*, *49*(5).

Brunner, L. S., & Suddarth, D. S. (1986). *The Lippincott manual of nursing practice* (4th ed.). Philadelphia: J. B. Lippincott.

Brunner, L. S., & Suddarth, D. S. (1988). *Textbook of medical-surgical nursing* (6th ed.). Philadelphia: J. B. Lippincott.

Felver, L., & Pendarvis, J. H. (1988). Perioperative risk factors for hypokalemia. *Today's OR Nurse*, *10*(4), 26–32.

Felver, L., & Pendarvis, J. H. (1989). Electrolyte imbalances: Intraoperative risk factors. *AORN Journal*, *49*(4), 922–1008.

Luckmann, J., & Sorenson, K. C. (1987). *Medical-surgical nursing: A psychophysiologic approach* (3rd ed.). Philadelphia: W. B. Saunders.

U.S. Department of Health and Human Services, Centers for Disease Control (1987). Recommendations for prevention of HIV transmission in health care settings. *Morbidity and Mortality Weekly Report*, *6*, 2s-18s.

STUDY QUESTIONS

1. Ms. Genuardi, aged 19, who was just admitted to OR from the trauma department, confides to the OR nurse about her daily induced vomiting and laxative use practices. From this information, the nurse would suspect that the patient is at specific risk for which of following nursing diagnoses?
   a. High Risk for Aspiration
   b. High Risk for Fluid Volume Deficit
   c. Altered Tissue Perfusion: Peripheral
   d. High Risk for Infection

2. Ms. Stein, aged 70, is about to undergo major abdominal surgery under general anesthesia. After the patient has been placed on the OR table, the nurse notes that ambient OR room temperature is 68°F (20°C). What would be the most appropriate nursing diagnosis related to this situation?
   a. High Risk for Injury
   b. Altered Tissue Perfusion
   c. High Risk for Altered Body Temperature
   d. High Risk for Infection

3. For an unconscious patient recently admitted to the PACU who has no contraindication to movement, which of the following represents the most effective nursing intervention to promote adequate respiratory function?
   a. Place the patient supine and perform jaw thrust maneuver.
   b. Turn the patient every 10 minutes from side to side.
   c. Position the patient on one side with a pillow at the back and with chin extended.
   d. Place the patient prone to facilitate drainage of secretions.

4. Mr. Russell, aged 56, underwent radical perineal prostatectomy 5 days ago. For the nurse evaluating Mr. Russell's psychological status regarding the postoperative impotence, which of the following statements by Mr. Russell would best demonstrate positive coping?

   a. "The doctor told me about penile prostheses; I'm considering using one."
   b. "Cancer runs in my family; I feel doomed after this surgery."
   c. "I'm going right back to my teaching job and act like this didn't happen."
   d. "How many men my age have you cared for who've had this surgery?"

5. Ms. Esteban, aged 37, is scheduled for an emergency vaginal procedure (D&C) under general anesthesia after experiencing a spontaneous abortion. The most therapeutic action on the part of the nurse, when she sees tears in Ms. Esteban's eyes, would be to
   a. Squeeze her hand and tell her, "There's nothing to be afraid of."
   b. Check her name band, and have the anesthesiologist give her a tranquilizer.
   c. Let her cry, and tell others to leave her alone until she is anesthetized.
   d. Stand by her side, and quietly ask her to describe what she is feeling.

6. Ms. Marsden, aged 32, is scheduled to have excess fat suctioned from her thighs for cosmetic reasons. When gathering preoperative assessment data, the nurse recognizes that this surgery is
   a. optional
   b. elective
   c. required
   d. urgent

7. Just after Ms. Jenrette, aged 65, signs the operative permit and the doctor leaves her room, she asks the nurse "When will this hotel bring me some food?" After the nurse verifies that Ms. Jenrette is confused as to her whereabouts, the next priority action should be to
   a. Report that the consent has been obtained from a confused patient.
   b. Teach preoperative exercises of moving, coughing, and deep breathing exercises.

c. Insert a bladder catheter and evaluate output.

d. Administer preoperative medication immediately.

8. Which of the following represents the most significant risk factor for postoperative physiologic complications?

a. pregnancy

b. hypertension

c. morbid obesity

d. age of 70 or older

9. Operating room personnel are required to wear specific clean OR attire and cover hair and shoes. What is the rationale for this clothing?

a. to promote a totally sterile patient environment

b. to exclude the environment outside of surgery

c. to provide uniforms that are non-static

d. to isolate the patient's diseases from OR staff

10. The OR nurse cautions the scrub team to be very quiet just as the patient is being induced with a general anesthetic. Evaluation of response to anesthesia at this point would demonstrate which of the following?

a. The patient has an increased risk of apnea.

b. The patient experiences noises as exaggerated in Stage I.

c. The patient may become excited and struggle.

d. The patient experiences an extension of time to get to Stage III.

11. Which of the following nursing interventions would be appropriate for a patient who develops malignant hyperthermia crisis?

a. Adminster iced IV saline solution and dantrolene sodium.

b. Begin monitoring heart rate and rhythm.

c. Insert a bladder catheter with temperature probe.

d. Type and crossmatch the patient for whole blood administration.

12. The circulating nurse refuses to let the consulting surgeon come into an OR wearing a sterile gown that was worn in another surgery. This action is based primarily on

a. value judgment

b. critical thinking

c. principle of asepsis

d. assertiveness

13. Mr. Daniels, aged 60, just underwent abdominal–perineal resection surgery. He entered the PACU at 11:00 A.M.; by 12:30 P.M., nursing assessment reveals that his blood pressure has dropped from 126/78 mmHg to 105/68 mmHg, his pulse rate has risen from 80 to 106 beats per minute, his skin is now pale and cool, and his urine output has decreased to 10 mL in the last hour. The perineal drainage reservoir contains 50 cc of bright red fluid—an increase of 20 cc since he entered the PACU. Based on a nursing diagnosis of Actual Fluid Volume Deficit, the nurse's best action at this time would be to

a. Notify the supervisor that Mr. Daniels is in moderate shock.

b. Increase nasal oxygen flow rate to 8 L.

c. Place Mr. Daniels in Trendelenburg position.

d. Notify the surgeon, and ask for increased IV fluid rate.

14. Later, Mr. Daniels is to be discharged from PACU to the clinical unit. Score points that indicate he has fulfilled minimum criteria are

a. one point each in respiratory, circulatory, consciousness, color, and muscle activity, for a total of five

b. one point in at least three areas—respiratory, circulatory, consciousness—for a total of three

c. a total score for the five areas of seven or above

d. two points each in respiratory, circulatory, consciousness, color, and muscle activity, for a total of 10

15. Mr. Daniels is now 36 hours postopera-

tive. The day shift nurse reports he needs much encouragement to use his incentive spirometer, cough, deep breathe, and ambulate. The evening nurse's beginning assessment reveals increased temperature and pulse, shallow, rapid breathing, and bilateral adventitious lung sounds. Based on these data, which of the following priority nursing diagnoses would be most appropriate?

a. Activity Intolerance
b. Ineffective Airway Clearance
c. Altered Tissue Perfusion: Cardiopulmonary
d. Ineffective Individual Coping

16. Ms. Parks, aged 43, underwent a splenectomy 7 days ago. She is morbidly obese and diabetic and has exhibited delayed recovery from the surgery. About 2 hours after the wound staples are removed, she tells the nurse "I felt something give and there was gush of fluid." On inspection, the nurse sees that the wound is separating. The most appropriate immediate nursing intervention would be to

a. Place Ms. Parks in a recumbent position, cover the wound with saline dressings, and call the surgeon immediately.
b. Leave Ms. Parks and tell her you will be right back with help.
c. Complete a head-to-toe assessment before calling the surgeon.
d. Place a sign on Ms. Parks's door for drainage precaution status.

ANSWER KEY

1. **Correct response: b**
   This patient is at risk for potassium imbalance (hypokalemia).
   a. The patient will not aspirate if her stomach is empty.
   c and d. These answers do not relate directly to the question and are not specific to vomiting and purging.
   Application/Safe care/Analysis (Dx)

2. **Correct response: c**
   Elderly patients are very susceptible to accidental hypothermia from the environment. General anesthesia causes vasodilation, which will further aggravate the situation.
   a. This is a possible diagnosis for all surgery patients but does not relate to this specific situation.
   b. This is inaccurate—decreased fluid volume would stem from NPO status and bleeding.
   d. This answer does not relate to the situation as presented.
   Comprehension/Health promotion/Analysis (Dx)

3. **Correct response: c**
   This is the correct intervention until the patient regains consciousness.
   a. This intervention would be appropriate for a patient with respiratory obstruction.
   b. During the immediate postoperative period, turning every 10 minutes is inappropriate.
   d. Postoperative patients are rarely, if ever, placed in the prone position.
   Application/Physiologic/Planning

4. **Correct response: a**
   Optimum psychosocial affect is manifested by the patient asking or discussing matters related to sexuality. A penile prosthesis may be an appropriate alternative for an impotent man.
   b. This response demonstrates possible depression.
   c. This response demonstrates denial

   of feelings, which can lead to psychological problems over time.
   d. This response does not address the problem specifically, although it may indicate the patient's willingness to possibly explore the problem further with the nurse.
   Analysis/Psychosocial/Evaluation

5. **Correct response: d**
   Therapeutic communication allows the patient to express fear or grief.
   a. This intervention is nontherapeutic and belittles the patient's fear or emotion.
   b. This intervention is nontherapeutic, because the nurse avoids the patient's expression.
   c. This intervention is nontherapeutic because the patient would be left alone in an anxiety producing environment.
   Application/Psychosocial/Implementation

6. **Correct response: a**
   Cosmetic surgeries, by definition, are most often optional.
   b, c, and d. These answers are incorrect according to definitions in text.
   Comprehension/Health promotion/ Assessment

7. **Correct response: a**
   Legal consent must be obtained from a comprehending patient or from a family member or guardian.
   b. This would be inappropriate until the legality of the patient's situation was assessed. If confusion makes her unteachable, the nurse should report this also.
   c. This usually would be done after the patient was anesthetized to minimize pain. It is not a priority.
   d. This would not be completed until the patient's legal status was clear.
   Analysis/Safe care/Planning

8. **Correct answer: c**
   Obese persons have been identified as

carrying the greatest risk for complications during the intraoperative and postoperative phases.

a, b, and d. Although pregnancy, hypertension, and advanced age are all risk factors, none is considered to be as significant a factor as obesity.

Analysis/Health promotion/Assessment

9. **Correct answer: b**
   The main goal is to protect patient from infection by eliminating outside hazards of dust, pollutants, and so forth.
   a. A "total" sterile environment is impossible to achieve.
   c. Nonstatic clothes no longer are required, as nonexplosive gases are now used in the OR.
   d. The patient is being protected from others.

Comprehension/Health promotion/Planning

10. **Correct answer: b**
    Hearing is extremely sensitive in Stage I, and noise reduction is important.
    a. Apnea will result from anesthetic drugs, but this is not a reason for quiet.
    c. The excitement stage is Stage II, not Stage I.
    d. Anesthetic, not noise, influences patient transition to Stage III.

Application/Physiologic/Evaluation

11. **Correct answer: a**
    Precise therapy is needed to decrease temperature and muscle rigidity. Supplies are usually kept in a special place; all OR nurses need to know the procedure and how to obtain needed supplies.
    b. A patient always has the heart monitored for every surgery.
    c. Temperature is always monitored in the OR either by rectal, esophageal, or other route before surgery starts.
    d. Whole blood is not the therapy for malignant hyperthermia.

Knowledge/Safe care/Implementation

12. **Correct answer: c**
    One principle of asepsis is the isolation of items for exclusive use for one patient. Therefore, a sterile gown worn by a surgeon in another surgery must be left in that room.
    a, b, and d. These answers are incorrect; however, they are characteristics that certainly assist the nurse in enforcing strict principles of asepsis.

Analysis/Physiologic/Assessment

13. **Correct answer: d**
    At this time Mr. Daniels could be showing early signs of hypovolemia and early shock and thus would require increased fluid. If symptoms should become more severe, the surgeon has already been alerted.
    a. This patient is in early, not moderate, shock.
    b and c. These measures could be appropriate later but would not be critical actions early.

Analysis/Physiologic/Implementation

14. **Correct answer: c**
    Seven points is the minimum score required for discharge from the PACU.
    a, b, and d. A patient is not considered stable for discharge with a score below seven, and ten points are not necessary for discharge.

Knowledge/Safe care/Evaluation

15. **Correct answer: b**
    Immediate nursing intervention could help prevent serious complications from atelectasis and pneumonia secondary to poor respiratory hygiene and immobility.
    a, c, and d. These measures would not be priority at this time.

Application/Physiologic/Analysis (Dx)

16. **Correct answer: a**
    Appropriate intervention would involve protecting the protruding intestine, re-

lieving abdominal pressure by positioning, and notifying the surgeon, who will
schedule immediate surgery.

b, c, and d. None of these interventions would be ap-
propriate for this patient.

Application/Physiologic/Implementation

COMPREHENSIVE TEST—QUESTIONS

1. A group of nurse leaders has developed a system of inter-related and interdependent problem-solving steps based on the science of nursing. Which of the following best describes the result of their work?
   a. a framework for nursing practice called the nursing process
   b. a universal language for nurses known as a taxonomy of nursing diagnoses
   c. a definition of nursing focused on human responses to health problems
   d. a social policy statement for the nursing profession

2. Which of the following questions would be the most appropriate as part of the "role and relationship patterns" segment of the nursing health history?
   a. "What are your ideas about health?"
   b. "Do you have any problems with mobility?"
   c. "How would you describe your family's health?"
   d. "How would you describe your strengths and weaknesses?"

3. Which of the following questions would the nurse *least* likely use when gathering data about a patient's health?
   a. "Describe how you care for your skin."
   b. "How would you describe your general health?"
   c. "You don't take drugs, do you?"
   d. "Have you ever had a physical examination other than when you have been ill?"

4. On examining the feet of Mrs. Bates, aged 79, the nurse observes pale and cold feet bilaterally, with no hair tufts on the toes and a circumscribed 3 cm lesion on the plantar surface at the first metatarsal joint. Which of the following would be the most likely source of Mrs. Bates's problem?
   a. insufficient venous circulation
   b. venous thrombosis
   c. expected age-related physiologic changes
   d. insufficient arterial circulation

5. Selected hematology and blood chemistry results for Mr. Rudzinski, aged 40, are as follows:

   ► Hemoglobin: 15 mg/dL
   ► Hematocrit: 50%
   ► Serum sodium: 140 mEq/L
   ► Serum potassium: 4.5 mEq/L
   ► Serum cholesterol: 160 mg/100 mL
   ► Serum triglycerides: 100 mg/100 mL

   Which of the following statements about these findings is correct?
   a. Two results are below normal ranges.
   b. All results are within normal ranges.
   c. Three results are within normal ranges.
   d. One result is above normal range.

6. When planning a teaching session for a group of patients with angina about energy conservation measures, the nurse could choose to use all the following in-class teaching methods focused on various learning domains *except*
   a. discussion
   b. practice of learned skills
   c. role playing
   d. self-monitoring

7. In talking with 73-year-old Mr. Abraham after a teaching session, the nurse discovers that he wears a hearing aid, has had some difficulty with the group discussions, and is a retired science teacher. Based on the nursing diagnosis

Answer sheet provided on page 727.

Sensory and Perceptual Alteration: Auditory, modifications to Mr. Abraham's plan of care should would most appropriately include which of the following?

a. closed-circuit television
b. computer-assisted instruction
c. videotapes
d. filmstrips

8. The inclusion of which of the following diagnoses on Mr. Abraham's care plan would indicate that he will need follow-up counseling after discharge to help ensure optimal health?

a. Anticipatory Grieving
b. Fatigue
c. Sleep Pattern Disturbance
d. Self-Concept Disturbance

9. When planning an educational series for adults, the nurse should keep in mind important differences between adult learners and young learners. Which of the following general assumptions regarding adult learners is *incorrect*?

a. Adult learners are self-directing.
b. Adult learners enter educational activities with a problem-centered orientation to learning.
c. Adult learners are motivated by internal needs.
d. Adult learners prefer a structured, lecture-style educational program.

10. Which of the following patient behaviors would clue the nurse that the patient is a tactile learner?

a. After listening to the nurse's explanation on using home oxygen equipment, the patient asks the nurse to write down the important information.
b. The patient reads printed instructions on home oxygen therapy carefully, underlining key points.
c. The patient picks up the oxygen tubing and begins attaching it to the oxygen cylinder before receiving teaching on the use of home oxygen equipment.

d. The patient listens to a discussion about using home oxygen equipment, asking questions to clarify certain steps.

11. In cellular injury, swelling of inflamed tissue results from

a. transient vasodilation followed by vasoconstriction
b. migration of white blood cells (WBCs) away from the site of injury
c. increased vascular permeability, with leakage of plasma fluids
d. irritation of nerve endings by fibrinogen

12. Ms. Garvin, aged 32, has been receiving radiation therapy for breast cancer. During a follow-up examination, she expresses distress over skin texture changes at the radiation site and complains of pain on swallowing. The nurse assessing Ms. Garvin's response to therapy could identify several nursing diagnoses that would be important in directing care. Which of the following most likely would *not* be a diagnosis specific to this patient's needs?

a. Altered Oral Mucous Membrane
b. Body Image Disturbance
c. Altered Sexuality Patterns
d. High Risk for Impaired Skin Integrity

13. Teaching Ms. Garvin about measures to help reduce her risk of complications and enhance healing most likely would incorporate instructions to

a. Apply heat to the radiation site to increase metabolic activity.
b. Eat a diet high in protein and calories to optimize tissue repair.
c. Apply cool packs to the radiation site to reduce swelling.
d. Drink warm fluids frequently throughout the day to relieve discomfort on swallowing.

14. In teaching Ms. Garvin skin care measures, the nurse would include all the following *except*

a. assessing the radiation site daily for signs of breakdown

b. washing hands properly after contact with infection sources (e.g., feces, urine)
c. avoiding clothes that rub the site
d. limiting daily sun exposure to site to no more than 1 hour of late afternoon sun

15. Pathologic cellular adaptation to excessive physiologic stress occurs to preserve cells. In evaluating this adaptive response in a patient, which of the following findings would represent hyperplasia?
a. The patient displays an enlarged heart muscle on radiograph.
b. The patient displays loss of cell substance resulting in cell shrinkage.
c. The patient shows evidence of changes in epithelial cells from habitual smoking.
d. The patient demonstrates increase in breast size during pregnancy.

16. Mr. Johnson, aged 49, was admitted with complaints of fatigue and muscle weakness. Laboratory studies revealed a serum potassium level of 2.8 mEq/L. Based on the physician's order for KCl, 20 mEq in 100 cc D5W over 2 hours, the nurse should take which of the following actions?
a. Teach Mr. Johnson about foods high in potassium.
b. Call the physician to clarify the order because KCl should be infused at a rate of 10 mEq every 2 hours.
c. Observe the ECG for peaked, narrow T waves.
d. Have laboratory results double-checked because low potassium levels commonly are hemolyzed.

17. Mrs. Fair, aged 77, is admitted with complaints of lethargy and confusion progressing over the past several days. Her husband reports that she has had a poor appetite over the past 2 weeks, with occasional nausea and vomiting. The ECG shows a shortened QT interval. Based on these data, the nurse

would suspect that Mrs. Fair is experiencing
a. hyponatremia
b. hypermagnesemia
c. hypercalcemia
d. hyperkalemia

18. The morning after eating fish at a local seafood restaurant, Mr. Sanders, aged 28, sought treatment for severe diarrhea (passage of 15 explosive diarrheal stools in the past 10 hours). When assessing Mr. Sanders, the nurse would expect to see which of the following group of abnormal laboratory values?
a. decreased blood urea nitrogen (BUN) and decreased hematocrit
b. decreased BUN and increased hematocrit
c. increased BUN and decreased hematocrit
d. increased BUN and increased hematocrit

19. Mr. Henry, aged 75, is admitted in obvious respiratory distress. His ABG values show a pH of 7.55, PO_2 of 68, and HCO_3 of 32 mEq/L. Belligerent and confused, he directs angry comments at his wife, who finally leaves the room crying. Which of the following reasons for Mr. Henry's behavior should the nurse explain to Mrs. Henry?
a. He likely is frightened by his breathing difficulty.
b. He is experiencing metabolic alkalosis, which causes mental changes.
c. He is experiencing respiratory acidosis, which causes mental changes.
d. He is exhibiting typical behavior for a patient in a respiratory crisis.

20. Mr. Johnston, aged 52, has been hospitalized for the past week for treatment of hypermagnesemia. He has a history of hiatal hernia and reports persistent heartburn, for which he takes antacids several times a day. Which of the following nursing diagnosis likely would be most appropriate to Mr. Johnston's care?

a. Impaired Physical Mobility related to magnesium loss from bone

b. Knowledge Deficit related to the role of antacids in increasing serum magnesium levels

c. Sleep Pattern Disturbance related to neuromuscular irritability

d. Fluid Volume Excess related to magnesium retention

21. Pain described as sharp and prickling and occurring after a cut finger is transmitted over

a. the smallest unmyelinated type C nerve fibers

b. medium myelinated type A-gamma nerve fibers

c. the largest myelinated type A-alpha and beta nerve fibers

d. medium myelinated type A-delta nerve fibers

22. Which of the following nursing diagnoses would be appropriate for a patient who "hates to bother the nurses" and so doesn't initially report intense pain he or she experiences when crutch-walking to the bathroom?

a. Powerlessness related to pain

b. Knowledge Deficit related to the need to call nurses

c. Fear related to pain

d. Self-Care Deficit related to the need to call nurses

23. Which of the following nursing interventions would be appropriate for a very stoic patient who refuses analgesics even when in severe pain?

a. Stay with the patient, and hold his or her hand.

b. Use patient-controlled analgesia, transcutaneous electrical nerve stimulation (TENS), distraction, and as many other psychologic interventions that the patient will accept.

c. Insist on analgesia, administering it in food or fluid without the patient's knowledge.

d. Do not provide pain relief measures until the patient requests.

24. Which of the following steps should a patient with periodic angina pain take *first* when pain occurs at home?

a. Take sublingual nitroglycerin and lie down.

b. Do mild breathing and range-of-motion exercises.

c. Take an extra long-lasting nitrate tablet.

d. Sit down and relax, using distraction and guided imagery.

25. Mr. Schmidt, aged 50, suffers from moderate to severe emphysema and is admitted in acute respiratory distress. The nursing health history, obtained after Mr. Schmidt is stabilized, reveals that he continues to smoke regularly and to mow his lawn weekly and refuses to use oxygen in front of his friends. Which of the following nursing diagnoses would the nurse use to address these behaviors?

a. Anticipatory Grieving

b. Body Image Disturbance

c. Ineffective Denial

d. Impaired Social Interaction

26. Lung dysfunction impacts physical and mental performance because of the lungs' critical role in maintaining the body's acid–base balance. Specifically, the lung plays a primary role in controlling

a. arterial O_2 and blood urea

b. arterial CO_2 and cholesterol

c. arterial CO_2, serum albumin, and pH

d. arterial CO_2 and pH

27. In planning care of a patient admitted to the thoracic ICU with pneumothorax, the nurse should recognize that an opening in the chest wall—whether due to a deliberate surgical intervention or to traumatic injury—causes the lung on that side to

a. expand due to intake of atmospheric air

b. collapse due to disturbed negative pressure in the pleural space

c. expand due to altered lung pressures

d. collapse due to disturbed positive pressure in the pleural space

28. Evaluation criteria indicating a patient's understanding of preventive measures important to respiratory care would include all the following *except*
    a. The patient avoids polluted environments.
    b. The patient abstains from smoking cigarettes.
    c. The patient balances rest, exercise, and proper eating habits.
    d. The patient uses a warm air humidifier at night.

29. Mrs. Roberts has undergone heart surgery for a valve replacement. When monitoring Mrs. Roberts's postsurgery, the nurse detects premature ventricular contractions (PVCs) on the ECG. The nurse recognizes that PVCs may be dangerous because they
    a. significantly increase cardiac workload
    b. may lead to ventricular tachycardia or ventricular fibrillation
    c. are the most common cause of myocardial infarction
    d. decrease heart rate and blood pressure

30. Mrs. Davidson, aged 63, has been admitted for unstable angina and is scheduled for coronary arteriography in the morning. When preparing her for the procedure, the nurse would do all the following *except*
    a. Provide emotional support, and encourage her to ask questions.
    b. Explain the procedure.
    c. Prepare her for the possibility of heart surgery.
    d. Discuss the prescribed medication regimen for angina.

31. On entering Mrs. Davidson's room to do an initial shift assessment, the nurse finds her crying. She expresses concern that she'll "have to cut back" on her activities and fears that she may become "a burden" to her husband. Based on this information, which of the following nursing diagnoses would be most appropriate for Mrs. Davidson?
    a. Impaired Verbal Communication
    b. Ineffective Family Coping: Compromised
    c. Knowledge Deficit
    d. Fear

32. In evaluating the effectiveness of patient teaching for home management of angina, the nurse would consider all the following *except*
    a. the patient's ability to recognize and avoid factors precipitating pain
    b. the patient's compliance with the prescribed nitroglycerin regimen
    c. the patient's knowledge of how to enter the emergency medical system
    d. the patient's knowledge of and ability to perform stretching exercises to relieve the pain

33. Mr. Sims, aged 68, is progressing well in his recovery from myocardial infarction; however, he complains of extreme fatigue at the end of the day. He states that he is kept busy with visitors and self-care activities. The nurse discusses ways to alleviate fatigue and plans all the following *except*
    a. limiting visitors and grouping his activities around rest periods
    b. backing up one step on the rehabilitation program
    c. encouraging his visitors to come in the evening so that he will have more time to complete his activities during the day
    d. allowing him to decide when activities will be done and when he will rest

34. Interventions to relieve the discomfort associated with chronic arterial occlusive vascular disease should be directed at
    a. improving venous return from the involved extremity
    b. avoiding narcotic analgesic medications

c. preventing edema in the extremities

d. increasing circulation to the extremities

35. On assessing a 69-year-old woman, the nurse notes that her left leg is swollen and warm, with palpable pedal pulses, an open wet ulcer above the medial malleolus, and thick, coarse, brown pigmented skin surrounding the ulcer. Based on these findings, the nurse likely would identify the probable cause of the ulcer as
   a. acute deep vein thrombosis
   b. chronic venous insufficiency
   c. chronic arterial insufficiency
   d. chronic lymphedema

36. In designing a nursing care plan for a patient released from the emergency room after initial care for a penetrating foot injury, the most important advice the nurse could give the patient would be to
   a. Call the physician if red streaking on the foot or leg occurs.
   b. Avoid crossing the legs at the knee or the ankle.
   c. Avoid smoking until the wound is completely healed.
   d. Notify the physician immediately of warning signs of anaphylactic shock from the tetanus toxoid.

37. Ms. Alton, aged 65, returns from postanesthesia recovery following surgery for an above-the-knee amputation. She has a large bulky dressing and ace wrap covering the stump. On vital sign monitoring, the nurse notes a blood pressure decrease from 174/84 to 136/88 mmHg; pulse increase from 88 to 92 beats per minute; respiration increase from 14 to 18 breaths per minute; and temperature of 98.2°F. The dressing has a 7-cm spot of red drainage at the distal portion. Which evaluation of these findings would be most appropriate?
   a. The patient demonstrates normal response to recovery from general anesthetic.

b. The patient demonstrates an early response to pain and should be medicated with analgesic.
   c. The patient demonstrates a response to excessive bleeding at the stump and should be reassessed at frequent intervals.
   d. The patient demonstrates early signs of respiratory complications; vigorous deep breathing and coughing should be encouraged.

38. Mr. Applegren, aged 44, has been diagnosed with primary hypertension and started on antihypertensive medication. During follow-up evaluation, the nurse inquires into Mr. Applegren's usual stressors and ways of dealing with them because
   a. The major cause of primary hypertension is excessive stress.
   b. Measures to reduce stress are part of any treatment regimen for hypertension.
   c. Asking the patient to describe his stress level will help him relax and foster a better nurse–patient therapeutic relationship.
   d. Stress must be reduced before learning can take place.

39. Mr. Burns, aged 47, has a healing gastric ulcer and is now being discharged. The discharge instructions presented to this patient should include which of the following information on medications?
   a. Continue taking antacids on schedule even if symptoms subside.
   b. Take antacids with other medications.
   c. Avoid magnesium-containing antacids if a cardiac problem develops.
   d. Take antacids with meals.

40. When caring for a patient with severe diarrhea related to Crohn's disease, the nurse should attempt to prevent complications by focusing care on all the following diagnoses *except*
   a. Altered Tissue Perfusion: Gastrointestinal

   b. High Risk for Fluid Volume Deficit
   c. Altered Nutrition: Less Than Body Requirements
   d. High Risk for Infection

41. Which of the following findings is *not* typically associated with appendicitis?
   a. referred pain to the right scapula
   b. rebound tenderness
   c. right lower quadrant pain
   d. nausea and vomiting

42. In evaluating large intestinal function following an acute episode of Crohn's disease, the nurse would assess for
   a. report of pain relief after eating
   b. evidence of adequate nutrient and vitamin absorption
   c. defecation of soft, formed stool
   d. absence of belching and acid reflux

43. When planning care for a 38-year-old man with ulcerative colitis, the nurse should keep in mind that a common complication is
   a. anal fistula abscess
   b. ascites
   c. nausea and vomiting
   d. anorexia with weight loss

44. Diabetic ketoacidosis most commonly is precipitated by
   a. overeating
   b. infection
   c. a missed insulin dose
   d. psychologic stress

45. The nurse should advise a diabetic patient with an open foot wound to
   a. Cleanse the foot, and observe for infection.
   b. Soak the foot daily, then bandage it.
   c. Cleanse the foot, and apply mercurochrome.
   d. Elevate the foot, and apply heat.

46. What emergency intervention may be necessary for the postoperative thyroidectomy patient experiencing hemorrhage?
   a. intravenous calcium
   b. oral airway insertion
   c. tracheostomy
   d. intravenous thyroid hormone

47. Evaluation criteria of a patient's understanding of prescribed glucocorticoid therapy would include all the following *except*?
   a. The patient states the need to wear medical identification.
   b. The patient states the need to increase the dosage when ill.
   c. The patient states the need to inform his or her dentist that he or she is on glucocorticoid therapy.
   d. The patient states the need to discontinue therapy if nausea and vomiting occur.

48. A 16-year-old diabetic patient exhibits the following behaviors: school truancy, five admissions for uncontrolled diabetes in the last 2 years, missed insulin injections, and isolation from friends. Which of the following nursing diagnoses would be most applicable for this patient?
   a. Knowledge Deficit
   b. Altered Thought Processes
   c. Altered Nutrition: Less Than Body Requirements
   d. Ineffective Individual Coping

49. Which of the following statements regarding impotence is correct?
   a. It almost always is caused by psychologic factors.
   b. It may be caused by a wide variety of vascular, neurologic, endocrine, and psychogenic causes, as well as by many medications.
   c. It may be related to various dietary factors.
   d. It occurs less frequently in elderly men.

50. A major complication of prostatectomy is hemorrhage due to
   a. pressure on the incision
   b. thrombosis
   c. clots obstructing urinary drainage
   d. infection

51. When teaching a patient how to do a self-testicular examination, the nurse should advise him that

a. Tenderness is an early sign of testicular cancer.

b. The testes should feel smooth and oval, with no masses.

c. Masses are difficult to find, and prognosis for cancer cure is poor.

d. A firm, pea-sized lump may be normal.

52. Possible complications of mastectomy include all the following *except*

a. infection

b. edema of the arm

c. thrombosis

d. headache

53. When caring for a patient who has undergone a hysterectomy, the nurse will perform urinary catheterization if the patient cannot void within 8 hours postoperatively so as to prevent urinary retention. Catheterization is necessary because

a. Surgical manipulation in the area of the bladder may cause edema and nerve trauma, producing temporary atony.

b. The bladder often is removed with the uterus.

c. Infection invariably results from surgery, making voiding difficult.

d. Surgical menopause affects urinary function.

54. Which of the following statements regarding allergic dermatitis is correct?

a. Reaction to the allergen is immediate.

b. Contact dermatitis always results from a chemical irritant.

c. Allergy affects rarely progress beyond skin rash.

d. The range and intensity of reaction varies depending on the causative agent.

55. The nurse is caring for an AIDS patient who is experiencing dyspnea. In evaluating his or her care, the nurse would include all the following criteria *except*

a. receives adequate hydration, 2.5 to 3 L/day

b. is encouraged to cough and deep breathe frequently

c. is maintained on complete bedrest to decrease dyspnea

d. paces activities to conserve energy

56. Ms. Shandra, aged 26, recently was diagnosed with rheumatoid arthritis. She understands that her disease is progressive and is worried that she will not be able to continue caring for her husband and young child. Nursing care for this patient would begin with

a. teaching her about the disease and its progression

b. making referrals to other health care team members as necessary

c. providing emotional support for her and her family

d. assessing her physical, psychosocial, and environmental needs

57. Based on Ms. Shandra's comments about the possibility of not being able to care for her child and her fear of being a burden on her husband, the nurse would consider which of the following nursing diagnoses?

a. Knowledge Deficit of the disease process related to lack of exposure to information

b. Self-Concept Disturbance related to loss of independence

c. Ineffective Individual Coping related to possibility of joint deformities

d. Impaired Physical Mobility related to the progressive nature of the disease

58. Mr. Williams, aged 62, has been hospitalized with an acute exacerbation of asthma. He is dyspneic, sitting forward in bed, and irritable. The admission history has been left for the nurse from the previous shift. After the nursing supervisor asks why it hasn't been done yet, the nurse decides to

a. Wait and try to obtain the necessary information from Mr. Williams's family.

b. Obtain the information from Mr. Williams.

c. Have the nursing assistant get the

necessary information from Mr. Williams.

d. Obtain part of the history from Mr. Williams now and the remainder later to let him rest.

59. According to the criteria set by the American Burn Association, burn injuries involving second-degree burns over more than 25% of total body surface area (TBSA) in adults or 20% of TBSA in children and burn injuries involving third-degree burns over 10% or more of TBSA are classified as
   a. minor burn injuries
   b. moderate uncomplicated burn injuries
   c. major burn injuries
   d. full-thickness burn injuries

60. During initial assessment of a patient with a major burn injury, the correct sequence of nursing interventions would be
   a. Eliminate the source of the burn, ensure airway patency, observe for and treat associated injuries, treat burn shock.
   b. Eliminate the source of the burn, ensure airway patency, cool the burn wound, apply topical antibiotic cream.
   c. Ensure airway patency, insert a nasogastric tube, insert a bladder catheter, start intravenous fluid infusion.
   d. Treat burn shock, ensure airway patency, put the patient in an isolation room.

61. Using the Parkland formula (4 mL of Ringer's lactate/% TBSA burn/kg body weight/24 hours), the nurse would calculate fluid replacement for a 70-kg patient with a 50% TBSA burn over 24 hours as
   a. 1400 mL
   b. 14,000 mL
   c. 6720 mL
   d. 700 mL

62. A 25-year-old man admitted to the emergency department following a house fire has a 25% TBSA burn that includes the face. He has carbonaceous material in his mouth and singed eyelashes. Nursing interventions for this patient would be based on all the following correct statements regarding smoke inhalation injury *except*
   a. Cellular damage prevents passage of oxygen across the lung.
   b. Smoke inhalation injury is the leading cause of death in burn patients.
   c. The goal is to promote healing of lung tissue and prevent pulmonary infection or sepsis.
   d. A chest radiograph provides the definitive diagnosis of injury.

63. A full-thickness burn injury may necessitate a free graft of the patient's own skin from one area to another. This homograph procedure potentially may involve all but which one of the following nursing diagnoses?
   a. Unilateral Neglect
   b. Body Image Disturbance
   c. Pain
   d. Self-Concept Disturbance

64. Ms. Landis, aged 42, has myasthenia gravis with moderate generalization. The mother of four children, ages 5 to 16, she has been active in volunteer organizations in town. As her symptoms progress, including increasing fatigue and decreasing mobility, which of the following nursing diagnoses most likely would apply?
   a. Sensory and Perceptual Alteration: Gustatory
   b. Decreased Cardiac Output
   c. Altered Family Processes
   d. Altered Thought Processes

65. Mr. Krysnewski, aged 67, is experiencing constipation following a craniotomy. An evaluation criterion that would indicate this patient's understanding of actions needed to achieve the goal of a regular defecation pattern (and avoiding straining at defecation) would be

a. The patient drinks adequate fluids and eats a fiber-free diet.
b. The patient drinks adequate fluids and asks for an enema.
c. The patient includes roughage in the diet and drinks adequate fluids.
d. The patient requests laxatives and includes roughage in the diet.

66. When ambulating a patient who has undergone surgical removal of a protruded intervertebral lumbar disk, the nurse should take special care to
a. Maintain proper body alignment, have the patient wear good walking shoes, and remove loose objects from the floor.
b. Administer pain medication 15 minutes before ambulation.
c. Maintain proper alignment, and provide a cane for the patient to use.
d. Provide prism glasses for the patient.

67. John Brensinger, aged 16, sustained a moderate concussion in a motorcycle accident 1 day ago. Based on John's current Glasgow Coma Scale score of 7, the nurse would include which of the following interventions in John's care plan?
a. decreasing noxious stimuli, monitoring vital signs and neurologic status carefully, and keeping the patient on his back with the bed flat
b. instituting a program of stimulation, monitoring vital signs and neurologic status carefully, elevating the head of the bed 60 degrees, and positioning the patient on his side with his body in alignment
c. encouraging the family to become involved in a stimulation program, decreasing monitoring at night so that the patient can rest, and keeping the patient on his back
d. decreasing noxious stimuli, monitoring vital signs and neurologic status carefully, elevating the head

of the bed 30 degrees, and positioning the patient on his side with his body in alignment

68. Ms. Pfautz, aged 63, has been in skeletal traction for 2 days following a dislocation of her C5–6 vertebrae. The most important assessment parameters for Ms. Pfautz would include
a. correctness of traction and amount of urine output
b. correctness of traction and movement and sensation in the arms
c. correctness of traction and movement, strength, and sensation in the toes and fingers
d. correctness of traction, range of eye movement, and strength of corneal reflex

69. Administration of miotic medications to treat glaucoma results in which of the following vision alterations?
a. impaired near vision
b. increased sensitivity to light
c. impaired night vision
d. diplopia

70. Which of the following postoperative assessment findings would point to intraocular hemorrhage?
a. temperature elevation
b. diplopia
c. visual floaters
d. eye pain

71. A person using over-the-counter nasal decongestant drops who reports unrelieved and worsening nasal congestion should be instructed to
a. Switch to a stronger dosage of the medication.
b. Discontinue the medication for a few weeks.
c. Continue taking the same medication, but use it more frequently.
d. Use a combination of medications for better relief.

72. The priority nursing diagnosis for the patient with eardrum perforation would be
a. Knowledge Deficit regarding general ear care and hearing protection

b. Sensory and Perceptual Alteration: Auditory related to hearing loss

c. High Risk for Injury related to infection

d. Pain related to vertigo, nausea, and vomiting

73. All the following nursing activities would be performed before a patient is discharged following total laryngectomy. Which one would be most important?

a. referring to the Lost Chord Club for group support

b. providing a medic-alert card explaining resuscitation needs for first-aid providers

c. teaching ways to prevent constipation since the Valsalva maneuver is no longer possible

d. discussing precautions to take when showering and shampooing

74. A patient with multiple fractures is at increased risk for a fat embolism. When caring for such a patient, the nurse should monitor for which early sign?

a. hematuria

b. mental confusion or restlessness

c. sudden temperature elevation

d. pallor and discoloration at the fracture site

75. When preparing a patient for magnetic resonance imaging, the nurse should

a. Obtain informed consent, and administer prescribed preoperative medication.

b. Scrub the injection site for 15 minutes, using aseptic technique.

c. Remove any jewelry, and inquire about metal implants.

d. Assess for allergies to seafood or iodine-containing substances.

76. Following application of a long arm cast, Mr. Johnstone complains of deep, throbbing pain in the elbow area that is out of proportion to his injury. After noting diminished capillary refill in the fingers and cyanotic nailbeds, the nurse should plan to

a. Notify the physician immediately, and prepare to bivalve the cast.

b. Cut a "window" in the cast over the elbow area, and check the area for drainage or infection.

c. Elevate the casted arm, apply ice packs, and assess every hour for symptom progression.

d. Administer prescribed analgesics, and notify the physician.

77. In the immediate postoperative period following a below-the-knee amputation, the nurse typically would be most concerned with which of the following nursing diagnoses?

a. Body Image Disturbance related to loss of body part

b. High Risk for Infection related to disruption in skin integrity

c. Pain related to phantom sensation

d. High Risk for Altered Tissue Perfusion related to hemorrhage

78. Which of the following patient behaviors would best indicate the patient's acceptance of the loss of an amputated limb?

a. looking at, touching, and caring for the residual limb

b. inviting friends and family members to visit

c. inquiring about methods to alleviate pain

d. expressing the desire to go home and resume work

79. Portal hypertension results from which of the following pathophysiologic processes?

a. obstructed blood flow from the GI tract to the liver

b. diversion of ascitic fluid from the peritoneal cavity back to the venous system

c. rupture of esophageal varices

d. obstruction of bile flow through the common bile duct

80. Which of the following explanations best describes why the nursing diagnoses Altered Body Image and Self-Esteem Disturbance may apply to a patient with ascites?

a. A grossly distended abdomen may make the patient feel obese.

b. Yellow-tinged skin may make the patient feel self-conscious.

c. Fecal incontinence may cause embarrassment.

d. Muscle wasting may cause weakness and mobility problems.

81. When caring for a patient following a large (2 to 3 L) paracentesis, the nurse should focus on monitoring for which of the following complications to ensure safe care?

a. respiratory distress

b. encephalopathy

c. bleeding from the site

d. vascular collapse

82. Which of the following represents the best evaluation criterion for assessing the effectiveness of treatment aimed at reducing aggravating factors related to cholecystitis?

a. The patient maintains intake and output within normal limits.

b. The patient reports no pain following a high-fat meal.

c. The patient maintains serum albumin within normal limits.

d. The patient displays improvement on ultrasonography.

83. When caring for a patient with pancreatitis, why would the nurse expect to administer meperidine rather than morphine sulfate for pain analgesia?

a. Meperidine provides more prolonged analgesia than morphine.

b. Unlike meperidine, morphine causes spasms of the sphincter of Oddi.

c. Meperidine is less addicting than morphine.

d. Unlike meperidine, morphine may cause liver dysfunction.

84. Clinical signs and symptoms of renal transplant rejection include

a. temperature over 100°F

b. weight loss

c. polyuria

d. decreased uptake of dye on renography

85. When teaching a patient about home peritoneal dialysis, the nurse should explain that the primary concept in prevention of peritonitis is to

a. Consume a high-sodium diet.

b. Increase the amount of dextrose in the dialysis solution.

c. Maintain aseptic technique throughout the procedure.

d. Add heparin to the dialysis solution.

86. The nurse should plan to check Mr. Jones's internal arteriovenous (AV) fistula because bleeding after hemodialysis usually is related to:

a. excessive urea in blood

b. heparin administration during dialysis

c. increased platelet activity during dialysis

d. increased hematocrit related to fluid removal during hemodialysis

87. Which of the following represents the most appropriate criterion for evaluating a patient's management of elevated phosphate levels in chronic renal failure?

a. The patient eliminates dairy products from the diet.

b. The patient increases dietary calcium intake.

c. The patient takes iron supplements with meals.

d. The patient takes phosphate-binding medications with meals.

88. The wife of a patient with chronic renal failure confides to the nurse that her husband has been confused, irritable, and paranoid and that, as a result, she has been thinking of divorcing him soon. Based on this information, the nurse most likely would make which of the following diagnoses?

a. Noncompliance with prescribed medication regimen

b. Self-Esteem Disturbance related to loss of kidney function

c. Anxiety related to the dialysis procedure

d. Altered Family Processes related to the effects of chronic renal failure

89. Which of the following statements regarding random donor platelet transfusion is correct?

a. Platelets generally should be administered over 3 to 4 hours.

b. Platelet transfusion is indicated only in patients who demonstrate active bleeding.

c. Fever may affect the incremental platelet count after transfusion.

d. An allergic reaction to platelet transfusion may include chills, hemoglobinuria, and hives.

90. Mr. Smithton received his first induction course of chemotherapy 10 days ago for treatment of acute myeloblastic leukemia. Complete blood count (CBC) results include: WBC, 300/mm³; Hgb, 10.4 g/dL; Hct, 31.5%; and platelet count, 35,000. He has a temperature of 101.4°F and is complaining of fatigue and general malaise but denies any other symptoms. Based on these findings, the nurse's first intervention should be to

a. Notify the physician immediately.

b. Administer acetaminophen to decrease temperature and increase patient comfort.

c. Continue monitoring temperature every 4 hours, and notify the physician if the patient develops any other symptoms of infection.

d. Move the patient to a semiprivate room farthest from the central activity of the nursing unit.

91. Ms. Matthews, aged 24, comes to the outpatient clinic complaining of feeling increasingly "tired and run down" over the last several weeks. Her past medical history is unremarkable. A CBC is obtained; findings are WBC, 4,300/mm³; Hgb, 6.0 g/dL; Hct, 25.3%; and platelet count, 175,000. In planning care for this patient, the nurse should keep in mind which of the following principles?

a. This patient will be very symptomatic because of her low hemoglobin level.

b. Hematocrit is consistently the best indicator of anemia because it is unaffected by the patient's hydration status.

c. Pallor should be assessed on the palms of the hands.

d. Packed red blood cells should be transfused at a rapid rate because of the low level of hemoglobin.

92. Mr. Morley, aged 44, is scheduled for lumbar laminectomy and discectomy to correct a compressed lumbar disc. He has a secondary diagnosis of "bleeding disorder." Several hours ago, the nurse administered an intramuscular injection of pain medication with a small gauge needle, held pressure over the site for 5 minutes, and noted no bleeding. Now, however, the nurse observes a large hematoma at the intramuscular site. Based on this information, a likely nursing diagnosis for Mr. Morley would be High Risk for Fluid Volume Deficit related to bleeding secondary to

a. coagulation factor deficiency

b. thrombocytopenia

c. vascular fragility

d. qualitative platelet defect

93. Follow-up evaluation of Ms. Callahan, a patient with sickle cell anemia, included discussion of self-care management to avoid crises. Which of the following practices would indicate the patient's poor adjustment to lifestyle changes necessary to prevent crises?

a. The patient demonstrates relaxation and guided imagery techniques.

b. The patient avoids ingesting alcohol.

c. The patient rests frequently to avoid fatigue.

d. The patient participates in a regular program of strenuous exercise.

94. Mr. Gamble, aged 29, has been hospitalized with a diagnosis of tuberculosis. He was actively employed in construction work until approximately 1 month ago, when he developed increasing fatigue, cough, chills, and hemoptyses. As the nurse discusses the plan of care, Mr. Gamble expresses concern about his future, including ability to work and his plans to marry. Which of the following nursing diagnoses would best address this patient's primary concerns?

    a. Health-Seeking Behaviors
    b. Anticipatory Grieving
    c. Ineffective Individual Coping
    d. Self-Concept Disturbance

95. In which of the following situations is it *not* necessary for the nurse to perform careful handwashing?

    a. before drawing blood
    b. following oral care if gloves are worn
    c. after emptying a patient's surgical drain
    d. after taking a patient's blood pressure

96. Ms. Lowrey, aged 71, has been admitted in septic shock. Her nursing care plan includes the diagnosis High Risk for Injury related to clotting disorder. Based on this diagnosis, all the following would be appropriate entries in the nursing care plan *except*

    a. Obtain an order for a stool softener.
    b. Administer packed RBCs, if necessary.
    c. Encourage the patient to rinse her mouth with mouthwash and scrub her teeth with an oral sponge.
    d. Dress venipuncture sites immediately to prevent infection.

97. The nurse is counseling a sexually active young woman who has just completed a course of penicillin for gonorrhea. Which of the following statements by the young woman indicates that she understands ways to protect against reinfection?

    a. "I plan to have all my sex partners use condoms."
    b. "I plan to avoid sexual intercourse from now on."
    c. "I will come to the clinic for periodic check-ups every 2 years."
    d. "May I have extra prescriptions for penicillin so that I may give them to my sex partners?"

98. Which of the following hospitalized patients would be *least* likely to acquire a nosocomial infection?

    a. a 30-year-old woman who has completed a normal vaginal delivery
    b. a 70-year-old man admitted for prostate surgery
    c. a 32-year-old woman with lymphoma admitted for chemotherapy
    d. a 3-month-old infant admitted for dehydration secondary to influenza

99. Mr. Kravitz, aged 32, will be receiving both chemotherapy and radiation therapy for treatment of Hodgkin's disease. All the following descriptors apply to both treatment modalities *except*

    a. One is a local treatment; the other, systemic.
    b. Both modalities alter the DNA of cells.
    c. Both types may be used for cure.
    d. Side effects are directly related to the treatment site.

100. Ms. Lesko, aged 39, is receiving radiation therapy to treat breast cancer. The nurse caring for Ms. Lesko has formulated the nursing diagnosis High Risk for Impaired Skin Integrity related to radiation therapy. Based on this information, the nursing plan of care would include all the following *except*

    a. applying moisturizer to the treatment site as prescribed
    b. suggesting that Ms. Lesko use her hot tub twice a day
    c. washing the treatment site with water only

d. avoiding clothes that rub or bind

101. Ms. Woods, a 36-year-old mother of four, has colon cancer with liver metastasis. As the nurse assesses her needs, which nursing diagnosis likely would *not* be appropriate?

a. High Risk for Altered Parenting
b. Anticipatory Grieving
c. Ineffective Family Coping: Compromised
d. Self-Care Deficit

102. Mr. Johns, aged 55, has recently received high-dose chemotherapy; today, his WBC count is 1000/mm³. How can the nurse best help protect Mr. Johns while he is in the hospital?

a. Monitor closely for signs of infection.
b. Place Mr. Johns in protective isolation.
c. Wash hands carefully before caring for the patient.
d. Restrict all visitors.

103. Hearing loss resulting from a large amount of dry, hard wax in the ear canal would be classified as

a. conductive
b. perceptive
c. sensorineural
d. impacted

104. Which of the following data would lead the nurse to establish falling precautions for Mr. Brown, age 78, an ambulatory hospital patient being treated for congestive heart failure and depression?

a. use of cathartics
b. chronic depression
c. excessive diuresis
d. slow ambulation

105. Which of the following statements by a 70-year-old stroke patient with right lower paralysis would indicate that she understands prevention of pressure sores?

a. "I'll shift my weight while sitting in the wheelchair, and examine my right foot every day."
b. "I'll spend the day in a reclining

chair, and apply lotion to my right leg every 4 hours."
c. "I'll wear my support stockings daily, and my daughter will give me a good back rub every night."
d. "I'll sit on an inflatable ring in my wheelchair and wear comfortable, nonskid shoes."

106. Which of the following would be the most appropriate goals of care for a hospitalized, terminally ill, cachectic 90-year-old man?

a. The patient will verbalize that he is free of pain, not hungry, and happy to remain in bed.
b. The patient will demonstrate effective coughing and deep breathing exercises, ability to feed himself, and acceptance of diagnosis.
c. The patient will be free of skin breakdown, demonstrate adequate nutritional intake, and be able to take part in desired activities.
d. The patient will exhibit no signs and symptoms of deep venous thrombosis, pneumonia, or urinary tract infection.

107. A 78-year-old confused and delirious man is brought to the emergency department on a hot summer day. His skin feels warm, but he is not sweating. His wife tells the nurse that he takes "water pills" for his high blood pressure. Based on this information, which of the following nursing diagnoses would be most appropriate?

a. Hyperthermia
b. Altered Thought Processes
c. Ineffective Thermoregulation
d. Ineffective Breathing Patterns

108. Which of the following is the appropriate route for administering small doses of narcotics to a patient with a major burn?

a. intravenous
b. intramuscular
c. subcutaneous
d. oral

109. Mr. James comes to the emergency

room complaining of abdominal pain after an automobile accident. The nurse places Mr. James on a stretcher and instructs him to lie quietly. The primary rationale for this action is to

a. decrease abdominal pain
b. decrease the risk of dislodging an intraabdominal clot
c. facilitate peristalsis
d. decrease the risk of peritoneal infection

110. Ms. Baker comes to the emergency department after receiving a bee sting. She is slightly dyspneic and has hives on her face and neck. After administering an epinephrine injection, the nurse should tell Ms. Baker to anticipate which of the following responses?

a. easier breathing
b. diminished pain at the sting site
c. drowsiness
d. increased itching

111. For a patient scheduled for surgery, the nurse should begin preoperative teaching by

a. assessing the patient's knowledge base related to the surgical procedure and its expected outcome
b. identifying standardized teaching plans to ensure consistency
c. describing the risks of the surgical procedure
d. having the patient read printed instructional materials

112. Ms. Angers, aged 27, is scheduled for a vaginal hysterectomy. Postoperative teaching for her should focus on

a. pelvic muscle strengthening exercises
b. turning in bed, deep breathing, and arm and leg exercises
c. availability of support systems (e.g., psychologist, clergy)
d. how to use a bedpan and call light

113. Mr. Henderson is admitted to the PACU at 9:30 A.M. following a partial thyroidectomy. Initial assessment reveals temperature, 96°F; blood pressure, 130/84 mmHg; pulse, 88 beats per minute; respirations, 14 breaths per minute; dry dressing, oral airway removed, and patient opens her eyes and responds clearly to verbal commands. At 10:00 A.M., however, the nurse detects vital sign changes—blood pressure, 108/72 mmHg; pulse, 110 beats per minute; respirations, 24 breaths per minute—swelling around the dressing margins, marked restlessness, and whispered speech. Based on these findings, the nurse notifies the physician because

a. The patient is exhibiting signs and symptoms of pulmonary embolism.
b. The patient is exhibiting signs and symptoms of internal bleeding.
c. The patient is exhibiting signs and symptoms of septic shock.
d. The patient is exhibiting signs and symptoms of electrolyte imbalances common in thyroidectomy patients.

114. Ms. Cunningham, recovering from cholecystectomy and common bile duct exploration, complains of increased upper abdominal pain 2½ days postoperatively. She states, "After I ate my first solid food, I seemed to blow up." Nursing assessment reveals stable vital signs, abdominal distention, and diminished but present bowel sounds. Assuming all the following interventions are available per physician's order, which one should the nurse implement for this patient?

a. Apply a hyperthermia pad.
b. Administer an antiemetic.
c. Insert a rectal tube.
d. Administer a narcotic analgesic.

Answer Sheet for Comprehensive Exam

With a pencil, blacken the circle under the option you have chosen for your correct answer.

	A	B	C	D			A	B	C	D			A	B	C	D
1.	○	○	○	○		21.	○	○	○	○		41.	○	○	○	○
2.	○	○	○	○		22.	○	○	○	○		42.	○	○	○	○
3.	○	○	○	○		23.	○	○	○	○		43.	○	○	○	○
4.	○	○	○	○		24.	○	○	○	○		44.	○	○	○	○
5.	○	○	○	○		25.	○	○	○	○		45.	○	○	○	○
6.	○	○	○	○		26.	○	○	○	○		46.	○	○	○	○
7.	○	○	○	○		27.	○	○	○	○		47.	○	○	○	○
8.	○	○	○	○		28.	○	○	○	○		48.	○	○	○	○
9.	○	○	○	○		29.	○	○	○	○		49.	○	○	○	○
10.	○	○	○	○		30.	○	○	○	○		50.	○	○	○	○
11.	○	○	○	○		31.	○	○	○	○		51.	○	○	○	○
12.	○	○	○	○		32.	○	○	○	○		52.	○	○	○	○
13.	○	○	○	○		33.	○	○	○	○		53.	○	○	○	○
14.	○	○	○	○		34.	○	○	○	○		54.	○	○	○	○
15.	○	○	○	○		35.	○	○	○	○		55.	○	○	○	○
16.	○	○	○	○		36.	○	○	○	○		56.	○	○	○	○
17.	○	○	○	○		37.	○	○	○	○		57.	○	○	○	○
18.	○	○	○	○		38.	○	○	○	○		58.	○	○	○	○
19.	○	○	○	○		39.	○	○	○	○		59.	○	○	○	○
20.	○	○	○	○		40.	○	○	○	○		60.	○	○	○	○

728

	A	B	C	D		A	B	C	D		A	B	C	D
61.	○	○	○	○	79.	○	○	○	○	97.	○	○	○	○
62.	○	○	○	○	80.	○	○	○	○	98.	○	○	○	○
63.	○	○	○	○	81.	○	○	○	○	99.	○	○	○	○
64.	○	○	○	○	82.	○	○	○	○	100.	○	○	○	○
65.	○	○	○	○	83.	○	○	○	○	101.	○	○	○	○
66.	○	○	○	○	84.	○	○	○	○	102.	○	○	○	○
67.	○	○	○	○	85.	○	○	○	○	103.	○	○	○	○
68.	○	○	○	○	86.	○	○	○	○	104.	○	○	○	○
69.	○	○	○	○	87.	○	○	○	○	105.	○	○	○	○
70.	○	○	○	○	88.	○	○	○	○	106.	○	○	○	○
71.	○	○	○	○	89.	○	○	○	○	107.	○	○	○	○
72.	○	○	○	○	90.	○	○	○	○	108.	○	○	○	○
73.	○	○	○	○	91.	○	○	○	○	109.	○	○	○	○
74.	○	○	○	○	92.	○	○	○	○	110.	○	○	○	○
75.	○	○	○	○	93.	○	○	○	○	111.	○	○	○	○
76.	○	○	○	○	94.	○	○	○	○	112.	○	○	○	○
77.	○	○	○	○	95.	○	○	○	○	113.	○	○	○	○
78.	○	○	○	○	96.	○	○	○	○	114.	○	○	○	○

1. **Correct response: a**
   This is Luckmann and Sorensen's (1987) definition of the nursing process.
   b. This describes the work of the North American Nursing Diagnosis Association (NANDA).
   c and d. These are not definitions of the nursing process but are self-explanatory.
   Comprehension/NA/NA

2. **Correct response: d**
   This question assesses self-concept, one of the factors associated with "role and relationship patterns."
   a. This is a part of the assessment associated with "health promotion and protection patterns."
   b and c. These are associated with the "health and illness patterns" segment.
   Application/Psychosocial/Assessment

3. **Correct response: c**
   This question imposes the nurse's bias and would tend to discourage an honest response from the patient.
   a, b, and d. These are all legitimate questions to ask regarding a patient's health and health practices.
   Application/Health promotion/Assessment

4. **Correct response: d**
   Along with the signs described, other indications of arterial insufficiency include delayed capillary refill in toenails; thin, shiny skin of the lower extremities; and diminished or absent pulses.
   a and b. These signs are not associated with insufficient venous circulation or venous thrombosis.
   c. Normal age-related changes do not include lesions on the feet.
   Analysis/Physiologic/Assessment

5. **Correct response: b**
   All results are at about midnormal ranges.

a, c, and d. No results are above or below normal ranges.
Analysis/Physiologic/Assessment

6. **Correct response: b**
   Practice would be more appropriate for at-home follow-up evaluation of a single patient than for group teaching sessions.
   a. Discussion involves the auditory learning domain and is appropriate for group teaching.
   c. Role playing involves the visual domain and is appropriate for group teaching.
   d. Self-monitoring involves the psychomotor domain and may be appropriate for group teaching.
   Application/Physiologic/Implementation

7. **Correct response: b**
   Given this patient's background and hearing deficit, computer-assisted instruction likely would be the most effective teaching tool.
   a, c, and d. These would not accommodate the patient's hearing deficit as well as the computer.
   Application/Physiologic/Evaluation

8. **Correct response: d**
   Perceived changes in role or self-image due to illness may call for counseling to help with problem solving and reality orientation.
   a. Grief would be an expected response to the diagnosis.
   b and c. These problems have the potential for short-term resolution.
   Analysis/Psychosocial/Analysis (Dx)

9. **Correct response: d**
   Adult learners generally prefer to be involved in educational activity and to share learned experiences.
   a, b, and c. These are all assumptions basic to the an-

dragogy model for adult learners.

Comprehension/Health promotion/Planning

10. Correct response: c

By putting together the equipment without waiting for instructions, this patient demonstrates that he or she is primarily a tactile learner.

a and b. These behaviors demonstrate a visual pattern of learning.

d. This behavior demonstrates an auditory pattern of learning.

Analysis/Health promotion/Assessment

11. Correct response: c

Tissue swelling results from increased vascular permeability and leakage of plasma fluids.

a. Increased vascular permeability results from transient vasoconstriction followed by vasodilation.

b. White blood cells migrate to the site of injury.

d. Nerve ending irritation by chemical mediators (e.g., as histamine) results in pain.

Comprehension/Physiologic/Assessment

12. Correct response: a

Radiation to the anterior chest wall may affect the mucosal lining of the esophagus, causing pain on swallowing. Oral mucosal changes would not occur because of the location of radiation.

b and c. Changes in body image and sexuality both should be addressed in caring for this patient.

d. The possibility of altered skin integrity would be great in this patient.

Analysis/Psychosocial/Analysis (Dx)

13. Correct response: b

A well-balanced diet high in protein and calories promotes tissue repair.

a and c. Either heat or cold applied to the radiation site could impair healing by destroying enzymes and causing

vasoconstriction, respectively.

d. Warm fluids would increase rather than decrease esophageal discomfort.

Analysis/Health promotion/Implementation

14. Correct response: d

This patient should avoid any sun exposure.

a, b, and c. These are all appropriate self-care interventions either to increase healing, reduce the risk of infection, or identify early signs of complications.

Application/Safe care/Planning

15. Correct response: d

Hyperplasia involves an increase in the number of cells in an organ or tissue, often related to hormonal influences.

a, b, and, c. These represent hypertrophy, atrophy, and metaplasia, respectively.

Application/Physiologic/Evaluation

16. Correct response: a

Because furosemide is a diuretic that commonly causes potassium depletion, Mr. Johnson should eat food high in potassium.

b. The stated rate of KCl infusion is correct (10 mEq/hour).

c. Hyperkalemia will manifest as peaked narrow T waves on ECG.

d. Hyperkalemia—not hypokalemia—can result from hemolysis.

Analysis/Health promotion/Planning

17. Correct response: c

These assessment data most strongly suggest hypercalcemia.

a and b. Although the patient's symptoms could also suggest either hyponatremia or hypermagnesemia, the ECG changes clearly point to calcium imbalance.

d. Hyperkalemia is marked by muscle weakness and paresthesias.

Comprehension/Physiologic/Assessment

18. *Correct response: d*
Due to increased loss of water and electrolytes from the diarrhea, this patient likely would develop fluid volume deficit (FVD). Laboratory values diagnostic of FVD include increased blood urea nitrogen (BUN) and hematocrit.
a, b, and c. These findings are not consistent with the scenario.

Analysis/Physiologic/Evaluation

19. *Correct response: b*
Metabolic alkalosis is marked by pH above 7.45 and HCO₃ above 26 mEq/L.
a. Nothing in the scenario indicates that fright is accounting for the patient's behavior.
c. In acidosis, pH is below 7.35.
d. The nurse should not assume that such behavior would be expected in response to a respiratory crisis; such an assumption could cause the nurse to ignore the underlying physiologic cause.

Application/Psychosocial/Implementation

20. *Correct response: b*
Because many antacids contain magnesium, indiscriminate antacid use may contribute to high magnesium levels.
a. Immobility leads to loss of calcium from bones, not magnesium.
c. Neuromuscular irritability causing sleep disturbance is a symptom of hypomagnesemia.
d. Fluid volume excess results form retention of sodium, not magnesium.

Application/Safe care/Analysis (Dx)

21. *Correct response: d*
A-delta fibers transmit pain faster than type C and therefore deliver the first sharp sensations.
a. C-fiber activation produces persistent, dull, aching pain.
b and c. Type A-alpha, beta, and gamma fibers transmit touch, pressure, heat, cold, and movement much faster.

Comprehension/Physiologic/Assessment

22. *Correct response: d*
This diagnosis would alert other nurses to the possibility that the patient may attempt to crutch-walk without assistance and fall.
a, b, and c. No information in this scenario suggests any of these diagnoses.

Analysis/Safe care/Analysis (Dx)

23. *Correct response: b*
These are noninvasive interventions that most persons will accept.
a. This would not be sufficient.
c. This would violate the patient's rights.
d. This would avoid attempting to meet the patient's needs.

Application/Psychosocial/Planning

24. *Correct response: a*
Anginal pain decreases with rest and the improved coronary circulation provided by sublingual nitroglycerin.
b. These measures will increase myocardial oxygen demand and exacerbate pain.
c. These tablets do not provide immediate symptom relief.
d. These measures will not improve coronary circulation.

Analysis/Health promotion/Implementation

25. *Correct response: c*
Continuation of behaviors detrimental to health are often a sign of ineffective denial.
a. Grieving over loss of health (rather than anticipatory) is very likely a part of this patient's emotional response, but it would not lead to this self-destructive behavior.
b and d. This scenario offers no evidence that the patient is experiencing disturbance of either body image or social interaction.

Application/Psychosocial/Analysis (Dx)

26. *Correct response: d*
CO_2 and H_2O, in differing concentrations, react to form carbonic acid (H_2CO_3), which in turn dissociates to form bicarbonate (HCO_3) and hydrogen (H^+) ions. This reaction determines the pH of arterial blood and the acid–base balance of the human body. CO_2 is blown off or conserved by the lungs as one variable in keeping this balance.
   a. Although the lungs do control O_2 intake, O_2 is not a primary mediator in acid–base balance.
   b. The mechanism for cholesterol control is not in the lungs.
   c. Urea and albumin are affected by the kidneys.
Application/Physiologic/Assessment

27. *Correct response: b*
Any opening in the chest causes pneumothorax (collapsed lung). As the pleura is incised or penetrated, atmospheric air rushes into the pleural space, which normally maintains a negative pressure to provide for lung expansion. Disruption of this negative pressure causes the lung to collapse.
   a. The lung will collapse, not expand, if any penetration of the pleura is made.
   c. Lung expansion is controlled by both lung pressures and intrapleural pressure. However, if intrapleural pressure is disturbed, the lung will collapse.
   d. Pressure in the intrapleural space is negative.
Analysis/Physiologic/Planning

28. *Correct response: d*
There is an increased incidence of respiratory infections related to bacterial growth in warm air humidifiers.
   a. Pollutants of many kinds tend to cause respiratory disease.
   b. Cigarette smoke is considered a pollutant, and research has shown it to be detrimental to lung function.
   c. A balance of rest and exercise and proper eating habits is of primary importance to respiratory health.
Comprehension/Health Promotion/ Evaluation

29. *Correct response: b*
PVCs can lead to lethal dysrhythmias because they indicate ventricular irritability.
   a, c, and d. These actions are not characteristic of PVCs.
Comprehension/Physiologic/Assessment

30. *Correct response: d*
This should be done after the procedure and before discharge.
   a, b, and c. These measures are all appropriate before arteriography.
Application/Physiologic/Implementation

31. *Correct response: d*
Mrs. Davidson is expressing fear over the uncertainty surrounding her future.
   a and b. No information in this scenario would point to either of these diagnoses.
   c. The patient may in fact have a knowledge deficit, but more assessment would be needed to confirm this.
Analysis/Psychosocial/Analysis (Dx)

32. *Correct response: d*
On experiencing anginal pain, a person should stop all activity to decrease workload on the heart.
   a, b, and c. All these measures would be appropriate to teach to a patient with angina.
Application/Health promotion/Evaluation

33. *Correct response: c*
This patient needs rest periods and perhaps curtailment of some activity, not prolongation.
   a, b, and d. These all would be appropriate for this patient.
Analysis/Safe care/Planning

34. Correct response: d
Improving circulation decreases ischemia, the basic cause of pain in arterial occlusive disorders.
  a. Venous return is not involved in the mechanism causing pain in arterial occlusive disorders.
  b. Narcotic pain medication may be necessary in combination with other measures.
  c. Edema is not the mechanism causing discomfort.
Comprehension/Physiologic/Implementation

35. Correct response: b
Chronic venous stasis causes chronically swollen legs; thick, coarse, brown pigmented skin; and nonpainful, wet ulcers on the ankles.
  a. Ulcers do not form rapidly enough to appear with acute deep venous thrombosis.
  c. Ulcers associated with chronic arterial insufficiency are marked by muscle atrophy, thin skin, dry painful ulcers, and diminished or absent pedal pulses.
  d. Ulcers rarely develop in lymphedema.
Analysis/Physiologic/Assessment

36. Correct response: a
Red streaking indicates lymphangitis and spread of infection.
  b. Although avoiding crossing the legs will help promote venous return, edema of the foot does not represent as serious a threat to health as does worsening of infection.
  c. Although avoiding smoking is an important health consideration, it will not have as immediate an affect on health status as will infection.
  d. Anaphylactic reaction to tetanus toxoid injection usually occurs immediately after administration while the patient is in the health care setting.
Application/Health promotion/Planning

37. Correct response: c
Blood pressure, pulse, and respiratory changes, along with blood on the dressing, are consistent with bleeding, one of the most common complications postamputation.
  a. Recovery from anesthesia usually is accompanied by a return to baseline vital signs, which are not known in this case.
  b. Although pain can be a factor in vital sign changes, the question does not address the patient's pain perception.
  d. Respiratory atelectasis following surgery often is accompanied by temperature elevation; although deep breathing is appropriate, vigorous deep breathing and coughing is not.
Analysis/Safe care/Evaluation

38. Correct response: b
Stress reduction represents one aspect of blood pressure control.
  a. A single major cause of primary hypertension has not been identified.
  c. The nurse's active listening skills and patient acceptance are essential to a therapeutic nurse–patient relationship; the patient's comfort level may or may not be significant.
  d. Stress may or may not interfere with learning. Most important to patient education in this case are the patient's understanding of the problem and treatment alternatives and his active involvement in the therapeutic regimen.
Application/Psychosocial/Analysis (Dx)

39. Correct response: a
Antacids decrease acidity and should be continued even in the absence of symptoms.
  b and d. Antacids should be taken 1 hour before or 2 hours after meals for best results and should not be given with

medications (which can alter the acid content and thus absorption of the drug).

  c. Sodium, not magnesium, content is of concern for cardiac patients.

Application/Health promotion/Implementation

40. Correct response: a
There is no evidence that tissue perfusion is an expected complication.

  b, c, and d. These diagnoses all represent likely complications of Crohn's disease.

Analysis/Safe care/Analysis (Dx)

41. Correct response: a
Right scapular pain commonly occurs with cholecystitis.

  b, c, and d. These symptoms are all associated with appendicitis.

Comprehension/Physiologic/Assessment

42. Correct response: c
Primary large bowel functions include absorption of water and elimination of feces.

  a. Relief of pain after ingestion of food is sign of duodenal ulcer.

  b. The small bowel is primarily responsible for the absorption of nutrients.

  d. Belching and reflux are symptoms of hiatal hernia.

Analysis/Physiologic/Evaluation

43. Correct response: d
Anorexia and weight loss are common complications of ulcerative colitis.

  a. Anal involvement is rare; an anal fistula or abscess is common with Crohn's disease.

  b and c. Neither ascites or nausea and vomiting would be expected with this diagnosis.

Application/Psychosocial/Planning

44. Correct response: b
Infection, causing increased stress hormones, insulin resistance, and in-creased insulin need, is the most frequent cause of diabetic ketoacidosis (DKA).

  a, c, and d. Overeating, missing a single insulin dose, or psychologic stress may increase blood glucose levels but will not cause DKA.

Comprehension/Physiologic/Assessment

45. Correct response: a
The open area should be cleaned with plain soap and water and observed for any signs of infection.

  b. Soaking the foot is not advised because of the increased potential for injury.

  c. Mercurochrome or any iodine product is not advised because of its potential to damage tissue.

  d. Applying heat also can increase the risk of tissue damage.

Application/Safe care/Implementation

46. Correct response: c
Hemorrhage in the postoperative thyroidectomy patient may cause compression of the trachea, necessitating emergency tracheostomy to maintain an airway.

  a and d. Calcium and thyroid hormone replacement may be needed but are not related to hemorrhage.

  b. Insertion of an oral airway would not be sufficient for this patient.

Analysis/Physiologic/Planning

47. Correct response: d
Any patient taking glucocorticoids, either for physiologic replacement or for pharmacologic treatment should not discontinue treatment abruptly for any reason.

  a. Medical identification helps ensure continuation of treatment at times when the patient cannot speak for himself or herself.

  b. During times of stress, dosages may need to be increased.

  c. All health care providers should

know of treatment in case dosages need to be adjusted.

Application/Health promotion/Evaluation

48. Correct response: d

The inability to continue usual social patterns is a sign of ineffective coping.

a, b, and c. None of these nursing diagnoses account for the antisocial and self-destructive behaviors described.

Analysis/Psychosocial/Analysis (Dx)

49. Correct response: b

Impotence can result from various psychologic and physiologic problems.

a. Psychologic factors are not the only contributing factors to impotence.

c. Although dietary factors conceivably could play a part in a physiologic disorder leading to impotence, they are not of primary consideration.

d. Incidence of impotence increases with age.

Knowledge/Health promotion/Planning

50. Correct response: c

Clots that obstruct urinary drainage and cause urinary retention can lead to hemorrhage from the prostatic bed given its high vascularity.

a. Pressure on the incision may cause pain, but not usually hemorrhage.

b and d. Thrombosis and infection are not usually associated with hemorrhage.

Knowledge/Physiologic/Assessment

51. Correct response: b

The testes normally feel smooth and oval, with no masses.

a. Tenderness or pain is not a common early symptom of testicular cancer.

c. Testicular masses generally are easy to detect.

d. With early detection and treatment, prognosis generally is fair to good.

Application/Health promotion/ Implementation

52. Correct response: d

Headache is not specifically associated with complications of mastectomy.

a, b, and c. Infection, thrombosis, and edema of the arm are all possible complications of mastectomy, associated with poor lymphatic drainage in the operative area and with reduced mobility postoperatively.

Knowledge/Physiologic/Assessment

53. Correct response: a

Surgical manipulation in the area around the bladder may cause nerve trauma and edema, which can affect voiding.

b, c, and d. These statements are simply not correct.

Analysis/Safe care/Implementation

54. Correct response: d

The causative agent determines the nature of the dermatitis.

a. Onset of reactions can range from immediate to as long as 21 days after exposure.

b. The dermatitis may be due to primary irritants or allergic sensitizers.

c. The inflammations may range from redness to ulcerations and is dependent on many factors.

Comprehension/Physiologic/Assessment

55. Correct response: c

Bedrest may exacerbate dyspnea by allowing atelectasis and pooling of secretions.

a. Adequate hydration will keep secretions viscous and easy to expectorate.

b. Coughing and deep breathing will maintain open airways.

d. Pacing activities will help decrease dyspnea by allowing adequate rest.

Application/Physiologic/Evaluation

56. Correct response: d

Assessment is the first step in nursing care for all patients.

a, b, and c. Although these all are important interventions for a patient with rheumatoid arthritis, none of them can be effective without a thorough assessment of Ms. Shandra's needs.

Application/Health promotion/Implementation

57. Correct response: b
This patient is expressing doubts about her ability to continue in her current role.
a, c, and d. Although these other diagnoses could be appropriate, they are not related to the patient's comments.

Analysis/Psychosocial/Analysis (Dx)

58. Correct response: a
Acute dyspnea will interfere with the patient's ability to talk; answering questions will tire the patient unnecessarily. Thus, the nurse would best wait until the patient can breathe easier or try to obtain the information from the family members.
b, c, and d. None of these would be the best approach to obtaining health history information for this patient.

Analysis/Safe care/Planning

59. Correct response: c
Major brain injuries are defined as those involving second-degree burns over more than 25% TBSA in adults or 20% of TBSA in children, or those involving third-degree burns over 10% of TBSA or more in any patient.
a. Minor burn injury involves second-degree burns over less than 15% of TBSA, or less than 10% of TBSA in children.
b. Moderate uncomplicated burn injury is defined as second-degree burns over 15% to 25% of TBSA in adults or 10% to 20% of TBSA

in children, or third-degree burns over more than 10% of TBSA without involvement of special care areas.
d. Full-thickness burn injury involves the epidermis, dermis, and underlying subcutaneous tissue.

Comprehension/Physiologic/Assessment

60. Correct response: a
The appropriate sequence of nursing action for patients with major burn injuries is: eliminate the source of the burn, ensure airway patency, assess for and treat associated injuries, and treat burn shock.
b, c, and d. The other actions may be appropriate during care of such a patient, but response a. represents the correct sequence for initial assessment.

Analysis/Safe care/Implementation

61. Correct response: b
14,000 mL is the correct number.
a, c, and d. None of the other fluid replacement amounts would be adequate.

Application/Health promotion/Evaluation

62. Correct response: d
A chest radiograph may not demonstrate immediate damage.
a, b, and c. The patient's clinical presentation calls for actions based on the presumption that smoke inhalation has occurred. All these statements are correct.

Application/Physiologic/Implementation

63. Correct response: a
Unilateral neglect is associated with neurologic deficit.
b and d. Body image and self-concept disturbances would commonly be associated with a large homograft.

c. Pain would be expected from both the graft and harvest sites.
Analysis/Psychosocial/Analysis (Dx)

64. Correct response: c
In myasthenia gravis, severe fatigue can significantly alter family processes.
a. Myasthenia gravis can entail changes that affect eating (e.g., increased salivation with difficulty swallowing and chewing) but is not associated with altered taste.
b. Cardiac output changes are not directly related to myasthenia gravis.
d. Myasthenia gravis is not associated with altered thought processes except indirectly related to fatigue.
Analysis/Psychosocial/Analysis (Dx)

65. Correct response: c
Ensuring adequate fluid and dietary fiber intake is the first step in preventing or easing constipation.
a, b, and d. Before resorting to a laxative or enema, fluids and diet modifications should be tried.
Comprehension/Physiologic/Evaluation

66. Correct response: a
Proper alignment will reduce pain and protect the surgical site; good shoes help prevent slipping and sudden jerky movements; removing objects also improves safety.
b. Not all patients require pain medication.
c. A cane would be needed only if the patient had suffered foot drop.
d. Prism glasses are not appropriate.
Application/Health promotion/Planning

67. Correct response: d
The autonomic nervous system is very labile; noxious stimuli would tend to increase intracranial pressure. Elevating the head of bed assists in venous return and in breathing. Positioning on the side helps facilitate breathing; frequent monitoring is needed to detect any adverse changes so that therapy can be implemented immediately.

a, b, and c. None of these sets of interventions would be appropriate for this patient.
Analysis/Safe care/Implementation

68. Correct response: c
Traction is needed to keep vertebrae in alignment because vertebral movement could damage the cord. Both fingers and toes need to be assessed because changes may indicate the need for immediate medical intervention.
a, b, and d. None of these sets of parameters would be appropriate for this patient.
Application/Physiologic/Assessment

69. Correct response: c
Miotics cause pupil constriction, impairing night vision.
a. Near vision impairment can result from mydriatics.
b and d. Increased sensitivity to light and double vision result when one eye is aphakic (without lens) and the other is phakic (with lens), not as an effect of medication.
Application/Physiologic/Evaluation

70. Correct response: d
Postoperative eye pain is indicative of increased intraocular pressure or hemorrhage.
a. Slight temperature elevation would be expected postoperatively as a manifestation of the inflammatory response.
b. Double vision results when one eye has a lens and the other does not.
c. Floaters are symptoms of retinal detachment.
Comprehension/Physiologic/Assessment

71. Correct response: b
Prolonged use of decongestant drops (3 to 5 days) can lead to rebound congestion, which is relieved by discontinuing the medication for 2 or 3 weeks.

738

a, c, and d. Continuing the medication or increasing the dose would worsen this phenomenon.

Analysis/Safe care/Implementation

72. Correct response: c
The eardrum separates the external ear from the middle ear. Perforation increases susceptibility to suppurative otitis media and necessitates special ear care.

a, b, and d. The patient may or may not experience hearing loss or pain and should receive general ear care instruction, but the priority concern with perforation is infection.

Analysis/Physiologic/Analysis (Dx)

73. Correct response: d
With a permanent tracheostomy, the airway must be protected from water and particulate matter.

a. Referral to support groups is important but not essential for safety.

b and c. Although the patient should carry a medic-alert card for special needs and should receive an explanation regarding loss of strength with Valsalva maneuver, these interventions are not essential for self-care safety in ADLs.

Application/Health promotion/Planning

74. Correct response: b
Mental disturbances such as confusion, irritability, restlessness, disorientation, stupor, or coma are often the first sign of systemic fat embolism. These symptoms are caused from hypoxemia and may begin very subtly with rapid advancement of respiratory, cardiovascular, and other systemic symptoms depending on where the embolus lodges.

a, c, and d. These signs and symptoms are not associated with fat embolism.

Comprehension/Physiologic/Assessment

75. Correct response: c
A patient undergoing magnetic resonance imaging (MRI) is exposed to a magnetic field approximately 15,000 times greater than the earth's magnetic field. It is therefore very important to remove all metal objects and assess for electrically, magnetically, or mechanically activated implants such as pacemakers, clips, staples, or shrapnel.

a. Because MRI is not an invasive procedure, it does not require informed consent.

b and d. MRI involves no injections or contrast media.

Application/Safe care/Implementation

76. Correct response: a
Compartment syndrome is a condition caused by either a decrease in compartment size or an increase in compartment contents. In this case, the patient has a cast applied and complains of pain over the elbow area, which is a site for pressure and resulting swelling. Common symptoms of compartment syndrome are pain out of proportion to the injury, pallor, pulselessness, paresthesias, paralysis, and poikilothermia. When compartment syndrome is suspected, the nurse should notify the physician immediately and prepare for immediate release of constriction, which may include bivalving the cast, cutting dressings, or performing a fasciotomy.

b, c, and d. This patient needs *immediate* relief of pressure inside the cast; none of these interventions would be appropriate.

Analysis/Physiologic/Planning

77. Correct response: d
Hemorrhage from a loosened ligature is the most threatening complication in the immediate postoperative period following limb amputation. The patient should be monitored very closely during this period for any signs or symptoms of bleeding either from the

operative site or in the suction drainage. A large tourniquet should be kept at the bedside to apply in the event of hemorrhage.

a, b, and c. Although these other nursing diagnoses also may be applicable during the postoperative period, none are of as much concern as the potential for hemorrhage.

Application/Health promotion/Analysis (Dx)

78. *Correct response: a*
A patient undergoing limb amputation typically experiences altered body image and must learn to accept the loss and a new image. It is important for the nurse to work closely with the patient and build a trusting relationship and encourage the patient to look at, feel, and care for the residual limb. Once the patient is able to do these tasks, he or she will learn to accept the loss and begin building a new self-image.

b, c, and d. Although these nursing diagnoses could apply to a patient recovering from amputation, Altered Body Image applies to virtually all such patients.

Analysis/Psychosocial/Evaluation

79. *Correct response: a*
Obstructed blood flow is the cause of portal hypertension.

b. Ascites results from portal hypertension; it is not a cause.

c. Esophageal varices are a result of portal hypertension, not a cause.

d. Obstruction of bile flow would lead to jaundice, not portal hypertension.

Comprehension/Physiologic/Assessment

80. *Correct response: a*
Patients commonly associate a dis-

tended abdomen with obesity, resulting in a body image alteration.

b. Ascites does not cause jaundice although they frequently do occur together.

c. Fecal incontinence is not generally associated with ascites.

d. Muscle wasting does not result from ascites.

Analysis/Psychosocial/Analysis (Dx)

81. *Correct response: d*
The removal of large amounts of ascites may lead to acute fluid shifts and hypotension.

a. Respiratory distress is not usually associated with this procedure.

b. Paracentesis does not effect ammonia level or alter protein status.

c. Bleeding from the site may occur, but it is not the most important side effect to monitor for.

Application/Safe care/Implementation

82. *Correct response: b*
History of pain following a high fat meal may lead the nurse to advise the patient to avoid this type of dietary intake.

a. Intake and output does not provide information regarding the aggravating factors of the disorder.

c and d. These criteria do provide important information about the disorder but do not provide keys to aggravating factors.

Application/Health promotion/Evaluation

83. *Correct response: b*
Morphine causes spasm of the sphincter of Oddi (at the end of the pancreatic duct), which may aggravate pancreatitis.

a. Meperidine is actually somewhat shorter acting than morphine.

c. Both drugs are potentially addictive.

d. Morphine use is not associated with liver dysfunction.

Analysis/Physiologic/Planning

84. *Correct response: a*

740

Fever is one sign of an active immune process.

b, c, and d. Fluid retention and weight gain, decreased urine output, and poor uptake of dye on renography are all characteristic of transplant rejection.

Comprehension/Physiologic/Assessment

85. *Correct response: c*
Aseptic technique is essential in all aspects of peritoneal dialysis procedure to prevent microorganisms from invading peritoneal cavity.

a. Sodium intake is not related to peritonitis.

b. Dextrose in dialysis solution is related to fluid removal; it is an excellent medium for bacterial growth.

d. Heparin helps prevent fibrin clots in the catheter.

Application/Physiologic/Implementation

86. *Correct response: b*
Heparin is added to dialyzer blood to prevent clotting in the dialyzer; the patient becomes anticoagulated and may bleed.

a. Urea level usually is decreased after dialysis and is not related to bleeding.

c. Dialysis does not affect platelet activity.

d. Increased hematocrit would not contribute to bleeding.

Analysis/Safe care/Planning

87. *Correct response: d*
Phosphate binding medications bind with phosphate in food and prevent its absorption.

a. Dairy products are an excellent source of HBV protein and calcium.

b. Dietary calcium has no affect on phosphate levels.

c. Iron intake has no effect on phosphate levels.

Application/Health promotion/Evaluation

88. *Correct response: d*
This patient's symptoms are disrupting his marital relationship.

a, b, and c. Nothing in this scenario would lead the nurse to formulate any of these diagnoses.

Analysis/Psychosocial/Analysis (Dx)

89. *Correct response: c*
Fever and infection may decrease the incremental count after transfusion.

a. Platelets should be administered as rapidly as tolerated by the patient.

b. Platelets may be transfused in selected instances to prevent bleeding.

d. Hemoglobinuria is indicative of a hemolytic transfusion reaction (lysis of RBCs).

Comprehension/Health promotion/Assessment

90. *Correct response: a*
Fever and infection in a severely neutropenic patient (neutrophils less than 500/mm^3) can be rapidly fatal if broad-spectrum antibiotic therapy is not instituted quickly.

b. This is incorrect because it would not be the immediate intervention.

c. Once the physician is notified, the patient should be monitored frequently.

d. The patient should be in a private room. (The location of the room should not compromise frequent monitoring.)

Analysis/Physiologic/Implementation

91. *Correct response: c*
Color changes are best assessed where capillary beds are superficial and pigmentation is minimal.

a. A patient may experience few symptoms if the onset of anemia has been gradual and there is adequate cardiopulmonary compensation.

b. Hematocrit can be affected by hydration (plasma volume) as well as RBC size.

d. Too-rapid administration of a transfusion in a patient with compensated anemia may produce circulatory overload.

Application/Physiologic/Planning

92. *Correct response: a*
Coagulation factor defects usually present with deep tissue bleeding after minor trauma, and bleeding may recur several hours after pressure is relieved.

b, c, and d. These responses are incorrect because delayed bleeding is rare in vascular and platelet disorders (either quantitative or qualitative). In addition, the patient stopped bleeding after 5 minutes of pressure initially, indicating platelet plug formulation (ability of platelets to aggregate and adhere).

Analysis/Safe care/Analysis (Dx)

93. *Correct response: d*
Strenuous physical activity is contraindicated because the physiologic stress can precipitate crisis.

a. Relaxation and other techniques would be encouraged to control emotional stress, which can precipitate crises.

b and c. Ingestion of alcohol and fatigue are both precipitating factors for crises.

Application/Psychosocial/Evaluation

94. *Correct response: a*
The concerns expressed show an interest in finding answers to maximize abilities in the future, which is characteristic of health-seeking behavior.

b. Although anticipatory grieving may occur, it is not evident from this scenario.

c and d. The scenario offers no evidence to indicate that the patient is coping ineffec-

tively or has a disturbed self-concept.

Analysis/Psychosocial/Analysis (Dx)

95. *Correct response: d*
Handwashing generally is not necessary following brief, routine patient activities.

a, b, and c. Handwashing is indicated before coming in contact with body fluids or mucous membranes. Wearing gloves does not eliminate the need for handwashing.

Comprehension/Safe care/Implementation

96. *Correct response: d*
Firm, direct pressure should be applied to the site for 3 to 7 minutes before final dressing because of a clotting abnormality.

a. Stool softeners will decrease straining, which could result in bleeding.

b. Packed RBCs will be ordered if the patient's hematocrit drops because of excessive blood loss.

c. The patient should avoid hard-bristled toothbrushes, which may increase bleeding.

Application/Physiologic/Planning

97. *Correct response: a*
Correct and consistent use of this barrier technique will reduce the risk of STD.

b. Although abstinence from sexual intercourse will eliminate risk of STD transmission, it is often an unrealistic expectation.

c. Periodic check-ups should be done at more frequent intervals.

d. Sexual partners should be examined and counseled for STDs. However, treatment without verification of disease is not indicated.

Application/Health promotion/Evaluation

98. *Correct response: a*
Although any hospitalized patient is at risk for nosocomial infection, the 30-

year-old woman admitted for normal delivery is least likely because she will be exposed to the fewest invasive procedures and will probably have the shortest hospital stay. Most important, however, is the fact that she, unlike the others, has a healthy immune system.

   b. The 70-year-old man is somewhat immunocompromised because of age and exposure to invasive procedures.

   c. The 32-year-old woman with lymphoma is compromised because of her disease and its treatment.

   d. The 3-month-old infant is compromised because of young age and debilitated state.

Analysis/Physiologic/Assessment

99. *Correct response: d*
Side effects from radiation are directly related to the treatment site, but those of chemotherapy are not.

   a. Radiation is a local treatment; chemotherapy is systemic treatment.

   b. Both modalities alter cellular function and reproduction.

   c. Both modalities are used for cure.

Comprehension/Physiologic/Assessment

100. *Correct response: b*
Heat of any type is a further insult to delicate skin in the treatment site.

   a. Use of moisturizers is allowed by some radiotherapists but not by others.

   c. Washing the treatment site is allowed if done gently.

   d. Clothes that rub can displace delicate skin with very little friction.

Application/Physiologic/Planning

101. *Correct response: d*
There is nothing to indicate a central neurologic deficit.

   a. Advanced disease commonly decreases mobility, which can impair parenting ability.

   b. Grieving would be an expected response to this diagnosis.

   c. Ineffective coping would be applicable with any advanced cancer; in this case, there are many people to take into account.

Analysis/Psychosocial/Analysis (Dx)

102. *Correct response: c*
The most important measure to decrease the risk from nocosomial exogenous organisms is proper handwashing.

   a. Observing for signs of infection is important, but prevention takes precedence over detection.

   b. Isolation may be done in some institutions, but handwashing is most important.

   d. Family members who are ill should certainly stay away; however, close family who practice good handwashing and wear protective garb can help sustain the patient through this difficult time.

Application/Safe care/Implementation

103. *Correct response: a*
Impacted cerumen is a leading cause of conductive hearing loss.

   b and c. Perceptive and sensorineural hearing loss involve the middle or inner ear.

   d. Impacted is not a type of hearing loss.

Comprehension/Psychosocial/Analysis (Dx)

104. *Correct response: c*
Volume depletion from diuretic use may increase a patient's risk of falling.

   a. Cathartics may cause problem with elimination, but unless the patient abuses them, leading to electrolyte imbalance, they would not increase the risk of falling.

   b and d. Chronic depression and slow ambulation would not be indications for fall precautions.

Analysis/Physiologic/Assessment

105. *Correct response: a*
Regular position changes and weight shifts can help prevent pressure sores.

The skin of the affected extremity needs to be visually inspected because altered sensation likely is present.

b. Regular position changes are important. Lotion can exacerbate skin breakdown.

c. These measures will not prevent pressure sores.

d. Sitting on an inflatable ring can impair tissue perfusion.

Application/Health promotion/Evaluation

106. *Correct response: c*

Cachectic older adults are malnourished and at risk for skin breakdown; goals should incorporate these factors. In addition, the nurse should encourage dying patients to participate in desired activities rather than just focus on disease treatment and prevention.

a, b, and d. These interventions are not as applicable as those described in response c.

Analysis/Physiologic/Planning

107. *Correct response: d*

This patient's history and signs and symptoms are consistent with hyperthermia. There is no evidence that respiratory function has changed although this could be a later consequence of unresolved hyperthermia.

a, b, and c. These all would be appropriate diagnoses based on the information presented in this scenario.

Application/Physiologic/Analysis (Dx)

108. *Correct response: a*

IV is the most appropriate route for this patient.

b, c, and d. A patient with major burns is in shock and therefore has poor peripheral circulation needed for absorption of IM or subcutaneous medication. Severely burned patients often develop paralytic ileus

and are NPO and unable to take medication by mouth.

Analysis/Physiologic/Planning

109. *Correct response: b*

Activity may dislodge a clot and start hemorrhage.

a. Decreasing abdominal pain should result from this action, but it is not the primary reason for bedrest in this situation.

c. Immobility will not facilitate peristalsis.

d. Immobility will not decrease the potential for infection.

Analysis/Safe care/Implementation

110. *Correct response: a*

Epinephrine acts as a bronchodilator and will relieve dyspnea.

b, c, and d. The action of epinephrine will not diminish pain, cause drowsiness, or increase itching.

Application/Health promotion/Evaluation

111. *Correct response: a*

Many fears related to surgery are based on inadequate or inappropriate information. Assessing the patient's knowledge and identifying misconceptions allows the nurse to tailor the teaching plan to the patient's specific needs.

b. All teaching should be individualized based on the patient's particular needs.

c. Explaining any risks related to surgery is the physician's responsibility.

d. Written materials only supplement preoperative teaching and do not supplant interactive sessions.

Comprehension/Psychosocial/Assessment

112. *Correct response: b*

Turning, extremity exercises, and deep breathing are important to postoperative recovery.

a. Kegel exercises would not be appropriate at this time and would be done only by medical orders.

c. Availability of support systems is not as high a priority as physiologic integrity according to Maslow's Hierarchy of Needs; teaching should be focused on the highest priority.

d. Teaching the use of a bedpan and call light are part of the patient's initial orientation to the unit.

Analysis/Health promotion/Planning

113. *Correct response: b*

Signs of hypovolemic shock and edema suggest internal bleeding.

a. Pulmonary embolism is marked by chest pain and hemoptysis, among other signs and symptoms.

c. This scenario presents no information to suggest septic shock.

d. A patient undergoing partial thy-roidectomy would not have had all parathyroids disrupted and would not likely experience electrolyte imbalance.

Analysis/Physiologic/Evaluation

114. *Correct response: c*

The patient is experiencing postoperative flatus and difficulty in expelling gas, which is common at this stage of recovery.

a. A hyperthermia pad will not help the patient expel gas.

b. The patient is not experiencing nausea or vomiting; thus, an antiemetic would be inappropriate.

d. Narcotics will decrease peristalsis and lead to increased abdominal distention.

Application/Physiologic/Implementation

Index

Page numbers followed by *d* indicate displays; page numbers followed by *f* indicate figures; page numbers followed by *t* indicate tabular material.